hindustantimes

antime

SUNDAY TIMES

Bennett, Coleman & Co., Ltd.

hrouds death tiger cubs

h, chief wildlife warden
Times of India on Tues-
hat the tigress and two
first spotted by Mr
gh, a former Member of
who also owns the
Farm House. The cubs
uld also have b
from the tigres
ly, died of star
pugmarks had
gh some ten da
f the tigress ha
ngh said. Post-m

though no suspects had been rounded up. Dr Rahul Shukla, an honorary wildlife warden, said that every year the presence of tigers in the sugarcane fields went unnoticed, and only when casualty struck did the forest department

Orphaned Tiger cubs in Lucknow Zoo

The Times of India News service

Baharaich found aban sugarcane village in village labo sugar field coming inces ... from a cluster. A closer search revealed two tiny fur balls lying hidden under an igloo shape formation of leaves. They were seemingly hungry and screaming in desperation. Dr. Rahul Shukla, a tiger activist who happened to be at the site for a personal investigation of cane tiger phenomena, learnt about their presence. Loosing no time, he hastily reached on the spot with foresters and made arrangements to send the cubs to Lucknow.

The cubs weigh around 8 Kgs each and are 7to 8 weeks old. It is more than three days; the villagers have not heard the tigress calling her cubs. Shukla fears that she has been poached.

AF659520

By Tarun Subhash

LUCKNOW: Two tiger worth more than Rs 20,00 recovered in a surprise catch in Aminabad on Tuesday ... Involvement gang in the ... anned ani- ... o revealed ... e woman ... while try- ... s. ... Dr Rahul ... warden, ... red hand- ... culprit who offered to sell the skins to him. He had earlier got information from a shopkeeper that a woman was looking for customers interested in buying wildlife items.

Dr Shukla met the shabbily- dressed woman carrying an expensive bag. Posing as a customer, he asked her to show the material. She showed him two tiger skins and demanded a measly price of Rs 2,000 for the skins.

Dr Shukla immediately informed the chief conservator of forest (wildlife), who instantly sent a forest police team to the spot. The woman was caught and brought for interrogation forest office.

During interrogation, revealed her name as La belonging to Karnataka. Ho

The Indian EXPRESS Newsline

LUCKNOW SUNDAY | JULY 10, 2011

Poachers attack Wildlife Wardens Patrol

The Times of India News Service

Baharaich - The maoists poachers operating on Indo-Nepal borders near Tikonia suddenly opened a burst of fire on a forest patrol, operating on the Indian side.

Dr. Rahul Shukla, Hon. Wildlife Warden and his six native henchmen, all reformed poachers immediately left the jeep and took position behind trees from where they returned fire with a pair of .12 bore shot guns and a . 315 rifle. The battle continued intermittently for nearly an hour in which an anti poaching activist Rumi Singh of Mahipurva villa shots from an AK 47 assa right shoulder. The seriousl has been admitted in Balra Lucknow for treatment

rmer

pur

ad killed two st
learnt that the
sed the tiger aw
us leaving him h
eturned to take t
r. Apparently, n
g an imminent d
the villagers mi

Two Dudhwa tigers poisoned to death

ver, no incident of killing tigers has been earlier re-

rming the news of death of ahul Shukla, wildlife warhjahanpur, informed that nvestigations showed that re no reports of tigers hathe local people. Interestukla informed, that he had recently concluded an orientation programme called 'saving men from tigers and vice versa' in that region. During the programme, Shukla said, the locals were taught to be environment-friendly and so informed about the ime of wildlife for the human

id that it was unfortunate me unscrupulous elements d the noble beast.

e official suspected the role nds in the killing the animals lefence or for protection of ttle, investigations were also the possibility of poachers the beast for their skins

Sunday Pioneer

ers Kill Recovered

er 5

elderly ta Singh ger in the eld near - Tanda covered. ere no around er, Rahul Warden, task of body. He uards to for the d with a Ultra the tiger es. and a ted with ong way

through sugarcane farms. Shukla moved between two buffalo's drawing them by reins till he finally found the remains of the dead Sikh lying inside a dense sugarcane plot. "The tiger was around but he leapt away at our arrival", said Rajendra Saxena, the ranger of Kishanpur reserve and a member of search team.

"The cattle are very useful in tracking destructive tigers, they invariably present an obstacle to the seizer of hunter", said Gyan Chandra Mishra, the Field Director of Dudhwa National Park. Billy Arjan Singh appreciated Dr. Shukla for the commendable job; adding that "the forest department will have to protect this tiger from poisoning".

Oldest Tiger of Kheri Jungles Dead

HT Corrospondent: November 30

Lakhimpur -Kheri: Reports reaching late at night confirmed the death of the oldest known tiger of Dudhwa National Park. It had been living around the cluster of Navarangpur villages in North Kheri. The rotting carcass of this tiger was discovered by village herdsmen on 26 November, lying near a ditch in the ravines of Sharda river. The preliminary examination revealed multiple wounds on the body and two fatal stab like wounds at the base of the neck. Dr. Rahul Shukla, the Hon. Wildlife Warden of Dudhwa, confirming the news told Hindsustan Times on telephone that the old tiger had been killed by another tiger in a territory duel.

"Known as 'Borhauoo' to the villagers, the tiger was supposedly nearly 25 years old", said W. Longwa, the deputy director of Dudhwa. "He lived largely by scavenging and was a very popular animal of the area"

SUGARCANE TIGER

The Phenomenon of Wildlife in Tarai Farmlands

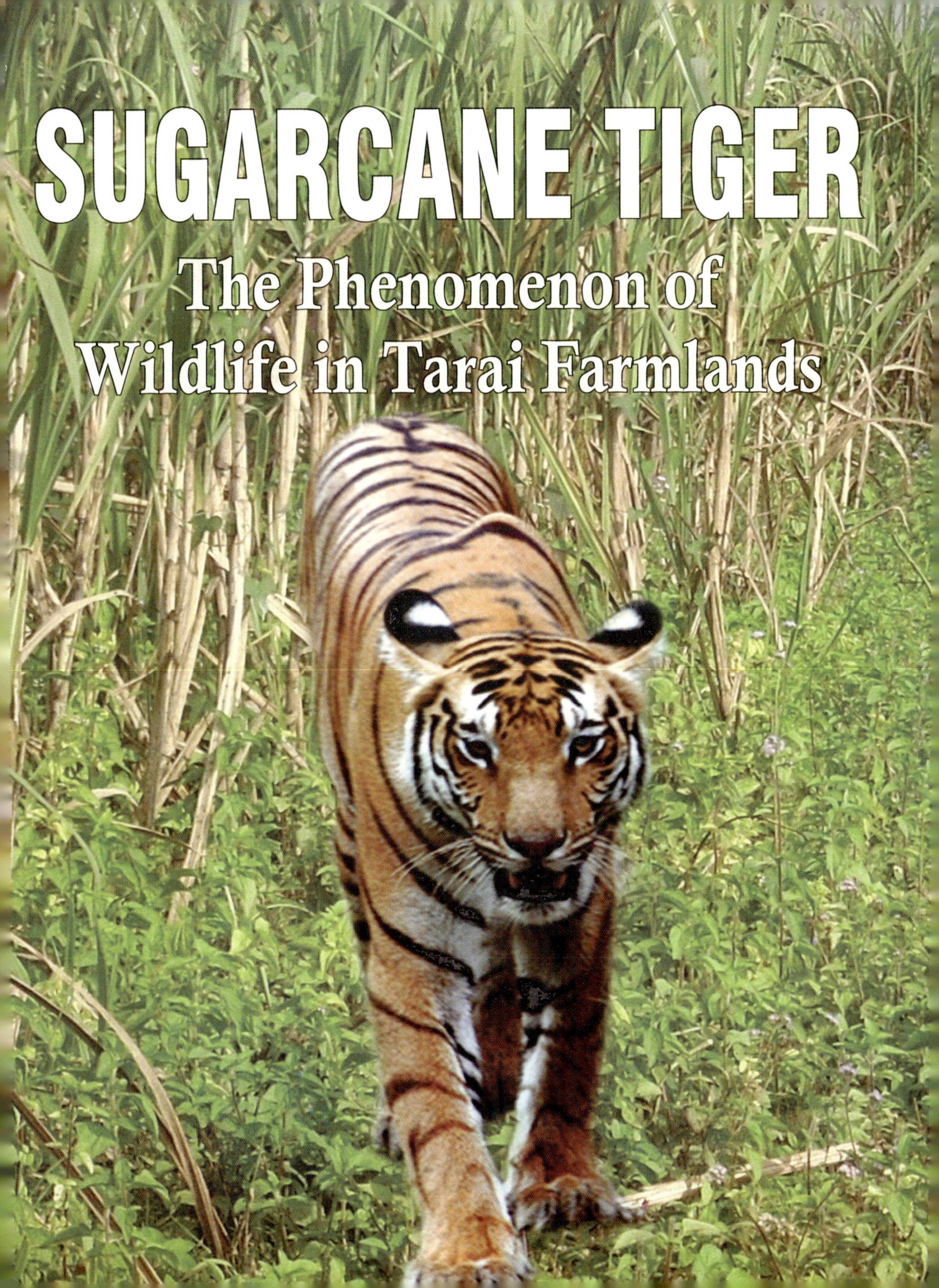

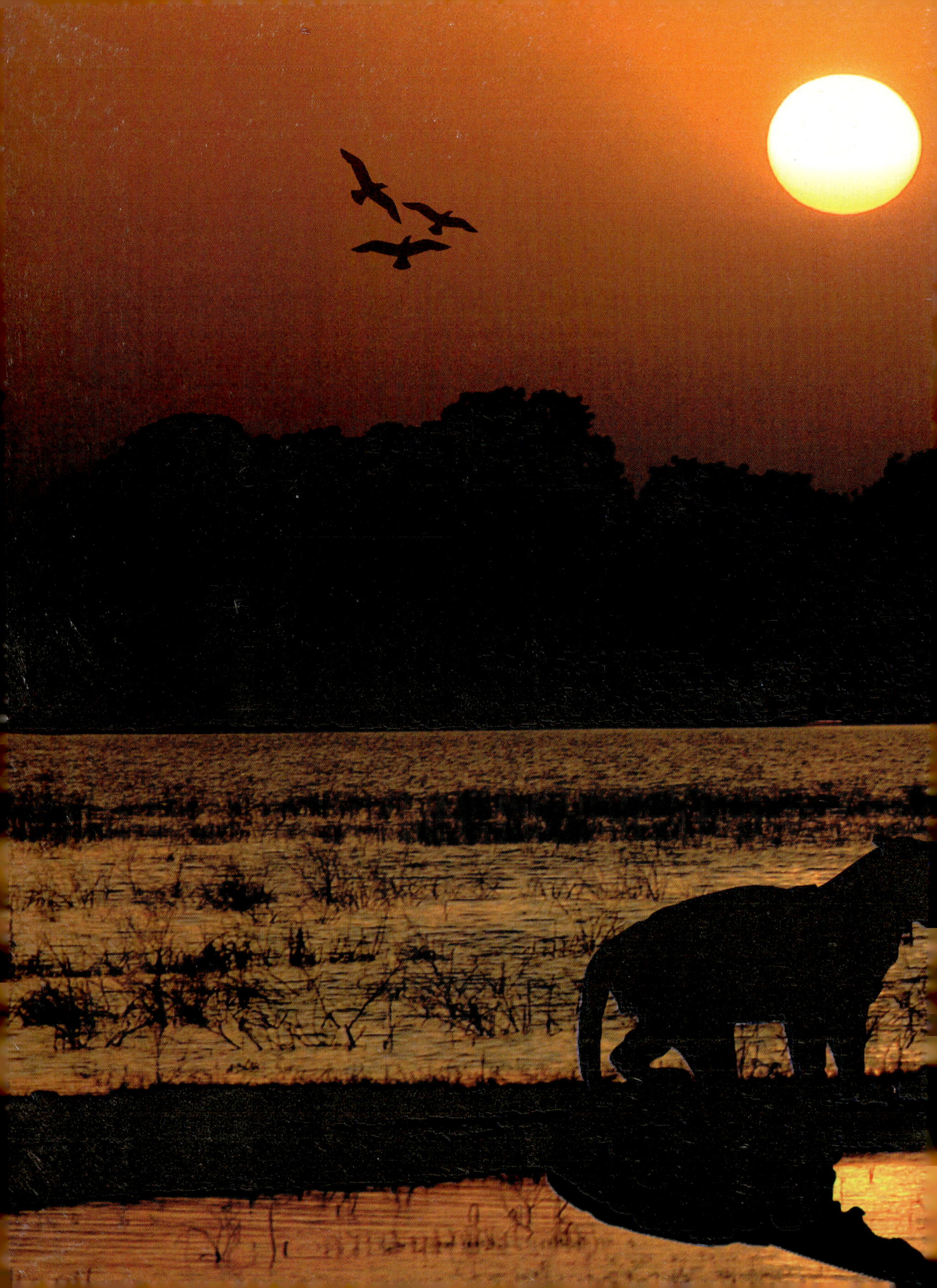

SUGARCANE TIGER

The Phenomenon of Wildlife in Tarai Farmlands

Rahul Shukla

**Edited & Assisted by
Shrivridhi & Samridhi Shukla**

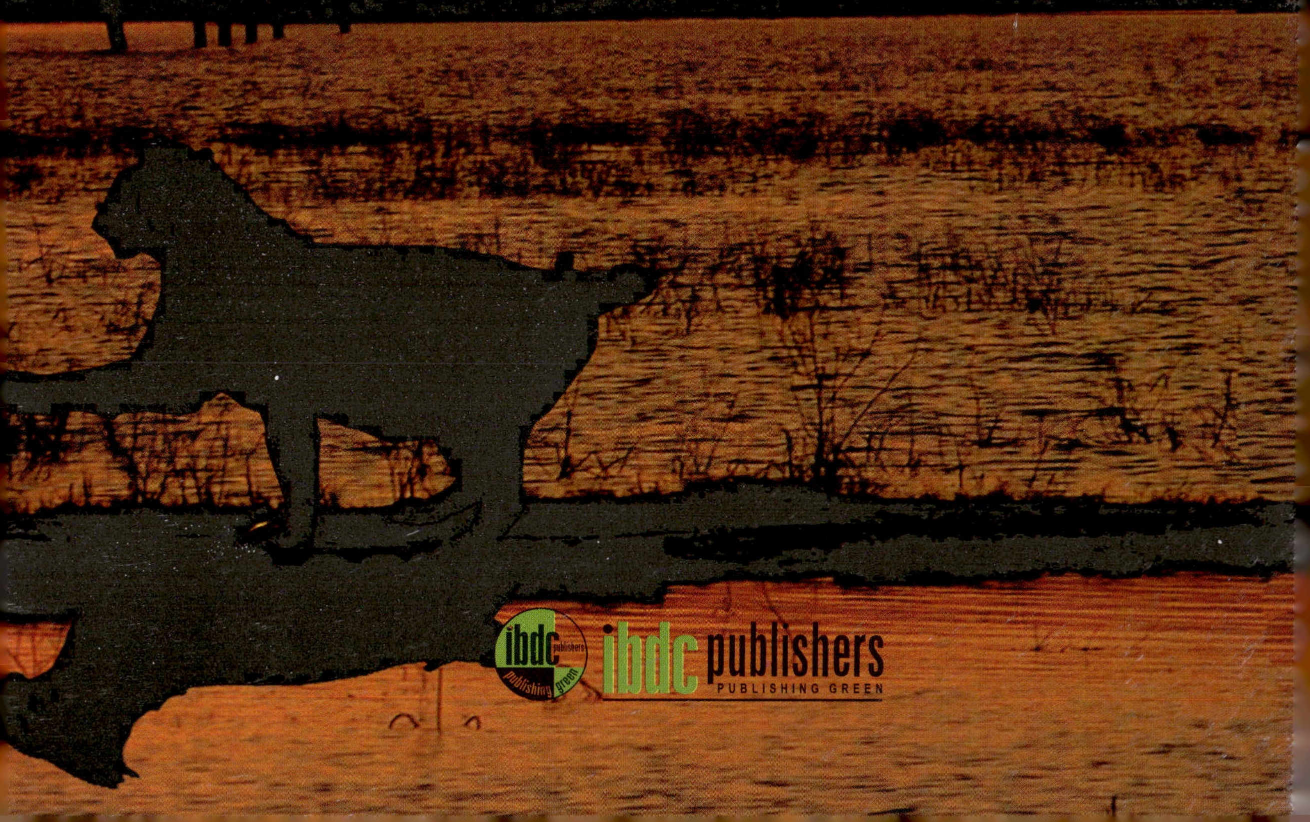

ibdc publishers
PUBLISHING GREEN

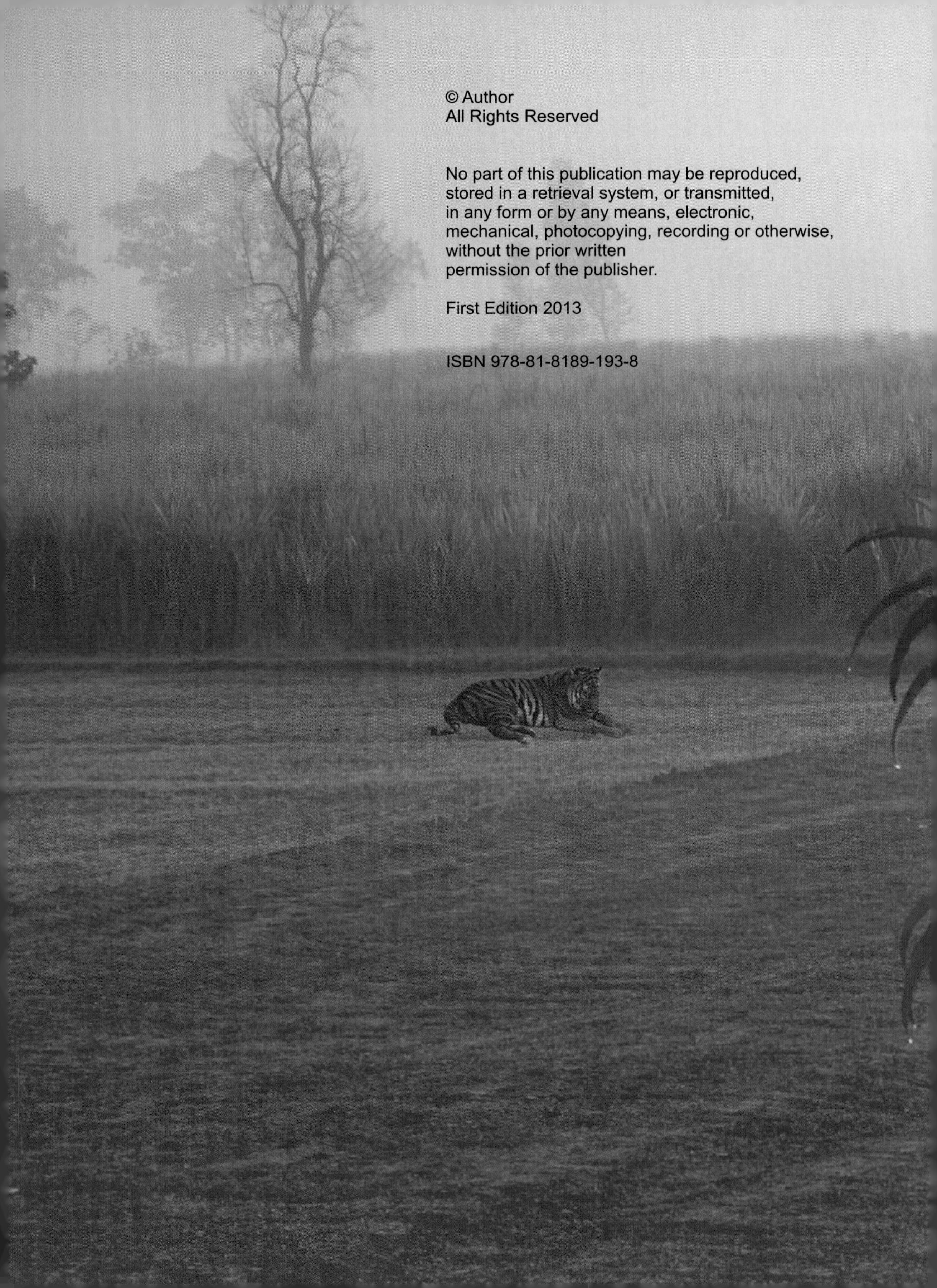

First Edition 2013

ISBN 978-81-8189-193-8

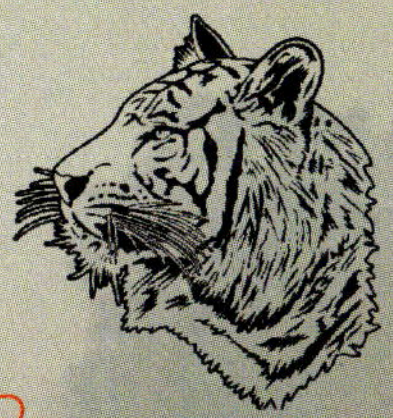

Contents

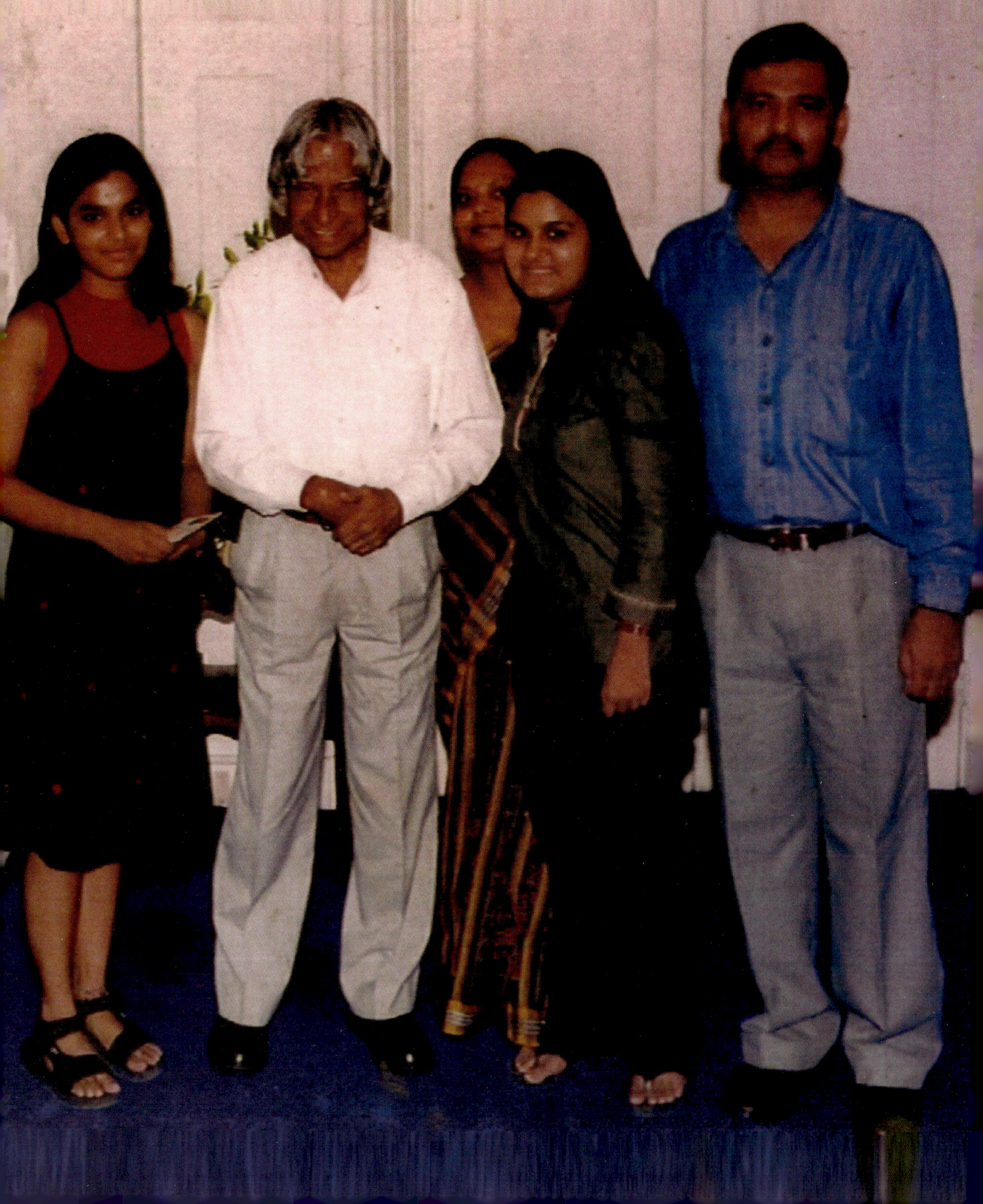

The Author and his family with the President of India
From L to R - Samridhi, HE the President, Anita, Shrivridhi and Rahul

Dr. APJ Abdul Kalam
Former President of India

10, Rajaji Marg,
New Delhi – 110 011, India

सत्यमेव जयते

Foreword

My first introduction to the author was through his book Tiger, which is indeed a very important contribution towards enrichment of our environment. When I read this book I get a feeling that man is becoming a liability for many animal lives including tiger and thereby the green forest environment. The environment and man have to work together. The story of Rahul Shukla's jungle partner Chotey Pasi is very interesting. The Chapter Heats of Fire is well written. The entry of Rahul with Phagunia and Dilli into the forest area of Larti during a fullmoon night and adventuring to witness the fierce fight between two tigers watched by the tigress is indeed thrilling. The Tiger Lair story is also very interesting to read.

When I saw his book and his unwavering commitment to the protection of nature, I thought of talking to the author. I spoke to him on telephone and I visualized his interest in Sugarcane Tigers and other types of tiger habitats about which he has collected substantial amount of information ever since he was just 22 years old.

Dr. Rahul Shukla has devoted three decades to monitoring populations of tigers in the sugarcane fields of the Terai while his vision of a new campaign called 'saving men from tigers' has added a fresh dimension in the field of wildlife conservation. We need to take his knowledge and attempt to find a way to use is for common good.

After reading the book, I have come to the conclusion that our Parliament and our Legislative Assemblies should have representation from Tiger Reserve areas. By giving representation to people of that area, citizens will be more responsible towards protection of natures' creations, the animal kingdom. I appreciate the idea of democratic rights for nature proposed by Shri A. P Singh, a Civil Engineer from Meerut. He also suggests Creation of a constituency called Natures' Constituency, which will be a motivation for conservation of the tiger and such a trend will spread in many other reserves.

The natural photography by author's daughters' Shrivridhi and Samridhi Shukla is very impressive with lot of messages. My best wishes to the author for presenting the case of silent animals like sugarcane tigers, which will go a long way in protecting the endangered species.

Dr. APJ Abdul Kalam
30 December 2008

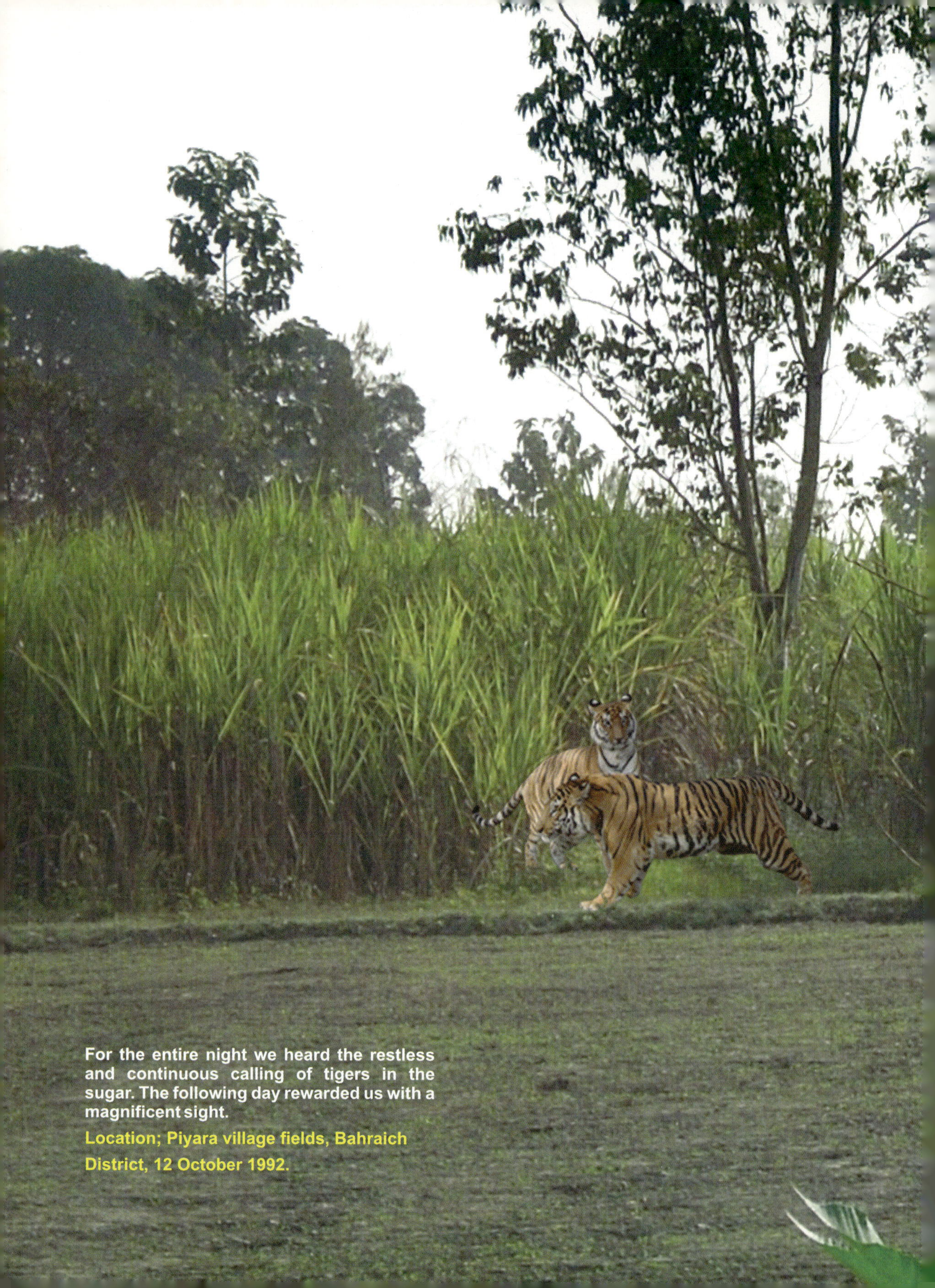

For the entire night we heard the restless and continuous calling of tigers in the sugar. The following day rewarded us with a magnificent sight.

Location; Piyara village fields, Bahraich District, 12 October 1992.

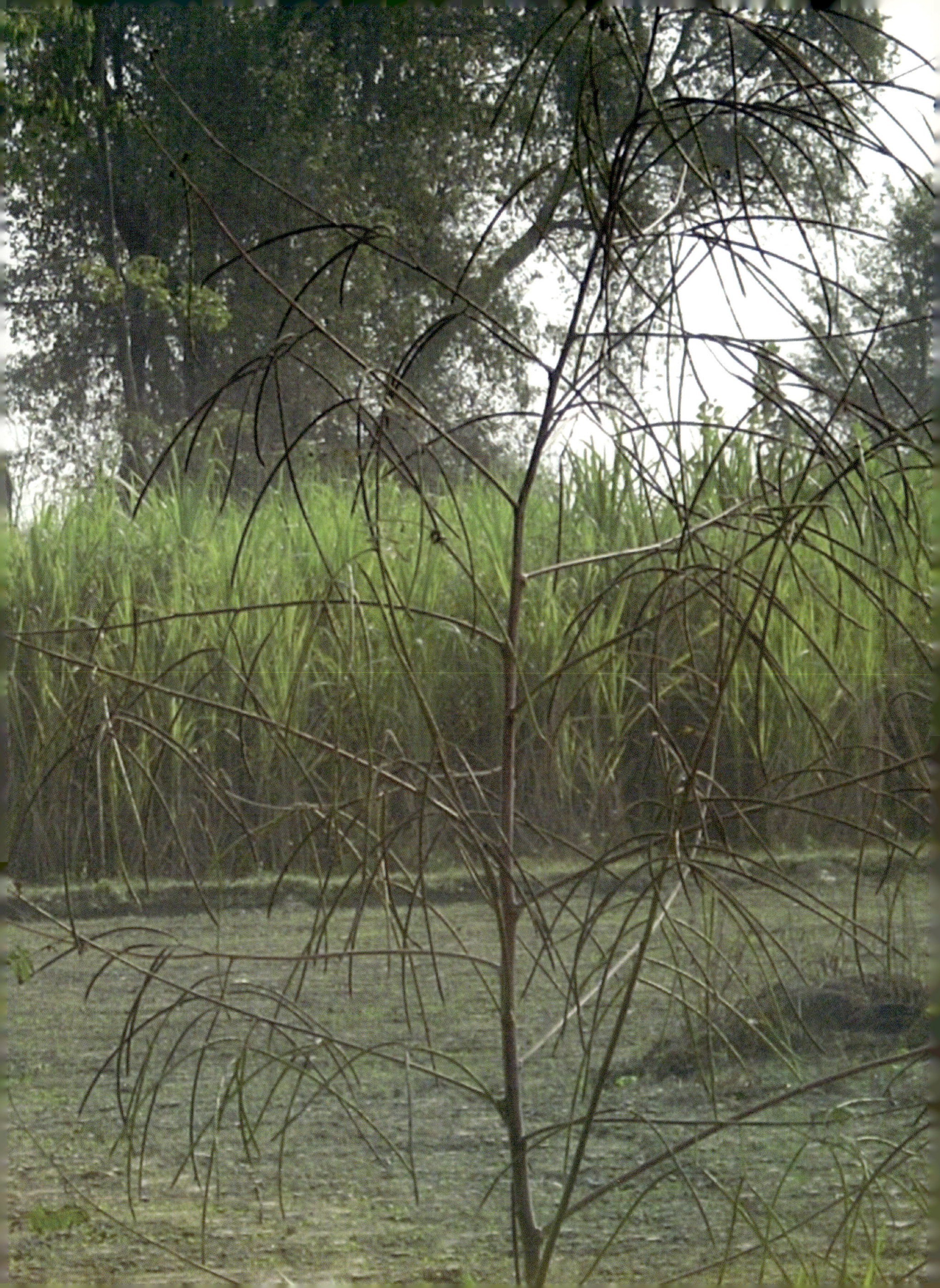

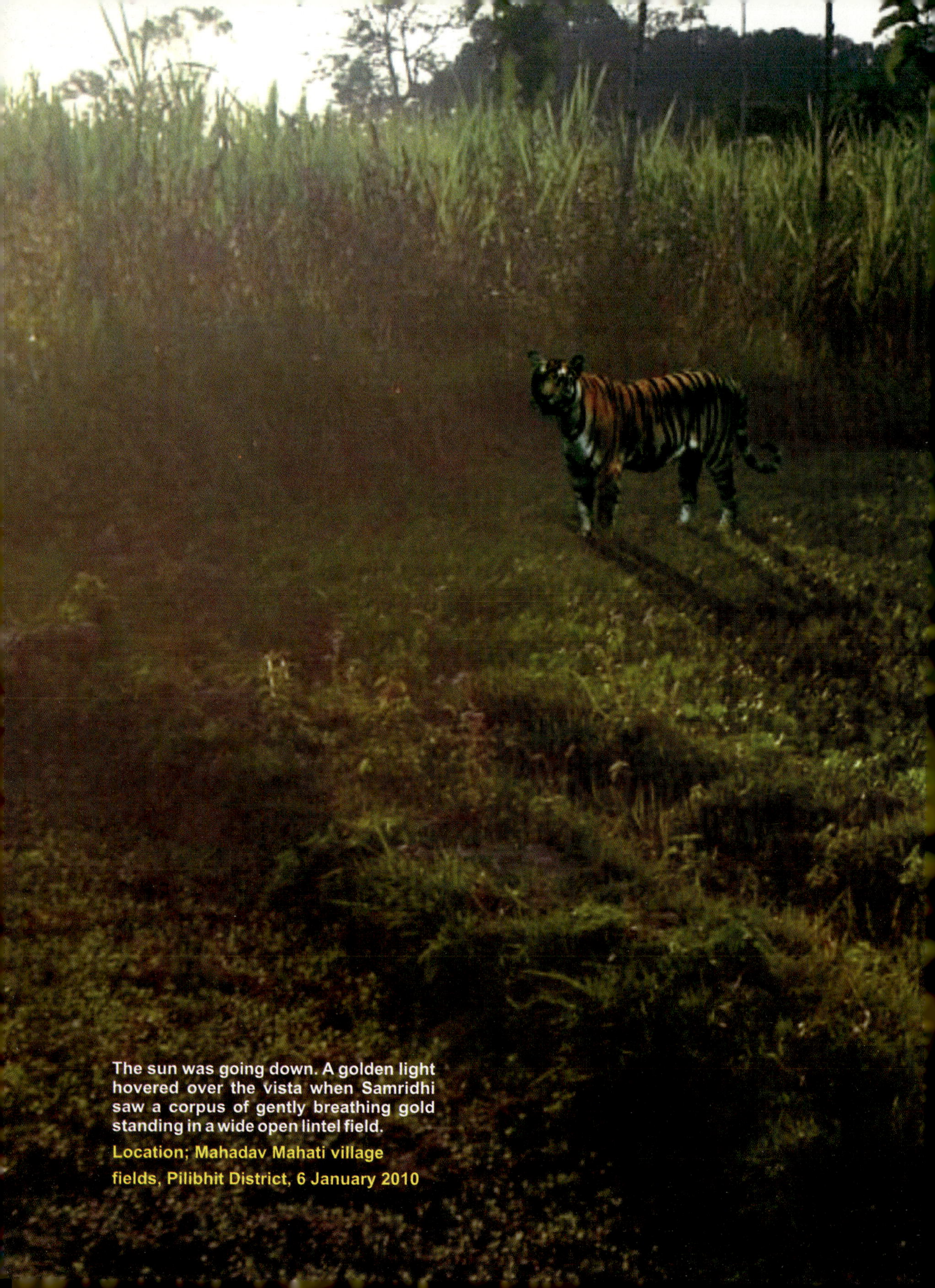

The sun was going down. A golden light hovered over the vista when Samridhi saw a corpus of gently breathing gold standing in a wide open lintel field.

Location; Mahadav Mahati village fields, Pilibhit District, 6 January 2010

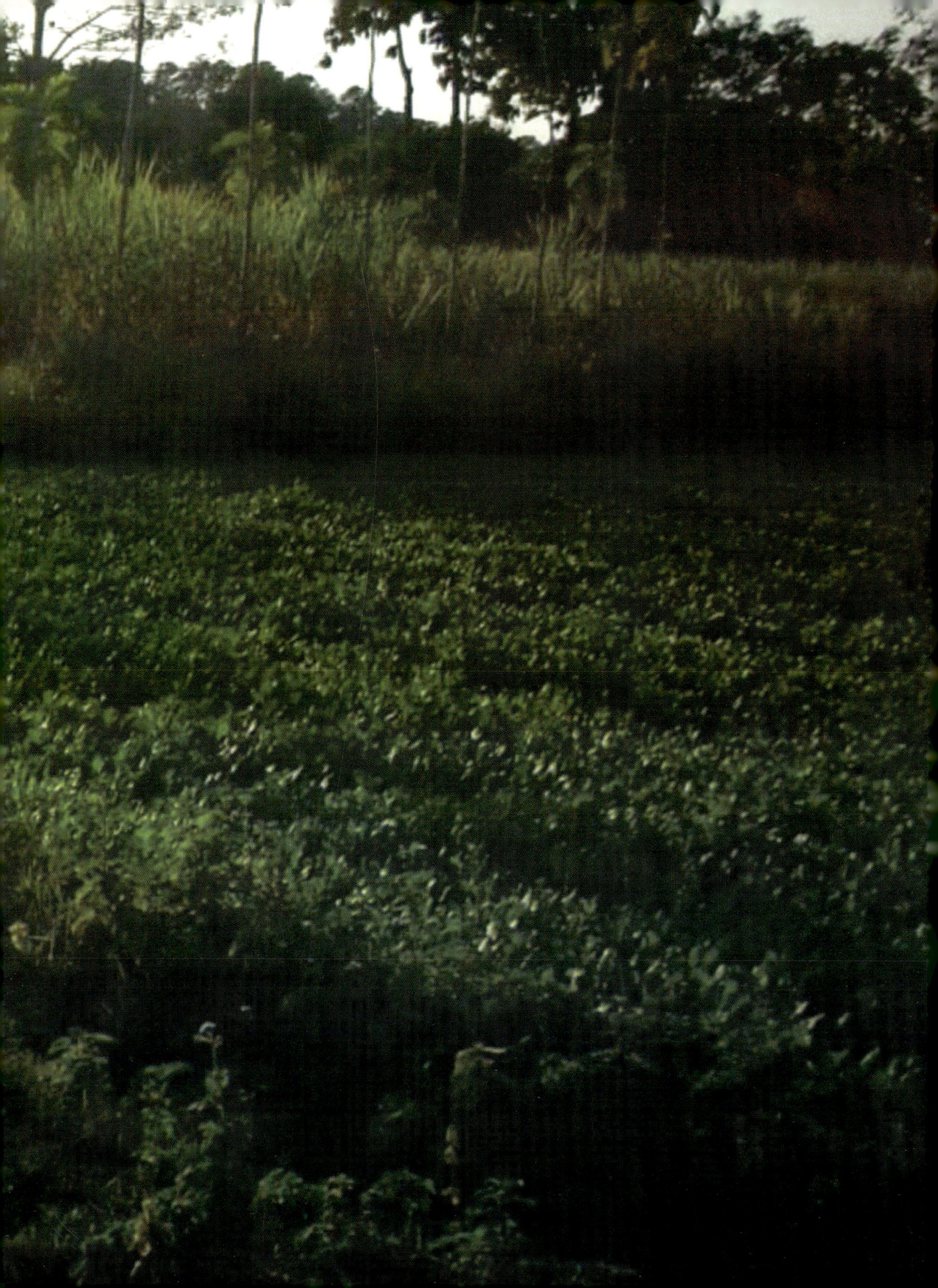

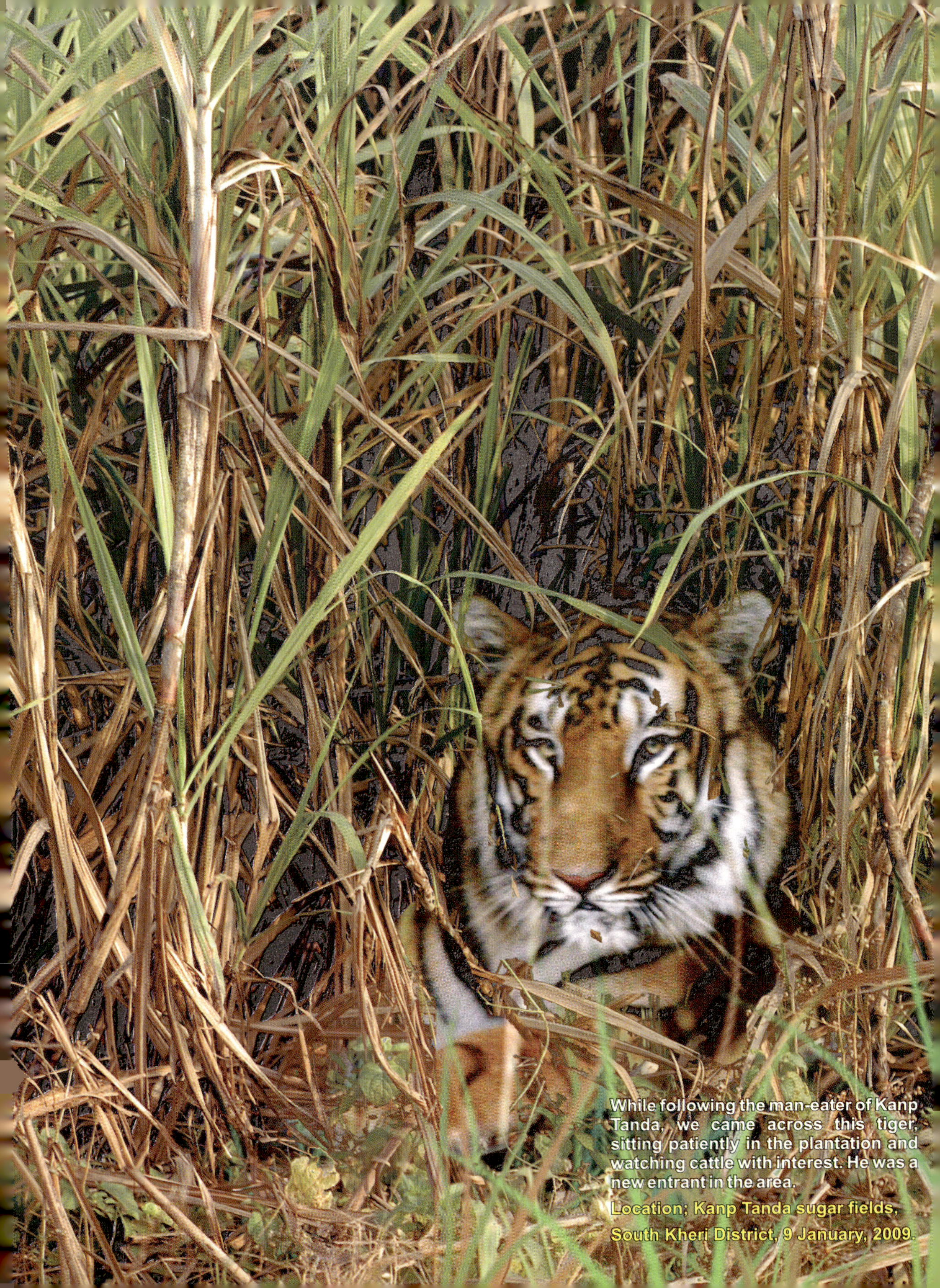

While following the man-eater of Kanp Tanda, we came across this tiger, sitting patiently in the plantation and watching cattle with interest. He was a new entrant in the area.

Location; Kanp Tanda sugar fields, South Kheri District, 9 January, 2009.

Author's Note

Having met Dr.A.P.J. Abdul Kalam with Padmbhushan Muzaffar Ali, the director of the much acclaimed film 'Umrao Jaan' at his residence, I reached New Delhi's Indira Gandhi International Airport in time to board the flight for Nepal. I settled on my seat giving a friendly nod to my co-passenger. The tall man, pleasant looking and very much in his late fifties, was with his wife, seemingly in her early thirties. The cheerful lady sat near the window with an awareness of her good luck shining on her face. They wore diamond studded wrist watches and gold rimmed spectacles, and the man, as a style statement held a golden cigarette case in his hands despite being in a no-smoking zone. The couple's affluence was very visible; perhaps they were on their way to have some fun at Nepal's Casinos.

Once the Kathmandu-bound plane became airborne, I turned towards my neighbor wondering if the magazine in his wife's hand would give me an option of chatting with them. It was the March 10, 2008 issue of the newsmagazine *India Today*. The lady started flipping the pages, thwarting my chance of borrowing it. Soon, I noticed that she had settled down to a news item. I could not help my eyes from peering down the page and saw that she was reading an item titled *'Preying on the Predator'.* The subject interested me and I found that I could read the article very well from across the man.

The report was about the startling figures released by the National Tiger Conservation Authority (NTCA) about the Indian tiger, suggesting that the number of this great predator had fallen from 3,642 in 2002 to 1,411 in 2008. It was a clear indication that the tiger was well on the road to extinction in at least Uttar Pradesh, where the number stood at a mere 109. The release of this report triggered a confrontation between the Uttar Pradesh government and the authority that had revealed the alarming figures. The forest officials never accepted the culpability for this shocking decline in tiger population, they rather pleaded that NTCA had got its counting all wrong, it had excluded the tigers living in the sugarcane belts, and therefore the results were unreliable. The Principal Chief Wildlife Warden maintained that that the numbers were much higher than the NTCA claim and instead stood by the 2005 census figure. NTCA also rejected the cane tiger theory as being unreliable and said neither do camera trappings show any tigers in the fields nor are there any signs of droppings.

Down the report I could even see my name quoted at certain places as the man behind the cane tiger theory, and then suddenly the lady asked her husband in a low voice: "Honey, what is this sugarcane tiger?"

"Cane tiger! Surely it would be the kind of tiger that eats sugarcane," replied the all knowledgeable man.

"Miserable," she said and next pointed at the standard photograph of a tiger printed with the news item.

"Look at this! The tiger seems to have stripes like sugar cane."

"Yes some tigers have such designs on their body. They are called sugarcane tigers," replied the husband, as though, in some measure, he was putting forward a new and original piece of information "...but I suppose they live in Kolkata and Mumbai zoos."

"Not in Delhi Zoo?" asked the lady, disappointed.

"No, they are not here", said the husband, breaking the news stoically.

The lady shook her head sadly as if she were sorry to hear of such a thing. "We must have one sugarcane tiger in our Zoo also," she murmured very possessively and sipped the drink that the air hostess had just brought.

Having heard the funny conversation I did not know whether I was glad or sorry. I said nothing although there was plenty I could have said. Just then the man asked me politely, "Sir if you don't mind, could you please change this seat with my sister-in-law who is sitting back there?" I had no problem and I duly changed places.

As I settled into the other seat, the couple's conversation stayed with me. I knew that people invariably ask ludicrous questions about wild animals but such great misconception about the sugarcane tigers was mind boggling. For me it was 'beyond a joke', something outside the boundary of a joke. I reflected on the hours I had spent in tracking these beasts, watching them and waiting for them in their favorite haunts, and the enormous efforts I had undertaken to establish this theory. I could have turned my energies to some other, less difficult goal, but I had instead chosen this less traveled road to soldier on and fight for their cause.

I was in an emotional frame of mind. Perhaps the time had come for me to put together my work and observations in the form of a book on this subject, if nothing then for shifting the focus from jungle tiger to this putative creed. I told myself I must take the opportune moment and tell the world the facts and trivia about these animals that I had witnessed with patience and resilience for over thirty years in the farm fields of the greater Tarai and so often in the rough-tough class room of experience.

There was a little annoyance in my mind: this was the thing I had tried to establish for years, so absolutely sure that there did exist a sugarcane tiger, and I was categorically told that I had built castles in the air, and I was wrong, quite wrong. However, being a naturalist myself, I knew that a true wild lifer is a man of great imagination, then how can it be otherwise if he comes to think of a new concept like sugarcane tiger? Imagination surely is more important than knowledge.

Sugarcane tiger was a paradigm-shaking development in the Tarai of Uttar Pradesh, which the Project Tiger officials found unpalatable before their own scientific dogma, which they in fact used as a shield for their incompetence and ecological ignorance. This proved to be a serious mistake on their part. The knowledge vacuum about this tiger led to chaos and an unprecedented outbreak in man-eating which took a toll of more than 400 human lives. The complex matrix of things rapidly brought the sugarcane fields of Tarai on par with the most talked-about tiger areas of the world, with Dudhwa at the centre point.

Today cane-tiger is no longer a debating point. The tumultuous phase of their existence and breeding in sugarcanes lasted for a good forty years around Dudhwa and its contiguous regions and then gradually faded out. The inexperienced forest officers and self-styled tiger activists caused an immeasurable damage to this animal. And now when the shades of night have already closed upon him and he has almost been decimated by poachers, crippled by trappers and poisoned by revengeful villagers, they are talking of this animal's identity, speaking my words verbatim, sanctimoniously. The carnage of the sugarcane tiger will always stand as a disgraceful and shameful episode in the history of wildlife conservation in Uttar Pradesh. When there was a chance to save it these very people had chosen to miss the bus.

Sugarcane tiger is the greatest of all adventure stories of the Tarai. Nowhere in the world did a similar scenario exist. Nowhere in the environs of human settlements had so many powerful predators ever concentrated and nowhere had so many human beings been killed by them in such a short time and nowhere had the notion of death itself grown as familiar as the flicker of lightening in the monsoon sky; something that a few would believe today.

The following narrative is drawn from my own experience and from the records of old cases that I have earnestly preserved in my study, mixed with accumulated information of a life time about these animals. The observations, on which this book is based were made entirely in the sugarcane fields of Tarai districts and apply only to those areas. Now there may be some interested readers who wish to read about the greatest chaotic era in India's natural history — the emergence of sugarcane tigers.

Rahul Shukla

Man is modifying the world so fast and so drastically that most animals cannot adapt to the new conditions... there are places that need help and have no scientists.

— **George B Schaller**

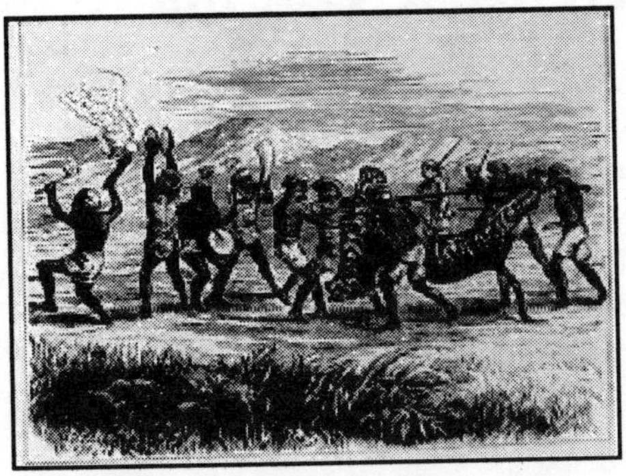

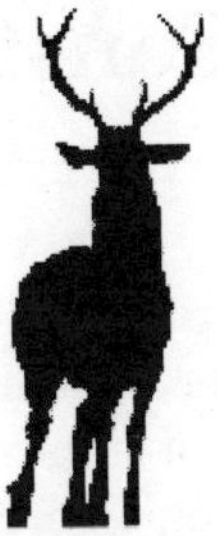

INTRODUCTION

The Constraints of Scientific Dogma

An Abstract of Sugarcane Tiger Controversy

Based on news clippings, articles, letter to the editor & interviews of the author
From
The Pioneer
National Herald
Blitz Weekly
Northern India Patrika
The Times of India,
Hindustan Times
Indian Express
India Today, Outlook
IBN7, Zee News, NDTV & Star News

"You can do the best science in the world but unless emotion is involved it's not really very relevant. Conservation is based on emotion. It comes from the heart and one should never forget that."

— George Schaller

The Constraints of Scientific Dogma

All the free ranging tigers of the Tarai, whether found in the primal jungles or perennial crops of sugarcane, are essentially beasts of the same strain. That is why the tigers of sugarcane farms share no less points in their favor than their kin from the jungle do. In their habits and behavior, they are but an altered copy of jungle tigers and thus a subject of utmost importance in wildlife conservation. This is what comes to my mind after having devoted much of my time and energies to learn more about these great cats. Any protection strategy will have to be inevitably drawn for both, but no excuse can be justified for not having a sugarcane-specific protection plan.

In limiting the conservation agenda only for the jungle tigers our forest managers have ignored the history of ecosystem functions.

-- Author in a Symposium of Environment Ministry, 1994, New Delhi.

Farmlands of Tarai adjacent to the jungle are indeed a country to warm the heart of a naturalist. This landscape harbors some curious compartments where the essentials of existence have still not been seriously vitiated; here the air and water, soil and the ecosystem, somehow still support the survival of great mammals and generate a pulsating rhythm of its own. Several rare to uncommon animals, like leopard, sloth bear, jackal, python, jungle cats and monitor lizards also intermittently frequent the place.

In their habits and behavior, sugarcane tigers are an altered copy of jungle tigers and thus a subject of utmost importance in wildlife conservation

It is the homeland of sugarcane tiger, a bizarre enigma, which carries on its precarious existence, by living on the phlegmatic cattle. The prevalence of droppings, tracks and other spoor indicate that they also prey on wild animals, such as occasional deer or boar that use the farmlands more regularly for their daily venture than the surrounding forest. These tigers live in the sugar crops so completely and so finally that their range only touches the ragged peripheries of jungles.

A life time devoted to the study of such an animal is certain to provide anyone a great deal of material of interest and value. As I trace these last 34 eventful

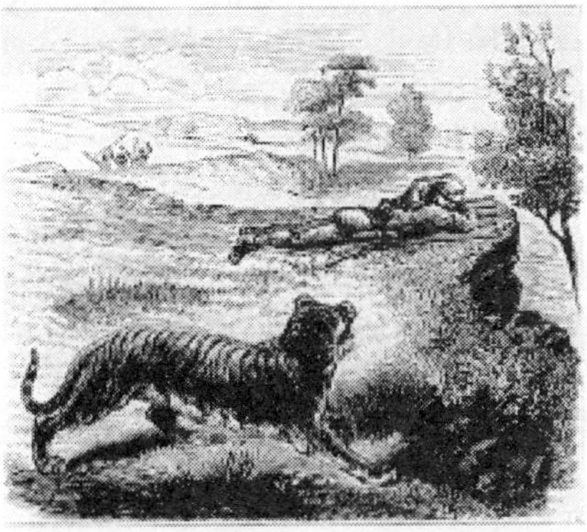

years of my in-depth research, I find this book is not merely about sugarcane tigers but it carries many vignettes and anecdotes which were a significant part of my struggle to establish the identity of this animal. The entire story had begun with my crossing of conventional boundary line about the perception of this animal. When I first expressed the possibility about the existence of sugarcane tigers, it was taken as a big joke. For conservative foresters, it was a weird and horrible conjecture. But seeing the series of my articles, which appeared in *The Times of India*, on the 'Joy of Stalking Wildlife in the Farmlands of Tarai', the interest of readership became deeper in the subject. The newspaper forays promoted my basic contention that the predominant expansion of sugar farms for hundreds of miles had created an artificial biome that offered ecological opportunities for large carnivores to expand their range. This brought the issue under the constant blaze of publicity and I was welcomed for providing a memorable, natural history record of this spectacular cat that eloquently proved its claim to survival.

Curiously enough in 1976, when I was a young bachelor and had embarked on this very project, I had everything to learn on my own. My earlier expeditions in the Tarai were an almost solo effort to comprehend the ecological needs of farm tigers. I had no infrastructural facilities and my operations were limited only to the outskirts of great jungles of Lakhimpur Kheri district. My first adventures with sugarcane tigers took place in the vicinity of Dudhwa National Park which soon caught me up with an unquestionable spirit of daring and an instinctive quest for the new and unexpected. My close observations of the farmland wildlife significantly enhanced my understanding about their stray into human dominated landscape, and I for the first time struck upon the hypothesis of sugarcane tiger. This hypothesis, perceived through years by an engaging equilibrium of focused study, conjectural rigors and comparative insights, gradually consolidated into a theory and the unflagging success induced a burning thirst to cover a large extent of Tarai and learn more about these animals.

Sugarcane tigers are a bizarre enigma that live in the sugar crops so completely and so finally that their range only touches the periphery of the jungle

Tiger science is different from canards of hunters and those who look at the animal with an eye of science hold such speculations as sugarcane tiger a figment of imagination. But as nature and its ways are concrete and material, the concept of sugarcane tiger rapidly expanded through fresh findings and so the cartel in the vanguard. The key idea was taken up by a few esteemed friends and acquaintances, who took up the campaign for this animal, and with abundant good intent, became my Rock of Gibraltar. Late Saroj Raj Chaudhary, Dr. Kailash Sankhala, Padma Shri Ranjit Bhargav, Dr. Ram Boojh and Raja D.P Singh, the trio of professional foresters Dr. R.L. Singh, G.C. Mishra and Uma Shanker Singh - all former directors of Dudhwa - J V Sharma and Rashmi Kant Shukla, to name a few, passionately argued in favor of my theory.

These wildlife protagonists, with decades of track record in scientific conservation interventions, acknowledged that the baseline component for the tiger's presence in the sugarcane was the inherent capacity of the crop to provide food and cover as grassland eco-system and the propensity of the tiger itself to multiply if adequate protection, food and cover are available. They affirmed that cane field tigers are generally known to local people but are often not known to foresters and therefore never find a place in national statistics.

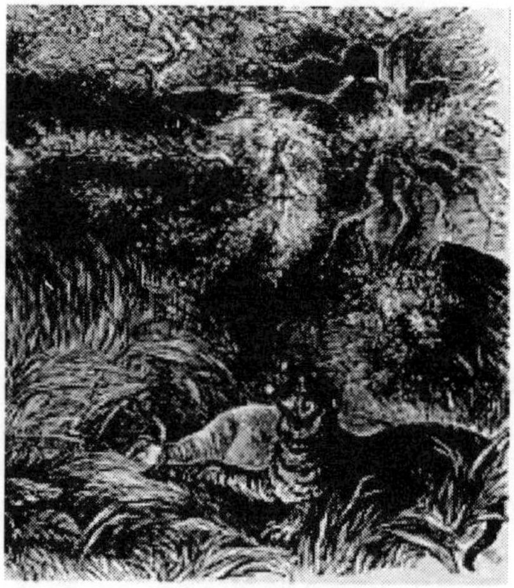

As I spanned the remote interiors of Tarai, my interaction with common men helped me to recognize native problems. Scores of farmers, erstwhile feudals and tiger buffs of repute reported about the presence of tigers in irrigated croplands adjacent to forests. They furnished me with local wildlife conditions and lent me a whole-hearted support for my research agenda. Though it was little harder to understand why people should save these tigers but there were many reasons why people tried to eliminate them. Some of them thought that these animals are not inherently dangerous, and though as with any other natural disaster, a threat does exist from them. They adamantly sought the government to take a hard protectionist view of this animal, while others who took them to be potentially dangerous towards livestock and human life advocated for their earliest capture or execution.

It is said if you do some work that is important for society, you want to reach society and show it. I say this with all indebtedness that the media editors lent me a generous support by throwing open the debate on this hypothesis, and like all men who try to break new ground, I savored my share of appreciation and criticism alike. I though feared that in a bid to champion the cause for this tiger, I may make matters worse by advertising the districts to organized poaching gangs. To this, the editors of The Pioneer and Northern India Patrika estimated that the feature is already known to too many to try and save it by keeping quiet. This attempt was rather in the hope to enlist the assistance of some appropriate influential bodies and individuals of India, who have interest in natural sciences and who could bestir themselves in time to get the necessary action before it is too late. I regret to say that though I could never generate even petite money to save this animal of unprotected areas but my writings slowly but surely assumed a greater significance for poachers than foresters.

Many cases coming into my knowledge proved that the trade driven poachers made a substantial capital from this goldmine of opportunity, which straightforwardly contributed to the terminal decline of this grand predator.

The first serious opposition of sugarcane tiger theory came in 1988, when in my struggle to prove the point by precept and example I submitted a report to WWF Delhi through Ranjit Bhargav, claiming the presence of four inveterate sugarcane tigers, in the remote farms of Kheri. I wrote "...because of the solid gravity of reasons stated above, I have successfully identified four well-established tigers operating between Pachperi-Ghat and Jhandi Riyasat area in Nighasan tehsil...... they appear fitting well into my idea of seasoned brand of sugarcane tigers. These are also known to forest rangers and the composition of their population as reflected by kill records shows them to be three females, one with dependent cubs and a male... It is an exceptional opportunity for experts to understand the matrix of sugarcane tigers and build a store of authentic information before they are poached or poisoned by some nefarious elements. All that is needed is to initiate a project to put a telemetric collar around their necks and monitor them. It would facilitate us to know for sure when they go back to the jungle or whether they do not go back at all and prefer to live in limbo with a compulsively altered life style".

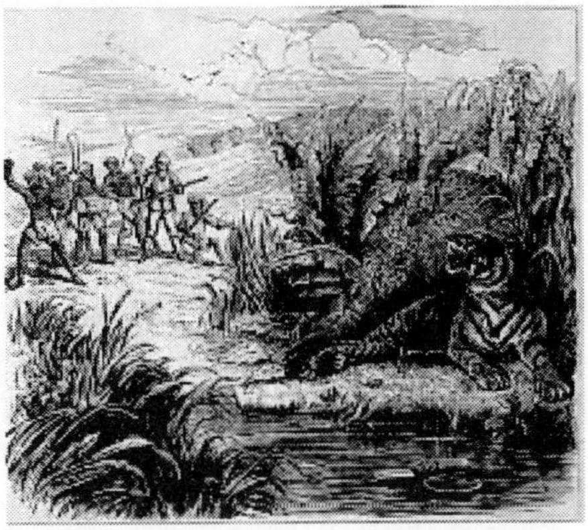

(It may be mentioned that the radio telemetry technique has been employed successfully for many years by Smithsonian Institution of Washington D.C, in its research programs on African and American wildlife reserves and was presently being used on tigers in Nepal in close collaboration with a team of scientists led by Dr. John C. Seidensticker. The Americans had initially offered the project to India, to carry out survey of Indian tigers but because of the unjustifiable fear of allowing unfettered access to foreign biologists, the Indian Inspector General of Forests and the Director of Project Tiger killed the valuable opportunity and Americans were constrained to transfer their project to Nepal.)

My initial desire to make the project a success was so great that I had weighed down my report with some academic professionalism that outlined a few distinctive traits of these tigers. To generate subjective romanticism, I had for the first time coined the term 'sugarcane tiger' to address these big cats, which however appeared too fantastic to some people in authority. Though government guidelines give preference to research which has visible and immediate implications for management of wildlife but the mandarins upheld that the lifestyle of tigers, I had corroborated in my report was entirely new-fangled and contrary to their conventional mode of existence.

Unmindful of the fact that a plethora of historical and contemporary factors has

The main deterrent in accepting my report was the incomplete knowledge about tigers and the old scientific dogma that wild animals cannot rationalize their coexistence with humans

contributed to the current state of affairs, and tigers have historically used farmlands as their ranges, their focus remained on protecting the wildlife within the physical boundaries of the reserve. They gave out a ready answer that the sugarcane farms were the borough of commercial operations, where the effect of human disturbance on local wildlife could be nothing but traumatic. The existence of any wildlife under these conditions was just an incidental by-product and it was almost ludicrous to press forward a conservation agenda for such wildlife. In conclusion the report dismissed my theory as unacceptably maculated and the word 'sugarcane tiger' as too avant-garde a neologism, for this deftly conveyed the dynamism and a great degree of 'unchecked-zeal' of an amateur environmentalist.

To my mind this unidirectional approach was accentuated by incomplete knowledge about farm tigers and their ecological history in human landscape. In the absence of baselines, measurable goals and monitoring, the staggering complexity of their survival in the farmlands had unfortunately always remained shrouded in mystery. Nobody had ever made a hard-hitting examination about the natural capacity of Tarai's welter of agrarian practices to attract and accommodate wildlife and a nuanced analysis of the tactics adopted by large carnivores to reside in maze, sugarcane and other tall crops. But now it was needed to be explored, to generate an effective conservation intervention for this tiger. **Conservation is no longer about creating a hard boundary between wildlife because people are ever increasing and there are hardly any workable isolation zones left for wildlife. It's about finding comprehensive and long-term solutions that benefit everyone involved. The singular idea that ph**ysically separating humans from wildlife is the only panacea is no longer applicable in majority of areas. This catch phrase hopelessly muddied the turbulent waters and became the main deterrent in the approval of my project.

Such obdurate attitudes have always diluted conservation initiatives in human operated countrysides, where much of the wildlife also lives. This has given rise to strong ideologies and entrenched conservation approaches that better work to neutralize -- rather than complement each other. That is why defining effectiveness of wildlife conservation within farmlands has remained so capricious. No wonder, real challenges to conservation of farmland wildlife persist in many prized areas and in many instances are not even acknowledged by experts. We must have a separate research wing for them, a flexible management system and a popular terrestrial wildlife conservation approach in human dominated landscape that is

Perhaps sugarcane tiger was too small a feature on the radar of these experts.

different from that of Protected Areas.

The opposition of WWF had another significant effect; it brought the term sugarcane tiger into universal circulation and equally fervidly its contradiction that amounted to a virtual forswearing. Furthermore it triggered an absurd wave of disagreement with my theory, both from the Project Tiger and the Big Battalion of Delhi-based wild-lifers. In the eyes of these leading combatants in the fight to save the Indian tiger my natural history annotations were of an entirely different quality, which were not only intriguing but some of these seemingly confronted biological explanations. For example when recent studies of scientists have recorded that tigers prefer larger species such as gaur and sambhar as prey and kill disproportionately more of them in comparison to much abundant chital and hog deer, the prudent predation pattern of Barotha tigers described in chapter 13 of this book, in which they killed jackals and eat was an abstruse situation almost corresponding to impossible.

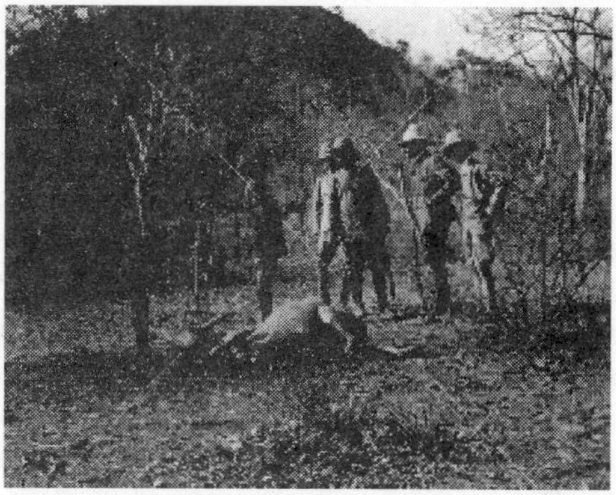

Perhaps the big battalion was more involved in the miasma of larger issues and the curious behavior of farm tigers was too small a feature on their radar. Their opposition to my observations was based on superficial checks, which could not help them think more deeply about a wide spectrum of carnivore survival issues in rural lands and advance their understanding of farmland wildlife. It took me time to convince them that tigers prey on animals that are vulnerable to predation and as a consequence of extinction of large predator from farm areas, prey may have lost knowledge about natural predators. Barotha tigers selectively killed jackals because they had effectively learnt to exploit their increased vulnerability, and continued to do so, before jackals could express behavioural adjustments at the return of predators.

I had observed and told what I had seen. I know the limitations of my statement and what are the boundary conditions for which statement is correct. Tigers' approach to acquire prey depends on various factors as different environments condition their behavior in different ways; now it was the job of a biologist to explain as what had carried tigers so far that the wretched jackal had suddenly figured strongly on their list of predation.

A recent documentation of environment ministry reveals that there is plenty of farmland wildlife in several states, yet no state has ever hosted even a single research to understand their mechanism of survival in such places, apart from participating and helping forest managers in the routine annual census of carnivores and ungulates inside the protected area. With due regard to the ego of these experts, I explained that the nature of my experiences was different because of the habitat specificity. My observations were made in the human dominated landscape. The circumstances here were not similar to those witnessed by somebody else in the deep, green woods, where tigers associate only with other wild animals. Moreover, sugarcane country is dense and often gives no indication where the tiger is likely to be. Here their behavior is invariably induced by anthropogenic commotion, which in some cases also causes damage to the tiger. This compels them to act in a manner contrary to the normal mode of existence and that is why, the term sugarcane tiger, is consistently conflated with opposition to the canon of modern tiger science.

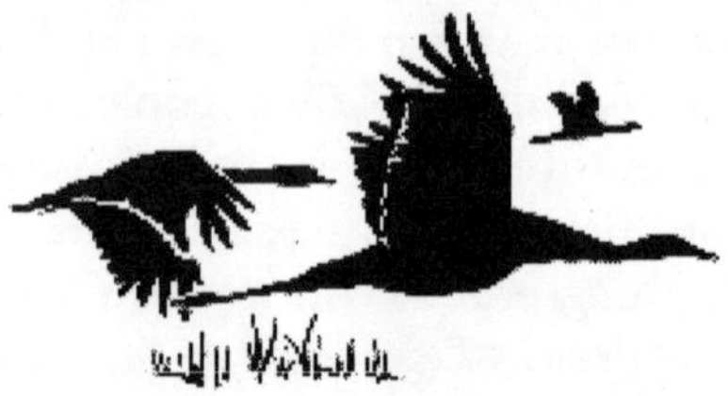

It was clear that for better or for worse the tigers had come to stay in the sugar-fields. They were here for good and that is why I had not only reported the reasons for their presence in the crops but also presented a comprehensive cinemascope view of the problem. My report also included many local details with honesty of purpose and dealing. Failure to appreciate these facts only showed a lamentable ignorance on part of the wildlife mandarins which led them to crass confusion and apparently accounted for many contradictions in their judgment and confutations.

I reiterate that my observations were based on wide experience of tigers in the farmlands and not in the jungle. However, it was hostility in the realm of concepts, where none of the Project Tiger officials were particularly anxious to count up and protect these animals or recognize the value of recondite knowledge I had discovered, by innumerable hours of sedulous investigation and exertion, skill and nerve. This knowledge was the key to the dreadfully unwholesome enigmas of the foresters -at least for the foreseeable future. Yet at no stage they opened any productive dialogue with me or called me to explain the applicability of my research in the management of these tigers and other farmland wildlife but rather scowled at my work with an inflexible scientific attitude.

Some senior authorities were so much bamboozled that they attempted to settle scientific question of sugarcane tiger by political affiliations.

Perhaps to the people who had in the least practical experience of the Tarai farmlands, the germane concept of cane tiger did not make any sense at all. It looked as if it would be a greatest fallacy on their part if they believed this nascent reality and stopped launching a gratuitous attack on my theory from a distance. Now I had no options left but to comfort myself in the feeling that whenever the new researches come out their findings are invariably doubted, and, if I am not on somebody's hit list or shit list, then I am not doing anything worthwhile.

Some foresters in authority, bamboozled by this ecological hypothesis, attempted to settle scientific question of sugarcane tiger by political affiliations. Some begged me not to create trouble for them by raising a ruckus in newspapers about sugar tigers. Some seniors even ordered me to stop this nonsense as they were answerable to man-tiger conflict and it was increasing their paper work. I consider both pleading and bullying signs of psychopathology. Argumentum ad baculum and argumentum ad misericordiam are both logical fallacies. If you do not like my arguments then disapprove and that is all. It is said that knowledge explodes when rules are broken. And a productive mistake in the knowledge that develops from rule-breaking reveals an entirely new world. Perhaps, I had not judiciously followed the old faithful rules that keep the body of knowledge safe and pure and I was relentlessly breaking them because they permitted me uncharted directions and fresh insights.

While the argument was in progress, I stated that the effective weapon of a conservationist is accurate information, and, for the most part I had studied the conundrum with this very notion in mind. It is a moral obligation of every tiger activist to do with the protection of the species, because often it is as important as the study of the species themselves. I had also stated that a great deal of my information is a matter of common sense; it does not necessarily include any specialized intelligence because the dynamic spectacle was obvious even without statistics. History is witness that common sense and dogma have always been at conflict, leading to many a confrontation.

Science is what you see with the bare eyes, and not what you believe in. It was not that the foresters were unaware of the quotidian phenomenon. Every DFO posted in the Tarai districts and every coming and going Director of Dudhwa Park knew that the tigers were seeking their living in sugar environs, without conflict and were responsible for attacks on people only when not treated correctly. Even the statistics confirmed what the eyes saw. For example in 1986, when 14 carcasses of poisoned tigers were found in cane fields, it was officially stated in Dudhwa's brochure that 80 tigers were residing inside the park and the residual population of 40-45 was settled in the farmlands. The estimate did not include an unknown number of casual visitors who crossed over from Nepal to India or to north from south Kheri, rambled for the time being and then went back into principal forests.

The predicament of miscomprehended nomenclature

The data clearly indicated that a majority of these tigers were peacefully living in the sugarcanes without attacking people and thus doing much to disapprove the negative perceptions of their tribe. Their presence also implied the existence of sufficient food to support and sustain them. Was my story something opposite to that, bearing little resemblance to the surprisingly positive facts? And if it was, then it was certainly the domain of a research scientist.

The nomenclature 'sugarcane tiger' sounded incredible to many yet it is fundamentally simple. An animal that has the characteristic elements of its cane dwelling ancestor and thus who represents the unfeigned line of descendents is a sugarcane tiger. But the real drawback was that nobody was ready to exercise his brains into the matter and analyze the causes for the continuous presence of tigers in the farms, which I had been doing almost single-handedly for years. Their ideas about these tigers were simplistic and incorrect. There were very few people who understood the inherent difference between the 'tigers in sugarcane' and a quintessential 'sugarcane tiger' which is the central thesis of this book. To repeat, the first category ranged partly inside and outside the park and visited farmlands only as transients whereas the second was using farmlands exclusively, where its graffiti blazoning of territory and daily routine was tempered by its understanding of humans and adapted to a rhythm amid their interruptions.

I felt sure that this tiger was here by a stint of natural selection and its sustainable natural history was a durable progressive trajectory in which its survival had never been at stake. Natural selection is a decisive seminal factor in determining the positive mode of things and as a professional historian I am even ready to face the fact that it was natural selection that determined the evolution of mighty cultures in the same manner as it did that of species. The idea that culture is mankind's ecological niche is still applicable

The widespread perception -that all tigers in cane were sugarcane tigers- continued to confuse some experienced masters of wildlife. The director Project Tiger Government of India, Dr R.L.Singh was more than happy to draw on the neologism of 'Sugarcane tiger' to address the plethora of tigers in the cane. He used it copiously in his books and made a great capital out of the fact, that at his behest, the first authentic count of sugar tigers was ever accomplished.

My humble entreaty was that a major chunk of these animals, to all intent and purposes comprised normal jungle tigers, taking a seasonal trip in the cane field and was not to be considered in study of a sugarcane tiger; whereas the latter that had evolved from historical farm tigers was the hardened sugarcane tiger by the process of naturalization. The difference between the two tigers was more real than apparent. The centrality of my idea was that the spread of immense sugarcane farms had tremendously rewarded this chronic animal. It was all comfortable in a separate ecological niche through ecological succession, and was a new ecological footprint in making. Thus despite sharing the same living conditions, the entire surfeit of tigers in the sugarcane farms, was not of the 'sugarcane tiger' kind, which I had instituted and advocated for years, invariably drawing a fine line that vindicated the difference between the two- the general and the prototypical.

> ***Putative sugarcane brand tiger was the one whose all corporeal and mental endowments were tending to progress towards aptness. On the basis of this thesis I had formed my concept of sugarcane tiger.***

Some foresters steadfastly ignored the part A of the problem -- that sugarcane is a pro-tiger crop and the tigers were convenient with it -- but reverted to the part B, the question of the beginning of a putative strain and then to its absolute denial and ultimately to the marginalization of the phenomenon itself to man-eating, which mired down the already jumbled socio-ecological issue to a parochial bickering. It was actually a reflection of whole new pattern of existence, a protracted exigency dictating the new ways of carnivores but no effort was ever made to corroborate this belief with on-ground scientific assessment.

An enthusiastic dilettante who thought of himself as a conscientious environmentalist and much ahead of his times even used the word sugarcane tiger in futuristic sense, imagining --there will be a day, when there will be no jungles but tigers may still be there and then they will have to live in sugarcanes; what a lame perspective it was, yet potent enough to extenuate the whole seriousness of problem in a humdrum fashion.

There were of course, two sides of this polemical subject, in which WWF Delhi, Project Tiger and some state forest officials occupied the opposite camp. In my opinion cane tiger is not an affair of logic than it is of circumstances and when even wildlife scientists also indentify such sites of sugar plantations, as having great potential to offer a second home to carnivores outside forest, the subject does not permit generalizations. I also read a few very ill-informed generalizations written by a vice chairman of State Wildlife Board. He considered wildlife scenario in farmlands as evanescent happening and not the eternal or evolutionary one and he had written at random, with great misunderstandings. He thought -not unreasonably then- that I was a protagonist in making, pointlessly hogged into limelight and needed to be cut short, something like half of my size.

Unfortunately, nobody could pin down how great cats had become crowded into a limbo of sugar-fields, to live cheek by jowl with human trespassers? No systematic judgment on the problem was ever sought while the local press, with little knowledge, advocated a wrong belief that sugarcane crops were the abode of exceedingly starved man-eaters, whose fear of humans was overridden by their hunger, and the other monsters at this base, full of ravening bloodlust, were just waiting for their appointed time to become man-eaters.

All this was asinine. My critics seemed to overlook the elementary fact that wildlife cannot be restricted into a limited space, which form our protected areas and especially the carnivores that have a mercurial temperament and very wide ranging habits, cannot be contained in the forests only. In the areas where no proper boundaries between man and tiger have been demarcated, the intricate mix up of such biology and ecology is to be regarded as natural hazard. Here much of wildlife is condemned to live in the farmlands; having trouble in grappling with environmental crisis, which makes their coexistence with humans a necessity. Simultaneously the inherent capacity of the sugarcane to provide

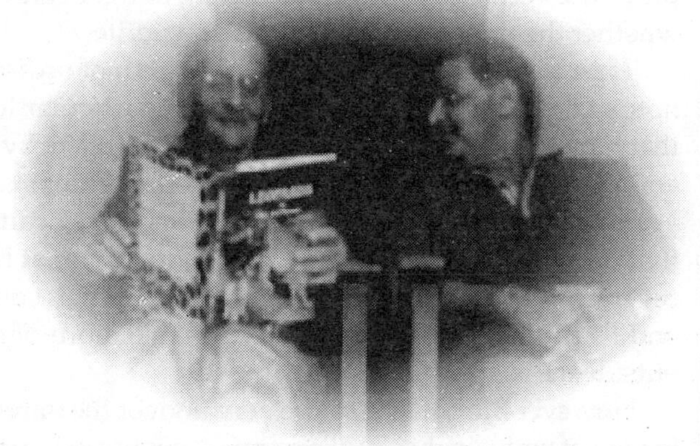

Billy with the author

food and cover as grassland eco-system produced a complex matrix, the net product of which was the emergence of sugarcane tiger; a new threat, trying to come to terms with his oppressor -- the human being.

This development was to be held up as a cautionary tale and treated as an ecological retort of nature and the outbreak of man-eating was the ultimate conforming demonstration of this ecological catastrophe. Still for many critics I was pulling a rabbit out of a hat. It was even alleged that the concept of sugar tiger was a phantasmagoria of my imagination. It was regrettable that I should have contravened the commandment of Project Tiger and fall out of it -fouled and sullied- despite working for the same basic imperative for which the apex body was designed.

Billy Arjan Singh also negated the cane tiger theory, for pseudo-scientific and sheer obstructionist reasons, he asked, "What a tiger will eat in the canes?" Billy was of the opinion that tigers do not like beef and generally do not go for it, they return to jungle in search of venison. The assumption was utterly unrealistic. George Schaller, whose first scientific study on tigers was conducted in Kanha National Park as early as 1964 stated that livestock has an important role in providing the cat with prey in many areas. It seemed ironic that Billy considered this finding as unempirical. The scientist wrote "With the drastic decline in India's wildlife, the tigers in most forests subsist partially to wholly on cattle, and buffalo. In fact it is likely that these two domestic animals are the chief source of food of the country's tiger population." Now when according to Schaller, a jungle tiger essentially depends on a cattle diet, then a sugar tiger has every reason to exploit this prey base because from the standpoint of tiger conservation, it makes no difference whether the prey consists of cattle or wildlife.

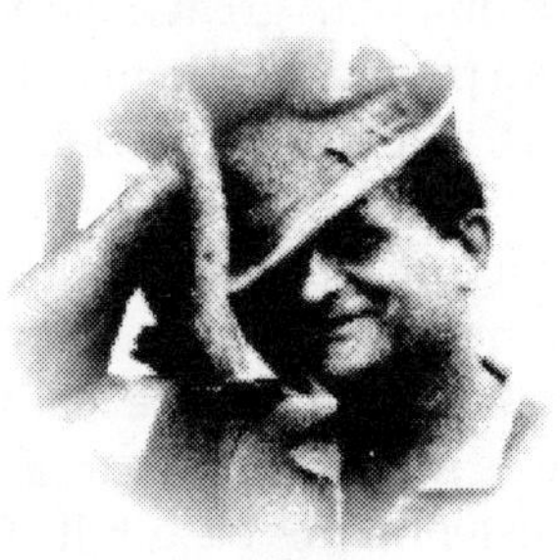

Billy in Young Days

Tiger's existence on cattle is nothing out of ordinary. Baker's (1890) emblematic note of a male staying for 14 years in a particular locality and killing 500 cattle in that time is endorsed by another exemplary claim by Sanderson (1912) that one tiger was cattle-killer for twenty years. Even Brander stated that one tiger remained 15 years near some villages on cattle diet. Moreover, cattle and buffalo are buffer species that help the tiger to maintain their population at high level. In such farmlands if revengeful killing and poaching is eliminated, it could speed their rate of increase, and this in turn would ultimately enable more tigers to inhabit the area that fall outside the rugged frontiers of forest.

However Billy, living by the very floor of the unremitting phenomenon continued to view it and -- in theory at any rate -- continued to differ with me. I do not know for what reasons he considered even Schaller's scientific statement erroneously wide off the mark, when once held responsible for degrading habitat and potentially out-competing wild prey, the cattle have now been arbitrarily elevated to the status of buffer prey by scientists in recent reports.

Ostensibly, Billy was more involved in wrangling with the Project Tiger authorities on Tara's death and the sentimental mush of publicizing the falsehood that his house pet was still alive in the wilds and was effectively proliferating the population of Dudhwa tigers. Though Tara did not exist anymore and he was on a shaky ground on this issue, yet he favored dissipation of his energies in efforts seeking to establish a prevarication, which involved him for the rest of his life. I think for the peace of his own mind it was imperative for him to see the soul and face of his beloved Tara in some other wild tigress and befall into drafting its biography as a canard of living Tara; and this he did acceptably and admirably by observing a surrogate Tara. Fortunately far from a blanket condemnation of my theory his writings do attach importance to an acerbic problem of special nature that does exist about tigers in sugarcane habitat; though nowhere in them does he try to decipher the deeply serious operational aspect of the problem or express concern about the future of these tigers.

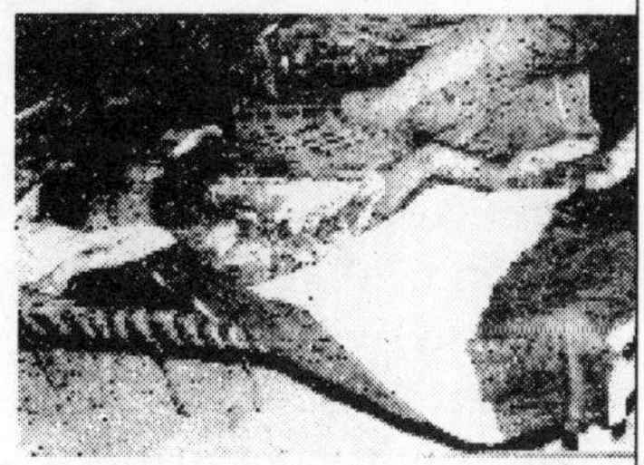

Tara's kill : Asgar's half eaten body

I may be pardoned for saying that Billy considered Dudhwa his own domain and guarded his interests as a resident tiger guards, believing in the cautionary chases of juveniles who time to time appeared on this terrain in guise of dedicated foresters and pollsters. Through his lofty international connections and prolific books, the old doyen successfully maintained his status of being an authority on Dudhwa tigers and never promoted any forester or naturalist to score a point over him or win advancement and challenge his supremacy. The mere mention of sugarcane tiger was enough to send him into delirious frenzy yet the apogee of the unrivalled feature that lingered as the cynosure of every naturalist's eye for good 40 years, (1960 onwards to 2000) remained a reclusive enigma in his life.

To my mind the stretch of sugarcane fields flanking jungles, hold the answer to many questions on wildlife which even Billy - who deserves respect as a knowledge creator and thinker- had yet not figured out to cotton on. Due to the lack of innuendo and stodgy approach- he rather continued to treat me as an unwelcome intruder. Perhaps for this reason, whenever I presented him with any of my newly published hardback, he retaliated to my accomplishment, burlesqued and lambasted me for trying to cozen with the puerile, flawed fancy of sugarcane tiger. He interpreted the scenario as an ecological disaster and the unending presence of tigers in the crops as crisis after crisis, which had no solution. He never appreciated the cross-fertilization of ideas on this subject to bring in new expertise and awaken the complacent scientist community to perk up the excellence of their research, instead he continued to chase me seriously for years, even seeing that I should be removed from honorary wildlife warden-ship of the reserve.

Project tiger is a much flogged example that explains that Indian conservationists, although are united in their dedication to the cause but because of their different priorities and ideologies, have always been divided in the choice of their conservation targets. The terrible part of this looming catastrophe is that people have been working on solutions for years yet nothing substantial seems to have been achieved. Moreover conservation itself is defined in so many different ways that there is no single overreaching agreement on what constitutes its effectiveness. That is why the great collective of dedicated people, represent a fractured conservation community, which has never been particularly effective in preventing or even slowing down, the ubiquitous decline of wildlife. The Indian wildlife scenario has now regretfully become a victim of the attitudes of supposed wildlife conservationists who would rather conserve their egoistical single minded choices than struggle for consensus for the conservation of their larger cause. Billy was just one in this basket.

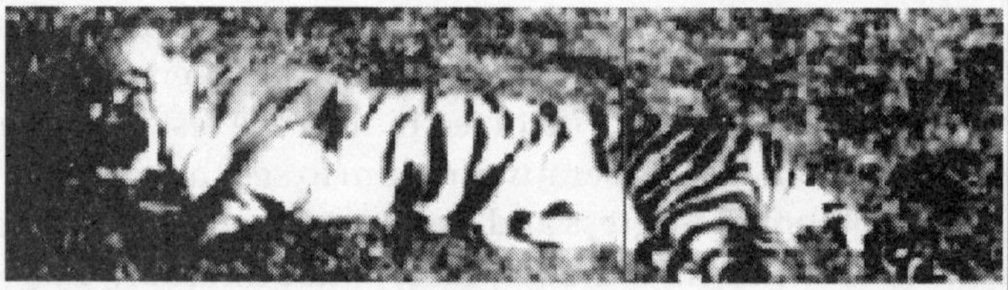

Dead Tara

Billy revealed the secrets of his heart very rarely. Once while sitting with him in the office of Ram Advani Booksellers at Hazratganj Lucknow, Ram and I heard spellbound his magical experiences , when Ram said, "Tigers are your prime concern, what is your assessment of this cane scene?" To this Billy pointed at me and said, "This kiddy has already listed loads of points on this line; now the very theory bears his signature. Let him establish it. To me the cane tiger has a vastly different meaning". When I asked if he could give some strategic inputs and solutions to save this almost universally repudiated animal? He never suggested any propitious means but to perorate, 'Less intensive production of sugarcane can reverse these trends. Remove sugarcane from the area'.

The permanent removal of sugarcane would thereby mean 'taking away the tiger's new lease on life' as the species would lose a substantial chance of sustaining itself on the buffer less borders of jungle.

His proposed cure to the malady seemed worst than the disease. Instead of putting his resources to protect this tiger, he seemed to have no sympathy for the plight of farmland wildlife. To my mind sugarcane is a unique wilderness; a replacement of grassland forest and a natural forest for some tigers, which had resuscitated their populace affectedly.

Needless to say, it is also an important zone for the mixing up of mammals, reptiles, birds and amphibian species. The permanent removal of this crop would thereby mean 'taking away the tiger's new lease on life' as the species would lose a substantial chance of sustaining itself on the buffer-less borders of jungle.

The constriction of predators' breathing space will create a woeful state of affairs for an animal which is listed as endangered species and the pressure on peripheral tigers will become unbearable. Then their numbers will again fiddle with themselves and the automatic system of population check, 'intra-specific aggression' will come into play, decreased production, decreased survival of cubs, abandoning of subnormal cubs, small families and fights will accelerate the process of their disappearance and thus qualifying for an immediate threat of extinction- a thriving biomass will shortfall by mendacious process of habitat reduction- a purported surplus will become a complete deficit- and all this will happen through human hubris, antagonism and parochialism.

Things have changed a great deal since 1948 when refugees deforested the great buffers of grass and scrub land to settle down. The past events have shaped the present. We cannot get those vanished forests back but instead we have overflowing sugarcane fields on the very land. The perennial crop, recurrent through the year or many years, happens repeatedly and provides water in lieu of desiccated jungle ponds serves as a superior substitute to grasslands. Its savannah environment supports many wildlife systems including that of big cats and helps to regenerate the tattered wildlife by providing a safe breeding space. At least for last sixty years, since post independence, this grassed real estate has been familial reproduction ground for much of Tarai's wildlife including that of tigers. This insinuates that sugar plantations are special places for special events and cannot be permanently removed without creating debacle for wild animals. It will amount to an acute poison pill, corresponding to a lasting deforesting this time that would aggrandize untenable habitat and push wildlife to its nadir.

Lest I be accused of being contemptuous of WWF, Project Tiger and a top set of experts; perhaps I never saw wisdom in guarding the sensitivity of personal human relationships with regard to sugarcane tiger conservation issues. This specialist subject remains of paramount importance for me and I am unable to comply with the authorities in charge of policy governing this specialist subject, who are willing to pay lip service to my sugarcane tiger concept but never learnt to honor the presence of tigers in farmlands. Their politically motivated operative discretions have played untold havoc with this animal and acrimoniously encumbered my commitment to preserve and protect it. In my renege and inability to sail the tricky winds; the farcical overtones and anthropocentric approaches, that override bio-centric priorities in the supposed interest of voting public, I have indeed fallen apart from my relationships with shock, despair and dudgeon, with many a 'recreant gentlemen' of these organizations.

The balance of nature is delicate, and once upset is not easy to set right again. Now when our wildlife and its habitat are so devastated we cannot run through the doctrine of laissez-faire and apply the old paradigms of wildlife management. We must go by proactive and pragmatic measures to help big cats to survive the crisis in any landscape wherever they feel contentedly ensconced and multiply, be it sugarcane or any other innovation.

It was difficult to imagine a more striking contrast. Yet in the changing times the sugarcane tiger better represented the spirit of the Tarai than the jungle tiger. And if there were indeed character differences, rooted in habitat differences, such as atypical prey composition, then which set of traits better embodied the survival mannerism was an interesting question. The essential pith of my project was to demonstrate the malleable capacity of tiger to adopt even the human dominated landscape as an ultimate mode of survival, often much 'rough-and - tumble' and much full of jeopardy. Thus our knowledge should not be restricted just to an ecological research of the habitat but studies of human dimensions of tiger conservation should be conducted in collaboration with social scientists to understand the vital factor effecting tiger recovery.

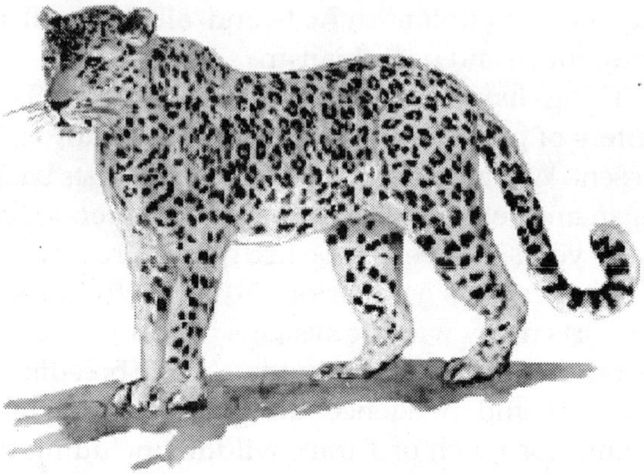

Sometimes I wondered when billions of dollars worth of resources were being poured into cosmetic tiger saving schemes and pseudo-scientific experiments by international agencies, this extraordinary story of sugar-tiger had lingered on so endlessly as dubious, and whenever I looked forward to any funding agency for my project, my proposals were stymied, undermining my confidence and forcing me to examine my motives and commitments for tiger protection once again. For example in1984, I wrote a letter to Dr. Bernhard Grzimek, the director of Frankfurt Zoo, Germany, seeking financial help from him for in-depth study of sugar tigers. This doyen, best known for establishing Serengeti National Park, along with his son Michael, thought it proper to take a feedback from Billy on this subject. He forwarded my letter to Billy, whose opinion never became clear and the things finally ended in a mess. A decade later same story was again repeated with John Aspinall Foundation in England. Though John was personally sympathetic towards the predicament of these tigers but due to the non-affirmation of big boss, he failed to release any fund to support my cause.

It was out of these failures and reactionary feelings that it grew into compulsion, perhaps an obsession for me to do more; to keep the secret fires burning and continue to map out more plans.

During this time, the leopard menace was raging at its peak in sugarcane farms in Maharashtra and a young scientist Vidya Athreya, a member of IUCN's Cat Expert Group was studying the causes. The problem was interesting. When these leopards were displaced and sent back to the forest they panicked and tried to return to the place where they thought they belonged. Many such cases were sighted in Ahmednagar, Junnar, Kolhapur and Karad districts and the most conservative estimate about the number of leopards in sugarcane area was at least 700 in

Maharashtra. Vidya was wondering whether these leopards were instinctively adapted to the crop and some particular niches that blandly favored their survival in contrast to jungles that were strangely unfamiliar to them. Sugar plantations were manmade ecological biome of their own kind and as per extrapolation there were 10 leopards per 100 square miles with four to six cubs. Vidya maintains if the natural 'agrarian rhythm' of the setting is not disturbed, leopards would continue to thrive interminably.

In the chapter 'Shifting paradigms', I have explained the basic factors that determine the presence of tigers in sugar crop. However, these apparent facts failed to gain much ground with the authorities, and the government failed to involve villagers strategically into tiger conservation. I think that instead of acknowledging what I had researched out in practical and inspired sprit, Project Tiger authorities were obsessed with their specific technical canon and conditioned mindset that believed in the all-time truth of old theories. At the root of this pedagogical approach was a firm belief in the vertical nature of science. You must know A before moving on to B; while I believed, even if you start with a clean slate and focus at any point of the phenomenon, the preceding and succeeding stages like alphabetical order will soon become clear to you.

I could even sense that there was also a basic spur of authority psychosis. Some typical Indian bureaucrats even raised questions on my nonscientific credentials that a professor of Ancient Indian History, with a doctorate in Buddhism and classical Pali literature should better talk about the cycle of rebirths and Nirvana, than to talk about land-ecology and tiger biology.

True community participation is important for continued success of any conservation programme. Sugarcane plantations are not a protected ecosystem like jungle where tigers can thrive at their will but an ecosystem where they are vulnerable and can only thrive at the will of human beings. I knew that my effort to save these tigers will neither prove sustainable without large funding, nor capable of eventual goal of expansion to cover other Tarai districts where cane tiger problem was growing.

True community participation is important for continued success of any conservation programme. Sugarcane plantations are not a protected ecosystem like jungle where tigers can thrive at their will but an ecosystem where they are vulnerable and can only thrive at the will of human beings.

In 1993, once again with the idea to attain some crucial financial support for the continuation of my research, I prepared a fresh proposal and sent it to Project Tiger. The officials, as usual, readily termed my report as unviable and refuted the hypothesis about the existence of a unique animal. Hypothesis is the first step in doing science and a wildlife scientist like George Schaller has probably listed some half a dozen really interesting hypothesis on his name, but it was unfortunate that my hypothesis could make no impression on the bulwark of dogma which defended the headquarters of apex body. Though I offered to appear personally before steering committee to answer their queries but the mandarins could not set aside their strongly held ideological positions to attempt a dialogue with me. My experience convinces me that in wildlife sector, ideology is a poor instrument in decision making and perhaps less absolute definitions can help us reach out better solutions.

This bogus, non realistic approach led the whole contention to an inane but mordant wrangle, which straight off went against the basic essentials of conservation; and the ultimate losers in this tussle were sugarcane tigers, who had no shield of political protection in a burgeoning democracy. They were vulnerable to human antipathy because the politician's electorate suffered from their depredations and the bureaucrats exploited their aberrant behavior as the best pretext to malign and shoot them. This also helped officers to score political points and oblige their bosses.

I wondered if only these guardians of our forests and wildlife could cultivate a commonsensical mindset and understand researchers better they would be able to share a new pool of knowledge and take advantage of it in their respective areas. But misfortune was heavy on farm tigers; they were blackguarded and rivaled and nobody was ready to welcome new facts. Like foresters, villagers too had adopted the irresponsible solution of their destruction to get rid of the problem.

As fate would have it, it was at this juncture of despair that Dr. P.L. Punia, the then Forest Secretary of U.P. and presently the Chairman of Scheduled Caste and Scheduled Tribe Commission of the Govt of India, sent a report to the Project Tiger office in Delhi, supporting my endeavors to protect these tigers, which struck a powerful blow at this crude perspective. It read, "Rahul Shukla is a competent observer of tiger affairs in the Tarai. This new concept of tiger guardians to conserve the noble heritage of this animal is a natural sequel to the original concepts to preserve, protect and manage wildlife and other natural resources. It comes out of the realization that conservation of sugarcane tigers now must of a necessity include the common man."

In the interim, three more tigers were found poisoned in sugar fields of Bankeyganj and Mailani areas. One had two newly-healed gun-shot wounds on him. The unhalting fiasco precisely illustrated that man would not generally spare living space to the great predator. Perhaps something was missing on my part too. I exceedingly thought that I had not been able to lay all my cards openly on the table and failed to plug the gap in the minds of officialdom. I had failed to orient them with the right knowledge, as to how the real tiger populations function in such habitats? In my inability to sustain a financially mammoth project all through these years, I could never put the venture on a fast track, using modern field techniques to work out scientifically. Otherwise, I verily believed, these tigers would not have met their nemesis in this blameworthy way.

Studying tigers and protecting them is an expensive hobby for an individual. No individual, regardless of how seriously motivated and how excellent a performer he is, could hope to arrest the process of decline of sugar tigers unless the slothful government machinery was not properly engaged. The authorities simply needed to understand that sugarcane is not just a strictly seasonal habitat, because the habitat loss created by harvesting is not of permanent nature. It is perennial, crop after crop, that carries all the four essential components, food, water, shelter and space and regenerates soon, paving way for tigers to come back and continue living there on the basic principle of existence -take a right prey and live well. Their selection of prey is the key to their comfortable sailing. To a predator anything that moves is a prospective game but it acknowledgment is controlled by proper judgment, such as an elephant is too large and mice too small and similarly a man is disagreeably queer and killing his livestock is also full of detrimental consequences, so a confirmed sugar tiger, self-oriented by treacherous expediencies, finds it better to steer clear of it and go for something unnoticeable, such as the feral cattle. I believe habitual farm tigers are also able to exist as scavengers for long periods.

It was an opportune moment for big cat Pundits to zero in on one of the greatest wildlife spectacles of the post independent India and understand inveterate sugar tigers. A realistic understanding on this line could facilitate them to quit the iniquitous 'naturalistic-fallacy' that tigers are exclusively jungle dwellers and prompt an innovative initiative to save this singular animal. If this tiger was to be saved, a reappraisal of phenomenon was de rigueur to recant the previously held beliefs but they showed no wish to face this reality and access the unsullied repository of knowledge hidden away in the coverts of Tarai farmlands; they rather preferred to condone the entire gamut of imbroglio.

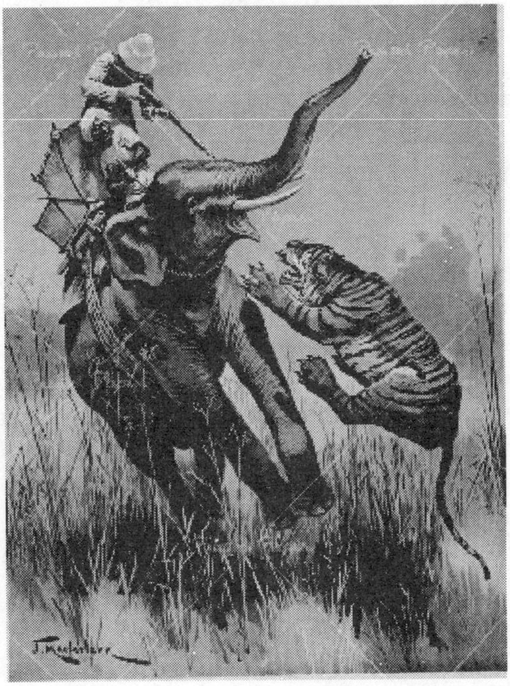

To my mind such an orthodox comprehension of tigers related to a particular place just as a vicar is related to cemetery, is only fit for babies and sucklings in the bureaucracy and not for experienced foresters, who have spanned the fields for years, watching ecological changes and who by the very nature of their job get opportunities for extensive travel and field surveys. They know for sure how much of infinite variety of wildlife lives outside the jungle, in farms and wastelands, odd areas, orchards with grassy herbaceous understory, abandoned fields and edges, riparian buffer strips, ponds, Fencerow/Hedgerow, banks of waterways, bush piles and snags, the standing dead trees that reptiles and birds use for food, shelter, and nesting; they know how to review and incorporate new information about it, as it becomes available, into all field operations, yet they mistakenly related tigers only to forests.

Now when many species are threatened by increasing habitat fragmentation and the gap between their survival and extinction is getting dangerously shorter, addressing these questions - as how fundamental niches differ from realized niches- would help us to understand as how in future the species will interact with the changing mosaics of habitat in their landscapes. To know is to predict and to predict is to control.

We lacked the systematic evaluation of the problem because it was unpalatable for many skeptics that the mega predators of the jungle were not only confidently holding their own by man's side, but underlining this was an elusive widespread 'throng', whose partiality to the sugar habitat was a weird genetic quirk. My rock-hard experience - a great deal diverse from inferences and conjectures - had imbued me with a cocksureness that most of the tigers operating in sugarcane were in broad terms just 'tigers in sugarcane' but a small segment amongst these that was doing arguably better, was the incorrigible 'sugarcane tiger'. In fact it was living there by the choice of habitat selection - accepted on ecological merits - and was not an inchoate signature in the making but was the obdurate dweller of canes. Here all the 4 basic habitat components for healthy communities were present necessary for nourishment and shelter against weather and predators. There was space for activities such as gathering food, attracting mates and raising young. This unique blend of elements created a sort of 'safety net' around tigers and sustained them so well that even if they were forcibly driven into the jungle, they came back in next to no time.

We lacked the systematic evaluation of the problem because it was unpalatable for many skeptics that the mega predators of the jungle were not only confidently holding their own by man's side, but underlining this was an elusive widespread 'throng', whose partiality to the sugar habitat was a weird genetic quirk.

The data emphasized five important points: (1) Perhaps, the sugarcane tiger was actually an 'ecotype-animal', strengthening in hitherto inaccessible and backward countryside; (2) perhaps it was not much capable of crossing the boundaries from farmlands into wilderness without fear of dire consequences; (3) the people seem to be unintentionally interfering with the natural development of this ecological foot print, which might be transforming into a putative strain (4) the buffer species of livestock constituted an important prey base and (5) that the last factor contributed in the increase and maintenance of high population, at times to the point of being artificial.

Tiger is a creature of remarkably open modes of life and they are at their best wherever they are - including sugarcane farms. I believe that the secret techniques of fortitude, genetically hard-wired in them were passed on by their ancestors who had also inhabited farmlands, because instincts are non-mental actions which, owing to their frequent repetition, become so habitual in the course of generations that all individuals of the same species automatically perform the same actions under stimulus supplied by the same appropriate circumstances. Here I may say that the tigers were living virtually unnoticed, so silently and secretly that the three tigers which I discovered in the neighborhood of five villages, between Jajmau and Sultanpur of east Pilibhit district were quite unknown to the inhabitants.

The discussion of the historical substantiation of sugarcane tiger is one of the central features of this book. Hence it is not in isolation to cite an instance which corroborate that big cats have the ability to go about their daily routine inconspicuously in human landscape for much longer periods than has hitherto been thought possible. Mullapur village lies under Pasgawan police station at the border of Hardoi district, where a tiger strayed in June 2001 and accommodated itself conveniently in the sugarcanes. The village is some fifty kilometers from regular jungle and the natives here had never experienced a tiger for generations. They came upon his pug marks almost daily on the banks of river Gomti but had no idea as which animal these belonged to. However, they were immensely happy at the sudden end of Nilgai menace, to which they could not attribute any apparent reason.

As per version of the herders who claimed to have seen the pugmarks of tiger for the first time in summers just before the start of monsoon season, the time period roughly corresponds to mid June 2001. The lonely tiger lived within the vicinity in a perfect placid state for nearly a year, with no record of confronting humans or killing cattle, thus escaping retribution, till one day it was unfortunately discovered. The poor beast had no idea as how determined people can be when they are afraid of a predator. The very idea that a large predator was nearby made the villagers feel vulnerable. The tiger was chased by a berserk mob, fired at and wounded by guns. For over a week, it carried several bullets in his flesh without molesting a single human soul and was finally shot down in April 2002 by Ashish Tewari, the deputy director of Dudhwa Park.

In latest incident of 2012, a male tiger arrived at the outskirts of Lucknow city and took refuge in the Subtropical Mango Institute. Perhaps a wanderer from sugarcane component and not directly from the jungle, it remains a mystery as how he covered 200 odd miles from Pilibhit, eluding observation, yet feeding on regular kills.

This animal understood the nuances of dealing with the people. It sheltered in the sanctuary during the day and moved out only in the night, taking round of some ten to fifteen kilometers but coming back home before the dawn broke. It gave a wide breath to the villagers by remaining silent at their sight, owing his power of concealment primarily to caution, noiselessness and capability to remain motionless rather than to any pattern of cover. Inside the mango orchards', it changed its locations repeatedly when labors moved about and retreated for the cover as soon they crossed the safe line of thirty meters. Once in the late evening, I saw him inspecting the ladder of the *Machan* where the dart shooters sat in wait, during day time. It moved around the cage set to trap him and despite temptation of bait, never entered it, only when shooters moved away after sun set it came to the tethered bait, broke the rope and took away the kill to eat in deep cover.

On 11 February, around Methepur village, I followed a drag mark and discovered the remains of a Nilgai calf. Surprisingly within hundred meters of kill, the people were working in the cereal fields and yet none was aware of the presence of tiger near it. We could only know that when some fishermen saw him crossing the Behta nala towards evening.

One day a minister arrived, accompanied by no less than fifty people and a big motorcade. His entourages chased the predator, threw bricks, shouted and abused and the beleaguered beast moved from cover to cover for the entire day. However the animosity remained only one sided as the tiger avoided responding.

It is the knack of animal that it learns to live by man without becoming a problem and it is the streak of man that he makes a problem of that presence. After this last incident I tagged this animal as 'No Problem Tiger'. It was finally darted by a zoo vet Utkarsh Shukla and relocated in Dudhwa jungles.

Broadly speaking our lack of understanding of the tiger's true nature and its fine-tuned mechanisms as well as our intellectual bankruptcy to rationalize the concept of sugar tiger has greatly hampered our effort to preserve these cats. The contradiction of wildlife conservation scenario is that we only talk of scientific dogmas replacing one with another even as reality takes its own course- often leading to wide-ranging fiasco.

However with the changing times, the old idyllic scenario of Tarai has rapidly transformed; the symbiosis of villagers and wild animals around them is slowly dying. The cause for concern is man-carnivore conflict and the continued indiscriminate removal of large carnivores from their rangelands by farmers; it is largely because a realistic understanding of human dominated landscapes and also its complex factors is yet not achieved. This aspect is reflected in the poor content of conservation plans that deal with large carnivore management and human-carnivore conflict mitigation measures. The failure to incorporate guidelines and scientifically sound conservation tools into conservancy management plans reflect the lack of a structured approach to solving this conflict on farmlands.

Baseline surveys conducted in recent past show a declining trend and threatened

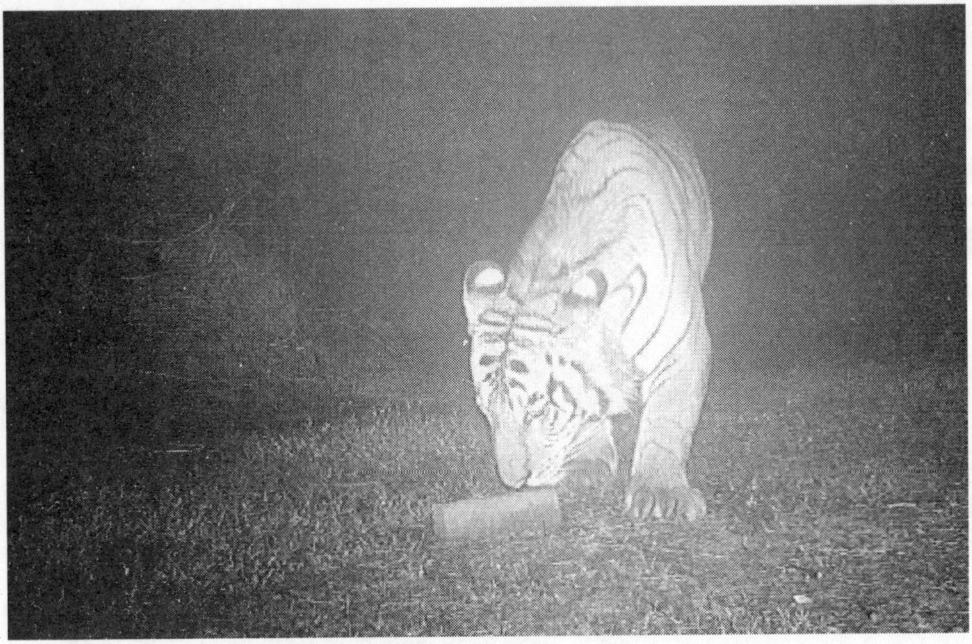

Rehmankhera Tiger, Near Lucknow city - January 2012

status of this tiger. We are practically left with no time to design a long-term research and await its results and then carefully plan a logical and legitimate action to save sugar tigers. It is believed that conservation is ultimately about creating and maintaining negotiated spaces for meeting ecological targets in human dominated landscape, where ad-hocism also serves the purpose as an acceptable way out.

This prelude sets the beginning of what is to follow in these pages. This book, however, is more than just about a theory on conservation. It is also about my life's struggles to overcome several predominant canards about tigers and their preservation. Many facts about sugar tigers are synthesized in these starting pages and as the intact gamut of information is cogently presented to readers at the very onset, one may wonder as what is to follow in coming chapters. All I can sincerely say is that having spent hundreds of hours observing sugar tigers, this is just a background to the repository of ecological and biological information that I have organized in this book. I would feel rewarded if something comes out of my work at any rate to save this inimitable creature.

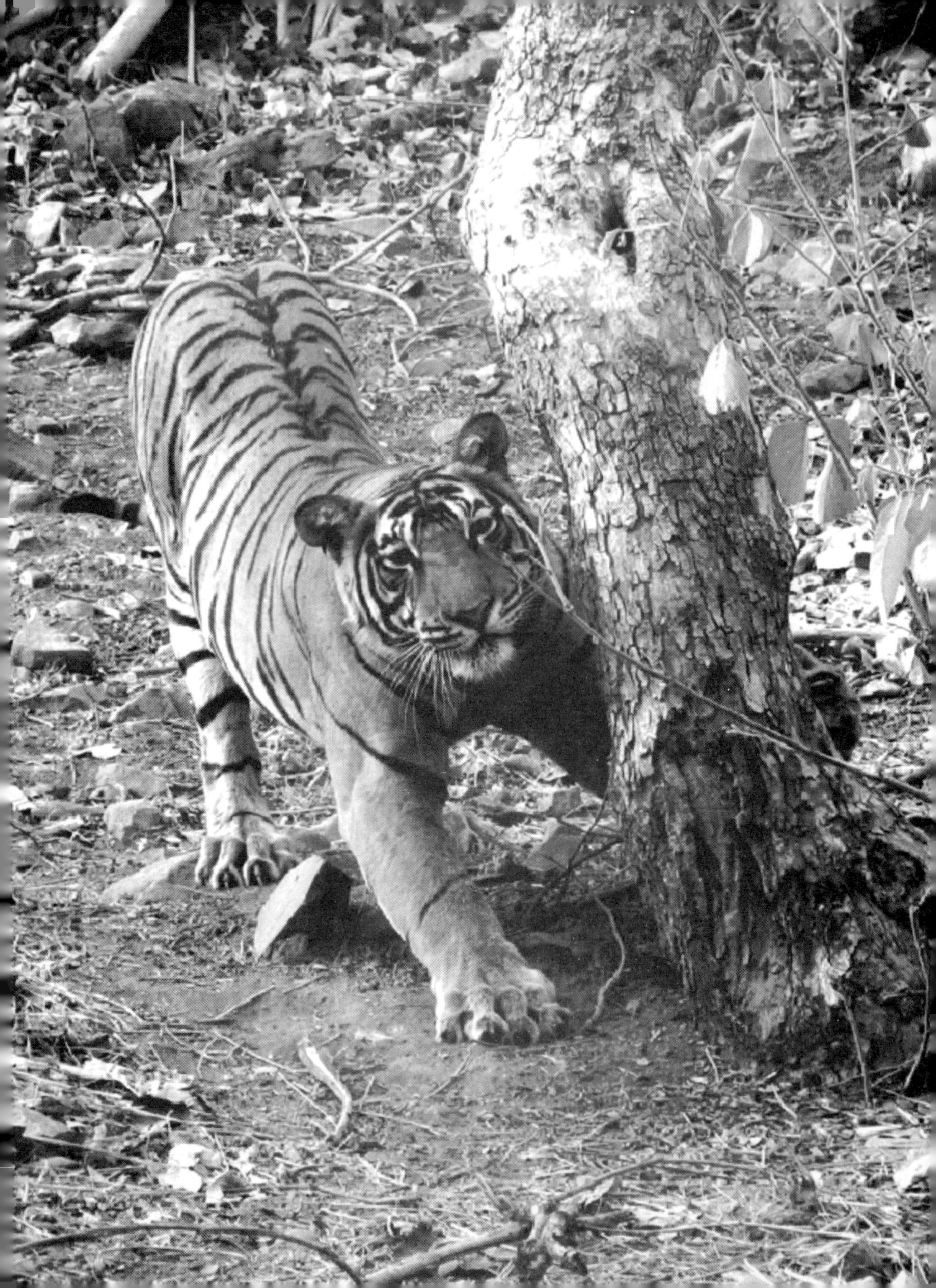

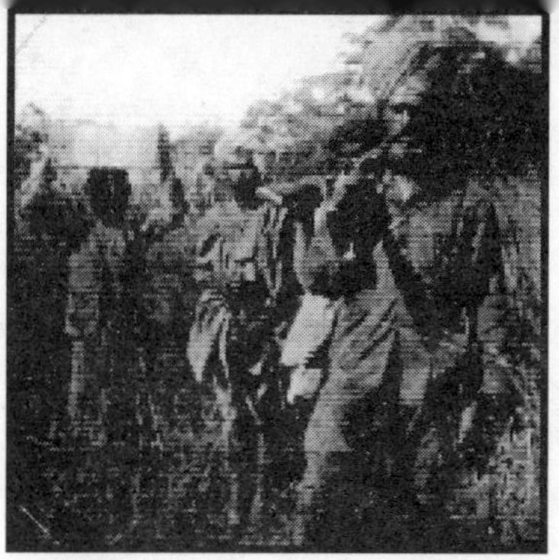

1

The Dawn of Independence

In some mysterious way, the woods have never seemed to me to be static things. In physical terms, I move through them; yet in metaphysical ones, they seem to move through me.

- John Fowles

The year was 1947. The joyful day in August that brought independence to India was indeed also a day of horror. The pro-partition Muslim leader Jinnah had declared that there were two Indias — one a Hindu India and the other a Muslim India. The Muslim minority did not want to live under the rule of Hindu majority because the Hindus stopped them from killing the cows it wanted to eat. The two-nation theory materialized on that day with the emergence of two nations — a secular India and an Islamic state of Pakistan. The partition brought in its wake an unprecedented wave of communal riots, first in Punjab and then in entire India. Amritsar railway station had become a camp for thousands of refugees that came in from the other half of Punjab that was now in Pakistan. They told horror stories about how their women were stripped, repeatedly raped and then paraded through the city.

This incited Sikhs in the Indian state of Patiala. They prowled the countryside pouncing upon Muslims and looting their property. The worried Maharaja of Patiala pleaded with them to return to their villages, "This is harvest time; you should be home, cutting your crops."

"There is another infected crop to cut first," replied the leaders slicing the air with their sword.

The holocaust on both sides continued for nearly a year, claiming the life of over a hundred thousand people and left ugly scars in the memory of those who had witnessed it. A large contingent of displaced Sikh farmers was living in refugee camps. Their properties looted, they were a poverty-stricken lot with little stock of food. They looked for a piece of land to settle down, if possible once again as farmers.

In the nascent government of India, the minister for home affairs Sardar Vallabh Bhai Patel was given the responsibility of identifying land for these troubled Sikhs. If he had his way, he would have made them settle down in the valley of Kashmir to 'correct' the demographic equation as a counter to the separatist challenge but Prime Minister Nehru would have none of it. He believed in a vibrant democracy.

Instead, he asked chief minister of Uttar Pradesh Gobind Vallabh Pant to look for a large tract of land in his own state.

The Himalayan Tarai, bordering Nepal, seemed to provide an answer to their problem. It was covered with jungles and the prime tiger range did not appear to be of much use to the government. A virulent form of malaria had until then prevented the encroachment of humans in this land. It was rightly considered to be the best place for the rehabilitation of refugees. Consequently, hordes of Sikhs were deported into this exigent land. They were asked to clear the forest and grassland for themselves. The decade of the 50s saw a major migration of Sikhs to this land.

The rights of the feudal chieftains administering this land were being gradually appropriated. Threatened by the Zamindari Abolition Act of the Central Government, they rather welcomed the settlement of the refugees and began to lease blocks of their surplus lands to the new arrivals. Their privately owned forests adjoining the government reserve forests had acted as a buffer zone to the latter and absorbed the biotic pressure from the adjacent village population.The feudal lords never waited for the government to acquire the land and pay them the compensation. Instead, they were happy with the jewelry, other expensive items and whatever cash the Sikhs carried with them, to pay for the land deal.

"They will give us indemnity bonds, what will I do with that paper? It will mature twenty years later. I want immediate settlement," said a feudal registering his land in the name of a refugee. It was a large tract of virgin grassland; a historical breeding ground of tigers. "We were cutting grasses when we met three young tigers in it. They were looking at us as if they had never seen humans. My brother shot one while the other two escaped," said the Sikh who had bought it. This arable land, once a section of tiger sward is now called Sarna farm. It is located on the metalled road between Palia and Majhra Singahi.

Life on the frontier was not for the timid. It was a challenge for the newcomers to adapt to the new environment. The humid and enervating climate was much different from the dry heat of their homes. Tarai was scantily populated. Here the people, rendered ambitionless by its hardships, had always lived a simple and frugal life. The new race of settlers soon showed that they were made of sterner stuff; though plagued at first by virulent malaria, which killed quite a few of them, they hung on grimly. This was the kind of spirit that had carved civilized towns out of wild and untamed territories.

The rugged settlers were not only handy with the axe but with guns also. Their taking up farms in remote regions meant sure death to the wild animals. Free issue of crop protection licenses made matters worse. Hunting degenerated from the status of a dignified and exciting sport to mass slaughter without any rules. They shot often for meat and killed many animals that destroyed their crops. Hundreds of *chital* and hog deer were slaughtered for their hides. The plentiful supply of

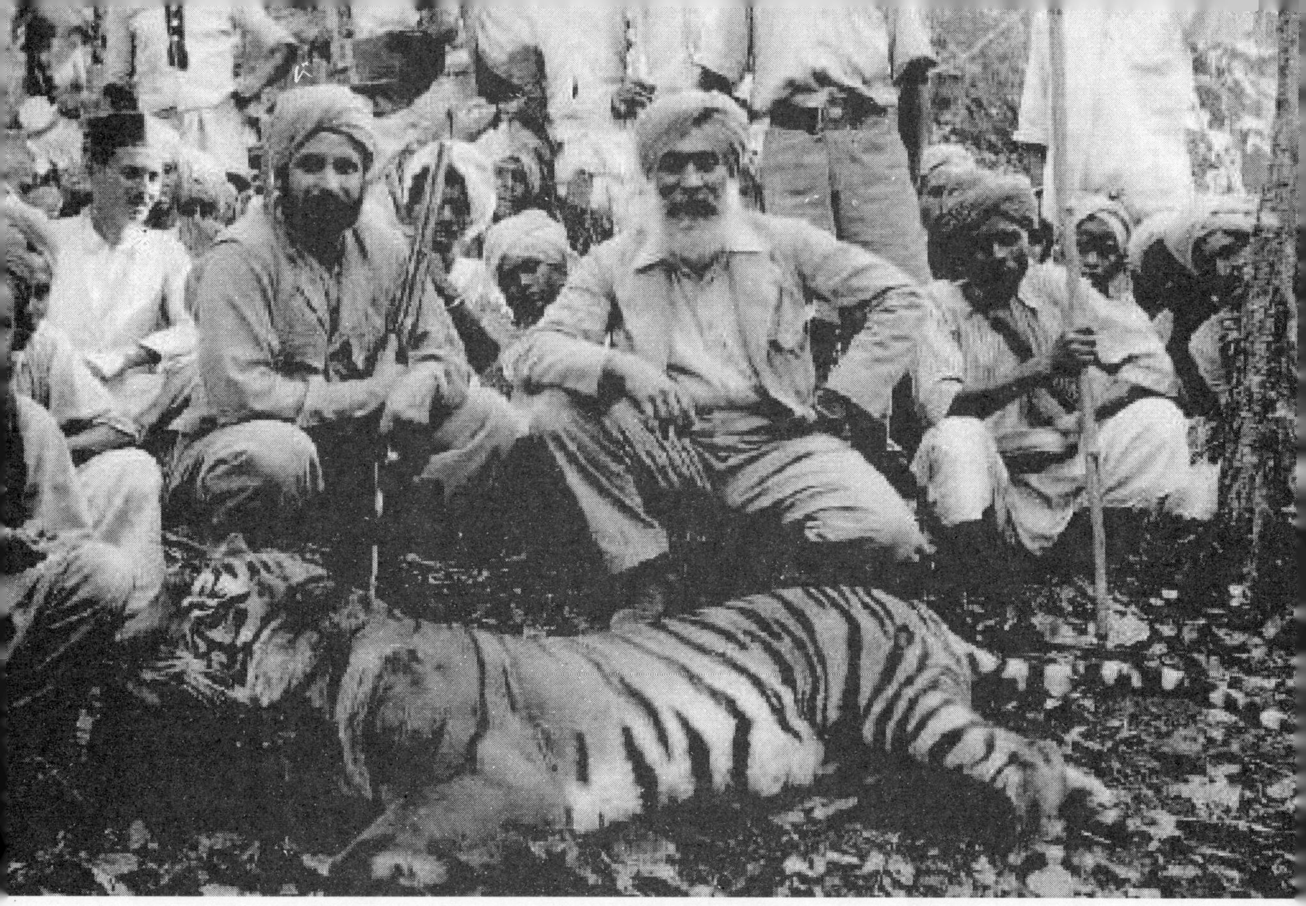

It was customary for the early settlers to shoot the predators which preyed upon their domestic stock.

game animals was an incentive to hold on to; the settler would at least not die of starvation. "It was certainly a different kind of hunting for us. The game came to you, instead of you going after it," recalled a settler from those early days.

Gradually, their farms began to open the grasslands all around. The wild Tarai slowly came under the influence of our so-called civilization. Deer competed with cattle for grazing lands and were heavily hunted; their meat served as food and their hides were turned into clothes and shoes. Each year the number of settlers and hunters increased. They felt no remorse over the killing of thousands of animals; to them it was a question of survival of cattle over wildlife. The game retreated before the march of human population. Gradually, the endeavor of settlers materialized and they began to make a decent living. Their ambitions succeeded where the apathy of the locals had failed.

The maternal side of my family belongs to Tarai; this way in some measure, I too, belong to this land. My maternal great grandfather was a *Zamindar* of high status. He owned an empire of over eighty villages in Kheri district. Most of these villages were nestled in the slots of forest abutting Kishanpur range which is now recognized as the second biotic complex of Dudhwa National Park. Comparable to Jim Corbett's home at Kala-Dhungi, a small settlement called Larti, stood amongst the magnificent stands of *Sal* trees, which served as capital to this empire. This ancestral village of mine was a thriving bastion of wildlife. Tigers roamed in its surroundings and roared in the nights. Paths leading to the village were ideal for the sporting purpose. I had an enjoyable fortune twice over — to grow up hearing the stories of family heroes and early settlers, and chasing the wildlife. I had seen my first wild tiger here at the age of eight years.

Near my family's feudal estate in Mailani-Khutar area, the great tracts of tiger paradise had begun to change. Threatened by the obliteration of feudal rights, the family too had begun to charter blocks to new comers to check the appropriation of superfluous land. A large company called 'Collective Farms and Forests Ltd' was entrusted with the job of clearing the forests. Mighty farms were forged out of the wilderness as men chopped, sawed, drilled, and plowed the serene and undefiled land. Hundreds of thousands of acres of wildlife habitat and waterfowl *Jhabur* that served as Tarai's 'duck-factories' were penetrated and gutted to make way for towns. The region of tamarisk brushwood, lining the bed of the Katna River where flocks of pelicans gathered in the season were reclaimed by agriculturists. Pelicans are not game birds, yet the settlers frequently shot the awkward looking

Painted storks nesting on a tree

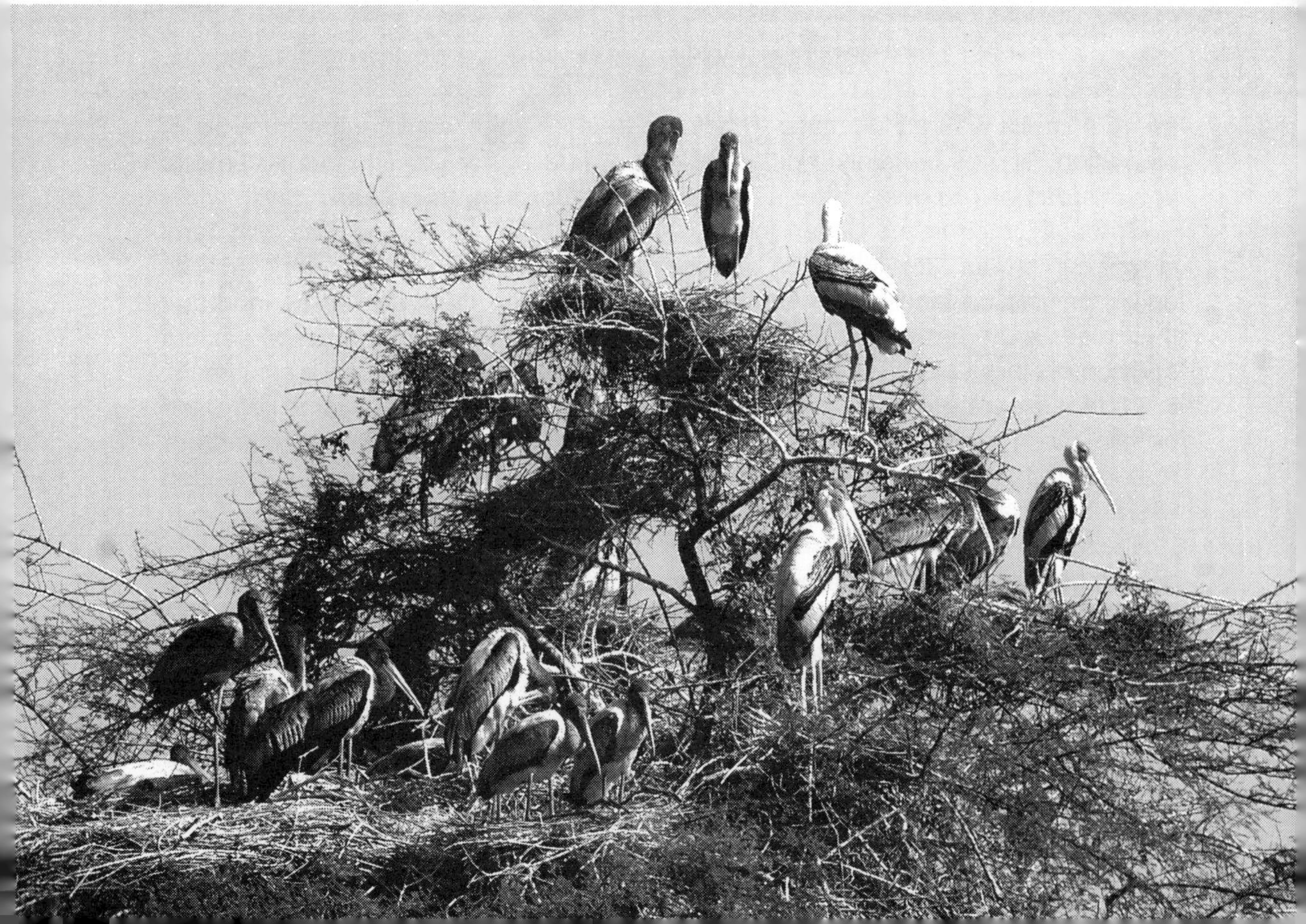

creatures with their suitcase like beaks just to see them fall and tumble.

When the pioneers had blazed the trail and tamed the wilderness, the less adventurous moved in, and townships and farmhouses sprang up overnight. Everywhere new settlers had only one thing to tell, that they often came upon the pug marks of a tiger approaching their *Jhala* in the night (*Jhala* is a temporary Sikh hutment). It was clear that the conversion of tiger forests into cropland on a massive scale had snatched away the old home of the tiger and compelled him to live an itinerant life. The ecological integrity of their homeland had been essentially decimated by agrarian expansion, and the species that is extremely shy and avoids contact with humans had no option but to accept human intruders into its own environment and adapt itself to live in closer proximity with them.

"I remember my father's oxen were time and again killed by a leopard which he could neither trap nor shoot. Once a doctor treated the remains of an ox with both strychnine and arsenic and left it out as bait. The leopard was never seen again," said Baj Bahadur Singh, an early settler in the area.

As the colonists dominated wildlife communities, the wildlife was forced into withdrawal first, and then into decline. Although, much of the virgin land had been cultivated, sugarcane farms were the latter human modifications to the hitherto inhospitable tiger habitats. The land use change offered an alternative form of cover to tigers, which was almost equivalent to grasslands. Sugarcane grows to a height of ten to twelve feet and remains a dense quiet shelter through the winter months. When the ancient land was covered with jungles, man was the intruder. Now as farms had come up in place of the jungles, the tiger had become an intruder, for him, it was a return to the long grass. Before long a unique accidental and unintentional relationship developed between the two species, which can only be aptly described as symbiotic. The tiger provided a strong protection to the crop from the nightly raids of herbivores. They instinctively ate the flesh of most of the crop raiding mammals and the villagers allowed him to flourish. The old theory that predators were 'bad' and therefore had to be destroyed was countered by the fact that predators had a significant role to play in the basic life support system of man. They were beneficial and served a purpose, cost-effectively.

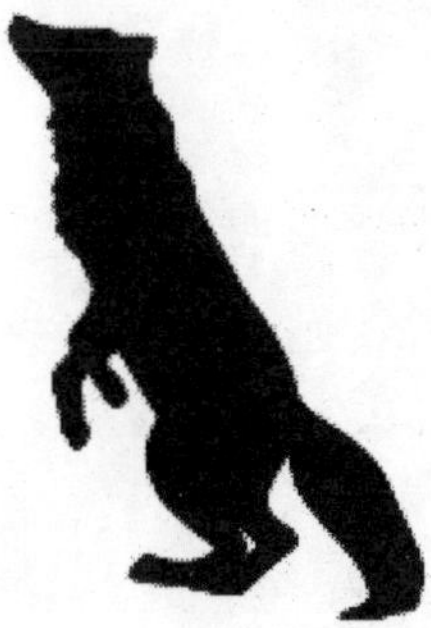

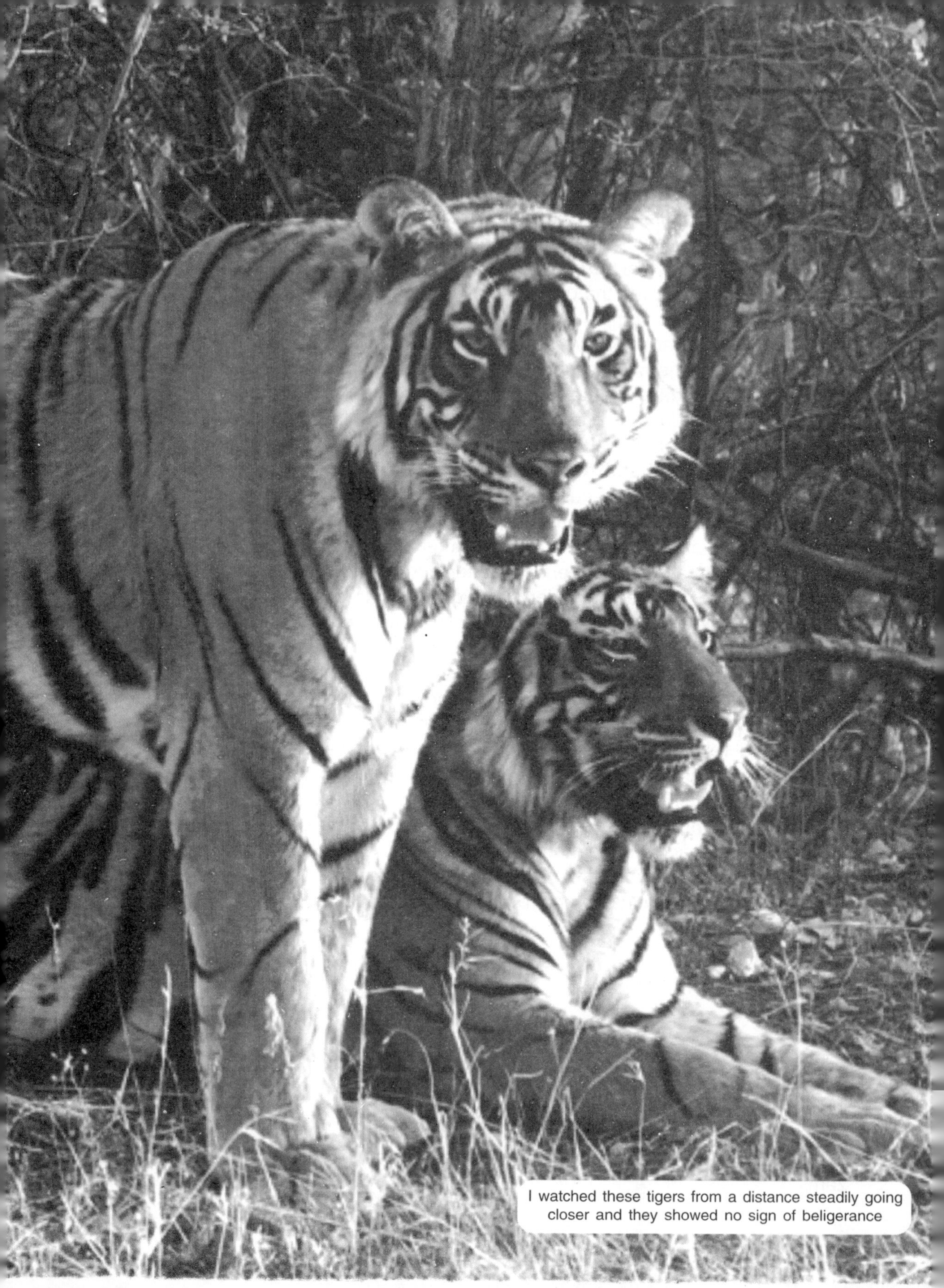

I watched these tigers from a distance steadily going closer and they showed no sign of beligerance

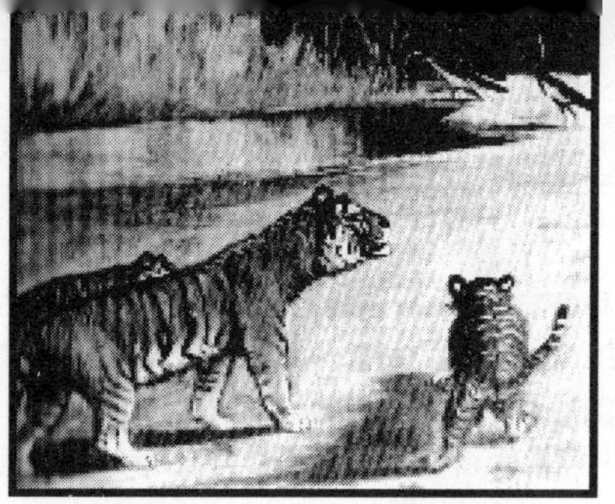

2

Arrival at Paraspur

I feel like I'm nothing without wildlife. They are the stars. I feel awkward without them.

- Bindi Irwin

It was well beyond midnight in early October of 1976. A passenger train screeched to a halt at Palia station of North-Eastern Railway. The darkness was warm and airless. The desolate platform was lit by a couple of wheezing pressure lamps each with a halo of swarming insects. Only a few people had alighted on the platform. I thanked my fellow-passenger for giving me good company through the journey and bade him goodbye. A minute later a shrill whistle pierced the stillness and with a loud puffing and clanking the train rumbled on its wounding way to Dudhwa. The red light at the rear of the last coach was soon lost to sight as it turned around a bend. Once again the station was shrouded in stillness.

A canopy of stars lit the beautiful night. I picked my rucksack and walked out of the platform. A short, plumpish figure emerged from the shadow of the station building. It was Vijay Singh, the driver sent by Mintoo Mama to pick me up. Mintoo Mama is a distant collateral on my maternal side. He lives in a settlement called Paraspur and owns some five hundred acres of farmland. I boarded the open jeep that proceeded for the village that was about fifteen miles away.

Removing my boots, I lay back in the seat and reflected on the turn of events that had brought me here. The death of my mother had orphaned me and I had just completed my post-graduation in History. I had much to worry about. The graph of my life had dipped to its lowest ever and future seemed bleak. Unemployment was rampant and there were no suitable jobs for educated young men like me. This outing was more like a runaway refuge for me from my problems and the insensitivity of a noisy city.

Sure that some change is better than none; I had come here to complete a contract assignment for a newspaper of Lucknow that required me to send field reports on tigers living in the farmlands of Tarai. I had grown up in a household which had its roots in the Tarai and regarded big-game hunting a normal part of life, and where the tigers had been kept even as pets.

Big cats were my passion. They were the focus of enthusiasm in my teens. In the zamindari forests of Larti, I used to follow them for fun with native hunters. This motley lot lived in a time warp – they had never sat in a train and could not imagine a country without tigers. In the company of such people, I had observed big cats on their hunts on moonlit nights from *machans* and blinds as they feasted on their kills. I had acquired some skills of the field crafts and traditional knowledge of wildlife. I had learnt from the Tarai and its milieu, understood its niceties, observed, felt and smelt it; often at an amount of danger and risk to life, hence reporting on tigers was not a very challenging subject for me.

The forest trail of Dudhwa National Park ran at a mile to my right and left. It was among India's oldest and finest protected areas that sheltered a variety of endangered species ranging from elephants to tigers. Full of giant *Sal* trees with massive trunks often rising to impressive heights, the park was said to be home to more than a hundred tigers. It was a part of globally significant tiger belt that included Kishanpur Reserve in the south and Katarnia-Ghat Wildlife Sanctuary in the east.

The sky was cloudless and dawn was breaking when we neared Paraspur. We occasionally passed a drooping, plodding donkey carrying a sleepy peasant on its back. I spent half an hour at a point to savour the grandeur of early morning. A little ahead, two large peacocks appeared on the edge of the road about a hundred yards ahead of us, heads down pecking grit and their feathers afire in the early morning glow. As the birds saw the jeep coming they ran a few feet and took off, flying grandly but quickly, their long tails flowering behind them.

We moved on a narrow dirt road that meandered through a thick young bamboo forest. Mintoo Mama's house was close at hand. In a little while it emerged as a neat and whitewashed building roofed with terracotta tiles and glistening in the morning dew. A cluster of Jamun trees grew around it. Mama was sitting in the verandah, half lying back in his armchair and holding a glass of *Mattha* with a smoldering cigarette held between his fingers. A bunch of his henchmen sat opposite him at the big table, relishing tea in brass glasses. The scenario was just what I had been expecting, since he had been holding this *durbar* for years – regardless of the weather. Mama's face lit up with a broad grin on seeing me. "Welcome boy, coming to study the cause of man- eating, eh?"

"You will surely get many chances to study them... there are many tigers here, more numerous than the leaves abounding the trees," he said with a stylish braggadocio even as he gestured me to sit. But then he was a little solemn. "Something has certainly gone awry. Their number has gone up like anything. Some of them just kill human beings but do not eat them."

"Well Mama," I said as I settled into a chair. "This is indeed alarming for these man-killers can later transform into man-eaters."

"You are right Hero, almost every week one or two people just vanish from their farms. It is only sometimes that their bodies are found. A male tiger is also visiting my premises these days. His pugs are marked in the vegetable garden. But he is harmless. A couple of days ago, he passed along the irrigation channel and spray marked the tyre of my tractor trolley," he said sipping his beverage. I was glad he remembered the affectionate term he used to call me since my childhood.

Meanwhile the driver brought my haversack in the verandah. Uncle's scruffy mongrel Fidoo was sitting on the stairs, watching him vigilantly with interest. The driver knocked at the door and Fidoo stiffened letting forth a torrent of deep barks. The driver asked Uncle if the dog would bite.

"Well," Mama answered with jovial sarcasm. "If it does not bite then it is a useless dog. His job is to do that only. After all I spend two rupees on him everyday."

The horrified driver threw the bag in the verandah and ran away with the jeep. Fidoo immediately galvanized into action and sped after the vehicle yapping vociferously. Some more dogs materialized on the scene swirling about the wheels and almost hysterical with anger. The laughter of farmers rang in the air as cheerful and full of life as ever. They feasted on the hot tea and biscuits while I turned my attention to the hot tea and *Pakori*, which Mami had sent for me.

The morning was cool with a rush of cold air and the exhilaration was narcotic. I felt a sense of freedom as the sun lifted over the horizon and the mist dispelled, changing the blue of sky to the purest gold. With no particular agenda for the next couple of hours and feeling completely relaxed, I went into a room and dozed off for a little while. In a vivid but short dream, I saw myself walking along a sugarcane field with a striped tale following me a short distance behind me.

I got up with a start, took a refreshing bath and towards forenoon I embarked on my job. Mintoo Mama's sons Om Bir and Shyamu volunteered to provide some succor. They had been my old acquaintances from Larti days. Om had once been a singularly handsome fellow but had now changed greatly. He was tall, his face was sallow and thin with prominent brown eyes but now he had hit the bottle hard and that had made him look like a pale faced, older and grimmer man.

I had brought along the old Ordnance maps of Kheri forests, prepared by the Survey of India. These high quality maps, four miles to an inch, folded in book form and mounted in cloth are so studiously primed that the topographical features including villages, groves of trees and even water bodies like rainy *nalas* and ponds are displayed in minute details. On the basis of authentic information gathered from print media and foresters, I had outlined at least twenty two villages on the map where the tigers had been very active during the previous months and several heads of cattle had fallen prey to them.

I had no idea about the movement patterns of these tigers or the spatial designs in which their ranges could exist in this human landscape that fell in conjunction with India's last optimum jungles of Tarai. A former hunter named Mahadev Lonia offered his services to assist me and map out the movements of tigers. Tiger movements are decisively linked to three main factors: hunting, fraternizing with their kin and avoiding the only enemy they fear — the man. The first factor, however, is a judicious determinant of tiger movement.

Mahadev was a sharp old man with a face lined with centuries of traditional jungle knowledge. With a pencil he drew rough semi-circles on the map, depicting the possible ranges of these tigers. I was amazed at his meticulousness. His approach to the subject was much on the lines of orthodox hunters who systematically planned the killing of a tiger by chalking out its route. Their basis was recording the points of tiger kills in the area. For example, a cattle lifting tiger has a habit of following a particular beat or route which may extend over even fifty miles and in case of man-eaters it can be even one hundred miles. Having secured a victim in the vicinity of villages and hamlets, it halts there for a couple of days and nights, until he has eaten out his kill and then moves on again. In this way, he not only escapes when things become too hot for him but he also arrives at fresh pastures of opportunity unknown to its inhabitants.

Such movements plotted over a period of months produce a definite pattern that is somewhat rhythmic. The most common of these is a rough triangle, the three points of which are flexible but generally four to seven miles apart. For the tiger works round the territory in a huge rough circle and according to the extent of his beat, surely returns to the vicinity of his starting point – it may be after a fortnight or a month or even much longer.

However, in the present case, I had no evidence of a regular beat of any tiger, yet theoretically Mahadev's methodology sounded so impressive that I believed in him. My problem was that the tigers were being reported from a greater part of sugarcane plantations in the Tarai, and their sightings were not always regular. They hid anywhere in the cane farms, lying in ambush besides village paths, confronted human beings and were even spotted during the daylight hours. There was no means to ascertain their actual number. I did not know that the marked 22 locations that covered nearly 100 square miles were being operated by just one adult tiger or two, three or four or as many as ten overlapping individuals, most of which were females, with exclusive sub-territories as I had anticipated.

We walked out a little and sat under a *gular* tree where a meeting of locals was called. Above the tree green pigeons conversed in bubbling flute like voices. In the course of the meeting that I learnt that within a limited area of 40 sq. km. about five tigers were seriously threatening the life of people. The situation was precarious as all were tagged as notorious with regular interactions among themselves. Plentiful supply of prey is believed to be a *sine qua non* for such a big build-up of tigers but I was doubtful if this landscape could offer anything like that. Could it be that they were taking greater interest in cattle as prey animals?

There were some leopards in the area too. I was told when the farmers were not visited by the stripes, they were bothered by the spots. A farmer named Pooran Singh, who had come to attend the gathering, had a unique experience with the beast. He lived in a hamlet called Belwa. One night he was startled by a tremendous commotion in the cattle shed but thinking it could be a tiger no one dared to go out and investigate the cause of disturbance.

"I stayed in my house and fired several shots in the direction hoping to frighten the tiger away but nothing happened and the noise continued erratically for over two hours before it finally ceased. Towards dawn I went into the pen and aghast to see my five pigs and over a dozen goats, lying dead on the ground. Their throats had been bitten through. It was only then I could realize that it was the work of a leopard. He had not eaten even a single morsel of flesh from any of the carcasses but just killed each victim all out of diabolical passion for hunting.

"The leopard had entered the shed through a hole in the mud wall and his tracks were made all over the ground. I hoped that he would return to make a meal next night and then I must have my revenge. Determined to do so, I set a strong rope trap near the entry hole and having secured it to a beam on the ceiling, sat in waiting with the gun. The dark winter night passed tediously. My family retired to the bed and I waited interminably but the wily beast never showed up his face.

"Towards dawn, I was getting half sleepy when I heard the beam falling on the ground. It was instantly followed by a growl and then a frantic roaring. I switched on my torch and the full view of a leopard appeared in the frame of the light. But holding the torch in one hand and the gun in the other was not a very comfortable position to fire a shot. My younger brother rushed out of the house carrying a lantern. As he approached the shed the leopard made a frantic spring in his direction but went only as far as the rope would allow him. My brother was so horrified by this attack that he lost balance and fell. The lamp broke on the dry Payra (thatch), which immediately caught fire and the flames began to leap. The leopard made another attempt and this time broke off the rope. Then like lightening, he moved within the shed, attempting to scale the walls. While feeling terribly frightened, I emptied the magazine of my rifle at the jumping and bouncing beast. He kept dodging the bullets and finally escaped out of a corner in the thatched roof of the shed."

The leopard had entered the shed much before the time Pooran became aware of him. Being caught in the knots, he was sitting patiently and chewing the rope to free himself. He had been doing it for quite some hours when in his noiseless effort to free himself he pulled the rope and the log fell down, awakening the hunter. But by then the rope had been pulverized enough to be severed by powerful jerks. He did that to escape away with a nasty knot still firmly tied to its right front leg.

"*Bhaiya*, he must have soon freed himself from knot too," Pooran said confidently as he concluded the experience. Indeed in my book, with all the 'ineffable malignity' and calumny leveled against leopards, they remain the finest cats beyond a doubt. Versatile and not selective about their habitat, they are equipped with the unsurpassed skills of survival and even if the misfortune of cataclysm strikes the big-cats, their kind will be the last to go extinct.

When all the excitement of story had died down we again returned to our subject of tigers. Then there was also the crucial information of a tiger killing a cow at a hamlet called Harkhapur. On hearing this occurrence I decided to go there, as the spot made an excellent starting point for an investigation.

It was midday before we got ready to start. Having selected our ammunition, a Rigby .350 Magazine for me and a shotgun and a revolver for Om Bir and Shyamu, we set out on a *Lehru* (bullock cart). Our intention was to examine some pet hangouts of tigers thus guns were only taken as weapons of defense. The air was bracing and the sky flecked with the white bulbous clouds that held the light like a drop of wine in a silver spoon. There had been some drizzle in the forenoon, so the climate was cool, not as hot as it can be in October. The rutted, muddy tracks led us from farm to farm. At a hamlet called Dukarha, we met three terrified laborers who had been recently mauled by a single tiger and had a miraculous escape. Their wounds were not very deep and seemed to cause little inconvenience. They emphasized on the enormity of the tiger's offensive and told us the strangest stories.

The track further led through a fairly dense cane country. On the way I was shown the favored spots of tiger attacks, where putrescent skeletons of two oxen still lay. A hog deer; warned by the approach of our cart, bounced away to the shelter of a thicket. At another settlement some natives claimed to know of a particular retreat where the tigers often concealed themselves during the day. They were eager to serve as beaters on a sighting-hunt but for a financial consideration. Their firm belief that a laborer is worthy of his hire, left me wondering that I could not even attempt to preserve their miserable lives without being expected to pay handsomely for this privilege.

An hour's journey finally brought us to the farmhouse, where the cow had been killed a couple of days ago. A tormented Sikh showed us the remains of the cattle, a square blotched mass of bones and skin, lying in a black pool of blood that had stained the earth darkly. A strong smell of decay permeated the air. I noticed that it had been killed in the open and then dragged near the well under a banyan tree. The killer must have been extremely hungry for he had demolished the carcass so fast that very little had been left of it. Now the vultures were finishing the work the tiger had begun. The owner of the cow told us, "Sahib, we have many sick and aged cattle, already close to death but the tiger does not go for them. He selects healthy and useful ones and inflicts a great loss to us."

Om Bir was high on booze. He becomes crazed and mean when drunk. He immediately caught the collar of the Sikh and said, "Don't you know that a tiger is a king after all and not a jackal who will be satisfied with a diseased bag of bones?" The man was so unnerved that with a sudden apology he made a ceremonial salaam and never argued further.

The farmer took us a furlong away to rain-fed nala. It had plenty of water at this time of the year with a narrow stretch of sand bank on its either side. A small bevy of peafowl, pecking bugs at its edge felt disturbed at our approach. They fluttered

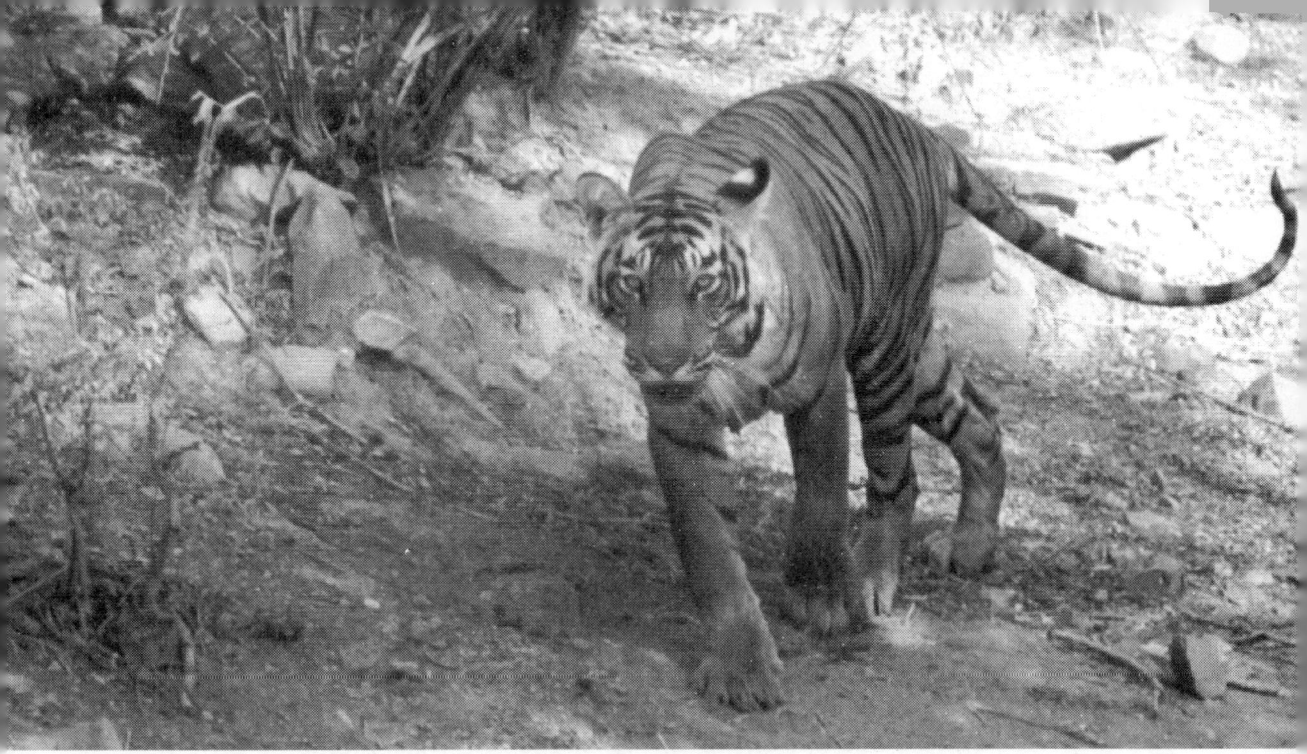

The lame tiger that roamed around Batihar village near Haldwani.

across the nala and stood in a curious broad line to watch us; females looking as vain as ebony peacocks. Now the sky had cleared and the midday sun, gliding over the land of fresh, wet green colors bathed it in a benison of light. We noticed that a tiger had indeed passed along the nala, from north to south a few hours ago. On favorable soil, the clearly cut square pugmarks of a male led far along the nala bed in a long dotted line. They were visible long before we reached there.

The pug had normal toes but a very large pad. As I stood looking down upon it, I figured that even allowing for exaggeration caused by imprints spreading in the squelchy sand, the animal that had made them was undoubtedly colossal in size.

Walking further along the banks of the river I came across the marks of another tiger. This one was of a smaller size. From some deeply-indented tracks, I could distinguish the signs of a territorial tension. The smears of dry coagulated blood and some tufts of hair showed that the visitor had been surprised by the local male and there had been a brief scuffle. Then bigger one had chased the smaller one across the river, and both of them had gone up the escarpment towards a small hamlet.

Genuine fights amongst tigers are very rare and confined almost entirely to wildlife films of a sensational nature. Intolerance amongst tigers is usually prompted by intense territorial tensions; it is assumed that such cautionary chases are part of nature's precaution against crowding.

In my eventful life as a teenager, I had seen very many tigers in the jungles of Larti. I had never thought that such fine and rangy animals that lived a solitary life in the cavernous forests could also make their home in the sugarcane plantations.

The sight of those great pads seemed to make all the exertion of the outing a meaningful exercise.

The day passed off in a whirl of activity. By sundown our inspection was over. We turned for home, making good progress on a virtually empty cart track. Here and there we passed by many temporary encampments of Sikhs set amongst crop lands carved out of forests. Darkness had fallen and the *jhalas* were illuminated by the glares of several bonfires, burning firewood with cow-dung, the ubiquitous fuel of the Indian countryside. All the men and children were gathered about them; their faces aglow as they sat sharing the village gossip with such inimitable gesticulations that every man broke into a laugh. I wondered at the will power of these families. As the night grew, the time was ripe for the super cats to go about their ghastly work in devastating silence, yet for these men, it was their normal state of existence.

We were nearing Paraspur, when a wild boar suddenly sprang out of the grass almost from beneath the feet of our oxen and quickly scampered on the road grunting. He had very fine and exceptionally long tusks, which prompted Shyamu to dismount at once and fire two rounds of ball cartridge from his shotgun. Fortunately in the fragile light of the night, without any flash of torch, he missed clean and to my great satisfaction I watched the porker quickly disappear, bounding away at a great rate.

Back home we took an early dinner and exchanging talks of adventure, sought the cool sheets of beds. I have very vivid recollections of that particular night; it was for the first time that after many months of emotional trauma, I was in a relaxed frame of mind. The day had been most delightful and interesting in every way. The change had been quite fine enough to monopolize my thoughts and prevent me from thinking of anything else.

Our cots were stretched in a row and lay closely in the open ground. Round the corner the pale grey cattle and buffalos chewed cud; fireflies flickered in the grass and night jars hopped on the trees. The power of nature that reflects itself in tremendous peace under the open sky had begun to take over. Shyamu blew vigorously at charcoal fires making them glow like rubies. The tropical night was gorgeous in its magnificence. The stars and planets blinked overhead and fluttered in their attempt to give off greater light. Man-made satellites hurried along on their journey through space. The moon floated up like a burnished globe with its rim cut clean for its trip across the sky.

Slowly the hours grew late. Then a muffled whir floated to our ears and a flock of flamingoes appeared above, flying the silent pathways of the sky at night. It was not the confused and hurried flight of fright, or the whirling darting turns of the birds at play, but a measured, stately pilgrimage through space. We lay and watched them flit across the moon. Past they sailed as fleeting specks borne in a current of soft whirring wings, bringing back to me a thousand boyhood nights from Larti.

I thought of geese in fixed formation in the sky, honking homeward toward the frozen North in prospects of their nests. The flamingos flew without a sound, under cover of the night. Where did they go? What was at their journey's end? Perhaps they were to settle in the moon's reflection in some far-off lake.

We fell silent as the excitement of the day came to a close. I crept under my blankets and slept soundly that night. It was a sleep of exhaustion. I finally awoke at an hour that appeared to be of late night, but as the jackals were yelping, I concluded that it was near dawn. The morning star hung over the dim dark trees. A chill, grey somber dawn was breaking in the east. A bulky shape stood motionless, casting a truculent inky shadow on the white dust of the moonlit road — it was a wild boar. I perceived it demurely, changed my posture and slept again.

(II)

I woke up quite late in the morning, watching the group of chirping sparrows fluttering in and out of the house. Shortly a Sikh named Sukhbir Singh arrived to meet me. An old acquaintance of uncle, he had a penchant for swear words and was like one of those you feel you have known for years even on your first meeting. He presented me a bottle of honey and a basket of fruits and immediately set on to recounting a harrowing experience he had had just two days ago. He was ploughing his field with a tractor, when he saw a tigress emerge out of a dense patch of sugarcane. On her trail was a pair of cubs who were completely unafraid of the tractor's sounds. They came near the machine and began to run around it. The Sikh was terrified. He dared not stop the tractor nor accelerate its speed to run away. He prayed to *Wahe Guru* and maintaining his calm continued to drive the tractor. All this while the tigress sat a little away unconcerned with the cubs' antics. A little misjudgment on part of the cubs could make them fall on the sharp-edged disk of the harrow and injure them. This could undoubtedly rouse the tigress into action with dreadful consequences.

But just then the mother stood up, coughed and returned to the thicket out of which she had appeared. The cubs followed her.

This experience, though nightmarish for the farmer, was most puzzling when viewed from the angle of tiger behavior. Sukhbir Singh was, however, emphatic on his narrative. "By God Sahib, I swear by my children, the tigers come and go. Original tigers. Sometimes they are here, sometimes they are there, but if we go to look for them, maybe we shall find them, maybe we won't," he said in his own matter-of-fact manner, and offered to take me to the place and show me the evidence.

We rode a tractor and reached the place that was about fifteen miles away. The blazing sun was already high in the heavens. I climbed a mound and surveyed the fields at length; it was a lonely point, an endless expanse of sugarcane crops running for miles stretched before me in every direction without a single distinctive feature. It was like a turbulent ocean of long grass over which the eye wandered, till it was lost in the dreamy indistinctness of the distance, where earth and sky blended in a cerulean silvery haze. And looming still beyond it was the panorama of snow capped mountains of Nepal, beautifully tinged in delicate rose colour. Here and there, throughout the course of luxuriant crop, the rainwater pools glistened, as the voluptuous sunshine, yellow as gold, poured over it.

I marveled at the immensity of the landscape as the light fleecy clouds hurried swiftly across the heavens, tinted of a wondrous blue. Such an uninterrupted habitat, though man-made yet without any sign of human presence as there were no villages or hutments in the sight, lies unattended for months, and is nearly a savage forest. This isolated, forlorn and undisturbed forest of sugarcane is certainly a prime habitat for wildlife, which can easily afford hundreds of prey and their various predators. A silence, deep as grave, pervaded the land. The snow-white egrets and a stately crane waded amongst the shallows, with their long necks outstretched, in attitudes of intense watchfulness. I felt impressed by the largeness of the scene I saw.

The Sikh, however, was accustomed to the scene and was therefore impervious to its splendor. For him, what was more memorable was the close shave he had with the big cat's family. He took me down to the harrowed plot of land where the ground was littered with tiny spoors and in midst of them various long checkered snakes were sunning themselves; the loathsome wriggly creatures lay over each other like mingled creepers. I penetrated a little further into the neighboring canes. With the sense of danger which becomes an instinct with the sportsman, my rifle was at the ready, and there, having walked for some 100 yards, I happened to discover a nursery. The place smelled considerably, a few splinters of bone that lay scattered around it showed that the tigress had been bringing small kills to this point. I found three hooves, a single horn attached to skull and the rib cage of a hog deer. There was no sign of the tigress as probably my arrival had alarmed her and she had moved away with her cubs. Or, she could be anywhere at all and difficult to locate and thus the tracking was left to the individual tracker's own skills.

It was this time that a *chital* started calling agitatedly in a patch of sugarcane. I came out and saw three does barking lustily some fifty yards towards south. Their sight was a good augury; for I knew that the tigress was somewhere around. I walked to that side and happened to catch a glimpse of a cub disappearing into a green plot of wheat; and the very next moment the tigress started to growl from an undergrowth close by. The deer fled away, and the natives, who had followed me, threw everything down and scattered like rabbits; some of them putting up a fine sprint to disappear among the trees. I quickly shifted on the mud path whereupon the bushes swayed violently and the tigress burst out at us with a series of coughing roars. She came through the thicket like a tornado and suddenly stalled as though she had applied a four paw break and stood facing us.

What a moment! What a magnificent animal she was! I watched her with my pulse racing. She had a large chest and broad frame, a portrait of power and strength as she stood there with her fangs bared in demonstration. She was at the edge of the track and only ten yards away from us. This was certainly one of the finest moments of my field life- the crown of all the joys of a tiger chase.

I had learnt to handle a gun since I was eight years old. There was no time to stop and think but I stood silent for some time with the safety-catch put at the ready and firearm carefully aimed between her green glowing eyes. The natural impulse is to shoot at once: a charging infuriated monster emitting terrific roars is likely to disturb the equanimity of the boldest heart but the life may depend on cool nerve and steady hand. I exercised utmost caution and withdrew slowly. Then lowering my gun, I deliberately walked a few yards along the road for the tigress to make sure that she had scared the intruders away and her cubs were now safe.

After a while as I had anticipated, she appeared to be thinking that she had admonished us enough; her look changed from one of defensive threat to that of unconcern. Her twitching muscles relaxed and she returned to her offspring.

I had held on to have a face-off with the tigress not to show off my daring, but because I know certain nuances of tiger behaviour that I had learnt in the wild surroundings of Larti. If this mock attack had been made on a non-naturalist, it would certainly have figured as an attempt on human life by a man-eater and a lot of furor would have been raised.

Jungle dwellers know that real aggressive threats of tigers are very rare. In them the mouth is closed, or partially so, the ears are erect and twisted in such a way that the backs almost face forward, displaying the bright white spot which the cats have there, and the pupils are contracted. It is followed by an intimidating growl and snarl as the tiger seizes its victim. On the other hand, in a defensive threat the canines may be exposed to, the mouth is fully open, ears are flattened and pupils are wide open and large. It gives the cat a fearsome countenance and makes it look larger then its original size. The rush is normally followed by a booming roar that continues as the tiger comes on and stops just a few feet from the target. I knew that this was a demonstration of annoyance and not an actual charge; but because I had adhered to the sound rules of sportsmanship that reduce the danger of a tiger attack to the minimum, things had not turned worse. However, I must admit that I had nightmares about this confrontation long after this incident.

We returned to Sukhbir's house. Our thoughts still dwelled on the tigress and her cubs. We found ourselves discussing the drama with amazement and appreciation. Anybody who thinks that a zoo tiger is like its wild counterpart has never seen a wild one up close. The power, the wildness and the fire of its eyes are so different from a captive animal. I knew that the place was no longer protected for the cubs and the tigress would now shift them away. The great cats as a matter of habit do not keep their young ones in any one place for long for security reasons.

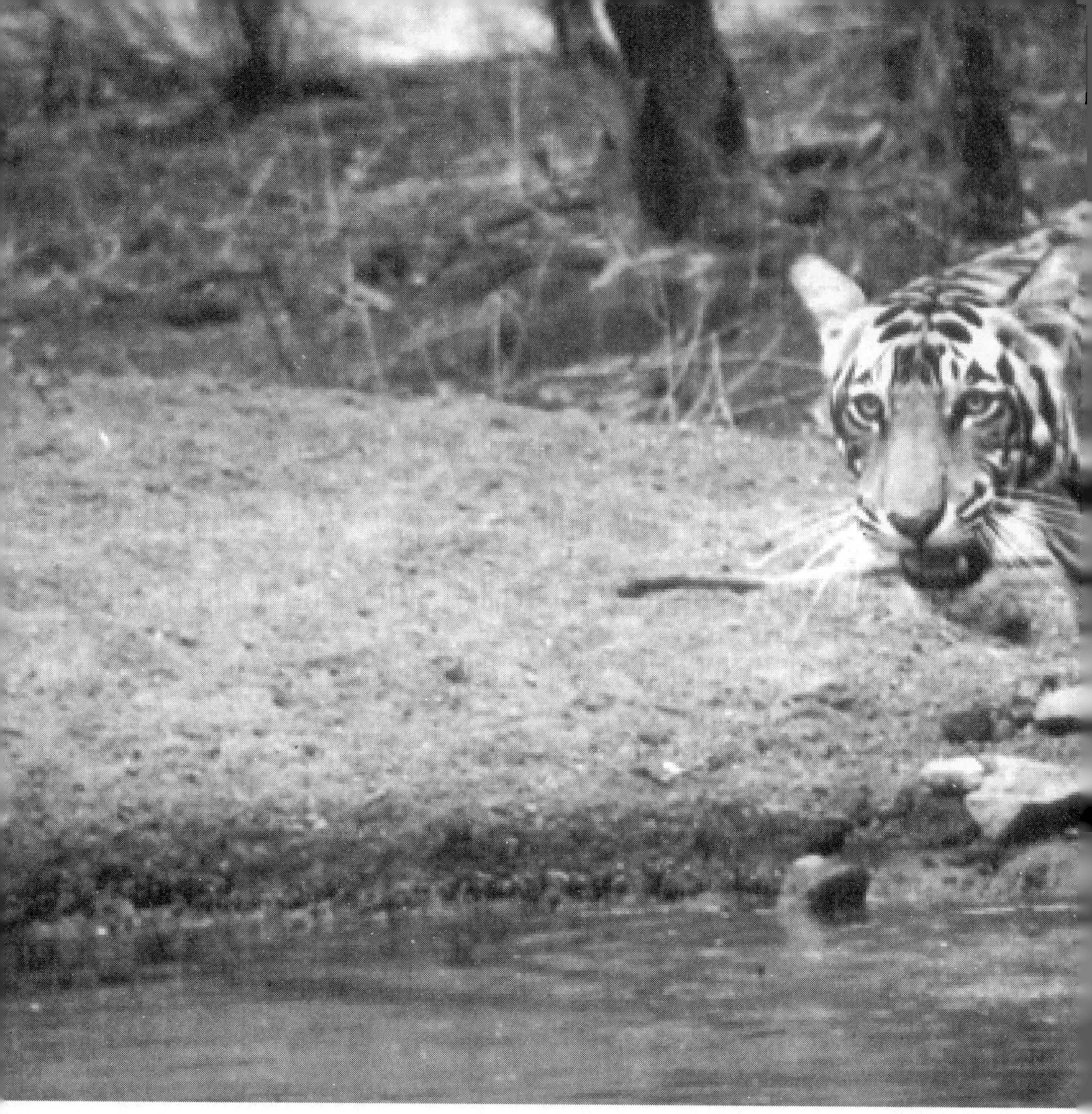

We had scarcely finished our meals when the driver informed us that the electrical circuit of the tractor had gone awry and was not responding. Sukhbir Singh was humbly apologetic to inform us that the diesel tank of his Jeep was almost empty. It was late afternoon and Paraspur was some fifteen miles away so it was still convenient to start on bicycles. With flourishing crops of sugarcane the character of the entire countryside had greatly changed and become confusing for a traveler, so two younger brothers of Sukhbir came along to escort us through the way.

We travelled at a good pace and within an hour had covered fully ten miles. Winter was already beginning to prowl over the expanses of Tarai and bird migration

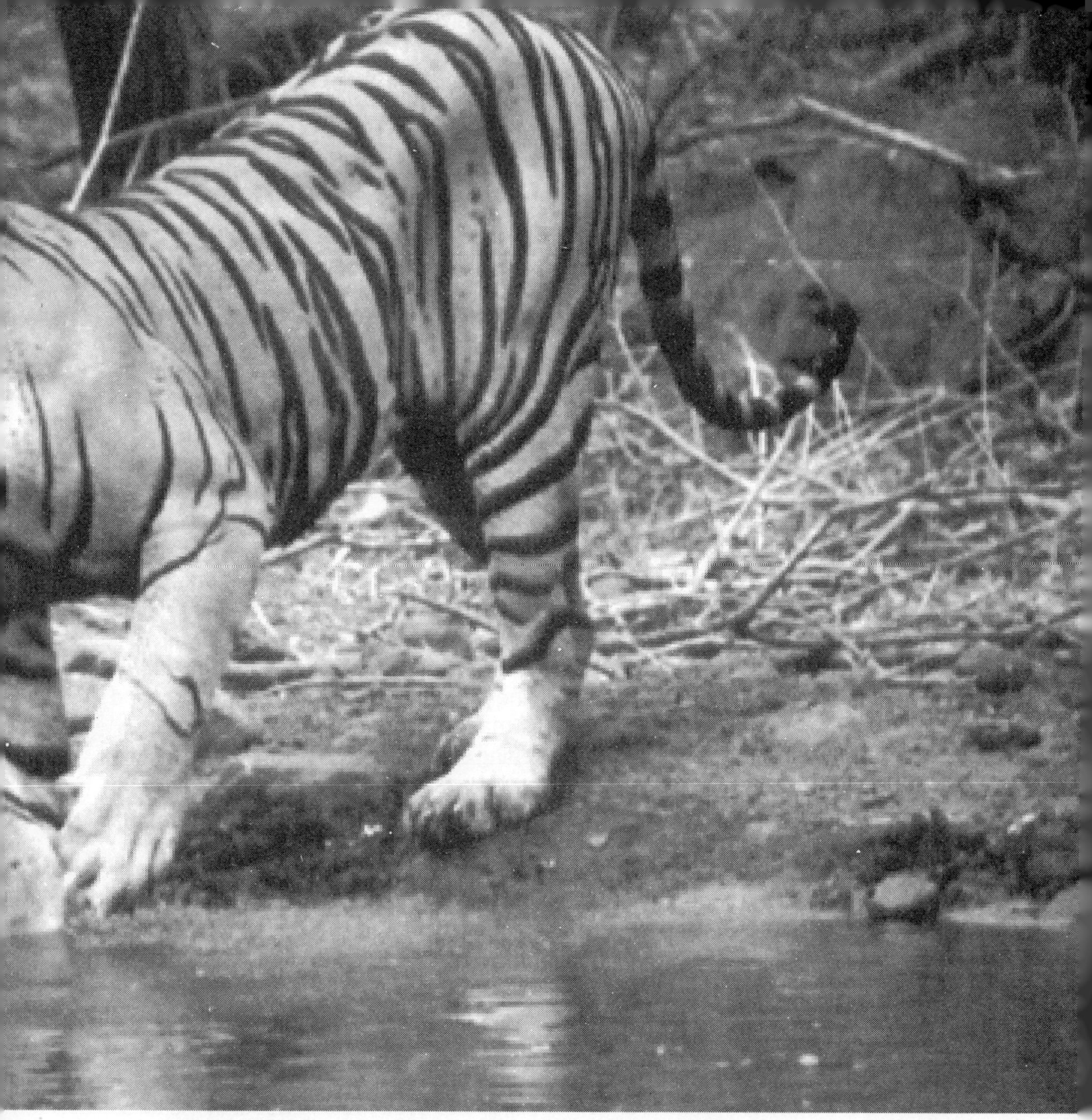

had begun. In the way, I saw the first flock of wild geese cross over the sky. The characteristic sound of ducks with their necks outstretched in purposeful flight conjured up the pleasant anticipation of time to come. Above and beyond the dusky jungle the fat dark clouds had compressed into an ominous inky mass. At one point I stood and watched the billowing clouds advance from the north east and slowly roll over the fields. Blinding zigzag flashes of lightning illuminated them in such a manner as if several gigantic electric wires had been hidden within them. But the birds were unaffected; they just drifted a bit, changed their course and passed the clouds safely. The sun was obscured but its refracted rays shed a ghostly half light over the huge flock which slowly sailed ahead and melted into the horizon.

Our day of thrill was yet not over. We reached near a place called Trikoliya and turned on a well defined cattle-path used by shepherds when all of a sudden I was overtaken by an uneasy feeling for no apparent reason. It seemed like a warning of the sixth sense, which people glibly talk about. I suspect it is probably no more than intuition supported by acute observation and shaped by sheer survival instinct in a dangerous and hostile environment. I slowed down the pace of my bicycle and very carefully examined the small lane running between two sugar plots from which I had to pass. A red fowl suddenly crossed the plot cackling cacophonously and some thirty yards away a pair of tigers suddenly emerged on the road and stood. The Sikhs moving ahead of me stopped singing and whispered '*Bhaiya , sher hai*'. We brought our vehicles to a sudden halt and stood rooted to the spot. We waited for them to move away but the tigers were seething with passion. They stood on the narrow lane and purred, signaled one another by facial expressions, body language and a wiggling tail, for want of better nuptial gestures. The female brushing provocatively against the male's head, flicked his face with her tail.

It was an astonishing and magical picture. We watched them making preliminary, flirtatious moves for some five minutes, when they took notice of us and crossed over to the other side. Soon their restless mating commenced inside the canes, with low growls and snarls breaking the evening silence. A peacock, whose roosting hour had been disturbed by the explosion of noises shrieked in protest whereupon we slowly backtracked the narrow lane and took another route to Paraspur.

It was amazing to see that tigers were infesting this part of the country to such an extent that they had made it almost inhospitable. It was wrong to say that the extension of cultivation and the increase of human population had driven them back to the forest. The check on the shooting of tigers showed how rapidly they would increase if protected by such immunity and how their domination would be restored even in the agriculture fields.

The evening was obstinately silent. The radiation fog that occurs at night and usually disappears after sunrise had begun to take over the tract. The sugar fields that were almost tenantless during the day suddenly appeared thronging with a multitude of wildlife and there were several pairs of eyes moving about in the torch lights. I could recognize these as wild boars and of course blue bulls, both favorite prey species of the tigers.

The dark had cloaked the land when we returned to the camp; all of us were dog tired and exhausted but feeling deeply contented. The two high voltage adventures had made the day something to remember.

I made an entry in my diary in which I addressed myself in a very different manner. "Red ink today, brother! The impressive show of feline fury made it something of a red letter day, but don't get conceited, lad. It is just the beginning. It seems that you are all set in for virtual experiences. Keep good judgment, son, keep alert."

The servants tended a fire in the open. The night was young. The stars blinked delightfully in the tropical sky. The dirt track leading to uncle's house gleamed like a pale ribbon, we sat round the fire chatting away unreservedly when Shyamu held up his hands and said sharply "Listen" and we heard a tiger roaring in the direction of the Sharda river. *Gharr..rr..r. hauom, hauom, hauom, auuungh, auuungh, aungh...*It started up like a soft throb of a motor engine and grew into a gurgle, like thunder. The sounds echoed back, amplified from the smooth embankments of river. These loud roars that carry as far as three miles through the forest in the silence of night are normally used by female tigers in estrus and males searching for them but often while mating or having mated well the male and female also indulge in a wide repertoire of sounds like nasal moans, hollow growls and grunts and full throated roars indicating an ultimate expression of besotted ecstasy- head over heels in love.

"Their mating is going full throttle", said uncle, adding dry sticks to the bon-fire, and we kept silent, listening to the awesome reverberations of a vibrant growling. I have heard these sounds quite a few times and these never cease to excite me. They make me realize that I am indeed in the midst of a favorite haunt of the king of beasts.

If it were not for the grave interests involved, the affair up to this point was almost insignificant. But I was to spend the next few weeks exploring the tiger infested crops of Tarai and somewhere in my heart I was deeply aware that all these happenings of the day were merely a curtain raiser.

Pleasantly weary from the day's work, I relaxed on a log in front of the fire. In the background there was an ethereal resonance of the tiger's call, which re-echoed sonorously through the encompassing escarpments of Sharda; sometimes so close that we felt physically effected by the unnerving acoustic energy. Om Bir and Shyamu even kept their rifles within an easy reach and cast many an anxious glance, out into the darkness beyond the circle of the firelight but I was in a different frame of mind, feeling imbued by the spell of Tarai -the grand scale of its adventure, danger and romance.

I let the feeling settel over me. It was glorious, intoxicating.

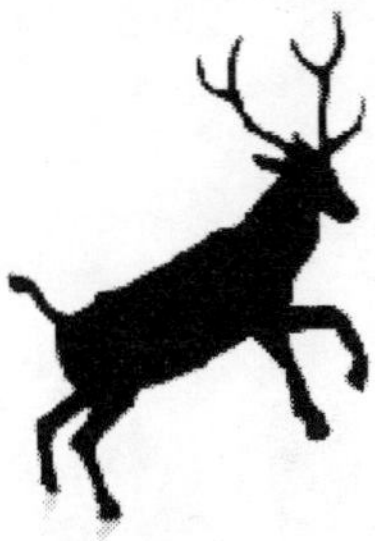

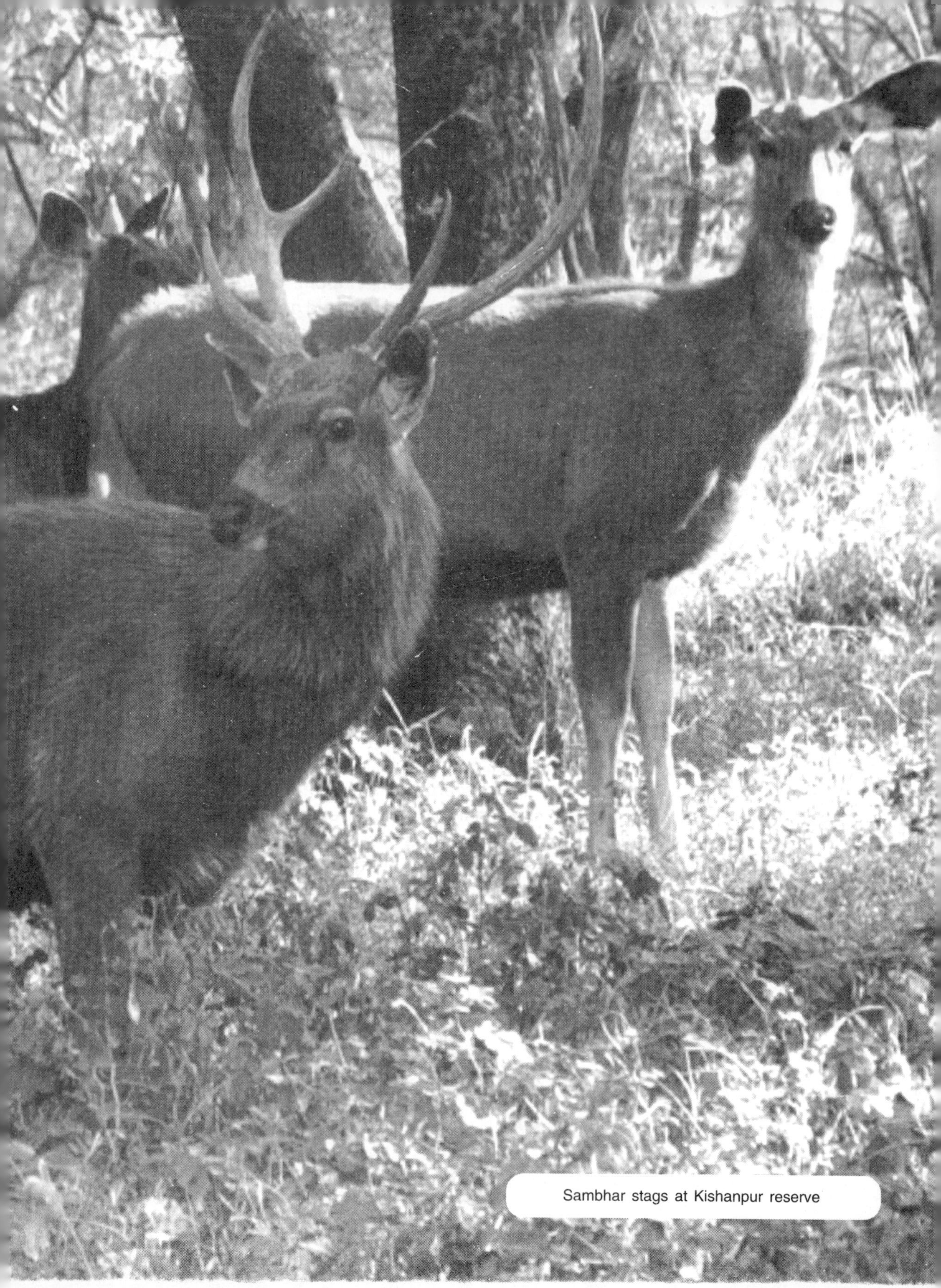

Sambhar stags at Kishanpur reserve

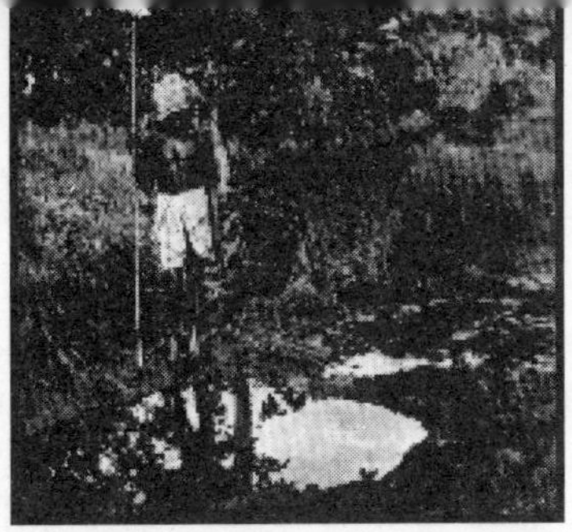

3

Trouble with Aberrant Tigers

The more we exploit nature, the more our options are reduced, until we have only one: to fight for survival.

- Morris K Udall

The full credit for my foray in wildlife reporting goes to Mr. Charles Baptista, the then Resident Editor in Lucknow head office of *The Pioneer.* This gentle, bespectacled old school journalist not only heard me out but encouraged me to come back with some stories from out there in the field. This opportunity of an assignment actually laid the basis of my research on cane-tigers. However, this enthusiasm was nowhere to be felt when I first expressed the possibility of the existence of such animals to foresters. To them, it appeared weird and something of a crude joke. I admit I too was initially taciturn but slowly as the phenomenon intensified, it started fitting scrupulously into the scientific scales of thinking, and this left no room for any doubt that there was indeed a specialized category of tigers, which preferred to live in sugar-fields than in the jungle. I had come to the *Tarai* on a journalistic mission, to take an assessment of situation, write and forget about it; but fate had lured me to tigers once again and little did I know then, that they were to become a part of my life, and that this was the beginning of a never-ending pursuit that would engage me for life.

Long back in 1877 Sanderson had sounded a prophetic warning about the tiger. "It is a pity to see the tiger proscribed and hunted to death by every unsportsmanlike method that can be devised, in response to popular outcries — chiefly in England – without foundation in fact, about his destructiveness. Trace out and slay every man-eater by all means possible, and at any expense; but ordinary tigers are exceedingly inoffensive, and have their uses. May the day be far distant when the tiger shall become practically extinct?"

Exactly a hundred years later, Project Tiger had been commissioned and was in full swing. Tiger population had stabilized and started to grow. A new cohort of tigers had replaced the older ones and had steadily come out in the open. These animals, initially believed to have spilled out of the perennial forests where their populations had become too high, were living and breeding in the sugarcane and marshes.

The Lakhimpur-Kheri district of Uttar Pradesh offered the most striking example of this anomaly. Tiger movements in many cane-farms of this region had suddenly grown high. Random sightings of tigers sitting, walking, laying, grooming or stalking cattle had become quite frequent to the villagers. This new existing generation of tigers did not have any cruel experience of man. They were unaware that their species had barely survived from extinction. Their sightings for long uninterrupted periods proved that they were oblivious of the recent past when their forefathers were considered a major hunting trophy in the world; and how they had adapted to a secretive nocturnal life to endure the pressure of hunting by humans. They never knew as how the dazzling spotlights, switched on over the fields were followed by a volley of shots and their forefathers, recognizing it as a signal of danger, went off headlong into hiding like a bullet. These new tigers were completely fearless of man and quite diurnal in their activities. Some of them had disposed off their initial shyness and were directly confronting human beings.

As far as I could gather from my observations, this was for the first time in history that such a fundamental change had occurred in tiger behaviour. It was unlike anything that Tarai had known before. Strangely enough the stage for this transformation was not set in the usual jungle home of tigers, but in an ersatz habitat in the guise of sugarcane, which is created and managed by man for his personal economic benefit. It was a delicate situation, liable to turn unwieldy and aggravate the problems for both man and the beast.

I kept pondering over these thoughts as I set about to my next meeting with Rana Omkar Jung, popularly known as Rana Sahib. It was a sheer delight to meet this old time manager of hunting camps who had witnessed a fair amount of shooting till the 70s. He told us that only till recently, the tigers were very retiring and it was literally impossible to glimpse them unless one systematically sought for them. "It's funny that now they are ubiquitous as if by magic." We were told many stories by the villagers of maneuvering massive 'beat techniques' for the hunters and tigers slipping out of hoop without being seen. A jolly Sikh, who had freshly returned from Canada, rendered one incongruous phrase that persisted in my mind, "God knows what has happened. At the moment our sugar farms are unquestionably the best tiger country outside the reserved forest".

Though contemporary developments symbolized the success of conservation programmes but the entire gamut had initiated many severe challenges. If man had saved tiger temporarily, he had also thrown himself straight out into a confrontation with it. There was no way to know for how long this win-win situation for both would last. Things seemingly appeared settled for the time being but the situation was definitely not genial, an ecological catastrophe was gathering momentum with terrifying conclusiveness and the tranquility, deceptive as it was, could not last for long. It is fundamental knowledge that young carnivores only need a hunger imperative to evolve into complete predators.

Fourteen kilometers south of Dudhwa abutting Palia-Nighasan road is located an old settlement called Sarkhana. It was the winter of 1976 when for the first time,

I had come to survey this area and stayed at a hamlet called Bhujia farm of Chaudhary Mahendra Pal Singh.

The farmer told me that only a fortnight back a tiger had created trouble on his farm. On that evening, he was sipping tea in his lounge when from the window, he saw a hazy shape enter into his verandah. The animal leisurely crossed over and went towards the cattle shed. Chaudhary took it to be a mongrel dog and did not bother but after a few seconds he heard choking, rasping sounds coming from the shed. They were followed by the brief sounds of struggle as if the bulls were frantically trying to break the ropes around their necks in order to run away.

The farmer cursed his bulls in anger; much in a belief that the rival bulls that intrinsically hated each other, had once again locked their horns. He went to separate them before they got down to serious trouble. As he lit a torch on the scene of commotion, he was shocked to see the bull lying dead on the ground and a tiger crouching upon it. Two reddish orbs gleamed brightly in the feeble glare of the torch. Indeed the tiger had sensed the arrival of human being, so he left his grip on the bull and retreating behind a small clump of straw, sat there to avoid further encounter with the interfering man. The farmer, not daring to attempt to rescue the bull, somehow maintained his nerve and retreated slowly. When he had entered the house he asked the women folk to sit in the drawing room and close the door tightly from inside.

Choudhary's youngest daughter Dr. Nirmala who works as principal in a local school, made an audacious attempt to get the gun. Despite the warnings of her father, she crossed the courtyard and reached an isolated hutment that was located beyond the cattle shed and where the single barrel .12 bore shotgun was kept. She locked the door from inside and fired four shots in the air from a window accompanied by the yelling sounds of women folk.

This intimidated the tiger; he came cantering out of the cattle shed. While in the process of retreating, he inspected all the closed doors sniffing and pressing them in his efforts to find the way out, till he finally reached the boundary wall and jumped out.

Choudhary's two brothers lived in farmhouses close by. Early next morning, the tiger killed a buffalo in one of the sheds and was brusquely chased away by the servants. Two day later he returned and killed yet another cow at his elder brother's shed. The alpha cat had killed more than it needed to satisfy his hunger but could not make a single meal out of the last three victims. Finally, he struck down a lonely dog and got his meal.

A week later the same tiger struck again, four miles to the south of Choudhary's farm. In this settlement, a poor peasant called Bacchu Pasi lived with his small family in an isolated hutment. The tiger apparently still hungry, wandered down into his area and set his eyes upon Bacchu's cattle, but here an extraordinarily interesting event took place that turned the tables on the tiger.

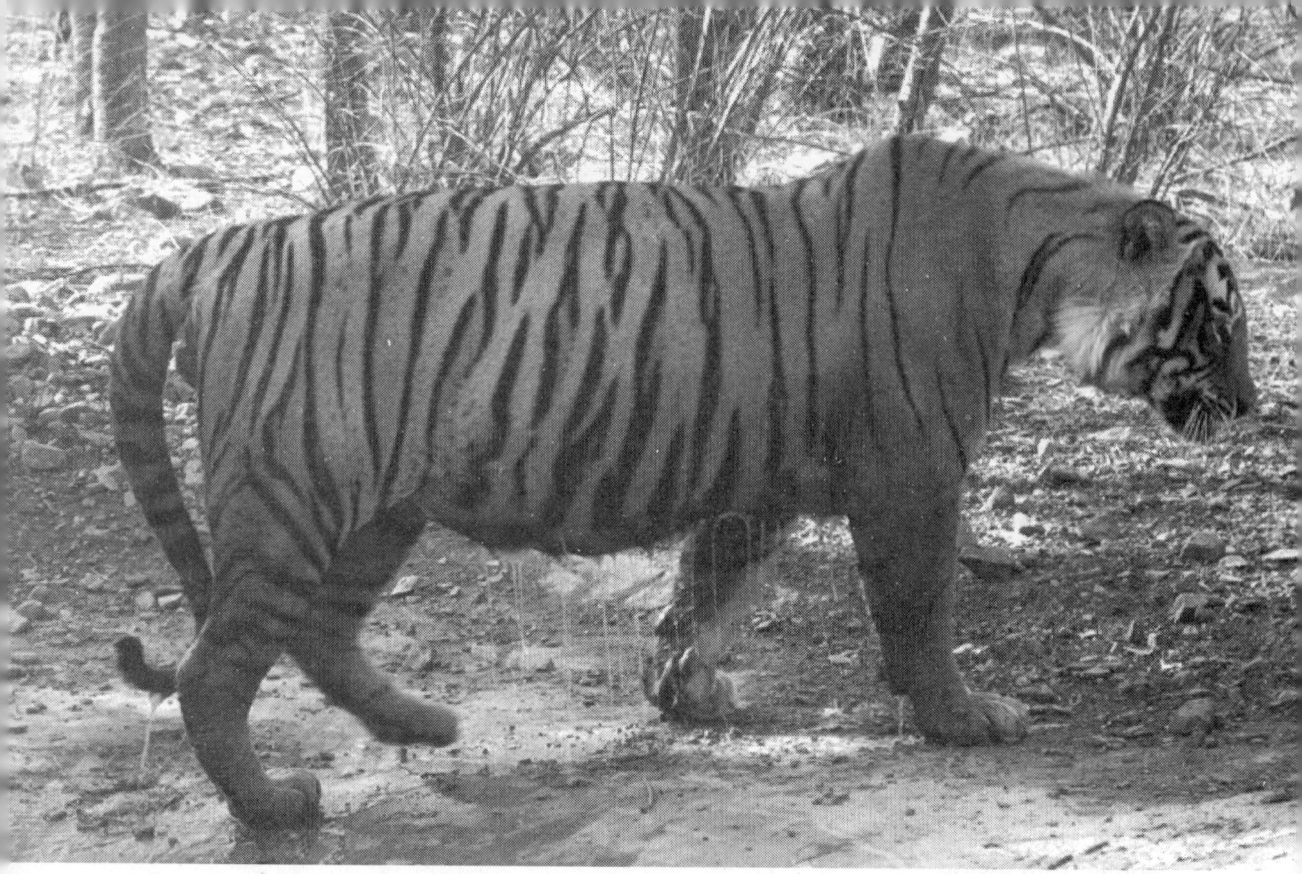

At our sight he got up from the small pool and walked away dripping with water

The poverty-stricken Bacchu earned a meager income from one acre of land and two milch cows, whose milk he sold to the local villagers. Just a week before this incident, a fierce and sturdy stud bull had come loitering to the area. Since it was the month of February and Bacchu's cow was in heat, the bull was taken as a welcome guest and he too settled in the area attracted by the cows. He often courted the cows in the grazing fields, but his wandering nature prevented him from entering their resting ground. When in the evening the cows returned, he habitually accompanied them up to the outer fringe of the settlement but then to spend the night at will he himself retired to some close by fields to browse in some unguarded crop. Bacchu did not have a shed for his cattle but this lapse was compensated by a shadowy *neem* tree, which stood just a few yards behind his shanty. The ground around it served as a provisional pen with several wooden pegs fixed on it. In winter the milkman usually covered his cattle with canvas and under the canopy of the tree tethered them in the open.

So that night Bacchu tied his cows in the open and went to sleep in his thatched hut. Towards midnight the same vagrant tiger happened to pass through that way in his desultory search for prey. Sensing the presence of un-barricaded cattle he stopped for an ambush and quickly seized a small calf that was tied close to the field. As the carnivore's fangs sought their way deep through the flesh of his prey, the calf desperately let out the last agonized bray. The sounds of death traveled in the silence of the night. They were heard by the stud bull who was hanging around the hutment. He became outraged and came thundering to the spot to investigate the cause and upon discovering a tiger involved in killing act, he instantly attacked him. The bull worked himself into such a furious anger that the tiger despite his minor demonstrations, soon found it difficult to stand against his formidable charge.

He soon fled into the darkness and the bull went after him to teach him a lesson. Meanwhile, the cow yard was disturbed and its all inmates created a boisterous din, trying to break their ropes from the pegs. A little later, having given a thoroughly defeating run to the tiger, the bull again returned to the shelter and with all pride stood there as guard as the calf lay dead.

Bacchu had awakened by now. He was utterly benumbed and paralyzed with fear, intently listening to the sounds of the duel, in horrible expectancy that the tiger may come crashing into his humble home. Sleep did not return to his eyes for the rest of the night, although the din had long subsided. The next morning Bacchu was greatly relieved to discover the benign gesture of the great bovine.

The rest of the day he spent in constructing a temporary shelter which he barricaded with barbed wire. But apparently the visiting predator had marked the spot as a definite store of beef, for that night he again materialized on the scene. The cows went wild upon sensing his presence. The tiger made persistent efforts to reach them but the barricade proved a tough obstacle. The attempts provoked the cows to cry hysterically, and in the silence of the night they were again picked up by the stud bull. He came crashing straight to the barricade and challenged the tiger. Discretion was evidently the better part of valor, for the tiger did not react to his defiant grunts and moved away safely.

Next morning, the tiger's pug marks imprinted around the cattle shed showed that cautiously avoiding the bull it had remained in the area in some fervent hope. Discouraged evidently by the security measures and the presence of a self appointed guard in form of a stud bull, the tiger had made no initiative for an attack. Later, the days passed off peacefully. The tiger maintained his distance and moved away for good showing due respect for the daring bull. And Bacchu, rid of the added discomfiture in his life, was left free to continue his battle against poverty without a shadow of a tiger.

The tiger was still hungry. On the night of October 14, he attacked the first human being near a settlement called Jamunaiya. Two Nepali boys were guarding their master's crop at the periphery of the village. They were sitting over a *Machan* (watch tower) under a thatched umbrella with a pet dog. Sometime during the night the tiger came slowly up wind, so that the dog could not get his smell and attacked the tower which came down trapping the boys beneath it. One of them was injured by a severe blow of forepaw on his stomach. As it ripped open, the entire haul of intestines fell out. The dog escaped from under the umbrella, the killer left the boy, and went chasing the dog in the dark fields. The skull of the dog was found the next morning about 500 meters away from the field. The unfortunate boy could not get any proper medical aid till morning and died of excessive bleeding.

The south Kheri landscape was also witnessing similar situations. During this very point of time, near the bustling township of Gola, some fifty kilometers away from Dudhwa, a new aggressive tiger was noticed in the vicinity of a village called Aheri. One fine morning some herdsmen were out on their routine work when they came across the pugmarks of a tiger near a big bamboo grove. Keen to learn more about the animal, they went inside the cluster and soon located a striped form resting amidst the thick bamboo shoots. Its pug marks, encircling the village showed that he had wandered around the settlement for entire night, but without success.

The men called out their fellow folk. Immediately, a mob turned up on the spot and everyone was impatient to have a glimpse of the beast. Among the keen watchers was a local Pundit named Amarnath who also carried a .12 bore double barrel shotgun. He was a sly poacher himself, and finding a good opportunity he set his mind to bag the tiger. He moved ahead and cautiously advanced up to three meters of the spot where the cat sat concealed. As he looked around to find the animal and aim the gun, the tiger suddenly emerged from his hide-out and sprang upon Pundit who did not have any time to move from his position. The man fell down on the ground, his gun being thrown away. The tiger mauled him and then stood upon his prostrate body, his jaws dripping with blood. Faced with this hideous sight, the rest of the men yelled at the top of their lungs, at this the startled animal turned and again retreated to his hideout.

A message was sent by a runner to the local police post and two armed constables duly arrived on the scene. The matter was then handed over to the custodians of law as they deemed fit to deal with. The policemen, feeling important, issued quick instructions much as the unfortunate Pundit had taken upon himself to deal with the tiger. The villagers were asked to collect dry leaves and scatter them in abundance around the thicket. Then the green cluster was set on fire. The two policemen took position at a safe distance with their guns aimed at the inferno. All of a sudden and with an amazing display of agility, the tiger sprang out of the grove and bolted blindly in one direction. By a singular stroke of misfortune another bystander Harkaran Bajpai who stood in the tiger's path was felled by the tiger. The policemen, denied the opportunity to fire the famed shots, took the poor man to nearby dispensary where he later died. The earlier victim was lucky to survive. Later the in-charge of Mikelganj police station arrived with a posse of policemen. They brought all available firearms and fired over 150 rounds into the grove. But by then the tiger had made its way into a further farm land.

This crisis in Tarai, particularly in Kheri district had been triggered by insensate plunder of environment and cultivation of sugarcane plantations. The latter had further caused enormous damage and fragmentation to the great grassland vistas. In fact, this new land use prototype had drastically changed the ecology of the place with dangerous consequences that no one could predict. There were tigers opportunistically using cane fields as their ranges, there were passing tigers, staying in the crops from a few days to perhaps a month or two, and then moving away. Then there were resident females rearing cubs, and there was wild prey to provide them nourishment.

When tigers tend to increase in numbers, it is almost inevitable that surplus animals will migrate into the surrounding areas. Abundant evidence showed that the big predators had taken up residence in the dense crops. Now these normally silent animals were announcing their occupation of ranges. Their scrap marks — the deep longitudinal cuts down the bark of trees, their chemical communications on trees and bushes and even occasional kills — were being reported in the fields. After dark, the travelers often came across them moving on the dirt roads near villages; in the beam of torches, their eyes blazing back an ambient light with awe inspiring intensity. The tiger's eyes, being the brightest of any creature on this earth, make them immediately recognizable to village folk. It seemed that the big predators had made a full return to their former ranges. Even a dilettante in tiger affairs could not have missed seeing the connection of things and its potential dangers.

It seemed incredible, yet it was true. These changes had naturally evolved in these tigers because of the circumstances which had been forced upon them. Far from habitually attacking humans, tigers prefer to give them a wide berth. They are known to go to any length to avoid contact with humans. Somehow now, all their actions and reactions appeared to be deliberate defiance of their tribe's very own special characteristics and the initiation of aberrational behaviour had come from the conflict with man. The prolonged comprehension of human relationship and appreciable need for survival and adjustment had inevitably brought them together to the detriment of both.

Tigers had once again occupied their previous legitimate home, now encroached upon by illegal human habitation. But humans were never ready to acknowledge that they were trespassers in tiger territory. In the light of the formidable fact that tigers are the largest of predators, five times bigger in size than a normal human being and are most exclusive meat-eaters, a disaster was impending. Shortly, some individuals of this giant tribe would be constrained to take a heavy toll of human life, not only just killing them by accident but also consuming their victims.

As a flash of lightning in the night shows up in an instant every detail of a wild landscape, so at one glance, I seemed to see every possible result of this tempestuous development.

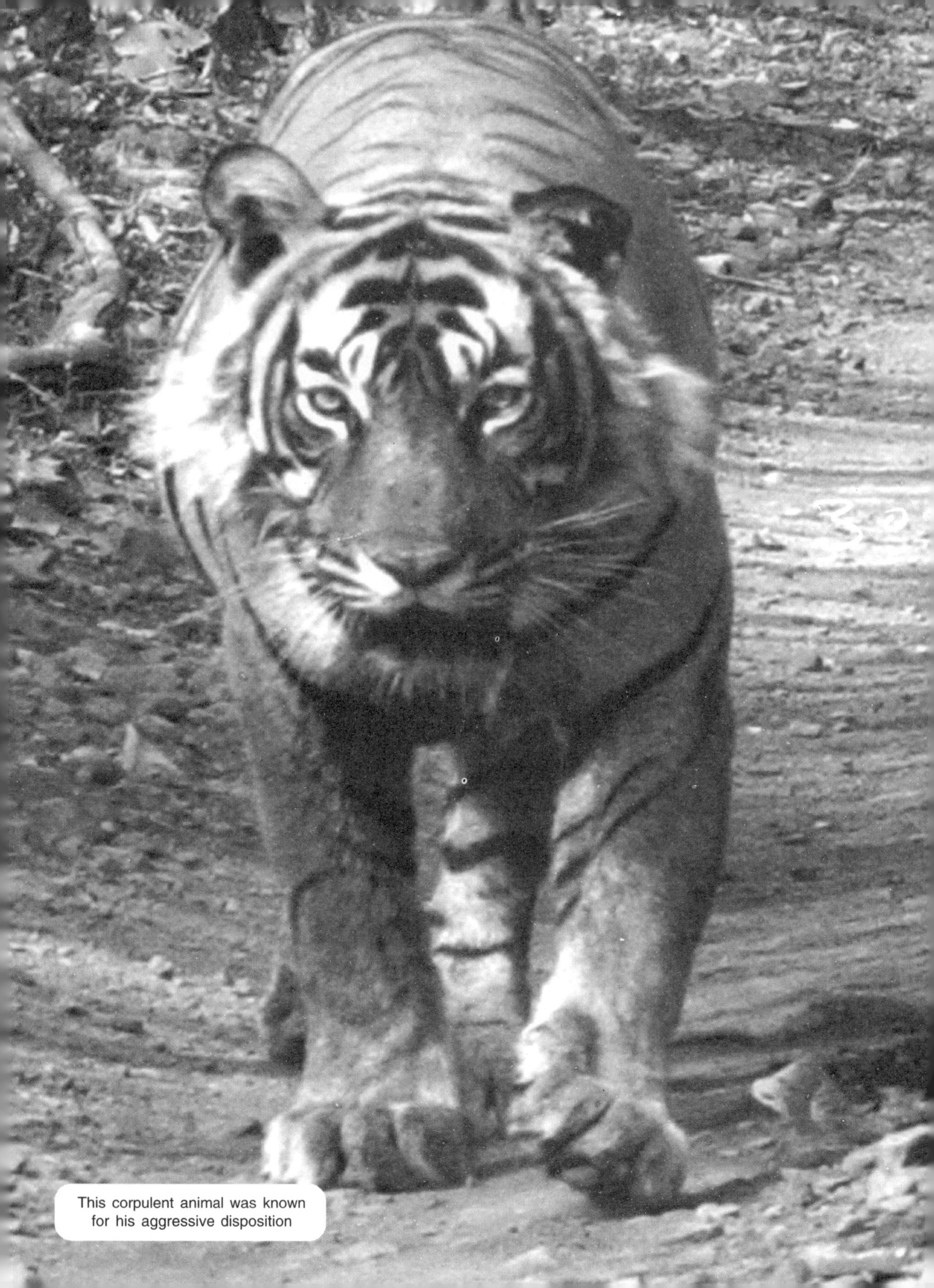

This corpulent animal was known for his aggressive disposition

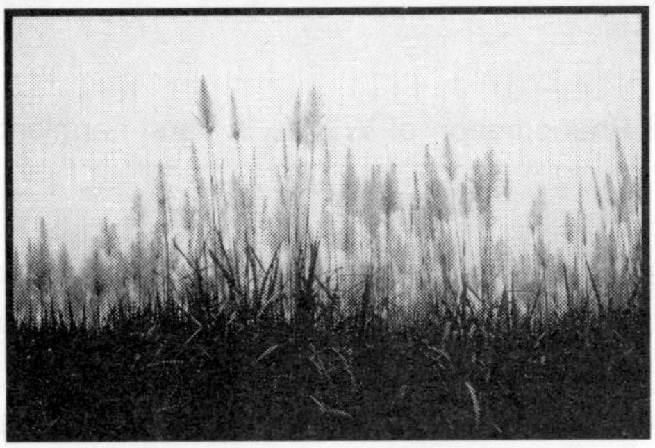

4

The Bio-network of Sugarcane

The difference between animals and humans is that animals change themselves for the environment, which the humans change for themselves.

- Ayn Rand

All events that form history need a time and place to unfold themselves. In the case of sugarcane tigers the platform happened to be the Tarai which is a belt of country in north India to the south of the outer foothills of Himalayas called the Shivalik range. The belt abuts the Indo-Nepalese border. This primeval forest is the original home of the tiger. It is a raw and beautiful country, full of sluggish meandering streams that emerge from beneath the porous southern flank of the Himalayan mountains and drain out in marshes and swamps. The water basins within it, created by the fluctuations of unstable riverbanks support the rich vegetation that is mostly covered with dense and tall grasslands. Great expansions of riverine forest line the river and stream courses for hundreds of miles; these are what ecologists call 'life-belts' or zones, and lush Sal forests cover vast expanses on the drier grounds. There were curious compartments in this landscape that were largely untouched by man since the first days of the world. This land was inhospitable to humans but perfect for wildlife.

At present the Tarai is no longer what it used to be even half a century ago. The pristine and impenetrable forests, with their towering trees and creeper clad undergrowth that were considered a microcosm of magnificent scenes from earliest India, now stand as a monument of raped environment. The old forest maps of United Provinces show that many woody landscapes that existed under British control -with their wealth of untapped natural resources- have now been completely wiped out from the face of earth. Nearly sixty percent of great grasslands, bush lands, sloughs, glens and waterfowl wetlands have been lost to make room for the flourishing agricultural farms and demographic dominance of human population. True wilderness is not a renewable resource. These were the very terrains that contained some immense tigers and where elephants were the best way of getting around. But in some islets, bogs and rank vegetation were so thickly intertwined, that even these beasts were known to concede defeat and relinquish pursuit.

Once these sprawling lands became farms, ploughed up and put into crops, a new segment of human civilization flourished, for which displaced wildlife was not the part of picture at all. The famed gubernatorial battus of swamp deer, where thirty to forty trophy stags were gunned down in a morning shoot by English crap shooters, became a thing of past. Soon a different but commercial agricultural pattern also came into existence. Sugarcane became the principal field crop of the Tarai. It was primarily grown as a source of sugar which is extracted from raw cane at sugar mills and crushers, and it gave rise to a flourishing sugar industry. Presently over a hundred sugar mills and nearly two thousand crushers are distributed throughout the region where the cane is shredded and the juice extracted by crushing. As a result, the major belt of this crop that runs through the state of Uttar Pradesh, at the moment makes it as only second best to Brazil in sugar production.

Sugarcane is a deep-rooted crop that unlike most crops remains in the soil all the year round and as a result consumes high quantity of water. This highly commercialized industry has resulted in agro-chemical and silt runoff, and also nutrient leaching from the fields that has affected the environment adversely where irrigation coverage has gone up from 40 per cent to ninety percent in the same period.

There is no doubt that the cane has destroyed most of the biodiversity in the Tarai or for that matter world-wide, wiping out several species. It has affected eco-systems yet in the context of global warming it is a vital crop which helps in de-carbonizing the atmosphere.

There is no denying the fact that cumulatively, more than any other factor, agricultural expansion had been the strongest force in shrinking the tiger habitat to present miniscule proportions in Tarai landscape. Amongst several problems posed by the crop, and the effects of an expanding civilization on wildlife, the sugarcane tiger is its latest and also a unique fall-out.

Botanically, sugarcane belongs to the genus *Saccharum L.* of tribe *Andropogoneae* in the grass family *Poaceae*. This tribe includes more than a hundred tropical and sub-tropical grasses, including the cereal genera Sorghum and Zea Corn. Just like the disproportionate annual grasses, it grows to maturity in nine months before it withers away. Often, some off-white and ochre looking flowers also germinate on certain varieties and the maximum flowering takes place from September to November. Although various strands of these species blossom at the same time, wherever they are growing, different species have different peak flowering time, and what triggers this flowering is not known.

It is apt to mention here that the form of the forest is not limited to big trees' vertical structure. There are different patterns and wildlife moves literally from one vegetation zone into another. Vegetation changes in the grasslands produce a mosaic effect. Consequently the sugarcane plantations apparently look like a bamboo tract to the tigers. The vegetation cover supports a diversified fauna, which includes several large prey species like blue bull and wild boar that thrive in it. And this makes an ideal country for the tiger to flourish in.

For a tiger, it is the extension of his habitat no different from reeds*. This ocean of tall grass, apparently an archetypical savannah forest, grows to the height of ten to twelve feet and stands all through the winter thick, cool and secure, quite familiar to the tiger for a residence. As the crop is owned and managed by farmers, it is inevitable that the tigers will come into contact with them repeatedly. This led to a familiarity that paved the way for him to lose his fear of man. Interestingly, whereas on one hand the government was planning to establish clearly demarcated reserves to save wild tigers with large buffer zones around them and also de-linking such habitats from the forces of market driven commerce, here was the paradox — a special population of tigers was flourishing on a man-made, ersatz and artificial habitat that rightly belonged to them as genuine jungle only 30 years ago.

In the post independence times, the Tarai, especially the particular area around Dudhwa National Park, has witnessed an unprecedented rise in sugarcane cultivation, which steadily climbed from 20,000 hectares to nearly 1.5 million hectares. According to official estimates, the state of Uttar Pradesh at present grows sugarcane in 2.12 mha, occupying 52% of the total cane acreage and contributes to over forty percent sugarcane production in India, where farmers harvest nearly 80 tons per hectare as crop.

To understand the reasons for tigers colonizing sugar plantations we must understand the cultivation pattern of this crop. In the Tarai the crop is taken by two methods; firstly from the ratoon rhizomes and secondly by the seeds. The ratoon occupies nearly sixty percent of the cane fields. Ratoon is a shoot growing from the root of the plant that has been cut and is a technique extensively used in sugarcane cultivation. It is regarded as a bonus crop and usually deprived of the normal cane husbandry practices.

The yield of ratoon crop is considered to be slightly less compared to plant crop but it has its many advantages, like the crops need not be managed at every stage. Even poor management and lower application of fertilizer does not adversely affect it and the cane productivity is good. There are enough gaps between the plants and the harvesting can be done in piecemeal. Besides ratoons raised from the crop experiencing biotic stresses viz., water logging, sub-optimal temperatures during stubble sprouting, late planted and late harvested crops, are invariably poor in yield as well as in sugar content.

Tarai farmers mostly use previous crop as a source of seed for planting or bring

* There is no satisfactory and universally accepted definition and classification of eco-systems since variations and gradations between ecological communities are yet to be adequately and properly understood. As such there is no unanimity in identifying eco-system boundary. In reality, there is no discreet bio-geographic region, or as small as natural habitat. And ecosystem diversity is considered at three levels:bio-geographic regions, biotic province and biomes. Sugarcane is a complex but fragile environment that needs a detailed study of the organisms that inhabit them, the forces that maintain them, and the agents that threaten them. In fact, it is a substitute to forest grasslands, the great savannah of coarse grasses that harbors much of the wildlife of the area.

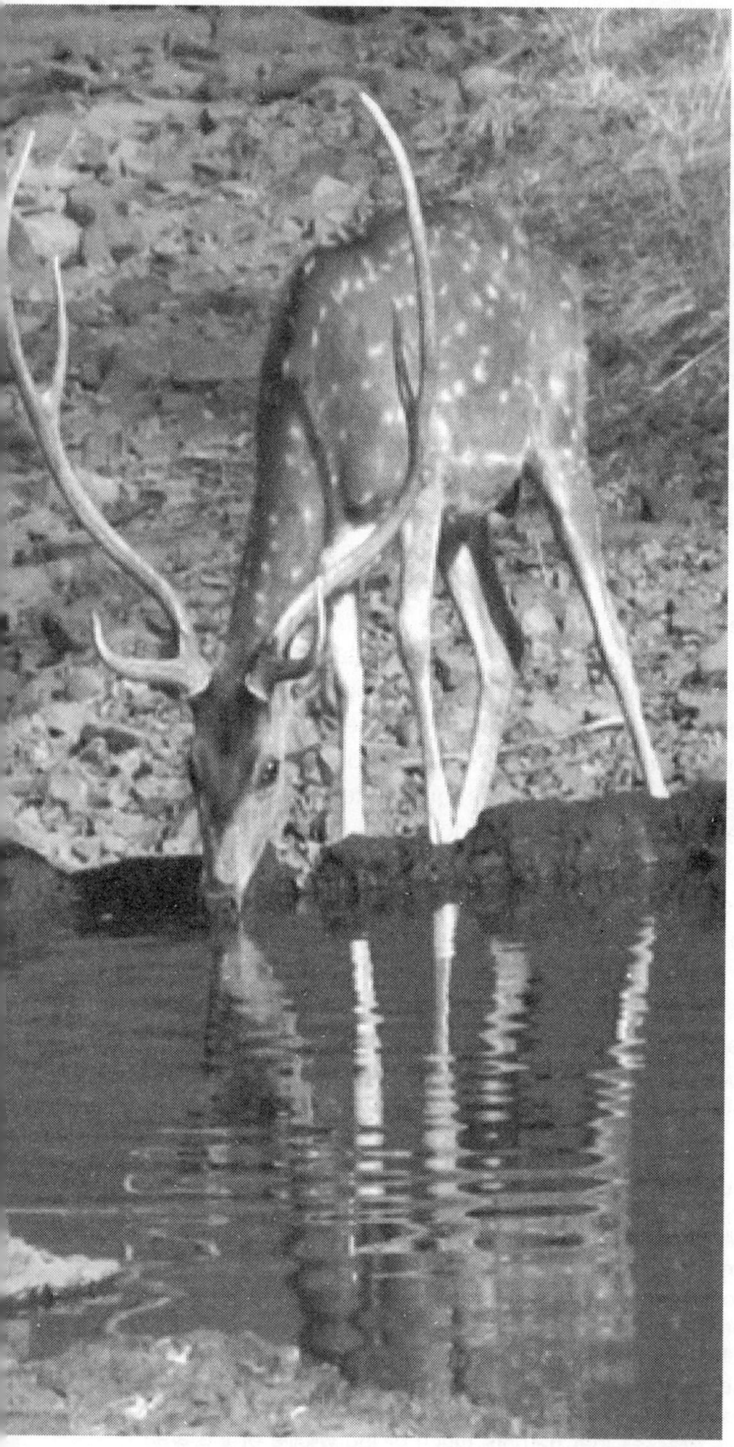

A typical sight in a pool of the Tarai

scientifically treated seeds from other areas. This helps them to get rid of many transmitted set of diseases such as red rot, smut, GSD, RSD, leaf scald etc, which bring down cane productivity. The constraint of low seed multiplication ratio which hinders rapid multiplication and spread of new varieties, does not apply here and the sprouting is good.

A large part of sugarcane acreage in U.P. is planted during February/March called spring planting and also in April/ May, which is late summer planting. This leads to poor germination resulting in poor stand of the crop. This subsequently affects its height, its strands tilt and fall upon each other and its green fronds cover the ground. This often creates some extra dense pockets like a canopy within the already dark cane field. This suits the tigers nicely and they adapt to it as their home.

The area under Early Maturing High Sugared Variety (EMV) in U.P is very low, thus there is predominance of late-maturing, mid and late season varieties. Thus, the cane fields are never really empty and there is never a real pinch period, though the cane yield of late planted crop is about half compared to spring planted crop. In jaggery (*gur*) and *Khandsari* dominated areas, a huge quantity of inferior quality of sugarcane is also consumed and the crop continues to stand even in hard summers.

Though, this traditional knowledge was at my disposal, I had no proper infrastructure to document the complex matrix of big cats in the sugarcane. However, I was sure a focused research was desperately needed to figure out as to what special adaptations had come to exist in these tigers. For instance, what was the composition of the sugarcane environment including the dependence of variety of life forms on it in certain situations and conditions, and the factors which generated differences in behavioral responses of the tigers that live in proximity of man as opposed to further away in the jungle, including their pattern of predation. There seemed to be no study of this kind yet in the country, or if there was, I was not aware of it. And eventually what animal communities inhabit them and what measures of protection were to be implemented if the species was to survive in the unreal surroundings.

By early February of 1977, the winter rains had set in earnest and it was time for me to leave Paraspur. I was happy with my findings, remembering somewhat thankfully that the temporary assignment was over now. Actually, I suspected I had overworked on it and generated more than sufficient material.

Back in Lucknow, I supplied some half a dozen articles to *The Pioneer* and with that my newspaper assignment came to an end. But brief as it was, the experience had rekindled in me a vital desire to know more about these tigers. I sometimes wondered how I had begun as a brash and unabashed explorer of the unknown, pushing on adventurously into unknown country and had come upon a novel phenomenon; perhaps a new brand of tigers in making. This development was also sounding a timely warning of danger, for grim portents were everywhere; and there was a premonition for trouble ahead.

I was still without a regular job and money was constant problem with me. My outstation trips were costing a terrific amount of money and I needed some funding agency to promote my studies or at least get some assignment to sustain myself. I hardly need to say that thus far all my trips, done for fun and making some money, had now acquired serious dimensions. Once I had set my cap on, I wanted to stay in the game. The more I thought passionately about the idea, the more it fuelled me. This was the thing I could really do in my life. So I decided to meet Ranjit Bhargava, a crusader of environmental protection in Uttar Pradesh to seek support from his organization.

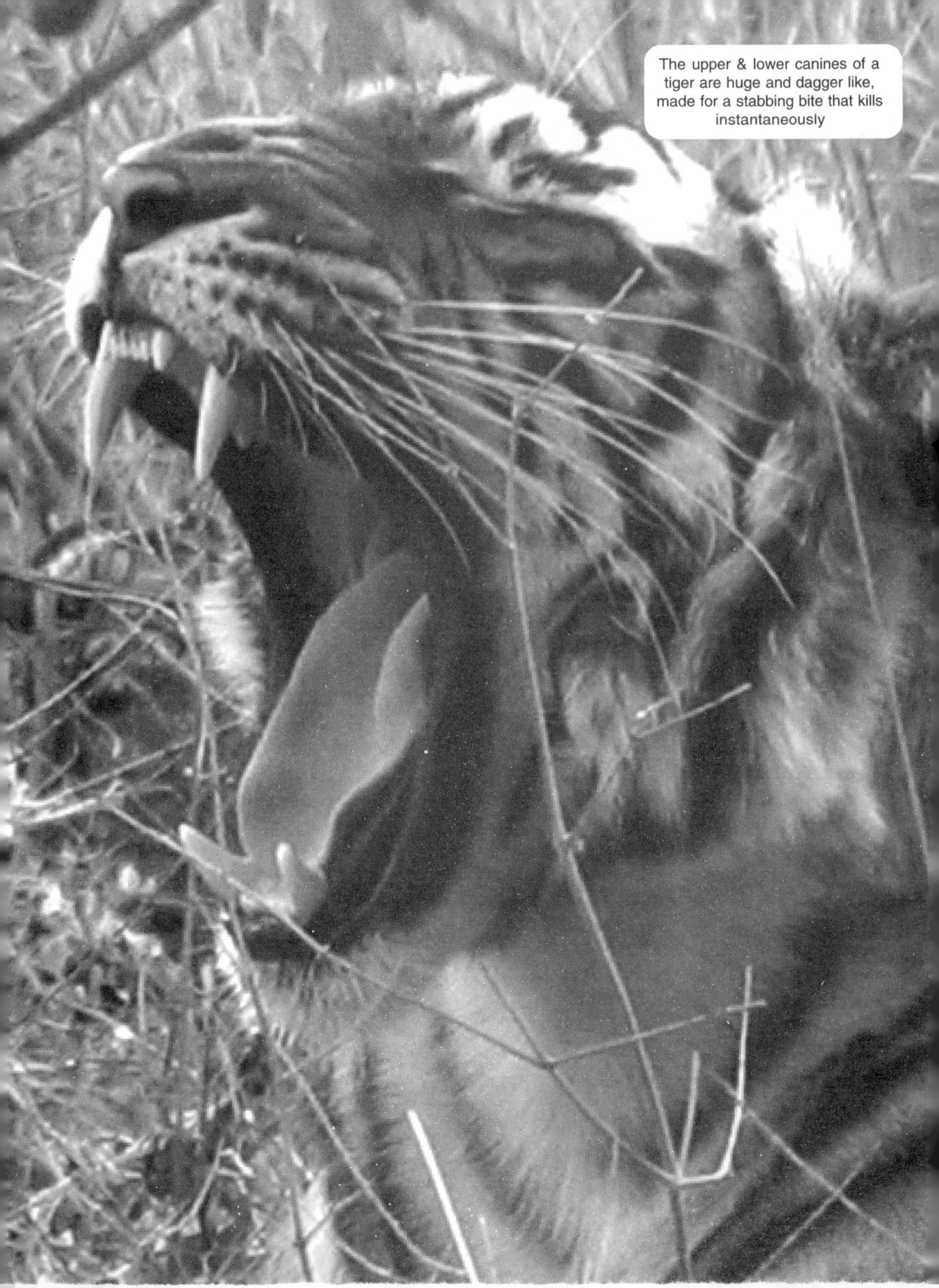
The upper & lower canines of a tiger are huge and dagger like, made for a stabbing bite that kills instantaneously

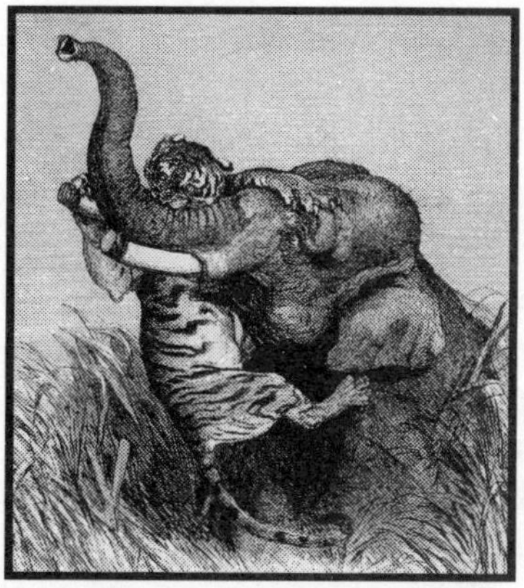

5

The Tiger Buffs of Lucknow

The ecologist cannot remain a voice crying in the wilderness — if he is to be heard and understood.

- M.W. Holdgate

Lucknow, the capital of Uttar Pradesh, is unique among all the mini-metro state capitals in India. Its proximity to New Delhi, combined with its strong roots in heritage, architecture and culture, gives it an aura that is difficult to find in other comparable cities. The city's association with the Mughal and Nawabi era of north Indian history makes it stand out as a pleasant mix of old and new.

In the heart of the city is Hazratganj, the most popular commercial soak of Lucknow. It is essentially a single broad road with well-designed footpaths on both sides and large stylish shops. A towering red building topped with a grand clock stands at its southern flank. This grand monument of imperial might, now over a century old gives the street it's most recognizable facial feature and belongs to the princely family of the Bhargava's. A small by-lane close to the building leads to the huge campus of a palatial house, built with grandeur and complacency. The most notable feature of this old home is that its composition is European while its structural elements are vernacular. The spacious portico, assorted columns and aggressive display of aristocratic veneer, gives it the ambience of a time gone by.

The eldest son of the family, Ranjit was a fine looking man and an uncompromising friend of wildlife. We had often met at India Coffee House and exchanged notes on conservation issues. Now over sixty, Ranjit lives in Nainital but despite the age he has retained a vigorous zest for life, bestowed on healthy mortals who are wise enough to live close to nature.

The old building was full of charm. One spacious section provided place for the trophies of chase as well as for interesting curios. Three large rooms contained several mounted heads of game that were arranged in the most admirable manner all over the walls. Ranjit's father, the late Raja Ram Kumar Bhargava, was an arduous shooter, having mowed down nearly a hundred tigers, and so was his wife Rani Lila Bhargava. There were trophies belonging to the early days of the Raj till

latter trophies were of such a high quality and so excellently superior that they looked almost alive.

On a table, in the centre of last room is the most valued trophy. It is an enormous male tiger measuring 10 feet 3 inches, shot by Rani in the middle of last century. It stands 42 inches in height and the girth of its neck measures round 2 feet 10 inches. These measurements all taken over curves, correspond very closely to those described by Rowland Wards in his 'Records of Big Game', allowing for two or three inches of difference, between pegs.

Ranjit's home was a rendezvous of many naturalists and tiger buffs. He had a Sportsmen's Club which put forth several aims regarding wildlife. The requirement for membership was that the applicant must be a well informed person, own a sport rifle and should have done some active wildlife protection work. During the hunting days, it represented gentlemanly sportsmanship, which meant fair play for the game. Now with the change of times, its attitude had undergone a radical change and the compilation of life histories of endangered animals and establishment of wildlife reserves had become its stated purpose.

Most of the Club members were old stalwarts, hunters, zoologists, ornithologists, and outdoorsmen, all with a genuine interest in Indian wilderness and wildlife. These included Mamman Khan, a professional shooter who had given 132 tigers to his clients, Sashi Raj Singh, the owner of a field outfitters' firm called Indian Shikar and Tours Private Ltd, which had the credit of shooting 300 tigers. Then there was

A tiger snarls at us from behind the rocks at the Panna National Park

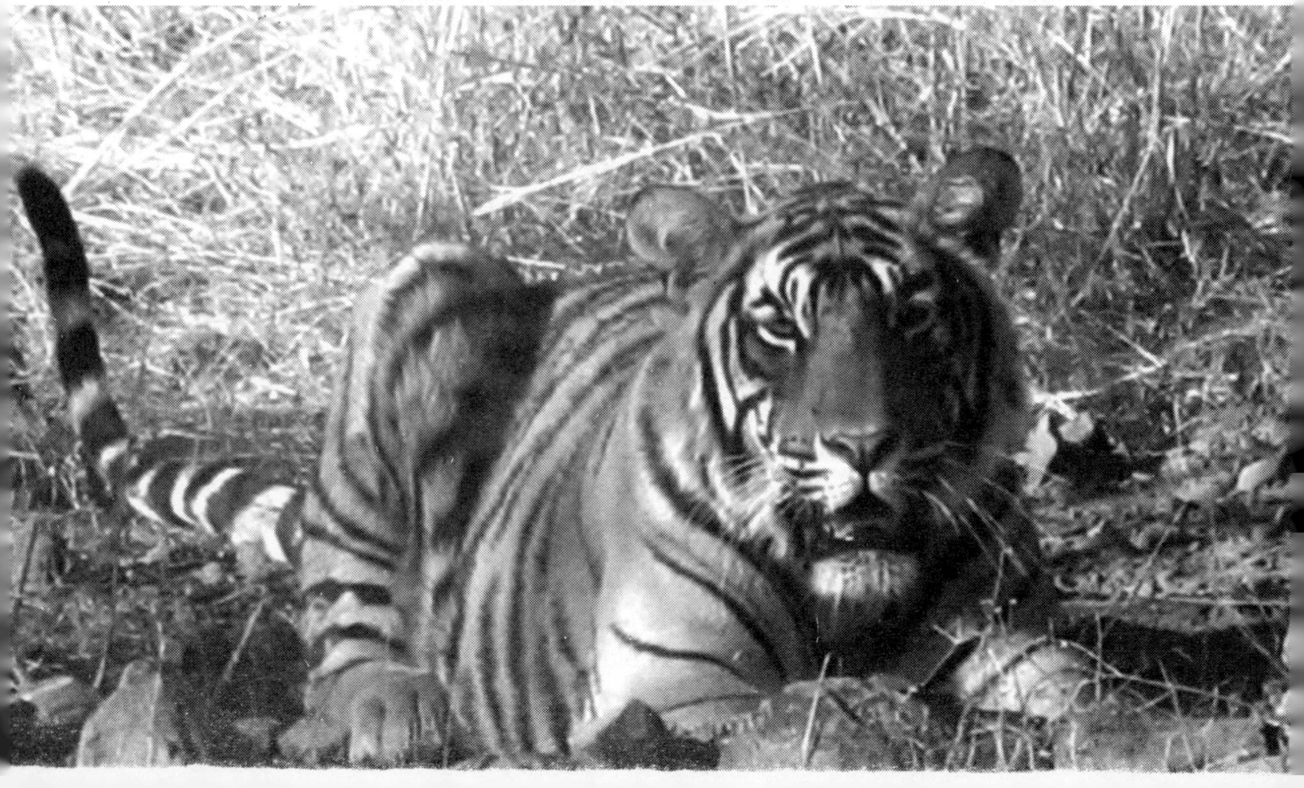

Bhushan Thapar, a field naturalist of eminence, Raja D. P. Singh of Balrampur, Raja Divyakar Singh of Kasmanda, Raja Yadavendra Dutt Dubey of Jaunpur (whose book *Tales of Shikar* is still going through repeated prints), Anup Sah, a celebrated wildlife photographer of *A Tiger's Tale* fame, Chandra Mani Kant Singh of Bhinga, and Dr. Ajay Rawat, later Honorary Wildlife Warden of Corbett National Park, and of course many forest officials.

That day, when I reached Ranjit's house, a meeting was going on. The weather was good, and I was in high spirits. Ranjit took me to a hall, where large tiger skins and tiger rugs were set up on the walls, laid on the floor, or flung luxuriously over the furniture, over which the guest patricians were seated. He introduced me to them and most of them had been reading my write-ups in newspapers with a critical point of view. They talked of wildlife with a classic literary fervor, and I got into some very illuminating discussion with them.

After the meeting was over Raja D.P. Singh called me by his side to have a drink with him and said, "Rahul, wildlife is an international subject and wildlife research is like literature, like novels that are never confined to their national linguistic boundaries. They transcend them. Dostoevsky was better understood by French and Ibsen by the Irish. Hemming and Faulkner were brought to light by the French. So is your sugar tiger, better understood by us than by foresters. Isn't it funny? All types of criticisms and denunciations are hurled at your idea. But forget bureaucrats and foresters, you are on the right track, the tiger buffs of the city are with you, we will bring your work to light."

Ranjit endorsed his viewpoint. Then with a captivating charm of his own, he put his arm over my shoulder and confidently said, "Don't worry man, great spirits have always encountered violent opposition from mediocre minds. You are an uncompromising teller of truth; Keep up your reputation, a reputation that is strengthened by your writings. We will see that you get a project from the state government."

As I heard these words, my frustration evaporated into dreams of monumental importance. Lofty thoughts swelled in my bosom. A project in the offing was sufficient to make me swallow previous disappointments but I well knew that this cane tiger was an unknown subject, how long do they live in the crops and where do they go when it is harvested? What kind of prey they eat, and how do they act in response to their man-made environment and adversative human factor? Although it is difficult and challenging to enter the world of a wild tiger, yet I must follow these cats in order to know the answer to some basic questions. Perhaps years of hard work were required before I could stretch leisurely on a rocking chair and claim that the sugarcane tiger was a reality, which indicated the emergence of a putative strain.

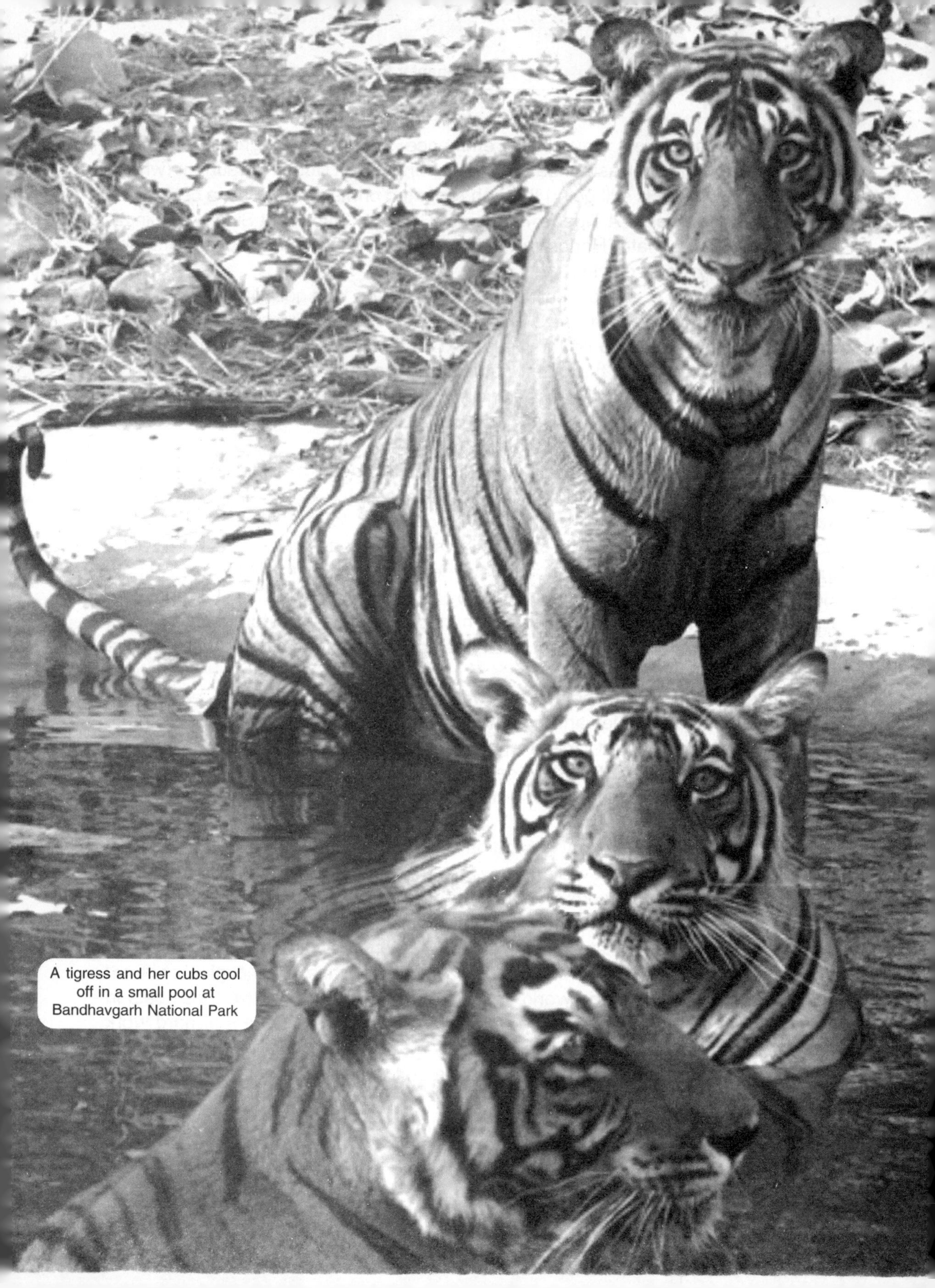

A tigress and her cubs cool off in a small pool at Bandhavgarh National Park

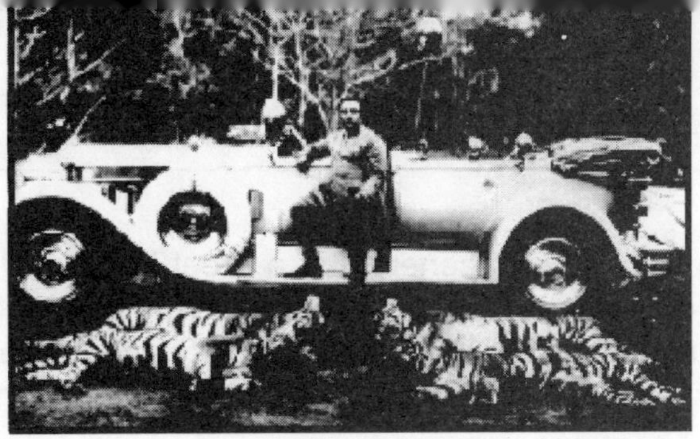

6

Born in the Cane: A Selective Breeding Ground

This is an ecosystem that has received very little attention.

- George Schaller

At the beginning of the 20th century, Major Hudson Rockwell of the Royal British Army, who shot 9 tigers in a fortnight at Sonaripur, had documented a telling comment in the register of the rest house, which is now preserved in the library of the forest department in Lucknow. He wrote, "The question of game depletion in Tarai is a complex one and while I hold that large government preserves are necessary, I do not agree with the conservation alarmists who would have us believe that Tarai game is in danger of becoming extinct in a few short years. This is puerile bosh, and those who think it is true have only to visit the country, particularly the interior, to see what I mean. There are thousands of square miles of wasteland, enormous swamps, and regions so unhealthy for human life that neither whitish nor brown man could live there. In vast areas, innumerable tropical diseases make life extremely difficult for both man and any domesticated animals he may try to raise. These enormous regions will remain stocked with game for untold centuries to come and will serve as breeding grounds to stock adjacent areas."

But now Hudson's predictions had been proved way off the mark. Leave aside centuries, the once-unconquerable Tarai has been fully tamed within two decades. On the one hand, I saw that the farms had pushed back forests at many places and areas once lost by tigers to the human settlements were gone forever, on the other there were several continuous stretches of crop-free and fallow lands surviving near the villages; the broken fragments of once flourishing Tarai forests where tigers were living by choice. There the tall coarse grass, dotted here and there by lofty banyan and *pipal* trees extended for several acres; and such terrain stuck between distant villages and cane farms, still served as small reservoirs for wildlife. But undoubtedly they were just a thin shadow of the past that Hudson had described.

My next visit to this region to investigate the sugar tiger was in March 1978. Ranjit helped make arrangements for my stay at Tikonia in the house of a Sikh named Harjinder Singh. This burly Sikh farmed on nearly 200 acres of land and bore a marked resemblance to Air India's mascot, the Maharaja. His face was lined and hard with a long sandy moustache that hid his mouth and droop with a curl. He had a big cottage with several generators, a great lavish bar and a fine library, abounding in encyclopedias of all types. His children were settled in the US and kept coming to him periodically, bringing lavish gifts and consequently their father lived an Americanized style of life in an area which is cut off from the mainstream of the country.

It was a heavenly evening, peculiar to the climate of Tarai when Chhotey Pasi, my old 'Tiger Guru' from Larti, and I reached the house of this Sikh gentleman. The amber sky was turning into the deepest bronze. As darkness fell a bonfire was lit and we sat with refreshments, chatting freely. Before long a kettle was steaming and rattling over the coals, and a hash of dried mutton, potatoes and onions was sizzling in the cooking pot.

An open fire, whether it is inside a fireplace or outside under the vast sky, seems to have a magical effect upon me, relaxing me to that point where I am completely at ease and conversation comes readily, peace begins to steal through me as I forget the fetters of civilization. Before the bonfire the Sikh sang with great gusto, dreary songs in a most tuneless voice while his nephew rendered some of the best old time favorites. After dinner, well lined with expensive wine, I pulled the cool bed sheet over my head and fell into a delicious slumber.

Towards midnight, I was roused from my drunken sleep by some disturbance. The moon had set and the clouds had obscured the stars. In the blank silence of the night, the clear muted calls of a tiger on the move from east to west were clearly audible. These were long plaintive-sounding calls, more a howl than a roar. I fumbled for the flashlight. Its batteries were nearly spent and its beam was too weak to penetrate the darkness. As I brought the beam slowly around I caught the faint glow of several pairs of eyes, dancing like stars. There were some thirty pairs of eyes, the animals standing purposefully in the shape of a vague arc around the yard. I swung the beam around and recognized a herd of Black Buck peering at us from no more than twenty yards. It was a clear case of wild animals seeking protection from predators near human habitation. I clapped and cooed at them and slowly, one by one, they disappeared into the night. I went back to sleep feeling plainly privileged to be in this magical land of promise I had come so far to enjoy.

Next morning, I woke to the clarion calls of peacocks resonating in the fields. The magnificent laburnums were in full bloom and during the night their petals had fallen over our mosquito nets, invariably covering their tops with a canopy of gold.

I took an early breakfast and made arrangements for the day's work. The warm pearly sky foretold a breathlessly warm day. Chhotey and I boarded a jeep with a driver and a local guide and proceeded for further investigations. I was rightly proud of Chhotey's company for there was always a professional touch to what he did while on the *Laati* of Shikar. He had spent much of his life in tiger territory. He was a wizard of wildlife craft, with solid comprehension of matters pertaining to tigers. He was familiar with twenty-two different types of impressions left by tigers.

His unerring knowledge of their every little peculiarity and even thought of the animal that he pursued- all these would fill a book from cover to cover.

To give an idea of his extraordinary sagacity, I recollect an incident. Once a mild west wind was blowing, when he went out hunting for pot in nearby Kishanpur jungle and got lost in the tangled intricacies of the deep forest. The situation turned serious when the sky became cloudy and with no idea of the sun's position, he became confused about the sense of direction. He now relied on the west wind but in the great expanse of greenery there was no wind; hardly any movement of leaves was perceptible, even the tropical ground was too damp to fling some earth up and test the direction of the wind. Finally, a black partridge rocketed up from the undergrowth, Chhotey shot it and intently watched how the feathers of the dead bird floated. This gave him a clue about the direction of the wind and he found his way out of the forest. Thus, what he did not know about jungles and its denizens was not worth knowing. I relied on his massive experience to deal with the lapses I may have made in my readings.

I spent the whole day in the fields and traveled more than thirty odd kilometers of sugarcane country. We passed by little thatched hutments, which cropped up now and then on both sides of the bridled road, inquiring about tigers and getting down at places to read the footprints of wild animals. The new trail was followed up rapidly, each step eliciting some cheering remark because of its distinctness. On the way, we passed a family of jungle fowl congregating in a rice field. An attention-grabbing black cock, with a glistening breast, had hopped up on a barren stump and was addressing his audience from there. He raised his head, which was crowned with his red comb, flapped his wings and uttered a shrill cry, which the other cocks repeated.

Our team made careful investigation of a low-lying, fertile area between Deep Nagar and Barsola villages. Like a hound on true scent, we counted the pugmarks of no less than three tigers and their cubs. The area held one male and two females with their six cubs. Chhotey's judgment was entirely reliable but to speak the truth, his findings baffled me. The heat was just too much and the burning wind blew without respite during the sun-up hours. Only a few pockets of mature cane crops were left standing in the field, apparently affected by top borer, the most damaging pest of sugarcane in the state. The irrigation supply to the canes had been stopped; hence it was too warm inside the cane cluster. The tigers had provisionally retired to the close-by thickets of *narkul* strands and ferns. They grew densely packed and tall, to the height of a full grown elephant and heralded the animals to a few places where large trees shaded the grasslands and where there were perhaps a solitary puddle or two, containing scarce water.

Clearly these tigers were breeding. The land use pattern was essentially tiger friendly. Their enhanced level of protection had enabled females to bring up larger litters with a greater degree of security and success. This increase in tiger population could be attributed not only to an effective protection but also to a greater prey base available in the sugar farms. A sizeable population of *Nilgai* and hog deer also abounded in this area. These animals belong to the same genus as *chital* and generally inhabit the outskirts of the forest; they live a solitary life, which naturally makes them exceedingly vulnerable to predation.

To our great satisfaction the villagers endorsed that a 'throng' of tigers was operating in the area. It was not surprising, for only three decades back, this tract was genuine jungle where for ages tigers had held an undisputed sway. Their return to this land-chunk substantiated that they had the propensity to respond to environmental changes.

The day passed uneventfully. Soon evening was at hand and from a coppice a pack of jackals rendered its eerie falsetto chorus as the setting sun fell below the horizon. It was time to go back home. We boarded the jeep and returned, watching the darkness take over the twilight shrouded landscape.

We returned next day to the same spot to resume our search from there. With a little help from shepherds we came across the remains of two hog deer recently devoured by tigers. It was obvious that the tigers were not facing a problem getting

A young juvenile tiger recently separated from his mother

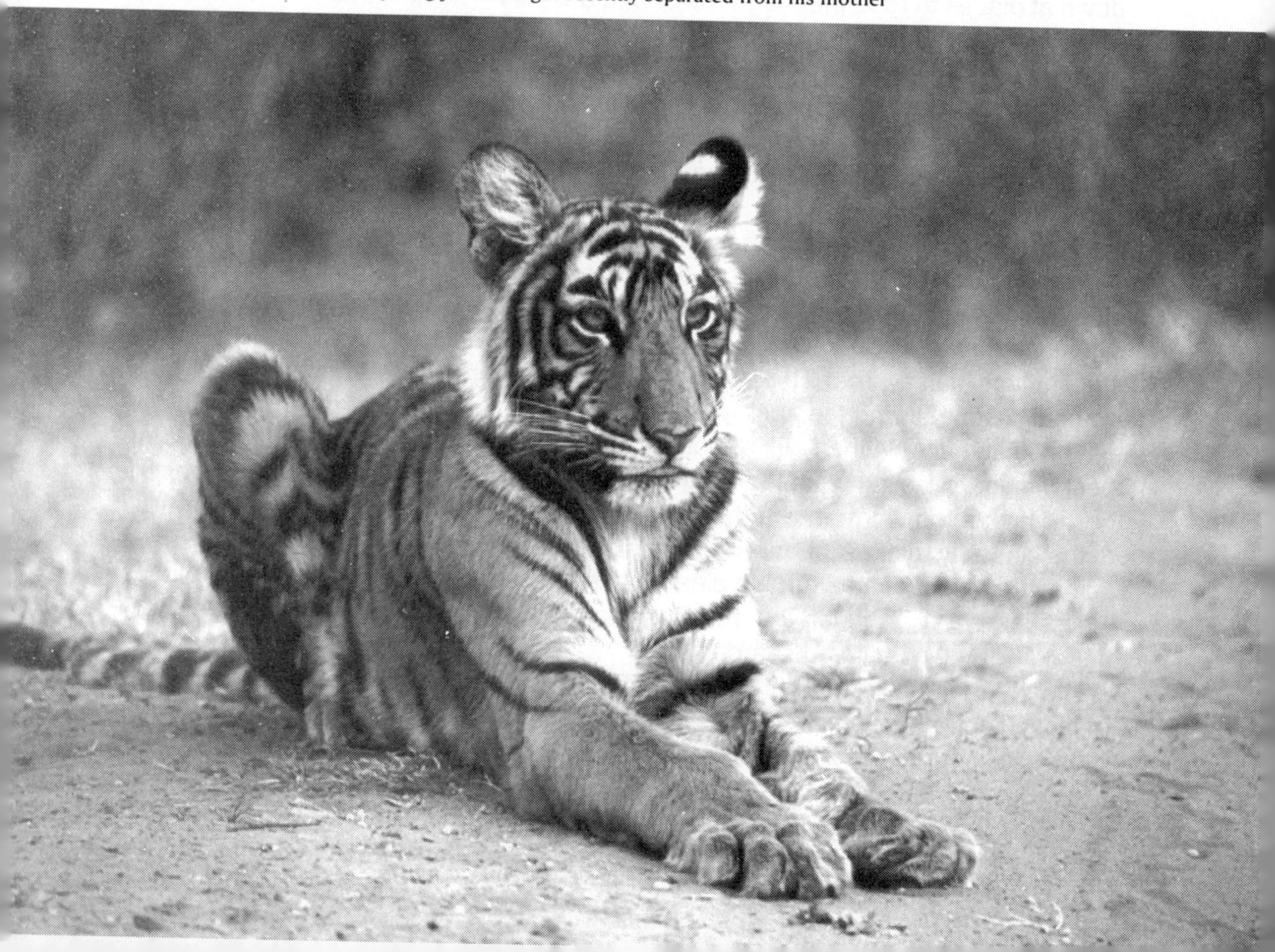

food. These were spots where they spent their day under cover to beat the heat and later prowled through the fields on their nocturnal journeys.

The heat of the day had become oppressive. Not a cloud appeared in the whole wide expanse of the blue sky to veil the splendor of the tropical sun, the vertical rays of which threatened to penetrate our body. To the south of Barsolā village, at the perimeter of the agriculture field lay a big water pond. It was bordered by some stretches of alkaline land, and still beyond that on the marshy soil grew a moderate block of grass and bush land. It was a mini forest, extending for almost two furlongs, and shrouded with stunted trees. We sought refuge near it to take a little rest.

After a quick lunch we took a stroll into the cool interiors of the block. We saw a civet cat, a jackal and the skeleton of a dead cow. The set of ribs was cleaned of flesh and visible through the chalky bones were fuzzy baby faces of two tiger cubs. Their tiny eyes were scrutinizing us with a penetrating stare.

We halted in our tracks and shifted behind a growth of grass. It was a time when nature seemed faint with heat, and every living thing had sought shelter from the merciless glare of the noon sun, save for the ever ravening vultures that swept through the air in wide extended circles seeking their food in the very light of the blazing sun. And at this time the jolly cubs were out to explore their world.

It seemed like the début venture of the cubs. They stood stiff legged in a dazzle of astonishment; they had never seen the outer world before; perhaps they had still not seen a human being around, the close environment of marsh had been but their second womb. A cool breeze blowing from the direction of the pond combed their yellow black hair and made the briars dance. After the scuffling in the stuffy nursery, it was a blaze of freedom for the cubs to toddle on their stumpy, unsteady legs, stumbling into one another and falling backward onto their plump fuzzy bottoms.

A silence, deep as that of midnight pervaded the land. Then the sudden realization that the mother must be somewhere close, took some of the pleasure out of the whole business and we hastily beat a retreat.

The experience left me in awe and astonishment about the success of tiger conservation. These cubs were not more than six weeks old. Nature's capacity to bounce back is remarkable. All this had happened in a relatively short period of five years. In fields conditions are very tough. Both pre natal and post natal mortality is very high and almost the entire first year of the cubs is fraught with many dangers yet the tiger population had been rising fast, indicating a strong survival rate. It was certainly a noteworthy feature.

(II)

The hearty Sardar was very lavish in his treatment and equally courteous. In his free time, he showed me his books and his private collection of cowboy items which were surely the finest I have ever known. There were old maps of the prairies and a variety of Wild West posters in his house. Everything was so closely set that there was hardly any space on the walls. There were many caps, jeans, shirts and leather jackets, with waist and shoulder gun belts. The Sikh was a well traveled man. He told me he had bought all of these items from Idaho and Buffalo in the USA where his children were settled. "I love this atmosphere around me. It keeps me charged with vigor and makes me feel smart", he said.

While on my look-out trip to Ballhipur near Majhgai, a laidback township near Palia, I had hardly awakened one morning when I saw two Tharu tribesmen pass close to my camp. They were carrying a twelve foot long python strung on a pole. They told me that they had killed the serpent in a banana plantation, as it had swallowed their pet mongrel. One could plainly see an enormous swelling half way down the reptile's body. The snake had been unable to escape with this load in his middle and the men were able to kill it with ease. They were jubilant over the fact that they now had enough food for their family and associates, for in primitive societies the meat of a kill is always shared.

These were relaxed times, though. The nexus between poachers and tribal communities, living in and around forests had not evolved so intensely; there were no clues whatsoever of organized gangs operating in the area. The district was not yet a hotbed for outside poachers.

During 1979 when I was staying at Majhgai, I met a couple of grazers from a hamlet who claimed to recognize some of the tigers in the area. They maintained that they knew of at least three tigresses that were raising cubs in the sugar fields between Majhgai and Badudhia Kalan villages. A man said that he had once seen two tigresses together, feeding on a feral cow, while the cubs were hidden in the crops. He promised to lead me up to them. I went out to investigate, knowing full well that to recognize a tiger by its appearance is one thing; but to know its movements and its range and dealings with other tigers is another, but as the movements of mother tigresses are largely localized, the chances of encountering them were brighter.

I started at sunrise and soon found the imprints of a tiger in the potato fields. There were multiple miniature tracks of cubs etched in the powdered earth. Dewdrops were shining on the edges of the prints, leading away into the sea of cane crops, where the big cats had gone just before daybreak. As I inspected the area for three days, I was amazed to know that even here the situation was much similar to the one I had witnessed at Barsola almost two years ago. Here, in an area of roughly fifteen square kilometers, I counted the pug marks of no less than three tigresses and six infants in the cane fields; a stage which biologists call 'saturation density' had been encouragingly achieved.

The home range of a normal tigress is believed to be ten to twelve square kilometers but here three tigresses were operating within that territory. This indicated that the home range of resident tigresses is related to the presence or absence of the young ones and tigresses with small cubs are restricted in their movements. The smallest areas are used by tigresses with cubs less than a year old. And within such an area the cubs are confined to an even smaller space; while the largest range is established by those without cubs.

Seven years later the tigers were breeding equally well. In 1986, I again came across a similar situation in Bilrayan area. These instances finally made me believe that the activities of tigers in sugarcane were to a great extent compatible to tiger conservation. The hypothesis propounded by late S.R. Choudhery suggests that reproductive dynamics in farm tigers registers a high increase in comparison to jungle tigers. Having noted, from time to time, three observations of the same kind I found the hypothesis was well on its way to becoming a theory.

S.R. Choudhery was a professional forester, a hunter of over fifty man-eaters and a tiger expert of international repute. He had come to Dudhwa as a member of a committee appointed by the Government of India to investigate into the causes of man-eating in the Tarai, when I had met him in the Park for the first and the only time. During a sitting we had debated many vexing questions. The doyen of wildlife conservation heard my experiences with interest and finally endorsed my viewpoint. He was the first person to have agreed with me, in principle, to the possibility of the existence of cane tigers as a new evolving putative creed of tigers. I filled his glass, and he, raising it, drank affectionately to the next meeting which, alas, we never had since he died the next year and India lost a great field scientist.

To proceed with my point; females attain sexual maturity at an age of around two or three years and become capable of conceiving. Male tigers also become capable of mating by this age but in the jungle they are rarely able to do so because of the presence of larger older males who accompany females in estrus and chase away any rival.

This had made sugarcane fields a potential production factory for the tigers. For the forest department, it was the most cost-effective way of raising wild tigers compared to raising expensive captive tigers that had little hope of finding suitable new habitats for reintroduction. A cursory survey had revealed that fourteen tigresses were bringing up as many as 23 cubs in the different cane clusters. Their movements overlapped but they tended to raise their cubs in separate tracts. The most important mortality factor in the wild is probably starvation caused by the mother's failure to hunt sufficient prey at regular intervals; but it did not seem to apply here as domestic prey was abundant.

The most important feature was that most of the cane tigresses seemed to be having cubs. The high percentage of litter is attributed to productive potential of females. Ironically, the young males who never got a chance to court a female in the jungle for the fear of their big daddies, were having a good time in the cane fields. At some stages, they were more successful here than they could have been against jungle tigers and their contribution to the next generation was of highest quality. With the genes of young tigers being stronger and healthier, the chances of the offspring's survival to maturity were relatively higher. If only mature tigers were to produce young, the risk of progeny containing a considerable portion of substandard genetic material is high. The young tigers had minimized this risk by transmitting their genes and the energy going through this fresh population was maximized in the canes.

It is highly probable that prolonged proximity of a male or an exposure to his strongly overpowering male sexual hormone or androus pheromone may make an unattached female impulsively inclined to go in for mating, thereby leading to a higher fertility.

Mating is not strongly a seasonal activity in tropical areas. Villagers have seen tigers mating in January, February, April, July, September and December. Consequently, population growth rate, contrary to the prevalent theory on population control as propounded by Malthus, is achieved in canes.

The substance in this conception is supported by observations of the fact that being the largest and most powerful of flesh eaters, tigers have no natural enemies. The top of the food chain is a lonely but comfortable niche. In sugarcane, the more important factor is the congenial condition for survival of their cubs, this being strictly controlled by the number of prey available in the human zones. The condition may turn critical in the absence of wild game when the survival of cubs may get deeply affected; but the presence of feral and domestic animals provides a dependable relief in favour of developing cubs.

Backed by recent researches, this might be another factor that compels a tiger to go in for unconventional food, such as mongrel dogs and with growing courage, even human livestock of cows and buffalos.

Chhotey used the pug mark tracks to follow the tigers. His interpretation of the marks was exhausting and exhilarating. It was rare for him to falter and I was taking every advantage of his experience. He was always calm and reassuring in contrast to my impetuosity. He was identifying individuals by their pug marks– talking about their gender, body weight and size with near mathematical accuracy. "This male must be over 200 kilograms" or "This tigress must be between 150 and 175 kilograms", he would say confidently. It was a treat to see him at work and I don't think I had much room to doubt his findings.

At a village named Pharasiya, natives reported of a tigress being accompanied by two cubs of different ages. The elder was said to be one year old and the junior one was of some four months. I examined the spoor and found this to be correct. An old English hunter Stewart (1928) had once shot a tigress with unborn cubs in her womb, and also having at her heels a cub about ten months old. If it was not an abandoned cub which had joined this tigress, this particular case could open up an interesting dimension of tiger's life cycle. Lions and tigers are biologically similar and lions have been known to go into estrus while nursing young ones. Estrus in most instances is held in abeyance while the tigress is rearing cubs. The lactation period is a hormonal shut-down mechanism, a natural phase for the female to enable her to provide parental care to the young, and automatically avoid cohabitation.

It is not known whether they may come into estrus when their milk formation stops, or the constant exposure to a male's sexual hormones brings them into estrus and stops their milk formation. The tigress is in full milk for two months and continues to lactate for another four months or so. However, lactation essentially stops by fifth or sixth month and any female, despite having cubs, if properly induced by a male with favorable temperature conditions can come into season. The males in such conditions do not need to kill her progenies as the female already seems inclined to mate. The killing of cubs is only done to bring a female into estrus. During such mating, the accompanying cubs maintain a safe distance from the male tigers or are probably temporarily abandoned by the mother or kept in a safe lair.

There are some indications that when a new male takes over the range of an old male he also tries to kill any cubs he finds. This behavioral trait is also observed among common *langoor* monkeys and lions. This practice of infanticide, apparently counter-productive, appears to be a product of deep evolutionary instinct. If cubs stay with the mother, she does not come into season again until they are one and half to two years old, and thus it delays a new male's chance of contributing his genes to the descendant line. On the other hand, by killing cubs that are not related to him, and of little genetic value as far as he is concerned, the male stimulates the female to go through her cycle faster, so that she can bear his own offspring sooner.

It is observed that a marked increase in cub mortality usually follows a change in the regime, when marauding nomadic males take a toll on young lives and females do not begin to breed again for several months. Infanticide is a system by which tigers have ruled for millions of years and the fact that this still survives in the wild is a proof that it works as nature's law.

The cubs are wholly dependent on their mother until they are about six months old. The survival instinct makes cubs learn fast and they already know the vital lesson of lying quietly hidden in a thicket, a patch of high grass or an overgrown crevice when their mother is hunting. Often the mother leaves a carcass of an animal for them to feed on for several days and goes out on longer periods of hunting. They remain hidden waiting for her return. During this time, the tigress may ally with a male for brief periods, may even share a kill with him but she seems to exercise a great caution to lead the male away from where she has concealed her cubs.

It is wrong to say that the female accompanied by cubs will neither come into estrus nor mate. In captive observation, females have been found coming into season even while raising babies. It is possible that in sugarcane fields the mothers come into estrus and practice the same procedure while mating with a male which is certainly their established partner and not a new entrant.

Charles Mac Dougal has observed that, "A tiger and tigress sharing the same range get to know each other individually over an extended period, a fact which probably favours increased breeding success." Once a cane-dwelling tigress comes into season, she alternates between periods of extreme restlessness, during which she searches for the male, and periods of remaining static, during which she is receptive. There are many factors working against her. The time of her maximum receptivity may not coincide with the presence of the male or she may have to go through her whole cycle again. Even if she does find a male at the right time, persistent copulation is needed to induce formation of mature ova.

As soon as the mating ends, the two go their separate ways. The mother comes back and joins her cubs. If she does not conceive she can come into natural estrus again thirty to ninety days later. It is therefore a remarkable biological fallacy to assume that tigresses do not conceive while they rear cubs. The only condition is that they should be the non-milk engendering mothers.

Even though definite figures in this perspective are not easy to obtain, yet the percentage of population increase in sugar tigers is certainly higher than in jungles. It should not be misunderstood as similar to that of lions who have confirmed reproductive advantage because of their social structure of prides, but to some extent it is on the same pattern. Sugar habitat has influenced the breeding dynamics of big cats. This may be taken as an explanation for the tigress being seen with the cubs of different size and ages; the two generations of cubs proceeding agreeably together. The senior cubs sometimes even babysit while the mother goes hunting – the pre-condition being that the father remains the same so that the older cubs are not in danger of being eliminated.

After all, lions and tigers are biologically similar; both have the same gestation period and parturition habits. Only their social structure differs. Unfortunately such hypothesis is almost impossible to test and an intelligent speculation will have to do for the while.

(III)

Having settled down at Harjinder Singh's house, I continued to conduct all my operations from there. Days turned into weeks as my quest for documentation of the striped feline took me into various farmlands. For this kind of operation, I used the minimum of equipment – what I call my 'commando gear'— some chocolates and roasted *channa* (gram), a water bottle, a paper pad with pen and of course a .32 Wesson & Wesson at my waist.

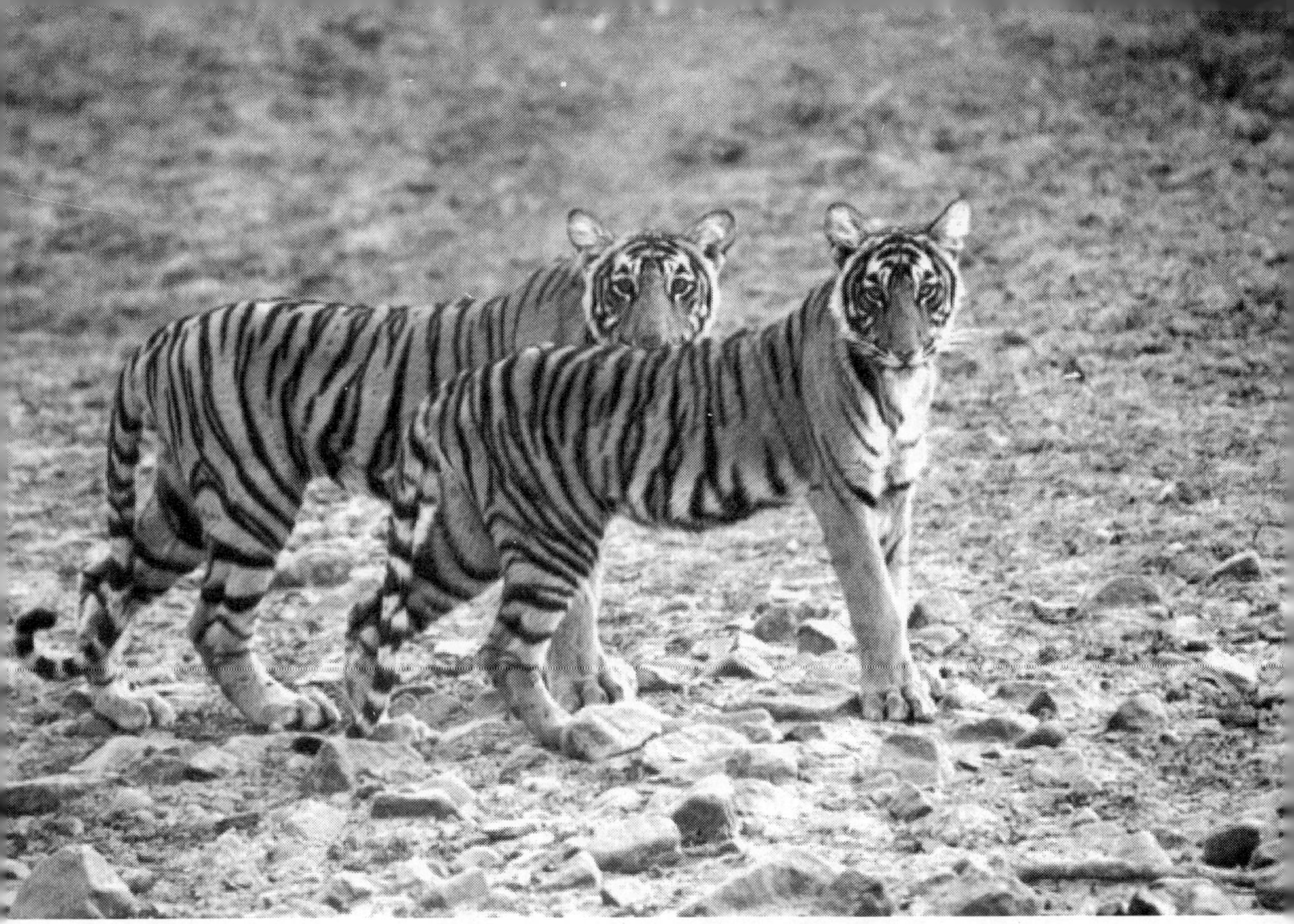

Young tigers on the banks of Ramganga river

It was rather strange to discover that many blocks of local forests were still intact in the Tarai, halfway between homes and cane fields. These bits of miniature jungles to be found in every rural block spread here and there in patches of 300 to 2000 acres, had a diverse assemblage of vegetation like grasslands, tall trees, shrub lands, sub-montane forests, thorn forests, swamps, glens and bamboo forests. Each of these patches had their own nuances and excelled in harboring a species-specific wildlife, like monitor lizards, hog deer, mouse deer or four-horned antelope. Here, the tigers could easily retreat during the interim period of summers and hunt the resident prey. Despite having been eroded by the growing demands of human populations, these diverse ecosystems were yet not exploited to the degree of corrosion by which the entire ecosystem is altered. These local jungles served as islands of conservation amongst overgrazed and over cultivated farms and still offered a reasonable cover to shelter wildlife. These were of added advantage for the cane tigers.

The menace of *Nilgai* raged almost everywhere around Dudhwa. These animals were quite plentiful and had become a nuisance. Their nightly raids on farms that often went out of control created a tense and uncertain situation for farmers. Some of the large bulls of the herd had grown audacious enough to intimidate the watchmen who guarded their crops. Their brutal attacks often resulted in death of a victim. This increasing nuisance of antelopes had made tigers a welcome entrant to the farmlands. The farmers did not mind the presence of tigers, they rather considered them as a benefactor and the best unpaid watchman they had ever had. The tiger was the best sentry against wild boars and *Nilgai*, for whenever they passed through the fields, none of these creatures came to damage the crops. Even their scats, lying here and there discouraged the antelopes for several days. It was indeed, for these tigers that sugarcane farmers had enjoyed a relaxed sleep for last many years.

R. L. Singh, in his book *The Cocktail Tigress* writes, "I found it hard to believe that 25-30 tigers were living next to human settlements, until I saw this for myself. The co-existence of humans and tigers was a special feature of this area. The sugarcane farmers would await a tigress to move into fields to deliver cubs, for the simple reason that a tigress with cubs stays on in a place longer than any other tigers."

It was early April and the dry season had set in. The sun shone in all its blaze of brightness and its warmth flooded the fields hardheartedly. During summer, the tigers orient their habits to remain within easy reach of water. But despite all the water holes having dried up, I knew that some tigers had still not left the area. Owing to the dampness of east wind that makes the cane so oppressively hot that they will not lie in it, they had shifted into a nearby reed bed, which was some two hundred acres in extent and surrounded by parched grass which had been burnt.

Only recently at dusk, a band of villagers had seen a female *Nilgai* being chased by two cubs in an inexperienced effort to make a kill and the very next night I had also heard a hog deer sounding his piping whistle in the plains to the south, supported by another in the south west. The dice of fortune was loaded heavily against them. My worry was whether they were getting enough water to live properly? So I became obsessed with the idea to support their existence and provide some water to the thirsty wildlife of the area. It seemed to me a job of moral responsibility, a culmination point of a unique experiment if I could afford a supplementary relief to hold the heat-oppressed animals in their old range.

One day, when the whirlwinds rose and swept across the heated fields, I gave a hundred rupee note to a farmer Kunj Bihari and asked him to profusely irrigate his scorched fields. I verily believe that the wildlife of farmlands recognizes the sounds of water pump as source of freshwater, and, as regards tigers, their extraordinary sensory perceptions enable them to discern moisture from miles. The man brought some twenty litres of diesel and worked his tube-well the entire night. Next morning when I reached the site, the overflowing water had formed a small pond around the tank where egrets were rejoicing and a colony of peacocks was pecking grit. I surveyed the fields and discovered the signs of many animals on the wet ground.

Towards early morning a pair of hog deer had drunk water from the irrigation channel that ran through an empty vegetable garden. There were also traces of a pig and a black buck and strangely enough, a four-horned antelope. By fortuitous chance the tigress with her cubs had also visited in the night. She had straightaway come to the tank, bathed and splashed in it, and then the whole family had lay down and rolled over the squelching mud. She had spent some two to three hours here and then as the careful mothers make sure of, had departed before light of the day.

It was but one water pump within many miles. As the examination of precincts revealed about the visit of tigers, the farmer's face gleamed with contentment. He was all jubilant that his effort had proved worthwhile in providing water to a concerned mother. Alongside, I was also conscious of a unique feeling of becoming a critical participant in actualizing the emergence of the cane tiger.

The very night I returned to Lucknow by a passenger train and got busy with some academic work. A month later, I received a postcard from Kunj Behari informing me that he was recurrently running his pump and the tigress was making periodical rounds, visiting the tank at an interval of three to four days.

It is an established fact that marked differences of habitat influence the breeding dynamics of an animal. If a tigress in the wild produces her first litter at the age of four years and raises on the average one cub per alternate year until she dies at the age of sixteen or eighteen, her total life time production is to the order of six to eight animals. The maximum longevity of a tiger under zoo conditions is about twenty years and I am sure that this age is probably not exceeded in the wild.

This potential can, of course be realized only under optimum circumstances, and under the conditions existing in cane, a tigress can go on mating almost every year. Giving some margin for her failure to conceive, dead litter, abortion and pseudo pregnancies (in which the abdomen and nipples of a female enlarge) her total life time production can be ten to fourteen animals —even half that number would do better than the average in the jungle.

George Schaller's studies reveal that in the Serengeti of East Africa a single lion pride lasts for generations. It has the same kin line, and at any one time, it has in its membership great-grandmothers, grandmothers, mothers, daughters, aunts, and female cousins. In such a sacrosanct, stable social unit, where infants are universal responsibilities, only twenty percent of the lion cubs survive to adulthood. Of those that do not survive, one quarter die of starvation, often because their mothers simply fail to lead them to kills. Another quarter die from predation or accidents, and one-half die of undetermined causes. So it is natural to presume that in the case of the solitary tigress, which raises its cubs all by itself, the percent of their reaching to maturity must be half of the lions' success rate.

In tigers, the prenatal and postnatal mortality rates remain very high. Some cubs are born dead and others die soon after birth. Still a free living tigress that loses her cubs in some mishap is potentially able to have a new litter within about five months.

It seems that in peninsular India, there is no definite season for courtship of a big cat but in the Tarai region, tigers seem to mate after rains and a majority of the young are born during December and January. Breeding females are the foundation of a secure tiger population. I was sure that a small breeding 'nuclei' population of tigers did live in the sizeable sugar fields that were relatively free from human disturbance. These prized tracts, not ones which simply made a pretty picture, but ones in which energy is flowing through numerous pathways, and in which materials are changing form continuously, would have been the storehouse of the lineage.

The population growth of such a magnitude is dramatic but could be expected of any population. The intriguing possibility was — if the prey density keeps increasing then the tiger number can also keep increasing. Perhaps the dynamics of nature communities had got significantly activated at both the producer and consumer level and this was ensuring the survival of the mothers in the sugarcane, and hence the baby boom.

The Rule of Ultimate Function says that the organisms which are better adapted to life in their surroundings will produce more young, bearing the very characteristics which gave their parents a survival edge. The benefits of differential fertility ultimately lead to conservation of a cluster of advantageous characters through their continued transmission from generation to generation. In this way, the environment is said to select the best sample for survival from the number of alternatives offered each time there is reproduction and recombination of genetic information. This defines a species.

It gave an impression that sugar crops had become the ultimate selective breeding grounds of tigers. I was sure that with each passing year, these tigresses were producing a generation that was more suited to the sugarcane habitat. Finally, there is natural selection — the most important concept of life in the natural world — that dictates that this novel order will also exist, along with that of the old order.

It seemed that over the years, these tigers had qualified the entire gamut of this parameter. If we could put aside some preconceptions and look at things objectively, the sugarcane tiger was a part of a much larger — perhaps many centuries old cycle of farm tigers that had always existed at the fringe of village communities.

F.W. Champion states, "A number of tigers occur outside the reserve forest (of Oudh) and it is possible that an average of about 25 tigers are shot each year... presently formed Hailey National Park is also breeding many tigers which spread out beyond the boundaries of the Park into farmlands." A British conservator of forests considered that the number of tigers shot outside reserved forests was certainly not less than within these forests.

It was the same class of tigers, which Champion described, that had now suddenly flourished to come into notice. Their essential characters belonged to this ecosystem, which was extended out of bounds by the arrival of the Sikh refugees from Punjab. They nourished and fostered this tiger by intense agriculture of sugarcane, made their function more operational, which in its own incongruity contributed in turning it back from the brink of extinction. At many a place the boundaries of huge sugar farms were congruent with the boundaries of swampy bogs and some left-out patches of forests; this feature helped the animals to spend their lean time and stay around farms all the year round.

This confirmed reproductive advantage of tigers in cane clearly demonstrated that human interventions can indeed play a greater role in wildlife manipulation. In a quite unpredictable way, the sugar cultivation had turned out to be decisively important in nurturing this latest capital of tigers. It was an event in natural history.

Sugarcane is a cash crop, and I was thinking — may be foolishly – if agricultural economic development projects could somehow be reconciled with tiger conservation or would it be most cost-effective to raise such habitats for the quantum jump of wild tiger population? We must pay compensation to cane farmers or reward them suitably, for their unwitting though catalytic role in tiger conservation. It had facilitated the bounce back of the species and that too in its own historical landscape.

Time and again, we have seen that the species which do not adjust with human beings' game plan start losing out and ultimately vanish. Experts believe if tigers do not find the peace and quiet which they need, they usually stop breeding, but paradoxically here the tiger was flourishing in a man-made environment and very much in the human zone, which was much distant from the real equilibrium of nature. Here, the area was disturbed by man and their livestock frequently as a matter of routine, yet the tigresses were sheltering their cubs and a viable tiger population had re-emerged after years of near-catastrophic losses.

We needed to explore this issue and understand its structural functioning. It is important to recognize that when the structure is functional, it releases energy and sets in a certain dynamics that effect the system in return. Perhaps the earlier paradigms of knowledge about these cats had reached their dead-end and new paradigms were required to understand this fragmented aspect of tiger behaviour; far away from the quantity and tome of the orthodox schools. The real barrier to their comparison was not necessarily the absence of common units of measure, but an absence of mutually compatible or mutually intelligible concepts, because the criteria of judgment depended on the situation and on the conceptual framework, which defined a new paradigm and gave it its explanatory value.

May be I was thinking far ahead. May be I was wrong, or maybe I was very correct. The fate of this tiger now seemed to be in the hand of private landowners, consisting of some 1,200 large-scale farmers only in Kheri district.

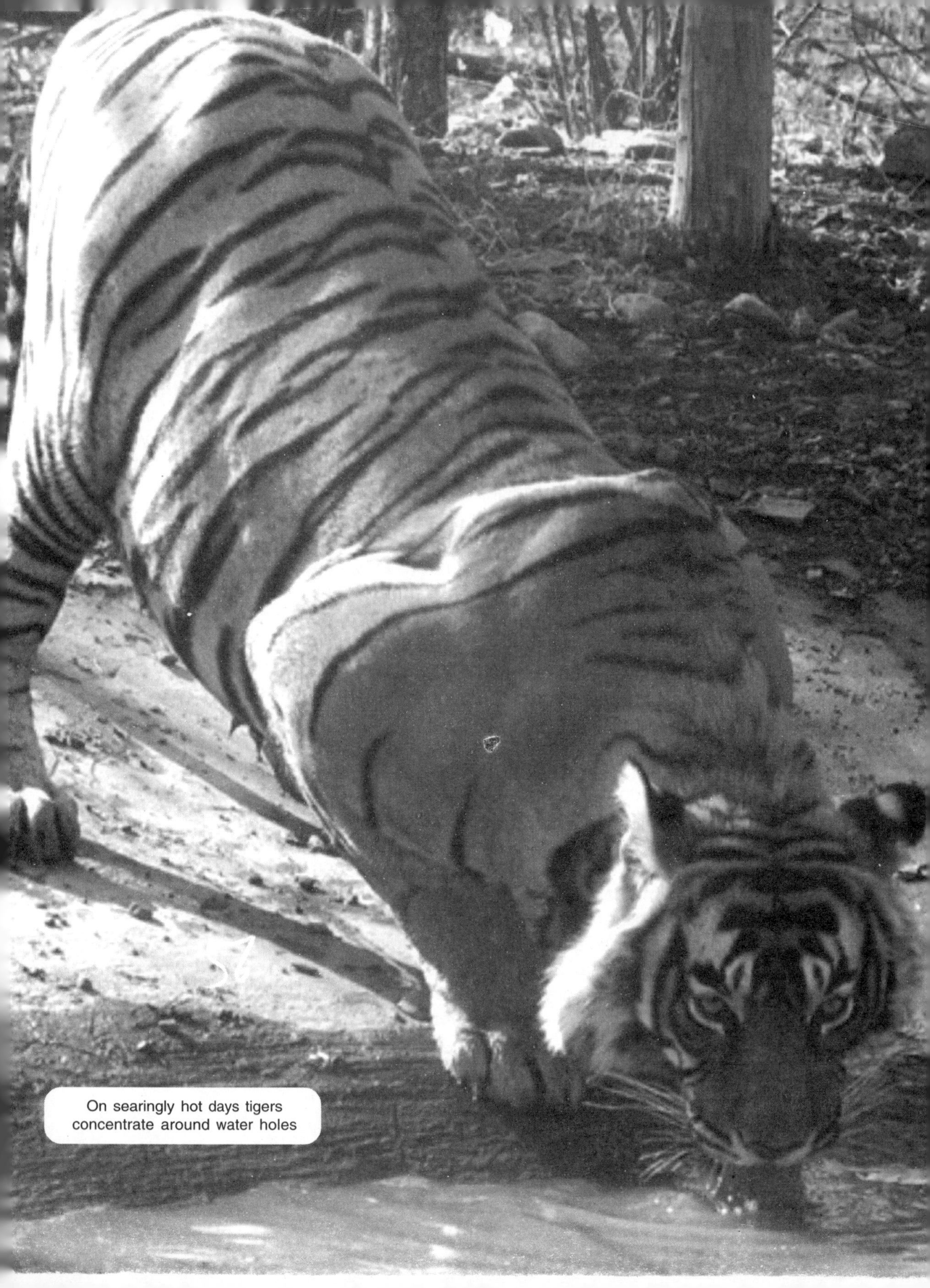

On searingly hot days tigers concentrate around water holes

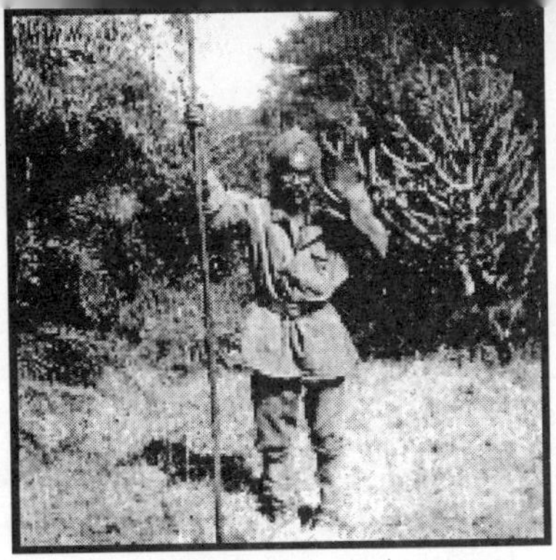

7

In the Tharu Country

There is a way that nature speaks, that land speaks. Most of the time we are simply not patient enough, quiet enough, to pay attention to the story.

- Linda Hogan

By 1980, having completed my doctorate, I had got the job of a lecturer in Christian College, an associated Institution of Lucknow University. My salary was over rupees eight hundred a month, an excellent wage in those days. I had a challenging future ahead of me and it boosted my self-esteem to know that I could push my project the way I wanted to. A thousand fancies chased each other through my mind. A reliable camera, a tape recorder, a good gun and a second hand vehicle –preferably a Willys Jeep, the celebrated World War II model that was still occasionally brought to the market for sale – these were the things I thought I must have for they were the tools of my trade. I went ahead and shortly acquired the first three things. As I swung my bag onto my shoulder and walked out of the railway platform of Palia, my thoughts went back to the image of the anxious young man that I was four years ago, when I arrived at this same railway station.

This was a sunny morning when my first singularly well-chosen expedition of Tharu country actually commenced. It was indeed good to move out of the city, into the folds of the countryside –to feel once more the grand unbroken solitude of native farms, to see the villagers working under the brilliant blue of the sky, to smell the resinous perfume of mustard flowers in clear air. And there were tigers too for asking.

Mintoo Mama's driver Vijay Singh and son Om Bir had come to the station to pick me up with a new Mahindra Jeep. The duo was as usual full of bonhomie and energy. This time, they were to take me to a village called Bisnupurva on Indo-Nepalese border; the country around which had once earned great name as a magnificent hunting-ground.

Driving slowly over meandering forest roads, we made our way to Bisnupurva. The village stands on a grassy flat bordering the river, which here runs over a wide terrain. Fresh dung and footprints of elephants, visitors during the night, lay on the wet sand at the river's edge. On the way, we stopped on a high bluff to look down at a sand bank where three crocodiles were basking in the sun. Lying absolutely immobile and slumbering with their mouths wide open, they looked like dead logs.

Bisnupurva was then considered to be among the best localities for cane tigers around Dudhwa. Soon after my arrival here, I was told that at least four tigers were living in the surrounding cane crops. There were three sub-adult males, a little more than one and a-half years old, and a mother. Like other social carnivores such as lions and wild dogs, a tiger does not normally move around with other tigers in groups but these being the litter of the same mother, despite having grown larger in size, were often seen hanging around with each other.

My stay arrangements had been made in a mud hut built on the traditional Tharu pattern. It was a basic framework of wood, thick heavy clay for the walls and thatch for the roof. The enchanting structure stood under a cluster of shady *Neem* trees that dotted a large bowl like area. It had an elliptical top and its tiny windows opened towards the bank of the river. The vast hinterland had a fascinating setting; encircled by rising mounds of golden mud, a ring of forest surrounded it in all directions. I felt completely at home in it. It is the way I felt I would like to live.

The rising ramparts of the Himalayan Mountains presented the most striking panorama, triggering a joy of solitude and comfort in me. By the afternoon, the clouds gathered and there was a blithe winter drizzle, settling the dust. The spectre of its crags happened to unfold itself. Range after range of snow clad mountains rose in their splendor, as the crown of the great Indian subcontinent spread out before me. In the gold of the sunlit evening they appeared on fire. The peak of Nanda Devi peeked languorously from the North-East over the vista, and slightly left to it was snow-capped Trishul, on top of which Lord Shiva is believed to support the sky.

After a quick bath and early dinner, we went out looking for tigers in the evening. The natives were well aware of the favorite resting places of this feline family and reckoned that they must now be near the water hole at a place called Khairatia. On the way, we saw plenty of tiger spoors which seemed to confirm their observation. We drove our vehicle leisurely and spent nearly two hours searching for the cats but without success, probably they were resting well concealed in some thick grass.

We returned through the dirt road along Mahona River when the sun went down. I had brought along a powerful searchlight which worked off the Jeep batteries. There was a very bright moon that night which rendered the dazzling beam from the torch far less effective. We drove slow and saw a number of spotted deer in groups of twos and threes and later a roaming band of jackals, which were quite unconcerned with the light. We caught a mother bear in the headlights with a tiny baby riding its back. For a second, it stood captured in the beam and then slinked away into a cane crop.

I wished to follow and take its photograph but Om Bir was of the opinion that bears are creatures of sudden impulses and when followed they do not seem to understand the difference between bolting and charging. When it hears you approaching it turns round and charges promptly, knocks down and scalps you with a few scrapes of its forepaw and then bolts. Numerous attacks of this nature are made and the uncertainty of the bear's character renders it by far the most dangerous animal an unarmed villager can encounter in the countryside. However, here the situation was trickier, for an attack could be triggered by the motive of maternal solicitude.

We moved along Mahona, Om Bir commandeering the Jeep. The river water flowed unhurriedly, glistening in the moonshine, when we saw two bright headlights coming down the northern bank of the river. It was a four-wheeler, fitted with a searchlight and somebody in there was manipulating the gadget with great dexterity. "It seems they are looking for tigers like us or can these be poachers?" said Om Bir as he left the steering wheel and worked on the bolt of his rifle and got it ready. "There are some crooks around always poaching", he grumbled, "It is not that I intend to shoot them but it is just a precaution. They are quite likely to take a pot shot at us and if this happens, I will blast their vehicle with my .416 D/B". He held the gun firmly waiting for some battle to begin.

The vehicle was an ancient Land Rover and its riders were equally curious to know as to who we were. They too had taken similar precautions. With the guns ready on both the sides we loudly asked for each other's introduction and it turned out they were the Nepalese patrol. We exchanged some information about wildlife and parted in good spirits.

Next day I got up early, rising to the booming call of a Caucal that announced the heralding of a new dawn. A bright star glittered on the eastern horizon. It was Lucifer-the morning star and bringer of light. We hurriedly gulped down some tea and went out again. The cultivation fields were thinly veiled in mist and a blue tinge of light added to the impression of coldness. We had hardly reached the green verdure towards the east of the village when the morning broke and the rim of rising sun, fiery red, cast its burgundy glow over everything. The tree tops caught a golden glint as the level beams ran like long, bright fingers through the newly awakened fields. While we drove on the Jeep, Vijay Singh happened to notice the spots of blood on the grass and the signs of a kill which had been dragged through a lentil field. It was the nocturnal work of tigers. We immediately decided to comb the borders of the sugar plot where the drag had been taken. There were no alarm calls and there was no mud for the foot prints, but the marks of vigorous drag were clear and sharp.

Om Bir saw the tigers first; what a beautiful sight it was, two of them sat in a sphinx like posture, rubbing faces. Steam rose from their mouths as they yawned in the cold air of sunrise. A few yards away from them, the third tiger lay surreptitiously behind a mud parapet where close to him a few cattle egrets were pecking the ground.

We halted the jeep and sat comfortably in silence. As the sun grew steadily in strength, from red to golden, they became clearly visible. These were remarkably large sub-adults, almost carbon copies of each other, pale-coloured and bigger in size than a mature male leopard. I speculated that they were brothers and the compact, athletic female that lay replete between the wooden stumps was their mother. Behind her lay the carcass of a large female blue bull, half of which was eaten up yet it still looked very heavy.

For an hour, we continued to watch them from a safe distance and they too looked curiously at us. I took out my diary and took quick notes. Their attitude displayed a confidence to disregard obvious danger signs, may be because they never had any bad experience with man to consider it their inveterate enemy. The tigress, having eaten merrily, looked round-bellied and there was much growling, rumbling and purring by cubs. By 9 O' clock the light became quite strong; when the clamorous trumpet notes of peacocks resonated in a small stand of mango grove near the Mahona river. Like us, the tigers turned instantly watchful. A juvenile got up and moved towards the cluster. His tail held horizontally in a classic pose of a pointer dog, he concentrated on the spot for a brief moment and then relaxed his caution. Moments later, a cattle egret drifted on the breeze and the tigress looked up as it flew over her and alighted near the blue bull carcass. The tigress stared at her and snarled. The egret flew away. Then one by one the entire family got up and strolled out towards the river bed.

It was a memorable morning to see these tigers for the first time. In later days, I

This tigress, a stray from Pilibhit sugar fields, arrived at Lucknow, 12th December 2009

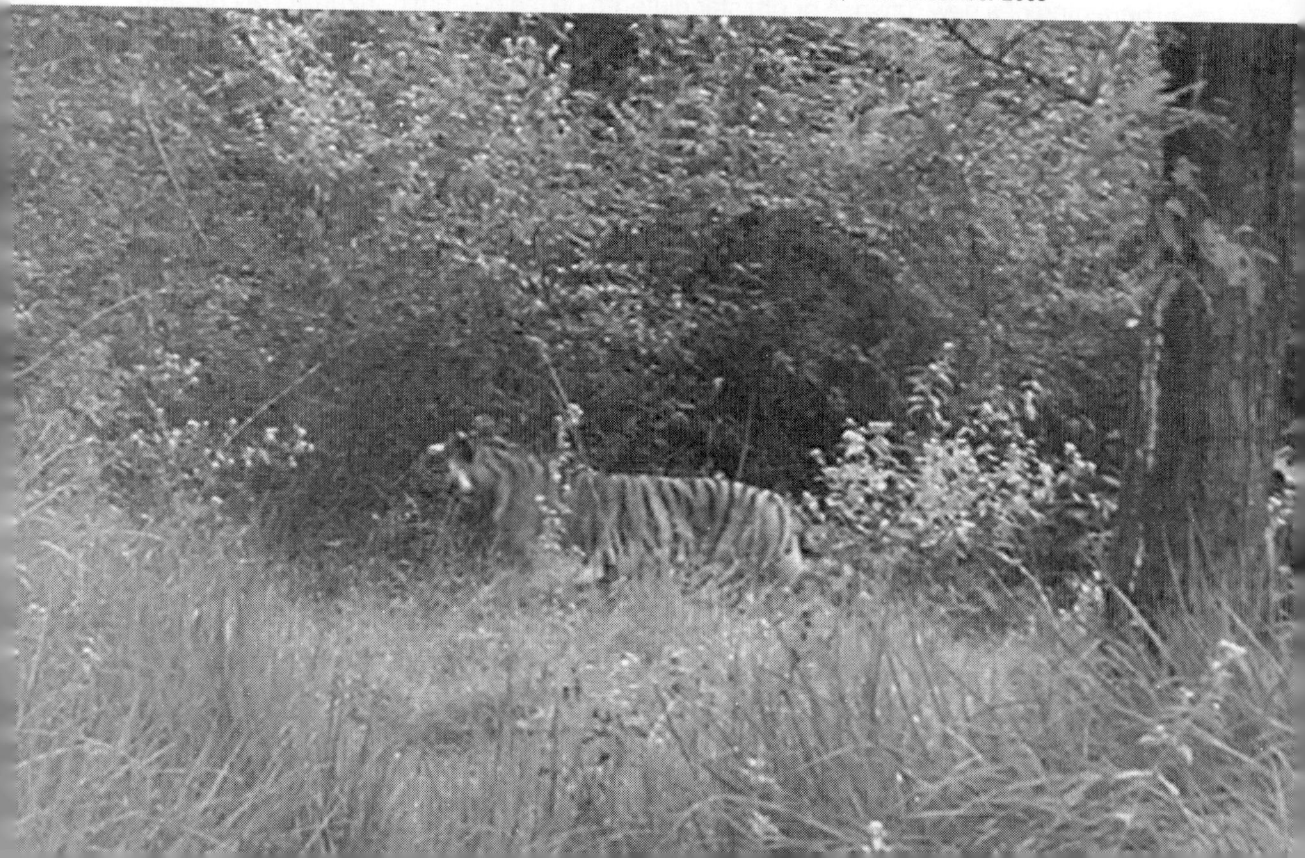

was to learn that their character was most interesting, and on the same wave length, most baffling as they stuck to a group most of the time. They moved around with a minimum distance of a hundred yards between them. This behaviour was either very bold as big cats normally do not advertise their presence or had evolved under the pressure of some circumstances which kept them in constant touch with each other, at least visually. For untold years, tigers have been living a solitary existence and their character and actions revolve round this dominant sense. Under what conditions do their habits and senses tend to become gregarious and this adaptability to changed conditions becomes acceptable is yet to be understood.

When the food is scarce, the under nourished cubs die and it appears uncommon for a tigress to raise a litter of as many as four cubs to adulthood but this one seemed to have done it wonderfully. For the next three weeks, I virtually lived with these tigers, coming to know about them well. There were many cattle in this area but the tigers were surviving quite well on wild boar, blue bull and hog deer. Surprisingly, the most important prey species was the peacock. Its quantum was high and young tigers seemed to enjoy stalking them. On many occasions, bevy after bevy of peahens crossed my path, followed by some isolated cock-birds, scattered to our right and left. Quite a few times, I came across the remains of a bird after a tiger had fed on it.

One afternoon in mid-April, Om Bir and I walked along the south bank of Majhoara *Nala*. The dry embankment was steep and thick with brush wood, with the sun blazing down over its nakedness and the temperature was well over 100 degrees F in the shade. On the far side of the *Nala*, a solitary Rhesus Macaque sat grinning in the dark nook of a sugarcane plot, avoiding the rays of the tropical sun. A pair of golden orioles flitted about in a mango tree and below it a male peacock was busy dancing with its flowered tail spread. His dance was being appreciated by a bevy of peahens when a tiger came out of a sugar plantation. As the monkey saw the cat emerge, it suddenly filled the air with its hideous screams; the peacock family responded and flew off rapidly in the opposite direction whilst the monkey began springing from plot to plot. The tiger charged the monkey in a hot pursuit. His sudden burst of speed was taken up in prodigious bounds. The dust rose as a bridled mass glided like a golden streak through the open space, closing upon the bouncing ball of the monkey.

Then suddenly two more tigers materialized on the scene. The shocked monkey abruptly changed his course and ran towards the dry river bed and it was here that the fourth tiger emerged from a clump of bush. In a fleeting sweep, he caught the primate midway; holding its nape with its fangs, muffling its dying shrieks and moved further to enter a thicket. The rest of the group followed him greedily, their saliva – coated teeth glistening in overhead sun, creating an effect akin to that of a pack of hunting wolves.

The thick bush waved for a brief second as the train of big cats promptly entered

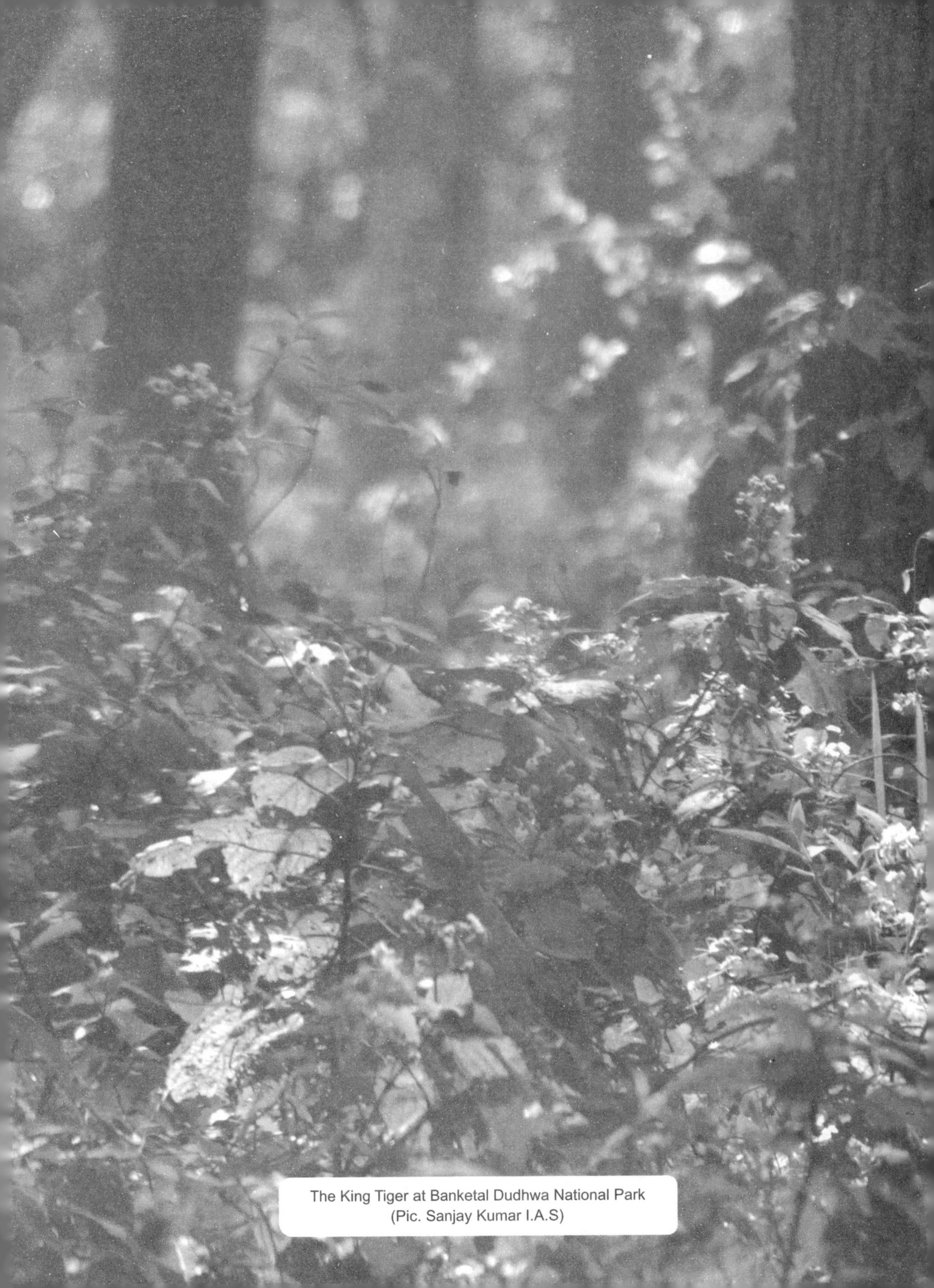

The King Tiger at Banketal Dudhwa National Park
(Pic. Sanjay Kumar I.A.S)

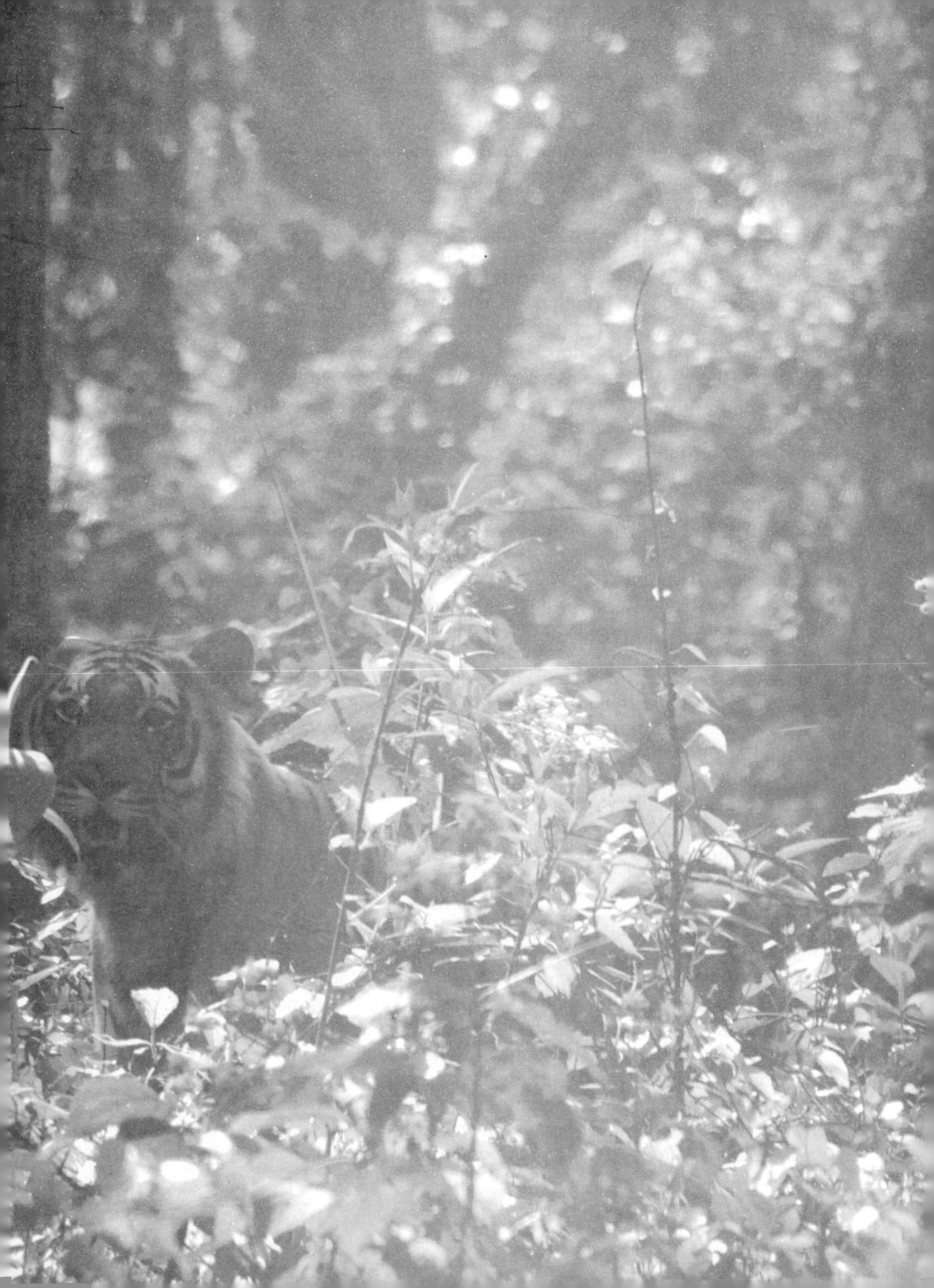

into it; leaping up in that peculiarly heavy lumbering way which so often misleads one into under-estimating the tiger's pace. The thicket recovered its wonted calm with extraordinary rapidity. An intense silence settled down as if nothing had happened; not even a bird called.

Such a stupendous scene, bursting so suddenly upon us was almost overpowering. Even Om Bir held his breath, and the remains of his beloved cigarette, not yet half consumed, dropped unheeded from his lips.

The incident was an impressive illustration of the fact of how these tigers were practicing group hunting. Though, their hunting ability was still amateurish yet they had learnt the art of troupe aggression and knew its advantages. The tiger activity patterns are shaped to meet their physiological needs of using the prey resources effectively and conserving energy. It certainly seemed that besides the purpose of self-protection, easy hunting was a significant part of group tactics, which conserved energy and used prey capital successfully.

Brander mentions that he once saw two adults hunting in a company; Baze watched a tiger and tigress stalk deer, and Baikov implied that in Manchuria two tigers frequently hunted together. Two or more tigers are also said to stalk pigs communally. To my mind these are more or less family groups who often rejoin and recognize each other by familiar filial smell which the tigers of a common litter carry all their life. But the evidence of this type of hunting is insufficient.

The key fact to remember is that the predatory patterns of tigers had evolved in dense forests, where hunting down a large prey provided them with several meals. The design of the group is such that the meal is shared, meaning thereby each member gets less meat from each kill. It is argued that group hunting does not bestow any advantage in heavy cover to a stalk-and-ambush predator like the tiger; unlike in the savannahs where prey can be located from a long distance and pursued relatively easily. Most of the tiger hunting is done in short surprise attacks, with little opportunity to co-operate. As per this line of reasoning, it was perhaps a family of three brothers and a mother that had overstayed together under opportune conditions.

I did not see these tigers until the following spring. It was some seven months later that I visited the place once again and was told by the villagers that the cubs had grown larger and had most probably separated. They had developed a habit of wandering off on their own and were last seen together in October last year. Presently, they usually focused their activities in different parts of the area which they naturally commanded as their mother's home range while the mother also provisionally used a marginal portion of the local jungle, to the north of Mahona river, moving across it to frequent the meadows of *narkul* grasses. This was believed to be the outer fringe of a strong male's territory, perhaps the father of these cubs. However, the tigress was keeping the cubs at a safe distance from the male and allowed them to roam the vista temporarily, only when their father was not there.

(II)

More then ever, tigers had got into my blood stream by now. But my teaching profession did not give me enough time to undertake repeated and prolonged trips to the Tarai. While I was in the city, my mind kept going back to the mysteriously swaying sugarcane; hiding within them the bravura images of tigers. This delightful terra firma combined enough excitement with personal danger to make it interesting. I wished to return there to feel in tune with my surroundings, without a jarring note from my principal who considered my wildlife stint as quite tangential to my academic pursuits.

The question of getting leave was a big one for me. The search for a tiger in sugarcane plantations is a time-consuming business. It could take several days and under odd circumstances even weeks if not months. They were rarely found in the same place for two successive days, unless they had made a sizeable kill. Thus there was nothing much to do than to await events and be prepared to waste time in fruitless efforts and return unrewarded when my time ran out. In those days the press had been giving little publicity to this problem and nothing much was known about the ravages of these tigers. The area being enormously large and remote, the news of accidents percolated late, often only in a brief paragraph informing the disinterested readers that a tiger had claimed yet another victim in the sugar fields.

Over the years, the problem acquired profoundly menacing proportions and yet no remedy was seriously thought about it. People with little knowledge approached the issue through the record of natural history that charts the eternal competition between top predators; the battle of man against carnivores that they coexist with.

Fruitless elementary discussions continued, and both the government quarters and ecologists, rejoiced at the increase in tiger population. It was taken as a hearty success of Project Tiger and indeed a tool to assess the effectiveness of conservation efforts. It seemed to some conservationists that in one of the world's most heavily populated countries, a balance between man and animals had been at last achieved. But what was considered a triumph by one group was read as an abysmal failure by Billy Arjan Singh. This doyen of wildlife conservation was skeptical about increase in tiger population. In his opinion, only recently in the bordering country of Nepal a large tract of sub-montane forest called Churia Range had been felled to pave way for the rehabilitation of retired army personnel and from here many tigers had crossed over to India and spilled out of forest in the cane crops. There was nothing like the cane tiger or any such phenomenon, rather it was just a temporary phase, created by an 'unnatural surplus immigration of guests' from Nepal, which the receiving country India, burdened as it was with similar problems of habitat destruction, could not cope. Now as the predators regulate their populations at a low enough level, it would soon be corrected by the lifestyle

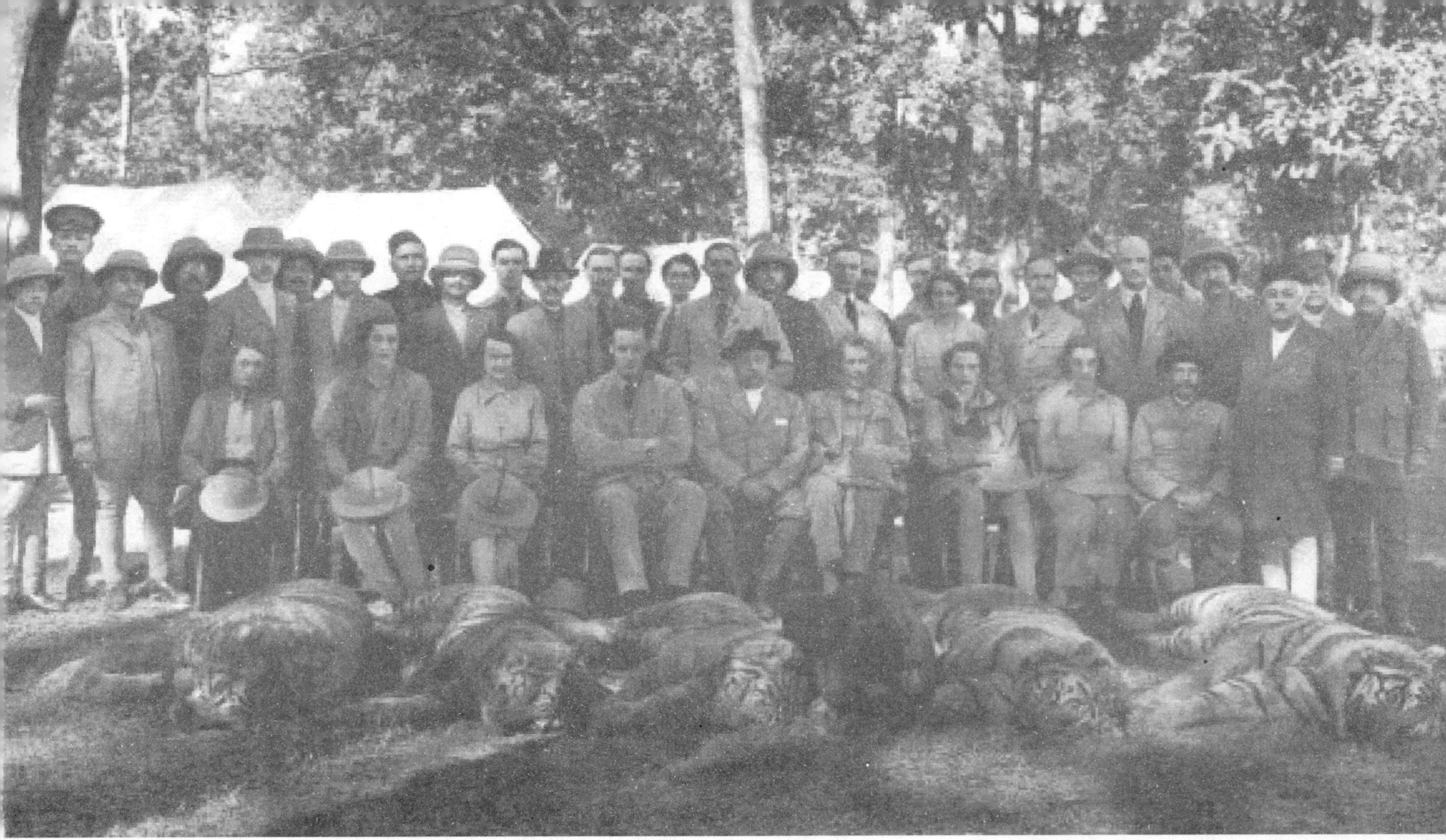

Recreational Murder

So tremendously powerful beasts, so bountifully and favorably endowed by nature, should have lived out their years in peace but were wafted to the brink of extinction by the erratic demands of human ego. Maharaja of Nepal with minor luminaries of British India.

of the tigers themselves.

Billy is undoubtedly a man of remarkable achievements, but his out of character priorities and ideologies with rigid definitions have invariably created too hard a basket of problems in the post-modernist pursuit of conservation. He could never have put forward a more baseless simplification of problem, which was in fact a statement about farmland tigers. Both halves of this syllogism were defective. Either the old man had failed to understand the glitch or it was just one more ideological stance -a willful blindness- that discounted the importance of biological understanding. Perhaps some less absolute definitions on his part might have furnished a precise answer for this problem.

During the years of Emergency, the Prime minister of India Mrs Indira Gandhi had placed wildlife on the Concurrent List by sacrificing revenue for the creation of several wildlife refuges and conditions were congenial for large predators to multiply. Thus in the contemporaneous circumstance, every kind of wildlife had increased. In the context of tigers, to avoid overcrowding their automatic number adjustment system had begun to impel superfluous animals into other unoccupied ranges. Thus as long as tigers continued to spill out of the forest into cane fields, they could continue to increase. It was indeed essential to understand that since this had happened; the system was working the other way round to reduce the pressure. True, this had laid the scene for conflict between tiger and humans, but equally true was the aspect that this threatening surplus of tigers would not be eliminated in natural conditions, until interrupted by man.

The resounding story of the big success was in fact an amassed impact of the abolition of sport hunting, ongoing conservation strategies, reckless deforestation in Nepal and availability of sugarcane fields towards Indian side as surrogate forest for tigers, which had brought back their population from the brink of extinction. This miracle had taken place in absence of ancient breeding grounds that were now lost to agrarian expansion. This reality was desirable to be understood at any reasonable depth but Billy was deliberately callous, unmindful to the sheer size, solitude and isolation of great sugar farms that provided sanctuary to this new generation of tigers, where despite the absence of anti-hunting measures, less rigorous government controls and the occasional reactionary activities of villagers, super predators and their prey had persistently managed to hold on.

The potential tiger carrying capacity of many sugar farms was considerable as the estimate of the secondary prey base was high. To create a similar ecological space, which these arable lands offered for free, ranging tiger conservation with minimal financial investment (save for compensation of cattle killed by tigers) even near less promising jungles would have cost a fortune to government. As a result a huge number of predators were living outside the protective umbrella of the park. The tigers themselves seemed to approve their increased population and the possibility of this unnatural expansion seemed in no way excluded from the future modules.

In the early seventies, when tiger hunting had been totally banned in India, it was still continuing in Nepal and consequently the Indian Shikar outfitters had shifted their attention there. During this phase I had once briefly visited Churia range and its adjacent Charkosia Jhari, (an eight mile forest, that consisted of the detritus wash down from the hills by the monsoon) with an American hunter Bum Garner. This shoot was conducted by an old family friend and professional hunter called M. Haider Mamman Khan. Of the tigers he has given to his clients 9 were shot by Bum Garner himself.

Churia was a sparse forest trail largely running on the low lands and partly on the second rampart of the Himalayan slopes known as Shivaliks. The very section of Churia range that Billy was talking about, called Hatti-khot, was hardly six by three miles in length and breadth, with five human settlements already existing within its core area, and some ten thousand people living with their thousands of livestock husbandry. (The fact was verifiable in the given context and scale.) They survived on forest products and practiced small scale agriculture in petite forest clearings. For years, incessant human movement had made the range biotic-ally damaged, the forest was denuded to an irreparable travesty of its former luxuriance and the normal life cycle of wildlife life was severely disturbed. Thus the place was no longer a source of permanent tiger supply for the more disturbed forests of India.

It may be mentioned that after the end of the despotic reign of the Rana's in Nepal, the era of old-fashioned tiger shoots conducted on grand scale, had ended and with that the longstanding protection offered to the forests in Nepal had also come to an end. Consequently, as early as in the middle of 1950's a large chunk of landless population had moved into forests and settled down there. Though Billy believed that it was still an ideal habitat with a variety of prey, where a natural sanctuary was being afforded for the tiger itself, but in my remembrance this was an undersized forest; exacerbated and disgracefully unsuitable for tigers. Even if I believed the old man's words that the artificial surplus had come from there, the small chunk could not contain more than two or three harassed big cats. I told Billy that at the most three tigers and may be a dozen leopards would have crossed over to India and not this imposing plethora that seemed to have spread out in the sprawling sugarcane belt of nine districts of Indo-Nepalese Tarai, including the neighboring districts of Bahraich, Shajahanpur and Pilibhit. Despite being surrounded by human populations, the steadily developing phenomenon of sugar tigers had literally outnumbered the tigers inhabiting regular jungles.

It is useful to understand that the entire 550 sq km of Dudhwa Reserve, 200 sq km of Kishanpur sanctuary and nearly 800 sq km of other forest ranges, in one district of Kheri only are bounded by no less than 5,000 square kilometers of cane crop cover. A similar situation also exists in the neighboring Tarai districts. Here the wild prey migrates into agricultural fields in search of food and the predators then follow them wherever they go. In addition, throughout monsoon months, water logging also degrades the habitat and presses the animals further towards agriculture fields. This primarily makes the sugarcane plantations a prey-rich habitat which offers the exploratory support to a higher number of transients and sub-adult tigers. Many of these tigers coming from the small pools of species that survive in small forest pockets and run the risk of inbreeding, now potentially affected the genetic exchanges on their own. This phenomenon was a classic example of the flagship which had brought out the species from the ambit of terminal decline and paved the way for the emergence of a putative creed.

It was true that some tigers, who were modest killers and also occasional consumers of human beings had created an ecological crisis but it needed to be ascertained whether they had chosen such a favorable place for their nefarious activities by discrimination -to deliberately stalk a victim, and thus, genuinely taking a wrong turn to the rifle or the steel cage- or whether their killing was the result of their disablement by age or injury or lack of prey or an accident or an outright reaction to human aggressiveness? The increased destruction of their principal prey species might cause a proportionate increase in the numbers of tigers to take to man-eating but seemingly, there were many more that beat a furtive retreat against man and tried to avoid him. Such animals needed to be valued emotively and protected.

Conservation forums believe that grasslands are the best mosaics of the jungle that sustain the highest number of tigers anywhere. In good habitats, like Kaziranga grasslands, tiger densities including those of cubs are known to go up to fifty tigers per one hundred square miles. This is the upper limit of tiger densities ever recorded anywhere in the grasslands of the world. On the same line of reasoning, it is not out of place to illustrate the example of sugarcane habitats. They also represent dense grasslands, where there is plenty of water and excellent stalking cover, supporting a density of ungulates. Thus it is natural to assume that it's potential to sustain tigers is quite high. The density of their population may be registered low because of the boundless extension of sugarcane and so many pressures built up against the survival of big cats, especially because human settlements are sparsely dotted over their terrain.

The statistics also showed that the number of females was much higher in the sugarcanes than males. It is a factor that high tiger densities are achieved, primarily due to female occupation of smaller ranges whose movements are restrained to a limited place due to their biological role of rearing the family, and when cubs are born, their chances of survival to maturity are better than in prey scarce habitat. This was the basic cause of the quantum jump in tiger population in farms. Thus this tiger like our farms of sugarcane, was the home-grown product of our soil. Billy has himself written about the feature on page 89 of his book '*Tiger Heaven*', "In 1969, for instance, five tigress were shot, eight cubs captured, and three burnt, all

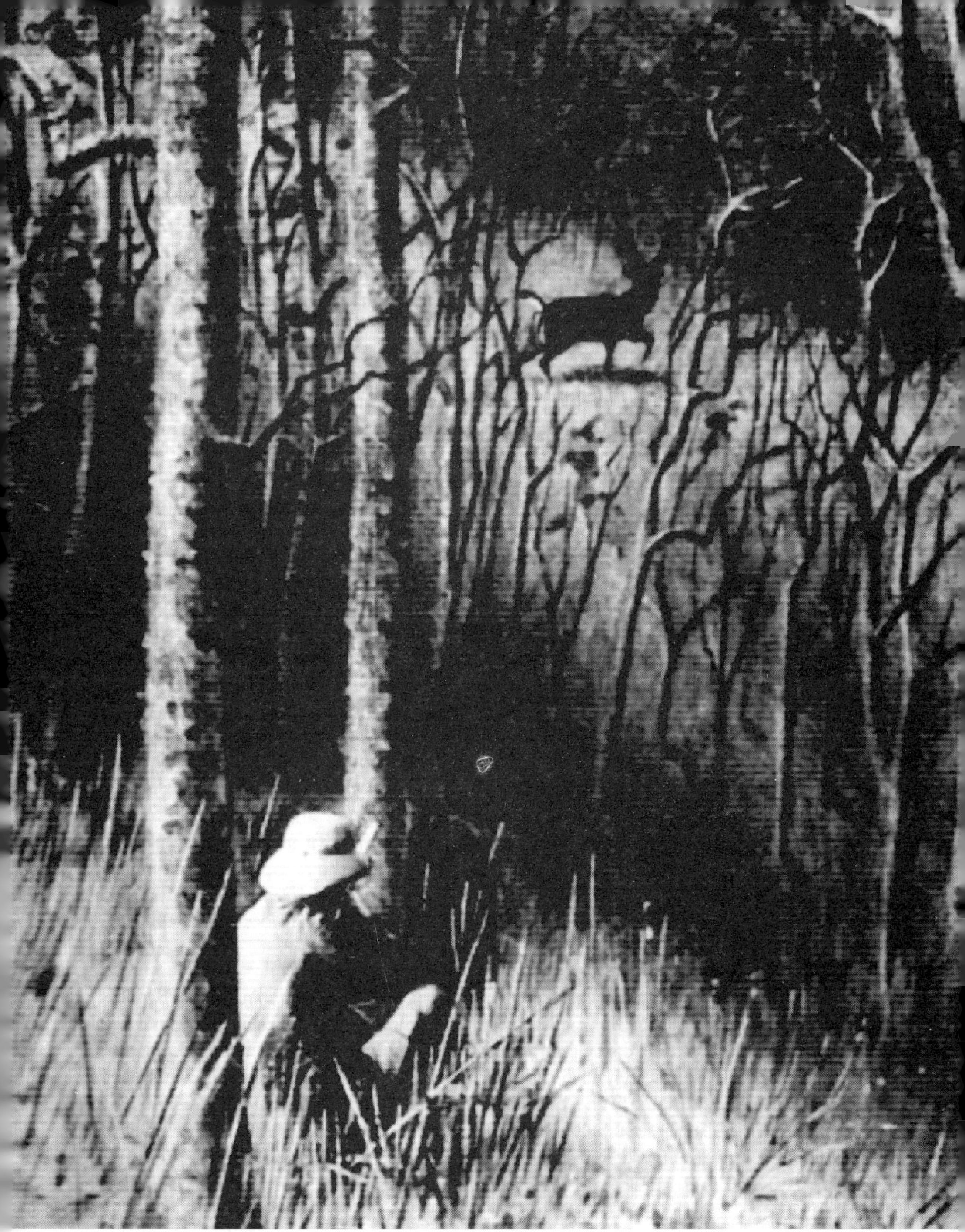

An arcive sketch from A.I.R Glassford

in local cane fields. Five of the cubs were found together in one place; the farmer who discovered them said that the tigress had run away, although no doubt she was shot."

In '69, Churia range was intact and the licensed massacre of tiger was open in India. It is while describing this phase, when a tiger still shied away from man, Billy in one sentence admits the existence of 21 tigers in the cane, meaning thereby that even then tigers were plentiful in the cane fields. The two diametrically opposite statements by Billy, where in '*Tiger Haven*', he describes local tigers as normal farm-dwellers and then, nearly 25 years later, modifies his opinion and calls them artificial surplus, (Billy for the first time used this expression in his book '*The Legend of The Man-eater*', page 91, 1993) show his deep-rooted self contradiction about this phenomenon, which is certainly ludicrous if not tragic.

The abundant power of malleability brings the tiger closer to a true cat than the lion. They agree to environmental changes with noteworthy ease and whatever habitat they have occupied, from Russian Taiga to Indonesia they have merged with it over generations. From record weight of 845 pounds of P.T. Altaica, that was shot in 1950, inside Siberian Mountains of Sikhote Alin, they have metamorphosed to a likely 200 pounds in form of P.T. Balica with much difference in size and weight and the color of their pelts. Thus their adaptability to sugarcane, with minute transformations is no surprise. It was neither the 'temporary surplus' nor some foreign material imported into India as a result of reclamation of the lesser tract of Churia range. It was all indigenous material.

"It is more probable," I told venerable Billy, that "tigers from the Indian side, overflowing Dudhwa have crossed over to Shukla Phanta, Royal Bardia and Parsa wildlife reserve in South Nepal, than for their tigers to have come into our canes. It is wrong to consider them as a surplus. Due to abundance of buffer prey in farmlands, the survival rate of tigers is naturally high, moreover tigers produce and nurture more young than needed to replace natural losses that is why in the halcyon days of battues they could take such a terrific bashing and still maintain their population. The great sugar plantations demonstrate the mastery of the man over his environment leading to the creation of improved man-made environment that is also -every so often- conducive to the wildlife. The farms should be taken as new emerging reserves of floating population which can readily plug holes when these occur among the residents, even in the jungle".

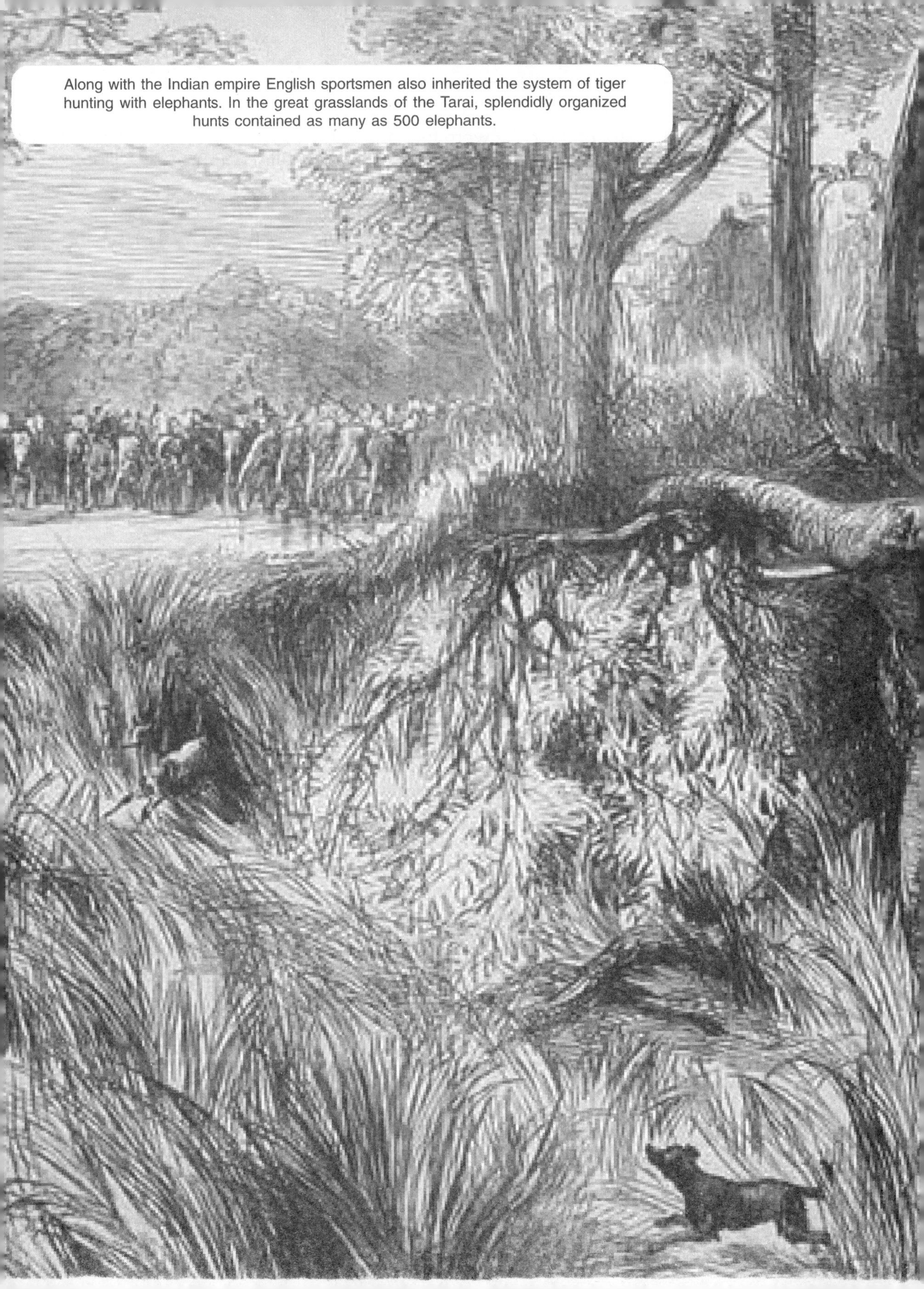

Along with the Indian empire English sportsmen also inherited the system of tiger hunting with elephants. In the great grasslands of the Tarai, splendidly organized hunts contained as many as 500 elephants.

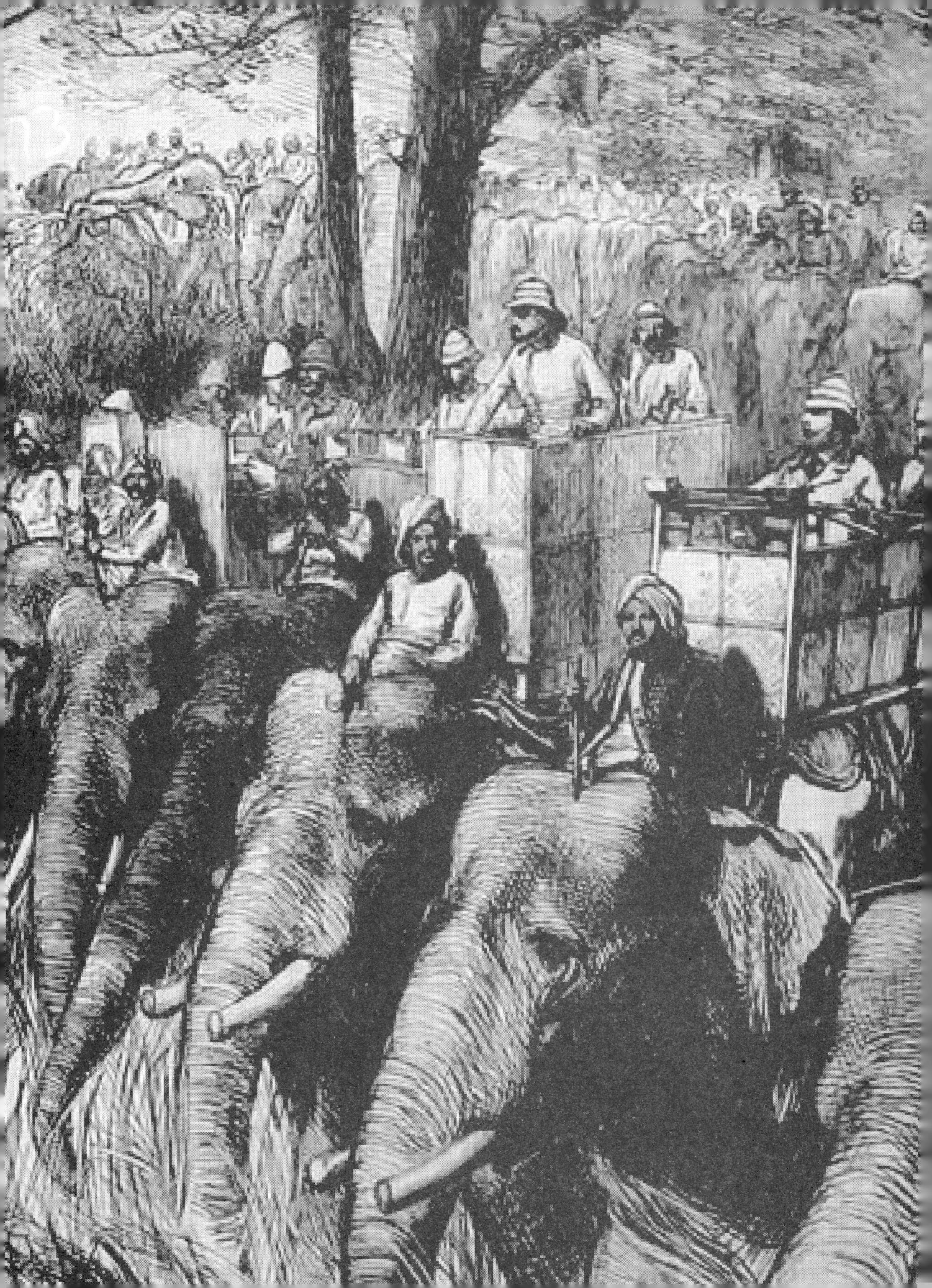

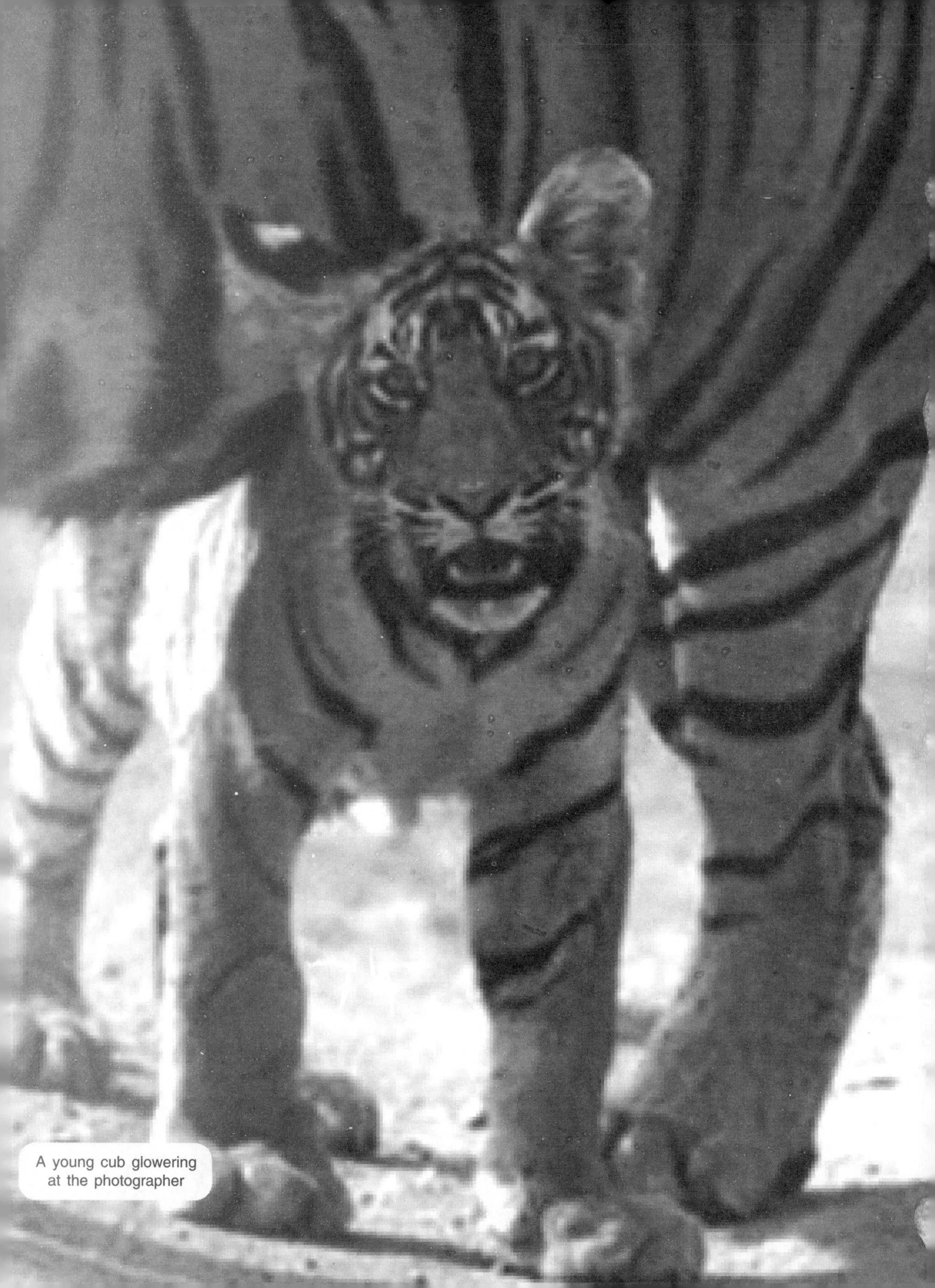

A young cub glowering at the photographer

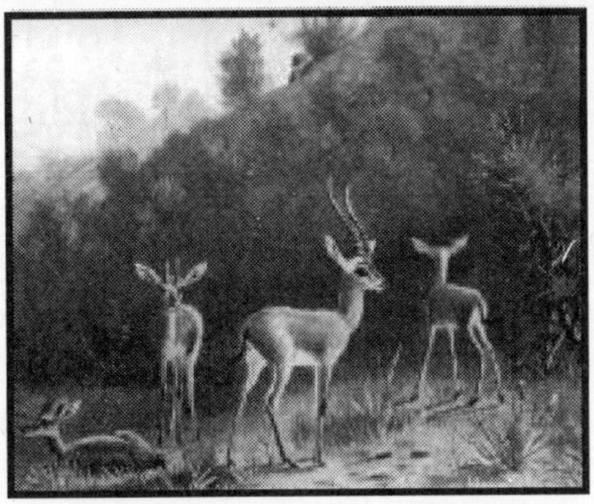

Katarnia Ghat Sanctuary

Top carnivores are predestined by their perch at the apex of the web to be big in size and sparse in numbers. They live on such a small portion of life's available energy as to always skirt the edge of extinction and they are the first to suffer when the ecosystem around them starts to erode.

- Wilson

The familiar combination of excessive hunting and loss of habitat in the Tarai region was responsible for the decline in the wildlife, especially tiger population. Wildlife is not an unlimited natural resource as our forefathers believed. But the comeback of tigers in the sugarcane had proved that it is certainly a renewable resource when preserved and properly managed.

Apart from the unpleasant brush with the wardens, who put useless obstructions in carrying out things smoothly, I was at last getting some success in my study. My hard practical undertaking required much travel and fieldwork. Any error at this level could result in a real catastrophe but the Wardens had a technical point that why I should not be arrested and prosecuted for disturbing tigers. It was a desperate allegation for which I was not prepared as I was not operating inside the jungle. However, I had learnt from experience that if you want to get something through, it is fatal to wait for permission, because the functioning of the bureaucracy is laggard and time-consuming. Wildlife is a subject of sensitive nature. Often holders of prestigious scholarships routinely face difficulties in getting clearances from respective departments. The best course of action for a conscious citizen is to get right ahead with whatever one is doing. As it happened some senior foresters wisely realized that there was no harm if someone else does day-to-day policing and takes a round at weird hours, and tries to keep a record of itinerant tigers which stray out of the jungle.

One day, a senior official named Narrottam Tripathi, who happened to be a friend of my uncle and was on the whole more sympathetic to my ventures, lambasted the lower echelons' of the forest administration in a meeting when they complained about me. "no researcher can be treated as intruder", he made things clear, "There are many poachers around, besides villagers and tribesmen. By all means this man has enough background in the area and is fighting the same war with poachers as we. So let him go ahead." Since then the Wardens who had made my life difficult began to co-operate though they still regarded me as an oddball who was keen on doing even their nightly duties for free.

Ranjit was not only encouraging but was also a helpful companion and this was important to me. One day, he planned to visit Katarnia Ghat sanctuary and take an assessment of the actual situation. This independent biotic complex lies at a distance of thirty five kilometers to the east of Dudhwa. The wildlife potential of this area is very high and in recent years, greater protection had led to an increase in prey species here. Ironically, the excellent quality of habitat makes the viewing of wildlife a rarity.

We arrived in the area in November of 1984. Our working team had nine members, including Dr. Ram Boojh, an environment scientist and presently an official at UNESCO. Our main interest was focused on a huge open tract, which fell between the two existing forests of Katarnia Ghat sanctuary and Bilrayan range of Dudhwa National Park. Seemingly unattractive from a tourist's point of view, the tract was primarily an agricultural frontier. Here, sugarcane was the predominant crop with human population densities honeycombed here and there. Though schools and dispensaries had sprung up in between, the region still harbored a number of fragmented patches of tree forests, which served as tenuous islands to wildlife.

In the olden times, Ranjit's father had led some daring expeditions in this region and every time he had associated with him as a growing teenager. It was an exciting privilege to camp once again in these wilds with an old stalwart. Our first evening was full of nostalgic recollections of early days; as we sat around the camp-fire he regaled us with stimulating stories, when these lovely lands were a continuous stretch of virgin forests and renowned for the wealth of big game, and where his father had achieved some unsurpassable scores in leopard and bird shootings. He thoroughly understood the nuances of tiger conservation, yet, as he had been an experienced eyewitness to immense hunting and trapping, he loved to talk like an explorer of pioneer times.

We found that both the forest ranges of Katarnia Ghat and Bilrayan harbored a fairly good population of wildlife but a concerted action was required to ensure the viability of reconnecting the fractured habitat again through a substantial corridor between the two areas. This sensitive landscape, abutting the international border, consists of nearly 22 villages in between and also the bustling township of Tikonia. The country is covered with thick and heavy sugar crops and intersected by numerous and much frequented bridled paths, where an infamous meter gauge railway line runs through it taking a heavy toll of wildlife each year.

The vista measures nearly fifteen miles in length and thirty miles in width. At present, as a mute indicator of silent demographic change, hundreds of encroachments, including illegal mosques and hutments have come up here in league with the timber mafia. The patronage of local politicians has also helped these refugees to settle down with legalized papers, and in turn they happily serve as vote banks to their guardians. This landless lot erodes jungles in search of living space -wresting away what belongs to animals- and sustains itself on forest products. They plunder timber and often hunt wild ungulates, thus exerting a great pressure on existing tiger habitats in both the directions. Lately, a Maoist movement has also started in the region ideologically driven from Nepal, complicating matters further.

A survey of the area revealed that this open tract was the end result of ecological catastrophe. This was actually a savannah land of coarse grasses, intercepted by glens and swamps that represented the richest genetic resource in the Tarai. Created by fluctuations of seasonal rivers this area was of incalculable value not only for the scientists but also for herbal medicine, animal husbandry, agriculture and arboriculture. The myopic government officers did not attach much importance to this savannah as in their imperfect definitions; the cluster of trees was forest, not grasslands. The fact was condoned and the tract was cleared for rehabilitation and agricultural colonization.

I think those who built up modern Tarai were fully embroiled in the immediate needs of the times. Even if they had paused to think about the depletion of the forest resources, it is doubtful they would have acted in any other way. Tarai still relied on agriculture for its basic needs and economy. People believed that more forest lands should be cleared and converted into croplands. But this was one of the greatest ecological disasters perpetrated by man and a substantial part of the once continuous forest trail of the Tarai was fractured and the extremely vigorous and potential grassland that served as a link between two great forest ranges of Bilrayan and Katarnia Ghat was completely eradicated. Nothing was even spared in the name of a corridor for the movement of animals.

Perhaps the entire history of tiger hunting by man had not caused so much damage as was caused by the destruction of its habitat. The widespread shrinking of forest ranges made tigers fight for survival, an exigent challenge that surpassed every other cause so far responsible for the decline in the numbers of this race. The endemic destruction of habitat drove tigers out in the fields; consequently many of them seeking cover were shot in the open. Deprived of shelter and food they backed away in smaller and smaller groups, which later got so isolated that they could no longer be considered as genetically viable breeding populations. Presently now, when even these are protected, it is feared that they would eventually degenerate and die out unless they can be moved to join other bigger groups, where they can re-establish a passable gene flow. The situation was no different in this land terrain; two big ranges, separated by a large gap were catering to their independent tiger population. This gargantuan task of marrying the two ranges -seemingly without a solution- had perhaps become possible here due to profuse agriculture of sugarcane.

This was November. The sugarcane crops were at their thickest, and a heavy movement of tigers was being reported between the two ranges. In fact, there were so many tigers moving about that it was a difficult period to locate them properly. Some transients had stayed and about eight tigers overlapped in between Banveerpura and Sarkoha area, living nocturnal lives. They were seemingly shy of human presence for they had come from the forests. Herders had seen their glimpses towards dawn and evening, some had even watched them spraying and scraping the earth in the manner of their tribe. These ritual activities insinuated that they were trying to create their territory in the croplands, which prevents unintended encounters in the territory that may be temporarily overcrowded.

A particular tiger had focused his activity around a water pond near a settlement called Majhegaura. One morning I started off in search of this animal, taking a .12-bore shot gun and accompanied by a group of villagers. The natives seemed to be quite certain of their way and led us across a large swampy *Baghar*, inside which, they showed me three carcasses of feral cows that had been gradually eaten from the rump. Their hides and part of skeleton were still intact but the carcass had been all emptied of its edible contents. Now the vultures were busy in transforming it into a clean thing, picking decaying flesh, ribbon by ribbon in their curved beaks until it would become a prehistoric carcass and then a pile of outsized bones.

We had not gone far from the last kill, when I happened to see something ruddy moving in a patch of green wheat, a good distance to our right. I set on my field glasses but by then the animal had moved on and disappeared. I kept my eyes on it and decided to approach the wheat patch and when I was some fifty yards, the object appeared again. Then I realized that it was the massive head of a tiger, peering over the standing crop. The natives also immediately saw it and whispered '*rukiye sahib, sher hai',* (In modern India, a sahib is not necessarily a European; it is almost anything in a pair of trousers and a cap.) but the object had again disappeared. By now my curiosity was at its peak. I approached still further, apparently oblivious of the ever-changing location of the tiger inside the wheat thicket but edging forward when it peered again to look grimly at our group that was ever drawing nearer to its resting place.

They walked to a small pool and after drinking entered in the water to play and rest

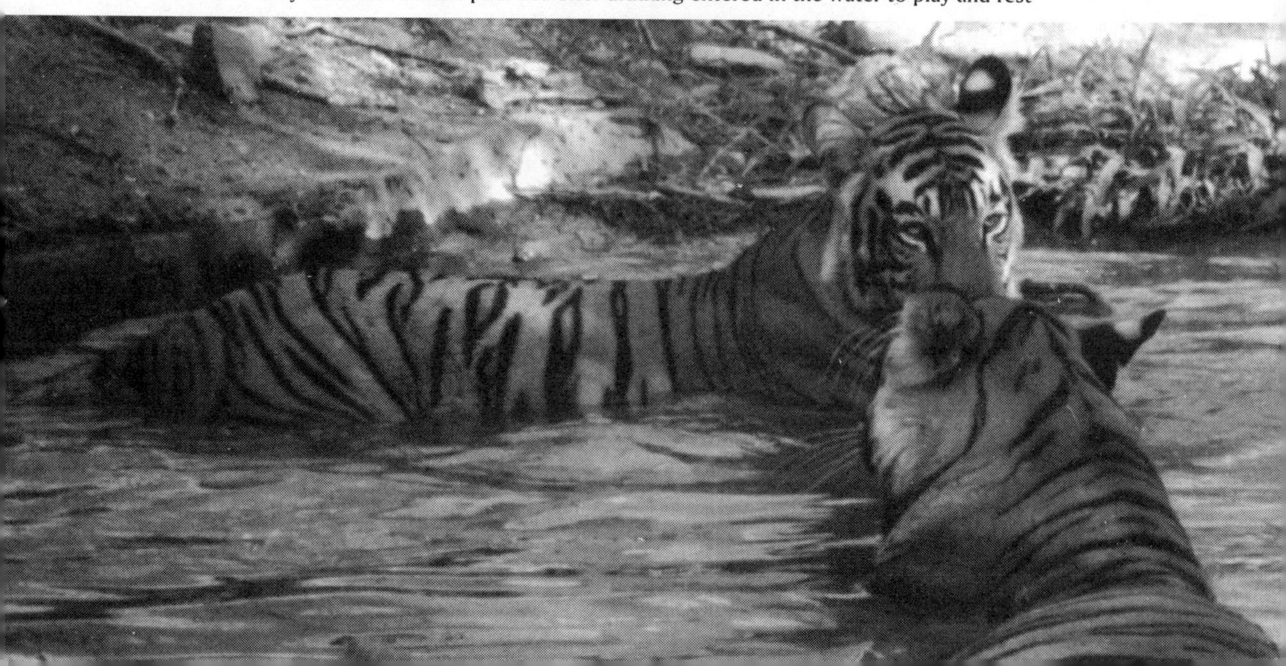

The big cat looked seemingly worried; I watched it carefully out of the corner of my eyes. It was a fascinating sight to see as how he slowly raised his massive head above the maze that was roughly three to four feet high, gazed steadily at us and then lowered its head and calmly shifted its position a few yards, and then again gazed to take a fresh appraisal of our position. In the meantime our party had also reached the parapet of the plot, where we stood watching him with great interest. Our eyes gazed into each other for a few minutes but he did not give us any impression that he meant to create problem. The large head suddenly backed into the crop and as the tiger turned I could faintly distinguish the outline of its body before it disappeared for the good. No doubt we had not provoked him and he too had allowed us to depart in peace.

Paradoxically, in this area I encountered some of the flabbiest tigers I have ever seen. Recently there was an outbreak of foot and mouth disease and many cattle that had died of this epidemic were thrown away near a pond where a tigress had come to enjoy the bonanza and stayed. One day late in the afternoon, a forest ranger took me to the place and tracked down the young tigress. He appeared very much happy when he found the beast was just sitting in the open besides a half eaten body of a cow and sunning herself in the evening light. She was seemingly overfed, lacking exercise and very obese. Perhaps she was also pregnant. She appeared quite unperturbed by our presence and looked at us quite unconcernedly when the ranger lauded his special words of praise for her. "This tigress lives on dead cattle, and she never hunts. She is very docile, like a household pet. She never reacts aggressively."

A considerable number of bones lay scattered around the place. They were certainly not of kills but were of animals that had naturally died and were subsequently consumed by her. It is said that so long as the tiger's meals are assured it gives no thought for the morrow. Since laziness is their tendency, they have no objection to an existence which requires no struggle. The ranger called her *Ghar Ki Billi*, meaning thereby a 'house cat'; as I watched her richly colored frame gleaming golden in the light of the setting sun, her eyes blazed back the last afterglow of the day. A single vulture glided silently down and landed near her. For minutes it stared at the tigress but there was no reaction. She was too full of food and too content to bother about a clumsy bird. Minutes later the sun set, the cicadas began to sing and the magic was extinguished.

In the light of a splendid full moon, the forester and I travelled back to the camp, we agreed that well-fed tigers are perfectly tranquil, but one should not to be carried away by their gesture of contentment, which is often temporary. Predators only need intense hunger to return to their radical instincts. This tigress was docile because she was getting food without effort. She had become addicted to cattle and did not contemplate looking for a fresh victim. But when her reserves would get exhausted, she would deliberately go after the cattle and what would happen then was an incommodious question.

(II)

The village of Banveerpura lies in a semi forested area. It is a picturesque country with miles of green paddy fields and thatched huts. This cluster of a hundred hutments intrudes into a small chunk of forest, practically cutting the southern edge of this tiger habitat between grasslands and forest. The population of the village is nearly a thousand and the people are poor. There is no hospital nearby and no electricity either and the villagers are almost entirely devoted to grazing big herds of cattle. Each year a modest number of livestock is invariably killed by the tigers and the leopards in this area.

My next visit to this village was in March. On one morning at about 11 a.m., we were tremendously impeded by a very high and continuous wind. It took us two hours by Jeep to reach our third camp against the current. The wind is well known in March, and goes by the name of *arahiya –wali* which means that it lasts for two and a half days. When we got the camp, we were perplexed by the constant flow of the people, past our camp towards a place called Sarkanda Beghar. They would not stop to tell us anything, but were evidently in great fright. We went out to discover as to what the trouble was and learnt that a grazer boy and his younger sister had been killed by a tiger. They were looking after their herd of cattle at the village boundaries, some two hundred meters from the cane fields, where a group of laborers was working. The ground was almost treeless and the duo could have a clear vision of the open pasture and their browsing cows.

It was this time when a tiger disturbed by the labour gangs moved out of the cane crops and went towards the cattle, completely unperceived and unseen by anyone. Later, investigations revealed that he sat in a little ravine and lurked in ambush. Unfortunately, the boy came near the place and sat on a parapet. The tiger charged at the boy and knocked him down with a powerful blow of his forepaw and caught hold of him. This caused commotion amongst the cattle and they ran haywire. A wild stampede of cattle with tails in the air attracted the attention of farmers. They rapidly located the tiger, which left the boy forthwith and dashed back into another cane retreat. The men gathered around the boy who was so terribly lacerated as to be beyond the reach of human aid. He had sustained deep canine injuries on the rear skull and nape. The rescuers took away the dazed little girl and dressed the boy's wounds. He succumbed to his injuries four days later.

There were many obnoxious but nevertheless inoffensive tigers around that had been destructive to cattle but harmless to their attendants. But this time, it was the other way round — the cattle were safe whilst the herdsmen were in danger. This tiger had been operating confidently for nearly two months and had attacked more than a dozen herdsmen, caught five of them, killed two of them and ate two of them partially. He had stayed by the last herdsman's body for over an hour, initially balking at the carcass, till hunger won and he ate a small part of the thighs.

All the attacks were made in daylight between 6 a.m. and 11 a.m. and in every case the victim was essentially alone. Some old hunters of village anticipated that the tiger was wounded and probably had a lead ball in his right foreleg. Nature had healed the bone but the limb had become shortened and twisted and he could no longer stalk his prey silently and effectively. His approach was noisy and method of attack was clumsy and even his ability to hold the prey was greatly hampered by his deformed limb. And it was not surprising if they often escaped.

The little experience I had of this tiger does not qualify me to say much about him but a fact that he was a two year old juvenile, who had perchance separated from his mother a little before time and launched on the critical process of independent living. During this phase of life the cubs grow somewhat larger and are relatively safe from threats posed by adverse climatic factors and predation but as their increased nutritional requirement makes starvation a scary possibility, it is also a high risk period in their life. This instigates them for additional hunting and they start chasing every sort of prey, even potentially dangerous ones which only a skilled male tiger would be capable of handling. Errors of judgment while hunting dangerous quarry are more likely to result in injury. The injury makes them incapable of any further hunting and thus nearly fifty percent juveniles perish, dying from starvation and suppurating wounds.

Apparently nervous of tackling full grown animals, he never made attempts on larger cattle. This made me believe that while on an early expedition of his own, he must have had a nasty experience in cattle hunting, which had dampened for good his courage for any such endeavor. The disability to hunt finally made this tiger emaciated and faced with starvation. Some villagers claimed that he was seen catching rats in a bamboo clump and even they escaped him. Perhaps his growing dependence on unnatural prey species also held some biological explanation for his attacks on humans. He grew weak and thin. One day a marriage party going on a tractor trolley happened to see him crossing the path and a self-styled sport killer let fly his gun. The L.G. pellets entered the right shoulder obliquely, seriously injuring the right flank. He leaped, clawing the air and growling viciously and then disappeared from the sight instantly in a sugar field. Next day the locals rigorously combed the area for a couple of days but the tiger was never traced again. It could not be ascertained whether he recovered from the effects of the shot or died.

In a hamlet called Damkuha, I met a grazer Bacchu Lal, his only tiger experience in life was one of the most unaccountable accidents of the Tarai. The animal had first growled at him ostensibly to keep him away from the place, and then coming out of the cane, gave him a bite on his posterior and went back into the clump. The only possible explanation for this was that the tiger, a sub adult cub was sitting with his kill and when Bacchu Lal had ignored its deep throated warning; he had later come out and bitten him. I have twice seen tigers bite at the rears of jackals to chase them away from their kills. I have begun to believe that this trick is tried against all interceptors, and sometimes even man is not excluded.

The philosophy with which the Tarai villagers take a tiger's presence near their home is interesting. At one village people were imperviously protecting and supporting themselves with magic and charms. Once I heard a tiger roaring restlessly during the daylight. And I was seriously told that the village priest had sewn the tiger's mouth with magic and the tiger could neither kill nor eat anything now and so he went about complaining because he was hungry.

In another village, I asked a group of people what they thought had caused the problem of man-killing tigers. They looked about thoughtfully for a while and then answered "Sahib it is a payback for our sins." They seemed to see a link between cosmology and governance. When I asked them what one should do to prevent such disaster, they said the government must dart such tigers with tranquillizing gun and put them into the zoos. I was flabbergasted, while one answer proceeded on the religious plane the other was based on the scientific reasoning, pragmatically instrumental. I then realized that the Indian mind does not work in consonance with the standard belief of science being opposed to religion, or science against superstition. It combines them in an intricate web of answers where categories mix to provide more complex messages.

Despite the presence of human densities, pressure of poaching, tree felling and cultivation, this open country still works as a wonderful passage for the tiger. The great feature of this land, which I watched with never failing interest, was the abundance of game animals. Both the prey and the predator species criss-cross the bucolic terrain to reach the forest blocks on either side. They travel through sugar corridors, instinctively sentient, that the jungle is there at the other end. I remember spotting the splendid horns of occasional chital or swamp deer, showing now and then above the cane plantations.

At the time I was there, the last surviving expanses of huge pastoral lands that formed principal grazing grounds for the immense herds of cattle owned by the villagers also served as potential coverts for a good stuff of wildlife. I myself saw wild boars, black buck, hog deer and *Nilgai* grazing peacefully within a few hundred yards of the railway line. I was lucky enough to get some fine views of leopards, pythons, porcupines, two small migrating herds of wild elephants, several big troops of langur monkeys and a host of birds too numerous to name, in these expanses. Having observed the phenomenon for a month, I was dismayed at the volume of wildlife that crossed the tract. It was the early eighties, conservation polices were being shaped and framed and Ranjit was then thinking far ahead of connecting the separated landscapes with a corridor. Such corridors widening up to about three kilometers are really life lines, for they help wildlife populations to recover not only from the attention of poachers but from disease as well.

It was this thought that later developed into a proposal and which laid down the foundation of The Tarai Arc project.

I also made a suggestion that a permanent game scout camp should be established in this area to prevent the poaching of migratory wildlife.

(Footnote - *The constitution of the Tarai Arc by WWF India has now been fully designed as another positive effort. The 11 protected areas within the Tarai Arc are not individually capable of supporting a viable population of tigers but connecting corridors could ensure their long term survival. The Tarai Arc Landscape includes the Parsa Wildlife Reserve, Bardia National Park, Royal Chitwan, and Shukla Phanta Wildlife reserve in South Nepal while Valmik Nagar Sanctuary, Sohalwa Wildlife Sanctuary, Katraniaghat Sanctuary, Dudhwa National Park, Kishanpur Tiger Reserve, Corbett National Park and Rajaji National Park, abutting the northern boundary qualify from India. The reconnection of disjointed protected areas into a single contiguous landscape will allow tigers and prey species to migrate greater distances, decrease inbreeding and increase chances of long term survival. But the process is not easy as it involves taking communities into confidence and using a mix of community forestry and revenue sharing to ensure the support and protection of these corridors.)*

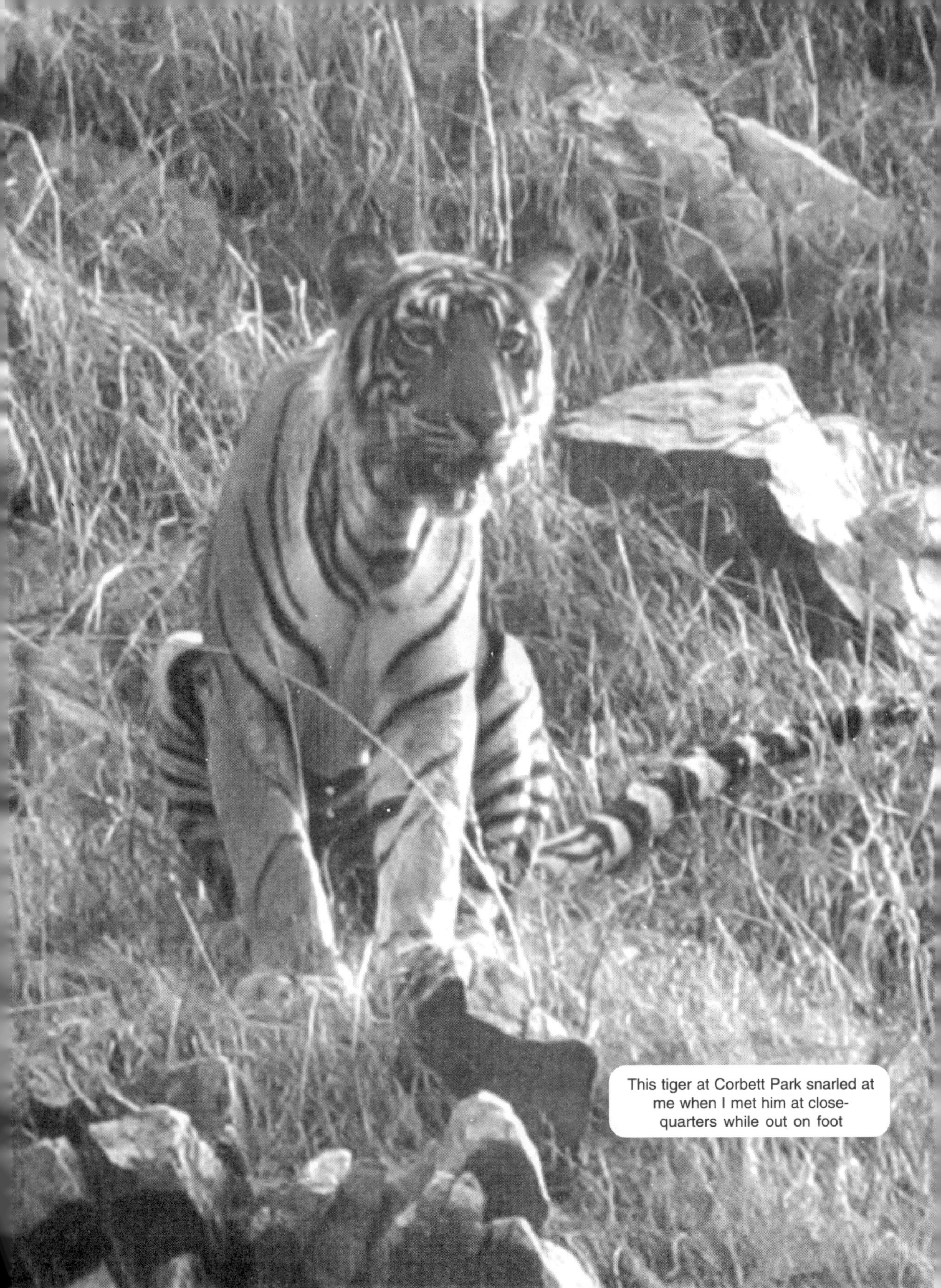

This tiger at Corbett Park snarled at me when I met him at close-quarters while out on foot

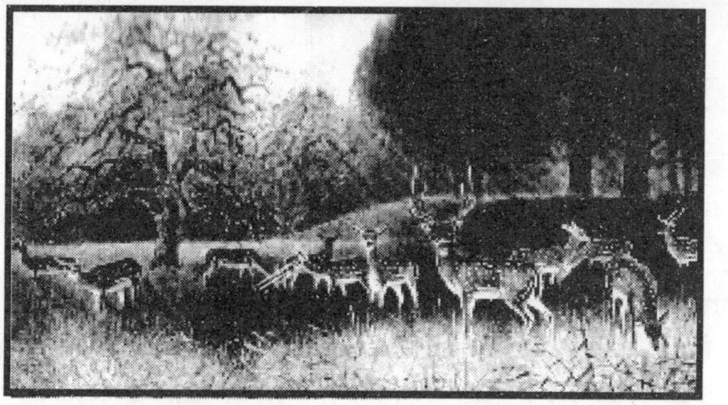

9

Shifting Paradigms: Why Wilderness

The survival of the fittest is the ageless law of nature, but the fittest are rarely the strong. The fittest are those endowed with the qualifications for adaptation, the ability to accept the inevitable and conform to the unavoidable, to harmonize with existing or changing conditions.

- Richard Dawkins

The existence of tigers in sugar crops was surely the most stupendous of all the dramas in the Tarai. The fact was that these animals did not seem to be distributed in space only but also in time. Tigers were breeding excessively, their number increasing at a biologically unrealistic rate. This overflow had led to the present condition where still more animals were shifting into sugar farms to find slots as resident animals.

In the last ten years, I had painstakingly observed this unfolding of events and gradually tried to theorize the existence of cane tigers. In spite of the imperfect state of my field knowledge, I had generated baseline data to make a few generalizations about the bio-ecological character of the entire cane tiger population. This quantitative data was free of the subjective impressions documented in early natural history. In doing so, I was aware that modern wildlife science is fundamentally different from the sporting records of past generations, and it needed explanation with extreme care, in the backdrop of some unfathomable dimension to this tiger. My investigations indicated that sugar farms were sensitive to wildlife needs and the tigers had adapted them for selective reasons which were complex and made an odd mixture of things but were common to all areas of the Tarai.

They are briefly stated as follows:-

1. Immensity and physiognomy of sugar plantations

The Tarai belt in Uttar Pradesh is some 500 kilometers long and about 6 to 20 kilometers in width (save for Dudhwa where the width crosses over some 40 kilometers of land span) whereas its adjacent sugarcane plantations extend by larger dimensions. By far, they are the largest single crop fields that run along the jungle trails on the Indo-Nepalese border. The physiognomy of the crop matches with the exact characteristics of *narkul* or reed grass habitat where tall stems of sugar provide an excellent cover for tigers to stretch out and relax. The thick growth of vegetation at all levels, and the flowering fronds at the top of the ten foot high crops prevent the direct penetration of sunlight within its environment. Thus, the cool and damp interior gratifies their extra needs of thermo-regulations.

2. The availability of free surface water

Tigers simply cannot live in arid environments where lions and leopards thrive. The availability of free surface water to drink regularly appears to be crucial. Sugarcane fields are profusely irrigated, so they remain green and there isn't much loss of weight and juice. Tolerance to water-logging and moisture deficit are the chief characteristic of new varieties of sugarcane. The dampness of the soil and the thin film of water that floats over it make it an ideal home for a tiger.

3. Congenial light conditions

Tiger is a crepuscular (active in half-light) and equally nocturnal animal (active in pitch darkness) with the retina of its eyes having an abundance of receptor cells known as 'Rods'. These cells are sensitive to low light levels, which enhance its ability to see even in pitch darkness. A hazy twilight that permeates the inner recess of the crop has an extremely soothing effect on nocturnal animals. It works as sun-goggles on the eyes of a tiger.

4. Protection from flies

Tigers are very intolerant to any touch on the ear and they being full of wax attract flies. In addition, being carnivores, the tigers' face, nails and body have small particles of flesh adhered to it. This constantly attracts flies and they hover around its forequarters and nostrils. The thickness of the crop deters the repetitive circling movement of all kinds of flies, especially the 'scarlet dragonflies', mango flies, blowflies and blue–bottle flies, they do not enter the crop due to bad light conditions; this keeps the animal free from the pest.

5. A perfect camouflage

The tigers are better camouflaged in sugarcanes than anywhere else. A motionless tiger standing in tall sugarcane almost dissolves from view, and the pattern of its stripes provides it with a surprisingly perfect camouflage; such camouflage is an essential element in the tiger's ability to pursue its prey unseen.

6. Advantage of stalking cover

Tigers are large, solitary, 'stalk and ambush' predators. All the intelligence they require is to be able to kill a game. The dense sugar landscape favors stalking predators rather than coursing ones. Tigers are at a constant advantage in a cover that enables them to get close to their circumspect prey.

7. Benefit of ample prey base

Sugar farms are compatible to the needs of wildlife and serve as a perfect combination of prey and cover for a tiger. Wheat, pulses, paddy and *chana* (gram) etc. grow simultaneously with the cane crops. Herbivores of all kinds are attracted by this staple food. Wild boars, porcupines, *chital*, hogdeer and swamp deer visit these fields and tigers having no option but to follow their prey wherever it may lead them, arrive in cane fields.

Besides livestock like cows, buffalos, horses, donkeys, goats and pigs roam about the vista. These animals comprising the routine prey list of the tiger are also slain by him with little effort in comparison to what they put up in the jungle. Besides, its propensity to scavenging also ensures its survival.

8. Healthy eco-system

Adding an additional input of solar energy, the sugarcanes are surely healthy eco-systems. It is wrong to assume that the food chain it sustains is inferior to the food chain of jungle animals. Sugarcane fields are more exposed to sun than canopy jungles where electromagnetic energy flows through light and heat and travels in the form of radiation, which the earth receives in enhanced quantum than jungles. Plants convert this electromagnetic energy into chemical energy and the flow of its extra dose in normal diet makes the ungulates of the open plains, such as *Nilgai* and blackbucks much more prolific breeders than jungle dwellers.

The health and productivity of tigers living in sugarcane demonstrates how a small increase of the incident solar irradiation on the biosphere can lead to enormous beneficial increase in the energy available in the food chain. Perhaps because of this reason the reproductive dynamics in farm tigers is much more prolific in comparison to jungle tigers.

9. Synchronous breeding

In the sugarcane plantations, tigers are able to communicate effectively, maintain social contacts and breed in a sustained manner. Presumably, the females easily come in estrus and breeding activity of young tigers is more pronounced as their stronger counterparts, the trouncing big daddy's are in the jungles. With strong healthier genes of young tigers; the chances of baby boom as well as of their survival to maturity are relatively high.

10. Stable ranges of females

In many Tarai districts, tigers feel as much at home in the sugarcanes as they are in the jungle. For here the immense terrain is interspersed with sizeable bogs and chunks of local forests and this factor appears to favor their survival. Tigresses are more stable in range occupations than tigers. Once they acquire the aforesaid ranges and start delivering cubs, they can use the particular centre for relatively long periods and may stay for several seasons. The occupation of a familiar locale by the female is liable to improve her chances of successful rearing of the young to an age when they are able to fend for themselves. This improves her chances of overstaying in the cane zone and in due course that is sure to generate a cohort of real sugarcane tigers.

11. Courting tigresses draw males from the jungles

It is contended that while females compete for land, suitable habitat, containing sufficient prey and other resources—in order to maintain themselves and to raise their offspring successfully, male tigers compete for females. The presence of cub rearing females draws male tigers from the jungles and often also accelerates the process of their adoption to canes.

12. Beneficial for parturient tigresses

In the Tarai, tiger mating becomes more pronounced after the rains and a majority of young ones are born in November or December. The normal period of gestation for a tigress is 103 to 110 days. As the parturition date approaches, the movement and the range of a tigress becomes restricted. "A long period of gestation with large fetus makes it difficult for mothers to secure food" as Brander comments, "and the danger of accidents and miscarriages would be great." Such parturient tigress, more pre-occupied with finding a safe home, readily takes to sugarcane and spends most of the time in the vicinity of the den, familiarizes herself with the movement of prey and water supply. Hunting upon a complex community of ungulate prey, they spend their last weeks of pregnancy there.

13. Safe nursery for the cubs

To give birth to young ones a tigress naturally searches for a dense patch of cover and the nursery should always be well concealed and have dark interiors. The spot should also be located in a position from where it can be readily defended. These preconditions are instinctively sought by the mother tigress, for tiger cubs are born blind and helpless. They are highly vulnerable to predation by scavengers. The hypothesis of dense foliage states that predation risk decreases with increase in the density of vegetation because greater foliage density inhibits transmission of visual, chemical, or auditory cues by cubs.

Canes serve as safe nurseries. From August to February cane crops are at their best and provide the mother with a perfect hideout to breed and the litter is relatively safe from the second and third order predators.

14. Availability of easy food for the nursing tigresses

During litter the tigresses are most localized. As they have to nurse and guard their cubs, their movements become restricted and their home range also shrinks to a fraction of its usual size, often to a minimum of 4 sq. km. and easy availability of prey becomes an important factor for a cub-rearing mother. This is a time of great risk for the nascent cubs. Their eyes open one to two weeks later but clear vision comes only after a month. The newly born demand constant attention from their mother and her body odor plays an essential role in this. For the first few days, she helps them to find her teats to provide them with vital nourishment.

The tigress is alone, without a mate to help her. While she is away hunting, the cubs may be found by random food searchers like jackals and foxes, and killed by them. The mother has to remain with them constantly. She can't afford to be away in search of food. In the event of disturbance she keeps moving them into new hideouts by carrying them in her mouth.

The focal mortality factor of cubs in the wild is starvation caused by the mother's failure to hunt sufficient prey, at regular intervals. Such times are tough for a tigress in the jungle. But in the cane fields big cats have the attraction of the feral cattle as

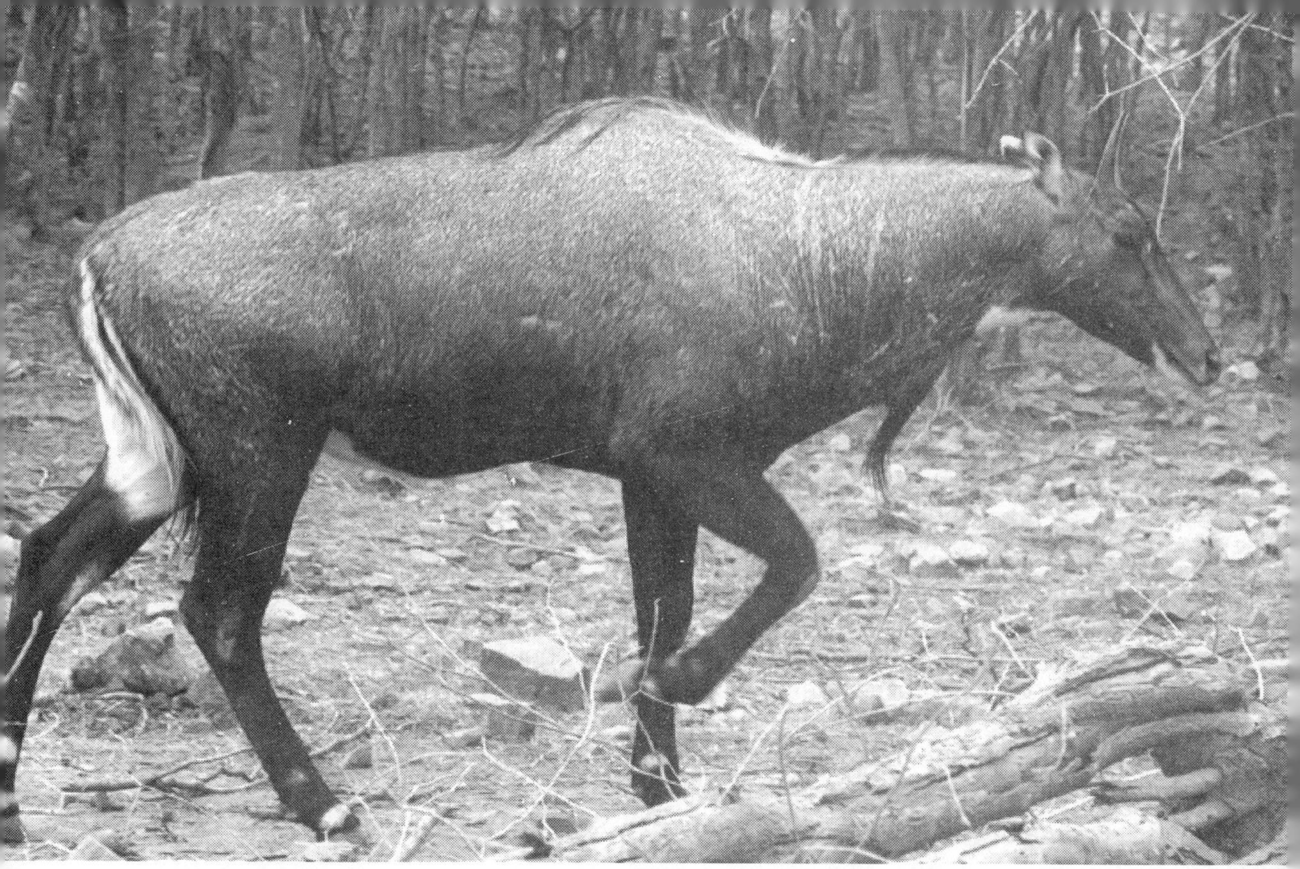

Nilgai (bluebull) is a strong and large antelope. Their nuisance has made tigers a welcome entrant to the farm lands

prey. Human livestock also provides an answer in emergencies.

15. Retreat for the sub-adult tigers

Sub-adult tigers steadily leave the area where they are born and raised. The reason for this deliberate dispersal is increased intolerance towards them by the resident adults. The father stops tolerating the actions of the young male and the mother acts the same way towards her female offspring. As a result, a segment of sub-adult population usually builds up on the periphery of prime jungle. Through con-specific competition, this segment is continuously enlarged as cubs grow up and begin an independent life. These emigrants to buffer zones later infiltrate into sugar-farms.

16. Dramatic carrying capacity

I can vouch for the fact that when human intrusions in forests have dramatically lowered their wildlife carrying capacity and water logging impacts have turned extensive primary Tarai forests into poor habitats of secondary forests, seasonal refuges of large sugarcane farms that are of a long term nature, offer a much better and a wholesome breeding landscape for wildlife. For example, the annual migration of hundreds of swamp deer of Sathiana-Dudhwa, into adjacent sugar fields of Ghola village to deliver their fawns, is a notable feature.

17. Crops as a biological corridor

The Project Tiger proposals to create corridors between forest blocks involve major decisions like land purchase, acquisition, resettling people and elimination of developmental programs, thus it is time taking and yet awaited. However, in the intervening time sugar crops continue to serve as temporary corridors for tigers to move from one place to another, whereas sizeable breaks in forest continuity caused by heavily populated human settlements have cut off the connectivity between tiger populations. For instance, there is a distance of 20 to 30 kilometers between Katarnia Ghat and Bilrayan, and between South and North Kheri forest divisions respectively but they get connected through uninterrupted cane corridors during the season.

18. Landscape connectivity promotes breeding

The extensive stretches of dense crops enhance the landscape connectivity and scope for tiger movements. This feature essentially improves the interlinking of populations and the status of sporadic meta-populations of the species that are effectively cut off from the forests and live in isolated spaces. Perhaps under pressure of creating post dispersal ranges, male tigers disperse further than females do. This way, often the unstable population of one or two females, destined to fade away may well resuscitate and breed.

19. Behavioral traits of sugar tigers

A. These tigers normally inhabit sparsely populated farmlands and avoid moving near villages.

B. Tiger activity is governed by the need to avoid human activity. In disturbed area with high frequency of human intrusions, they tend to become entirely nocturnal and act diurnal when frequenting undisturbed farm lands.

C. Due to the pressure of human activities in sugar farms, the naturally diurnal wildlife such as hog deer, *chital* and wild boar also become nocturnal. If tigers are predominantly preying upon wildlife they prefer nocturnal activities and if on domestic livestock, they tend to become more diurnal.

20. Peculiar features of behavior

A. Tigers have evolved as killers of large prey in a closed habitat where ambushing and hamstringing are preliminary methods of subduing a prey. In sugar habitat tigers seem more natural with the hamstringing method of pulling down prey. Out of 32 ungulate kills I had so far discovered inside the sugarcane fields, almost all of them whether big or modest had been caught from behind or hamstrung.

It seems that the denser crops often make it difficult for a tiger to target the animal for a frontal attack and it finds easier to seize the prey from behind by grabbing its hind leg. During winters, the tiger kills discovered in sugar fields show a high percentage of hamstringing and then crushing the windpipe, instead of neck breaking. Perhaps in working out a series of permutations in killing a prey, where they have to judge distances accurately and in split seconds, this is a major difference amid the tigers of sugarcane and the jungle. Perhaps canes are more advantageous to the standard style of hunting.

B. The jungle tigers seem to dislike the strong pungent odour of ammoniac gases emanated by excreta of vultures and the kills bleached white by them are usually abandoned. But sugarcane tigers do not appear to have such dislikes. They eat vulture operated kills without a qualm. In nature, scavenging birds are essential creatures to the operation of the tropical grasslands, so my conjecture is that the tigers of sugar grasslands — like lions — have to meet the terms of their functioning too.

C. Besides the soil and grass tigers also relish sugarcane. I could discover this important observation many years later in 1997 when to my astonishment, some villagers from Chaltua informed me that they had noticed a tigress with a pair of cubs eating sugarcane, after she had finished off a wild boar. She pulled out soft stems, and sitting in a squirrel like posture munched them with the support of her forepaws. Presumably, sugarcane juices aid the tiger's digestive system. Frank Simpson, in '*Sport in Eastern Bengal*' (1886) writes, "that they catch fish, turtles, crocodiles, and large lizards. I believe they will occasionally eat sugarcane and maize".

I may add that eating grass is not of any nutritional value. Grass is mainly fiber and is pretty indigestible to cats and also low in nourishment. Carnivores eat grass, maze or soil specifically as an emetic substance -that induces vomiting when administered orally- to discharge the toxic contents of their upset stomach. I do not think that the obligate hyper-carnivores like tigers whose intestines lack the micro flora and bacteria designed to absorb carbohydrates and break high cellulose diet, can ever transform into facultative-carnivores and munch through a quantum produce of sugarcane, such as meso-carnivore or hypo-carnivore like jackals and foxes do in emergencies. But still in view of their diverse diet, this may be an 'out of the ordinary reason' that prompts the tiger's adaptation to farmlands.

Joseph G. Brand of the Monell Chemical Senses Center in Philadelphia, believes that though cats have no ability to taste sweet as they harbor a genetic mutation that renders the sugar detectors on their taste buds inoperative but still they need some sugar, in form of glucose, to transport cellular energy. It seems that such exceedingly subtle adaptations are not only temporarily revitalizing to a tiger in sugarcane areas but are more practical in their final consummation.

D. Jungle tigers are known to discard innards of prey and eat solid meat from rump and thigh first but I have noted in two kills, made by sugar tigers, one of a feral cow and the other of a Nilgai bull that when prey was killed and ingested, the first bit of the carcass eaten was the intestine. The explanation I can give for this is that the intestines contain lots of nutrients needed for good health and some tigers who value such parts do go for it.

It may be also partially true for grass. Although, mainly an indigestible fiber lacking almost everything the cat needs in its diet, grass does have a lot of moisture, some trace minerals and the vitamins A and D and folic acid, a required nutrient. Grass also contains chlorophyll, which before the discovery of antibiotics, was a remedy for pain, infection, ulcers, skin diseases, and anemia. Tigers, like most other animals, are very skilled in controlling their needs for particular nutrients and finding healthy diet supplements, some of which can come from grass.

21. General features

A. The area of sugarcane tiger roughly deals with territory of nine contiguous districts of Terai, namely, Nainital Plains, Udhamsingh Nagar, Pilibhit, Kheri, Shajahanpur, Bahraich, Gonda, Basti and Balrampur. The secondary data provided by the forest department showed the distribution of livestock attack sites. The incidents were clearly restricted to within 10-15 miles of the nearest jungle and not spread all across the area. The households sampled on this basis did not report any depredation by tigers from further off lands. This helped me to conclude that the phenomenon starts from the periphery of the jungle and gradually extends southwards, maximum up to a width of 10-15 miles in agricultural land. The extension or contraction of area depends on the number of tigers inhabiting different pockets, which involuntarily regulate their space requirements according to seasonal needs.

This also indicated that any beast floating down further south could be treated as having strayed. Such floaters transgress their eco-system, cross unacceptable terrain, and emerge in the most unanticipated places.

B. Besides hunting, the movements of tigers are intensely linked to fraternizing with their own kind. The range expansion of a tiger, as to how far a tiger has to move in sugarcane in search of a prey or to avoid inter or intra-species tensions and then get back into his natal range, depends on the constraints of ecological factors and also the maintenance of chemical communication with neighborhood tigers, especially females. A tiger advancing in a sugar zone might continue to exploit the rich prey base of domestic livestock, but a complete breakdown of the social communication network with other tigers is a critical determinant in the straying of lonely tigers.

C. Influx of dispersing animals from jungle into population and vice-versa -- the influx of animals retreating from it -- is the factor that affects the size and dynamics of sugar tiger population.

D. The invasive alien species of plants have deteriorated the ecosystem of Tarai forests, posing a threat to its biodiversity. Inedible vegetation like Lantana, Congress grass (*Parthenium*), Carrot grass, *Saccharum munjha*, Ban Maura, Castor and Water Hyacinth have drastically exacerbated the forest. The aromatic oils and exudates of leaves and roots have an anti-biotic effect on natural edible species. It retards their growth, suffocates and prevents their seedlings from germination and finally eradicates them from the area. Hence herbivores run out to agricultural fields and tigers follow them, accelerating the progression of the sugarcane tiger phenomena.

E. The northern area of the Tarai forests has now ceased to be a prime habitat of tigers because of unbridled deforestation in Nepal and subsequent human pressure on the Indian side. Their illegal intrusion, unsustainable collection of fuel wood and cattle grazing has laid waste huge tracts of forests, resulting in the shift of major tiger populations towards the south, which unremittingly nourishes the sugarcane tiger population.

F. Sugar harvesting does not seem to produce an acute forbidding impact on tigers. The crop is harvested smoothly without causing much damage to wildlife, save partial poaching, whereas in the jungles the erosions of grasslands, through fire or inundations are prone to be catastrophic; resulting in colossal loss of bird eggs and the near wipe-out of reptilian life. (For example when Kaziranga grasslands are annually battered by excessive flooding, a great number of ungulates drown and die, including rhino calves and tiger cubs.) But no such big toll of life is sacrificed in erosion of sugar habitat; harvesting is the mildest method of habitat erosion which the tigers and their prey easily endure.

G. Sugar-fields should not be confused as a strictly seasonal habitat for tigers. Even after harvesting, the loss of habitat is not of permanent nature. It is a temporary phase of three months, in which rhizomes speedily regenerate and pave the way for the tigers to come back, demonstrating more or less the durable nature of the crop which offers all the four basic habitat components for healthy communities — food, water, shelter and space.

H. The duel characteristics of sugar crop -- cool in summers and warm in winters -- support tigers well and properly. Frost is created at about zero degree temperature. During the frost season, the non-irrigated dry patches of sugar crops become ideal spots for tigers. The essential soil heat in form of radiation is constantly emitted. It is high in the night and low during the day. The canopy of frond is too heavy and continuous; it does not let the heat escape, which facilitates the creation of a green house like effect. During the sharp bouts of frost towards January tigers live here, (as prior to harvesting irrigation is discontinued) and these develop into warm spots.

I. The expanse of tall crops does help the tiger to inhabit areas in numbers that is not possible in the jungle and would not have been possible earlier when the area was jungle.

J. And finally tigers, like other cats, are quick learners through observations. They exhibit defense and caution against wandering bands of people that share their range. They show distrust to human taint and rely more on their keen vision to preserve themselves from dangerous proximity of human enemies. Thus they thrive better in the country where the lives of people and wildlife are intertwined with mutual respect and tolerance. (These traits are indeed select for fitness to survive in a given environment. Survival of the fittest is often misinterpreted to mean survival of the most aggressive. Fitness is a much broader term.)

K. Even in the dry period, when the fields are an empty waste of charred and smoldering desolation, the tiger's presence in them had been proved. For example in the summers of 1979, the officially documented fifteen attacks on humans were mostly from these tigers. The partially eaten human bodies, which were recovered from Mohamdi and Mailani area of Kheri in the months of March, April and May and June, proved the presence of sugar tigers. The latest attack in this series had come in July when a youth from Ayodhya village in Mohamdi was attacked about eight miles away from the forest area.

L. Repeated surveys have revealed one more key factor for the presence of tigers in sugar crops. Human interference and grazing by cattle have degraded many areas on the outskirts of reserved forests in the Tarai. The herdsmen with their hundreds of cattle, cross the threshold of forest, going three to four miles inside in search of fodder, with the result peripheral tiger population prefers to move out into sugarcane plantations, using it as a day-time lair, to lie down and snooze than to face constant disturbance in the jungle.

In this case, even the presence of huge buffer prey population entering the jungle is not an inducement enough to hold them inside and not to transgress the imposed barrier of their natural home, where they are presumably safer.

M. It is argued that sugarcane plantation is not a pleasant habitat. The edges of saccharum have silica deposits (silicon-dioxide, used in production of glass) which makes full-blown sugar leaves unpalatable. In some varieties of cane,

This young powerful male is ready to take over a prime range

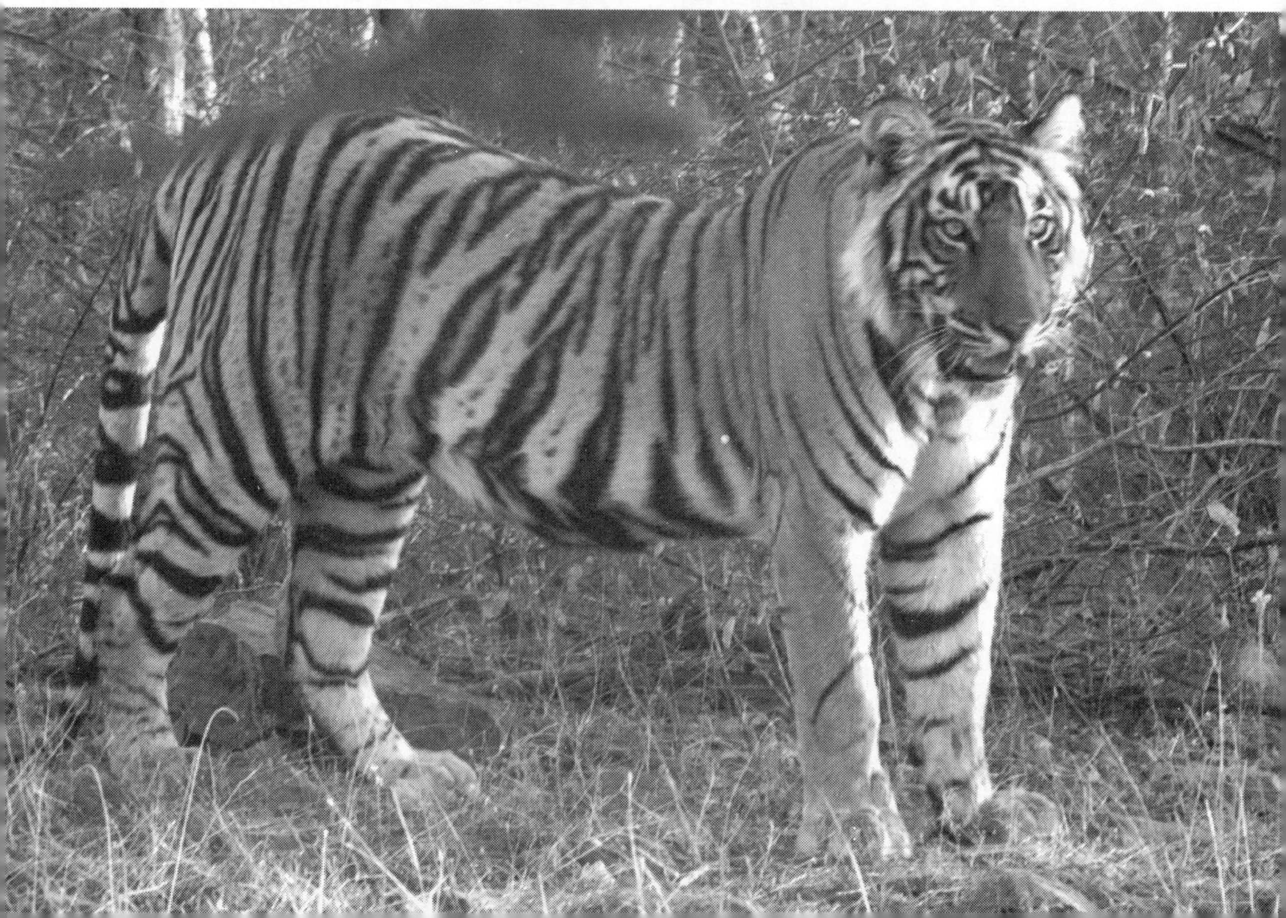

leaves tend to become crudely rough and knife-edged and worry the cat by disrupting its movements. Yet, as tigers take to this habitat, it is possible that the gradual physiological adaptation to undulating fronds of sugar cane creates conditions which make a tiger's tactile adjustments with plant communities almost effortless.

N. Sugarcane plantations are an important land use in the Tarai and are a food resource for many omnivores but this landscape is of low conservation value, for it does not fit into the way ecosystems are valued and governed. Moreover in agricultural landscapes no conservation strategies can be applied to protect the habitat loss for the wildlife that takes place at harvesting and becomes dangerous for these animals including exposures to roads and vehicles and exposure to poisons such as rodenticide, but a modicum of protection given to waste lands, patches and expanses of local unprotected forest, where various animal groups migrate during desiccated period is sufficient to make cane tiger survive. These forests outside the proteted area network fall under the legal jurisdiction of Gram-Sabhas and play a critical role in conservation of farmland wildlife by providing important additional habitat for animal and plant species.

Now the whole inexplicable tangle seemed to have straightened out before me. Although a further knowledge of facts was necessary before I could venture to give a full and final opinion on the subject but nevertheless these were the aces up my sleeve, the subtle stepping stones on which I hoped to get across to solid solutions. The pursuit of tiger, conducted on such lines, will afford ample scope for breaking new ground regarding their supplementary habits and the character in sugarcane fields, where they lived on a completely different scale from jungle tigers. I wondered as I always did, as how such a simple thing -so strikingly obvious- had not been obvious to foresters in the past. Obviously one needs to be more attentive than natural to notice such facts?

The only obstacle in the growth of this tiger was the tremendous anthropogenic pressure they endured. The involvement of this factor in petite percentage might serve as a component, adding to the improvement of ecology but the increasing percentage essentially creates a diametrically opposite effect and perpetrates crisis. This absurd and self-contradictory juggernaut interestingly happens to be a key factor in determining the etiology of a tiger's adaptation to the farm lands. Tigers living here are forced to live in an area surrounded by humans because the sugar-crops are an entirely man-made environ planted, watered and harvested by none else than the human agency, yet paving the way for tigers to walk in. Thus, human agency is a mandatory component of this feature, which maintains essential ecological processes and life support systems, to ensure the sustainable utilization of species and ecosystem.

It is my gut feeling that when the habitats supporting larger breeding populations have already shrunk to a minuscule of about one percent of their former range and are also biotically messed up, then in order to survive, the species has to harden against anthropogenic pressures or eventually lose the battle. Thus, many a tiger seemed most responsive to change that determines the qualifications of fortitude at much stronger levels than the jungle tigers because behavioral adaptation is a top quality trait which can happen far more quickly. The more intelligent the animal, the faster it can learn to make behavioral changes in order to survive.

The species with useful adaptations to the environment are more likely to survive and produce progeny than those with less useful adaptations, thereby increasing the frequency with which useful adaptations occur over the generations. Along this line of reasoning, sugar tigers are definitely more equipped to absorb multiple pressures. The concept should not be confused with rhetorical tautology of survival of those who are better equipped for surviving; but it also contains an independent criterion of fitness for a segment of species to turn into a putative creed.

However, it is not as if the tigers' presence in sugar is all plain sailing. It accelerates man-tiger conflict, which goes against the complex rules of survival. In Kheri district alone, records show that between 1978 and 1984, the mortality figures due to man-tiger conflict had rocketed to 1586 domestic animals (not including dogs) and more disastrously, 169 human beings. How much more the figure would have been in this eternal war raged by tigers is anybody's guess. Social mechanisms to address people's grievances were inadequate and almost non-existent in many areas. Thus, many instances would have gone unreported and thus not included in the list. In many cases, the affected local people were not compensated adequately and this had caused such a widespread panic and distress that villagers had lost their confidence in normal living. Over the years, nearly thirty tigers were held responsible for this chaos and all were eventually done away with, either by officials or by natives.

With this train of reasoning in my head, the theory behind the phenomenon had roughly emerged but one part still remained unclear. When the mother tigress brings up her cubs in sugarcane nurseries and as they mature they get to know their home and its laws under the tutelage of their parents, triggering their steady establishment in the land. So the question was – whether indeed just a miniscule part of this population could be acclaimed as a compulsive creed of sugarcane tiger; the hard core dweller of this exclusive habitat. Because when the cubs are almost fully grown and the tigress leaves them to prepare for independence, some individuals are presumably more familiar with the habitat where they are raised and where they feel naturalized, and thus are better able to take on. It was incredible and challenging, yet it was always a possibility; a potential horizon of a ground breaking biological significance. Why should I not test it to the full?

A simplified analogy for *paradigm* is a habit of reasoning on old lines or thinking inside the box that is analogous with normal science. The box encompasses the thinking of normal science and thus the box is analogous with *paradigm.* And on these lines there cannot be the sugarcane tigers. But I was thinking "outside the box", this is what science historian Thomas Kuhn calls revolutionary science. It is usually unsuccessful, and only rarely leads to new paradigms but whenever it is successful it leads to large scale changes in the scientific worldview.

The fact that the tigers were living in the canes for years could be a tentative demonstration of the hypothesis that could help me arrive at a comfortable conclusion. The more I browsed my field notes, the more convinced I became of the challenge to discover such beasts and establish their identity. The beasts were capable of absorbing utmost pressures generated by humans like animal husbandry, developmental projects, poaching and habitat loss at the same time. It was vague but –man is a creature of reason – to my mind the problem lay with the behavioral adaptation of some animals, which repeatedly made their progeny return to the same environment and place.

An ideal example of this can be found in sea turtles. Of the five species of marine turtles in this region, four nest on Indian beaches. Their real nesting extravaganza takes place in Tamil Nadu and Orissa where over 200,000 Olive Ridley turtles come to nest for a week between February and March. Humans, dogs, birds, jackals and monitor lizards know when the laying season starts and where the eggs will be laid. Despite the colossal destruction of eggs and their hunting, turtles always return to the same beaches. In the way, they pass by several uninhabited islands, which might serve as safe havens for egg laying and also keep the turtles protected, yet they travel to a disturbed zone. Their problem is their behavioral adaptation for the place and they can't get rid of it.

During the 80's, a similar situation existed in the western state of Maharashtra, whereas per estimates, around 600 leopards were reported in sugarcane farms alone. They lived there as they found ample food in form of sheep and goats. These farms served a good hiding place for them too and according to forest department if these leopards were displaced and sent back to the forest, a region foreign to them, they panicked and tried to return to the place where they belonged. Was it that they found survival difficult in the forests?

Much later, in 2002, a report of forest department showed that 103 leopards were trapped and released in the forest, most of which later lost their way and strayed into other places. Leopard attacks were often reported around 60-70 km distance of a release site. The repeated return of these leopards not only signified their penchant for the sugar habitat, but it was the problem of behavioral adaptation which despite my point blank assertion made in a WWF seminar at Mumbai, the foresters had failed to understand.

Vague notions soared in my head. I felt that I had not only sneaked into the sugar tiger's dominion but had also attained some understanding of it. Like the vorticist painters of Europe, whose unadulterated futuristic images were conceived on the basis of enduring reason, I too had the *raison d'être* that was to set the direction of my research for years to come. I had to develop my knowledge base. I had to test my theory.

It was an ambitious idea, which might fail easily, but at that time it seemed better than giving up. Perhaps I had reached the next bend of the road.

(II)

I believe that tigers living under stressful conditions have a curious perception of human emotions. The fearful man with his sweat ducts betraying his fear is more likely to invite an attack than the one exuding his normal irrepressible body smell. For the tiger or indeed any killing beast seems to realize at once that the intruder before him is in fact trembling with fear and will make an easy victim.

On an occasion, I too had nearly ended up as a victim myself. On 16 February 1981, not because of fear or foolishness on my part but because of those incidents that crop up in any job and cannot by any means be anticipated, I escaped a pair of tigers, entirely by luck and not by any skill or judgment.

One day, I had gone to conduct a spot investigation into the death of an old tigress. It had apparently died in an inter-species fight; the carcass was mutilated and filled with crawling maggots. The primary autopsy revealed multiple deep puncture wounds in the neck and thoracic cavity that had finally killed her. Two severed claws were also found within her mouth. The nails were wedged deeply in the victim's mouth, including the tongue and the lower jaw, which she had bitten off from the frontal forepaw of the antagonist in her death struggle.

When the foresters had taken the body to the headquarters, Bhai Lal Pasi, the chief of a nearby village invited me for tea with him and we set out to his village on foot. It was a gorgeous winter afternoon and we were walking on a dust road when we looked back and saw two tigers following us at a distance of two hundred yards. We were quite alone, without any weapon and there were no climbable tree within reach. We could not make the mistake of running away for then the tigers would have come after us in a matter of seconds.

We kept our head low and kept walking, quickening our pace, but the tigers also did the same and began gaining on us. Once more when we glanced around they were actually trotting, eyes keen, ears erect and their tails swishing from side to side. But they never uttered a sound, for tigers are one of the most silent predators on this earth. Eventually, when they closed the distance to about thirty yards we could actually hear them breathing, like dogs. Their mouths were partially open and the tip of the tongue moved in and out as they panted. They looked fully-grown to a normal size but were perhaps young and inexperienced as killers; otherwise they should have taken us long ago.

I had not hoped to surprise the tiger duo in this way. I was completely at a loss to ascertain whether they intended to charge us or just wanted to threaten us so that we clear out from their area. By these days, under somewhat peculiar circumstances, the forests of north Kheri were getting infested with man-eating tigers, and rightly so, sixteen operative man-killers had already accounted for several human lives. In such conditions, every tiger that haunted the environs of village communities was a suspect. It occurred to me that here was probably a duo of man-eaters, showing ingenious and courageous discrimination in choosing such a favorable place for their nefarious activities.

However, the point had been reached when we felt they would wait no longer. So, we started yelling for all we were worth. Bhai Lal's nerves were nearly gone and he was shaking with fear when to our intense relief we saw some travelers coming from the opposite direction. They had realized what was happening and they came waving their staves and shouting. The tigers just turned tail and bolted into a bush but continued to growl from there with glaring eyes and a hellish expression on face.

The incident hovered over my mind for many days. It was rare and unusual behaviour on part of tigers; their complete lack of fear was astonishing, for every predator is basically shy of humans since man is not their natural prey. A later analysis showed that this duo was the litter of an aberrant tigress that by some eccentric idiosyncrasy had specialized in removing the occupants of cycle rickshaws. She had inhabited this territory for a good length of time and was also known for her unprovoked demonstration against travelers, till it was netted by a group of *kanjars* (traveling nomadic tribe) and mowed down.

These cubs, obviously born in the sugarcane fields had started the very first day of their lives in the pronounced proximity of man. My observations put the extent of such association as being 30 to 60 per cent of total human sightings by the cubs. The experience gained by this informal association had removed their initial inhibition of man. The familiarization had impelled them to chase us.

Moreover, they were some two years of age. This is the age when predators show a greater interest in prey animals and run after them, as a dog does, rather than stalking them in the true cat fashion.

I am in the habit of reading something before I go to sleep. That night as I lay near the warm blaze of campfire and read Forsyth who hunted in the Central Provinces way back in 1889, I came across a passage recounting the time when tigers were abundant. "At the outset of one's experience of forest life it is impossible to avoid the belief that the tiger of the story is about to show himself at every step one takes in the jungle; and it is not till every effort to meet him has been used in vain that one realizes how very rarely a mere rambler in the jungles comes across a tiger. During ten years of my pretty constant roaming about on foot in the most 'tigerish' localities of Central Provinces, I have only come across a tiger when I was not shooting and only twice more when I was not searching for tigers to shoot. In truth excepting in the very haunts of a known man-eater, there is no danger whatever in traversing any part of jungles of this, or any other part of India."

Ninety years after Forsyth wrote this passage, Tarai, a wild part of India, was witnessing the worst of man-tiger conflict. Never in the annals of wildlife history were so many humans killed by so many tigers in such short a time. The brave old Forsyth must be turning in his grave now. "Had you been there, old hat, you would have revised this statement," I muttered in deride as I closed down the book and settled to sleep.

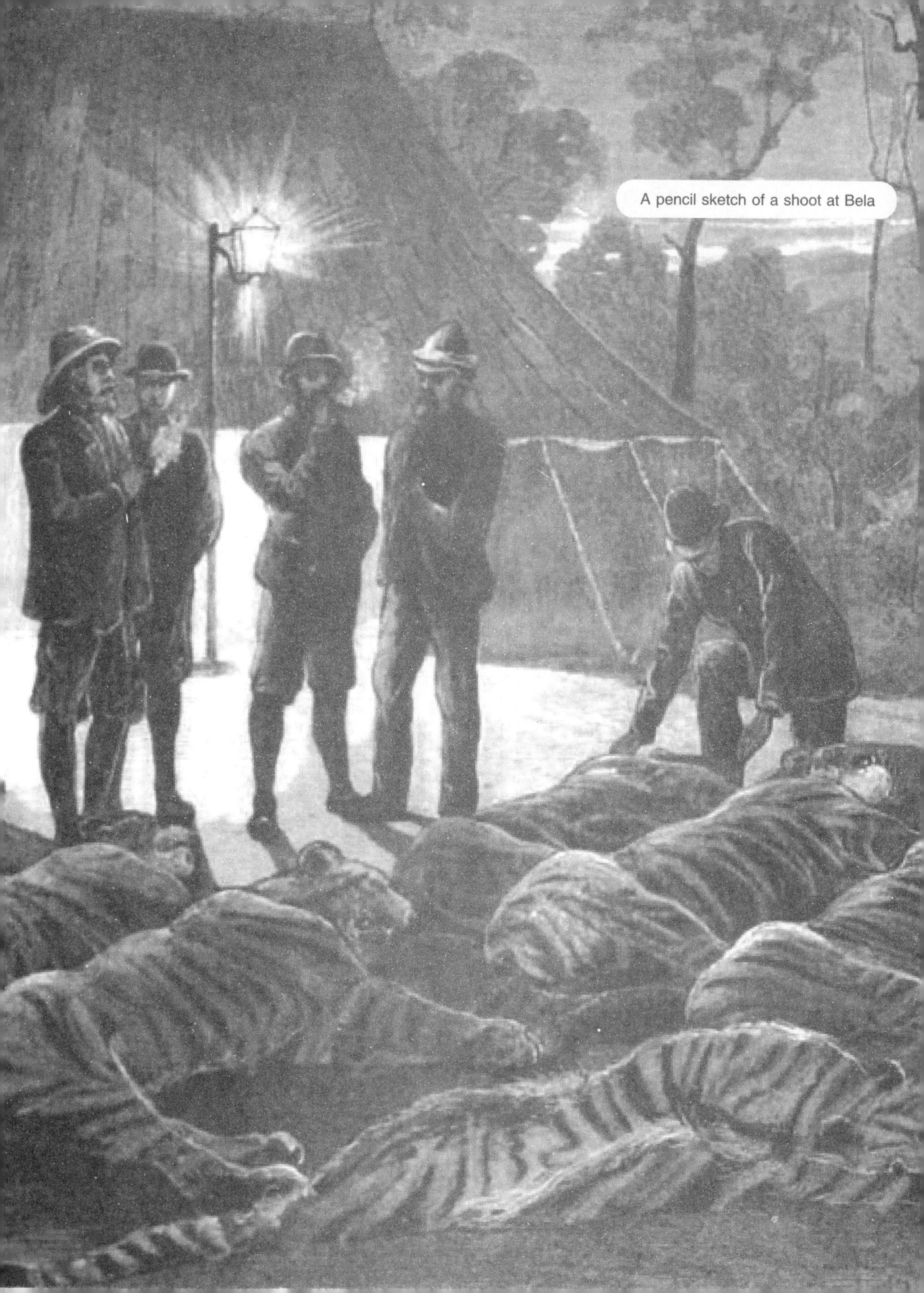

A pencil sketch of a shoot at Bela

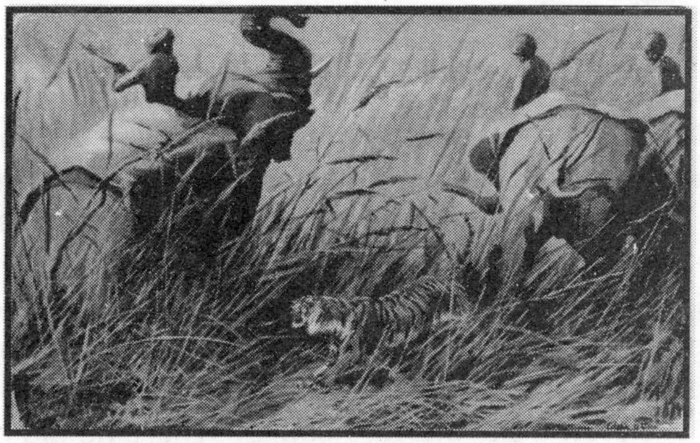

10

Singahi Bela

Nature has been for me, for as long as I remember, a source of solace, inspiration, venture, and delight; a home, a teacher, a companion.

- Anderson

While traveling in the countryside, you do not carry all those trappings needed for any other travel. On this particular expedition, I was traveling as light as possible. I had not brought along any game rifles while tracking tigers on foot. But after the last life-threatening experience, I was determined to get one firearm for myself. There was a great arsenal of light and medium bore rifles preserved at Larti. I first thought of fetching my favorite Purdy and a .375 Holland & Holland from there, but as the place fell some seventy miles away from my camp, I decided to borrow a weapon from some local feudal chieftain, many of whom had been old associates of my maternal family. Here, I must introduce Raja Mahendra Shah, a descendent of a princely state called Singahi which at one time, had great power in lower Tarai and arranged shoots for British officials. He was a tall and fine looking man with broad shoulders and essentially a simple personality. He has an enviable command over the English language and amazingly knowledgeable about the hunting history of India and Africa. I have yet to meet a man who knows more than him on this subject; he indubitably represents a vanishing breed.

I visited Mahendra Shah the same evening. He was sitting alone in his verandah and reading a worn-out book on Africana; the first illustrated, original edition on President Roosevelt's Safari in British East Africa. He was more than delighted to see me. After the preliminaries were over, he politely smiled and promised me every type of co-operation for the subsequent weeks as I stayed around Dudhwa as his guest.

Raja's aged citadel called 'Singahi Palace' reeked of a glowing veneer of antiquity. The forlorn structure had many spacious rooms lying unused and locked except for the half a dozen which the Raja was using. I was ushered into a spacious but dimly lit room with fans whirring away from a high ceiling. The southern wall held half a dozen old-fashioned showcases made of teak wood; where an exquisite selection of firearms was meticulously displayed. It belonged to the days of his grandfather

A photograph stared at me – a sepia vignette of a smart young man and his wife from 1941. This was Maharaj Kumar of Vizianagram, a leading patron of cricket known as Vizzy to his fans. He was also among the relatives of the princely family, and one who excelled as a great slayer of big game, supposedly having killed 406 big cats. Once charged by a wounded tigress in the sugarcane fields close to Majhra Singahi —his famous stamping ground in pre-independence times and now a great farmland— he was thrown off by the bolting elephant, damaging both his kidneys; he was brought to Lucknow's Balrampur hospital, where he did not survive long. It is said that with his passing the sport killing of tigers in the Tarai virtually came to an end. The Maharaja had a great array of sport guns and many of his class rifles gifted to the family are still decorating the showcases of Raja Mahendra Shah and his brothers.

The furniture was archetypal English memorabilia. We reclined on a luxurious relic of a Victorian sofa that had been kept in the courtyard for cleaning. A pint of beer marked the occasion this evening and after dinner, served in Edwardian crockery, I lounged on a Georgian rocking chair to enjoy the comfort of relaxed swings. It was sheer delight to renew ties with Raja after such a long gap. Amidst reflective recapitulations, we sat conversing warmly about sport rifles and shotguns. He loved his guns, as much as ladies love their ornaments. He pointed to a pair of .275 and .256 caliber rifles displayed separately in a single glass case and said, in accented english "My grandfather shot thousands of swamp deer at Mirchia Jheel with these first-class guns. They are light but dead accurate," he told me with gratification. The gleaming weapons looked as if they had just been supplied by a gun dealer.

An allied subject to the section of rifles is the important question about where to hit big game animal and old timers still talk about it with interest - for the heck of it. "Rahul, those who are familiar with the history of African hunting always recall names of three legendary hunters Frederick Courtney Selous, old Karamojo Bell and Mickey Norton. All these three were astonishing shots," said the Raja. "Bell was quite arguably the greatest elephant hunter that ever lived. All of them were the principal advocates for the use of the small-bore rifles for elephants that would only seem suitable for deer in today's hunting circles. They believed that the size of the bullet was not nearly as important as the placement of the shot."

He told me how the old masters' accomplishments with the rifle continue to be the standard by which all others are compared. They had mastered the art of piercing elephant organs with .275 and .256 caliber rifles. Thoughtful and skeptical men of an experimental turn of mind, they cross sectioned elephant skulls to find out just how to reach the brain with shots from various angles. Bell often butchered the whole of the animal to trace the bullet paths and the results of his shots. The brain of an elephant weighs about 10 lbs compared to its weight of 6 tons. This method had given him tremendous knowledge of all the vital spots of elephant anatomy, as a result his shots were so reasonably well placed that he needed no heavier weapons.

It may be mentioned that of the one thousand and eleven elephants Bell had shot, over 500 elephants were shot with a .256. The tusks of these elephants averaged about 80 pounds. But he had earned his nickname by his remarkable feats in the lion holds of Karamojo in the north western part of Kenya where he had scored 27 pachyderms in a day, and all shot stone dead with one bullet each. Later his great successor Mickey Norton had scored exactly a dozen elephants with a similar bore in one hour.

Yet, I am conscious of the fact that I am talking about the men who will forever fill the top niche in the history of hunting and who could not only pick and place their shots but who also knew all the tricks in the trade of stalking animals at zero range. Otherwise, all comes back to one established fact that even the finest rifle is rendered impotent by a novice's lack of experience and poor marksmanship.

However, the gun he finally selected for me was a U.S. Army 30 Springfield, fitted with a Lyman 48 rear peep-sight. He had tested it on the range and sighting in at 100 yards, was able to place the 240 grain bullets in a five inch circle from this distance. It was a reliable rifle, its barrels felt thicker and when I fitted it to my shoulder; I knew immediately that it was a tool for a serious job.

"The old days of hunting are gone forever, where choice of stylish weaponry was a classy crutch for egoistical demolition of the biggest and strongest, now these guns are for emergency – an insurance against the worst, in case something goes wrong," the Raja said crisply and lit a fresh cigarette. He took a paper and pencil and started drawing on it, the outline of a plan he had made for me — his pampered guest — to travel in his erstwhile kingdom.

I thanked the Raja for his concern and together we walked out in the open. The Tarai night was cool. The harvest moon was upon the harvest fields. It cast its sheen upon the empty landscape, and the deserted and lifeless walls of the old palace stood out grey blue or softly black. Our conversation was tempered by the screech of *Gubars*, the tiny spotted owlets that had their nest in a crevice of a wall. They sat demurely side by side and set up their little paroxysms of vociferous chuckling at short intervals.

I was told by the Raja that they were generations-old residents of this building and their job like their forefathers was to keep people merry on moonlit nights. Suddenly the owlets detached themselves from the darkness of the crevice, swooped down into the moonlight and went away; now white against a shadow, now black against the moon. The quiet night was lit by a soft silvery splendor and there was something about this panorama that suggested the fantasy of a strange romantic dream.

The night had intensified, when we heard the sound of a Land Rover halting in the premises. Mahendra Shah's son, Deep Shah arrived from Bela. He had a big news to convey that the very evening a stud bull had been brought down by tigers in cane fields of his village. He gave us an exhilarating account of the fight that

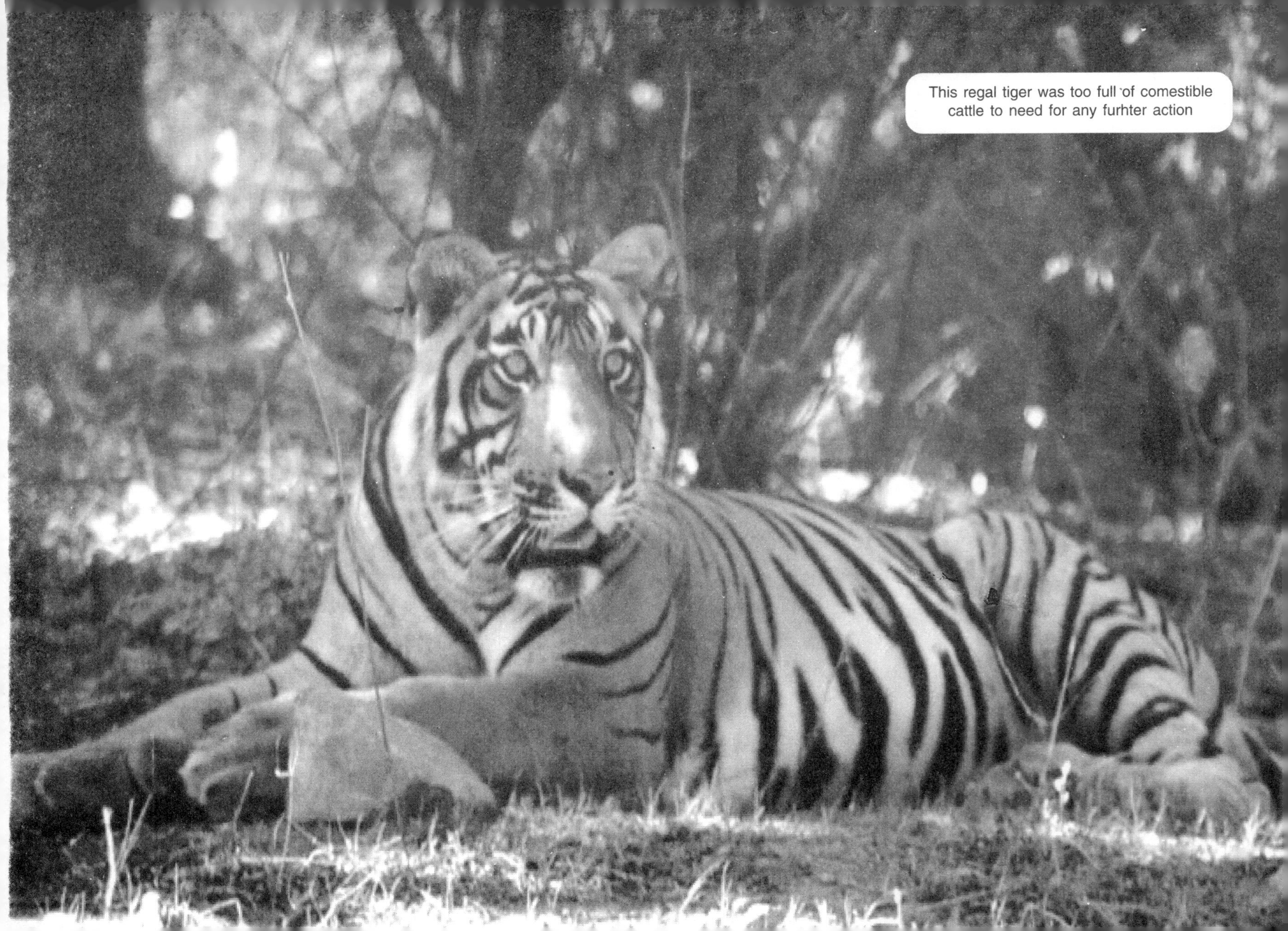

This regal tiger was too full of comestible cattle to need for any furhter action

appeared beguiling on the line of reasoning. He told us that the bull was first attacked by a mother tigress. She caught him by the neck and drove him towards her waiting cubs, injuring him more. The cubs too then attacked the bull to take their share in the killings. A protracted fight ensued on the outskirts of Bela village. The bull in his mortal fury bellowed grunts, so fearfully wild and rushed again and again upon his antagonist. His body was soaked in sweat and blood and that grueling pace and strain of the fight was telling upon him. Froth drooled from his mouth and splattered on the tigers.

The fight raged for some half an hour; the maddened brutes crashed the tangled masses of sugarcane like whirlwind and heavy cane stems two inches thick splintered like matchsticks. Looking like massive prizefighters, they slashed at each other; great cords of muscle stood out like steel cables across their backs, till huge effort drained all the energy of the bull and it succumbed to the loss of blood. An unwise cub that had approached the bull from the front had also received a severe stab from the horns and was in a bad plight.

"You know Dada", said Deep addressing me, "the tigress usually intervenes, but here she had apparently permitted her cubs to make fools of themselves. She never came forward to protect them".

"This happens," I endorsed him, "Some novice mothers, training their cubs for the first time, often do not teach them as how to exercise discretion".

The story was grand and I was more interested than ever. The next morning, Deep and I reached Bela by his automobile and accompanied by a crowd of villagers reached the site which was less than a mile away. Indeed the place looked like a rank arena. There were signs of a titanic struggle all around. The ground had been torn up by straining hooves and claws. Great gouts of flesh were sprayed on the sugarcane in all directions, which were red with dried blood and flattened by the weight of the contestants. The dead bull also lay there but was not eaten by the killers. Instead a sheet of pushing and shoving Bald-headed Sarcogyps vultures covered it. A crowed of expectant Egyptian vultures also sat importunately around, waiting for their chance.

At our approach, the two-dozen-odd repulsive birds stopped quarreling for a moment and looked at us, with their snake like necks turned in our direction. Their hideous faces were bloodstained and smeared with fleshy tissues; they stared at us for brief moments than drifted back to the skeleton and continued to strip fresh chunks of red meat.

We passed the kill and proceeded in the search of the tigress. There were splotches of blood and tufts of hair outside a cane retreat, and something resembling a bulky bag also lay in a ditch. I picked up the bag and examined it, these were the testicles of the stud —impressively outsized and neatly cut away from the root— and surprisingly all intact. As per description of a witness, a violent cub had caught the gizmo in his mouth and snatched away at the very start of the fight. "Sahib, thereafter the bull fought for an hour without his testicles."

By this time, a large crowd had already moved about the ground and most signs of the event had been obliterated. Foolish, as it may seem, I began the unpleasant task of trying to locate the wounded cub. Mine was a party of six guns. Every man made a good check of his weapon and ammunition because it was too dangerous to follow injured tigers on foot, and expose ourselves to an attack when the visibility inside the crop was almost as good as zero. I knew from experience that even the best rifle shots cannot always be exact and those who have been good marksmen at a hundred yard target often miss wild animals at very close ranges. In addition since tigers stay in concealment and move quickly over jagged grounds, it is often difficult to home in on them.

The gunmen were reluctant to proceed, and being an amateur I too was suffering all the sensations of intense excitement, despite knowing the risks of such a follow-up, when luckily someone happened to spot a striped form in one of the lanes to my right. It was a cub, lying on his side in an irrigation furrow that crossed through the plots. He was half submerged in the cool running water. The slanted sun rays made stripes of light and shade through the cane that so closely resembled the tiger's pattern that it was difficult to make out his presence.

Tigers may be beautiful but their deadly power is to be respected. Their power belongs to the rugged terrain of Jungle, where they have been created to live. In such conditions there invariably is an actual LOC (line of control) which should never be crossed unless you are hunting them. We stopped in our tracks and took an appraisal of his condition. There was a raw scratch of a stab like wound on his left cheek and left forepaw and the skin was completely gone exposing a part of jaw bone. He looked dreadful but still had enough life in him. He demonstrated a couple of times but we kept at a respectful distance so that he no longer considered us a threat and relaxed. The cub could never convalesce sufficiently and later died of gangrene.

The men who had watched the amazing combat told me that the cubs, despite being eight to ten months old, with little or no previous experience in dispatching such a large animal, largely confined their attack to biting and clawing around the rump, back and belly rather than grasping the throat. They pounced again and again on the stud and bit at it with all the strength of their little jaws; warm blood seemed to have stimulated their senses. They tore little pieces of flesh and as the stud attempted to get up they threw it down repeatedly. They were reasonably adapted in pulling it down, but they failed to kill efficiently.

Rearing family is a difficult time as mothers have to kill an adequate amount of prey to feed ever more hungry cubs. Perhaps this explained the irrational impetuousness of the tigress, she must have been very hard pressed for food or else cub rearing mothers don't meddle with large animals. Mac Dougal observes, "Any serious injury sustained by a solitary tiger, dependent on its own efforts to obtain food, can ultimately prove fatal… the tigers that stay out of trouble keep their skins the longest."

A week later a cyclist, pedalling on a mud path came across the tigress standing on an exposed ground along the river course. She was on the other side of the river bank sniffing the soil and the bark of a tree repeatedly. Even now there were dark stains of clotted blood on her neck where she had been gored by the bull. The tigress was alone with no cub and she was probably trying to pick up the scent of some male or may be of her second surviving cub. The cyclist was at a safe distance from the animal so he stopped the bike and stood in his saddle with one foot on the ground to watch the animal.

Tigers have scent glands around their cheeks, toes, tail and ano-genital area, which aid them in imparting scent marks by rubbing their bodies on trees and bushes. They also leave behind 'cologne scents' mixed with their urine and feces, called 'odor fields' in cat lexicon. Scent is a medium of communication. A tiger's sense of smell plays a greater role in learning about the whereabouts of their own kind rather than being used for any other purpose.

This animal had perhaps hit upon a scent trail. She circled the tree quite a few times, turned back and began to climb the bank. Obviously, attracted by the scent she kept her nose to the ground. She would have disappeared in the cane fields in a couple of seconds when the cyclist out of fun, got down from the bike, hurled a mud stone upon her and started to abuse loudly but this tigress stopped, looked backwards over her shoulder and gave a blood curdling snarl. At this the man hopped on to the cycle seat and took a frenzied start for his village.

After this last news, the tigress was not seen anywhere. I stayed at Bela for a week, all the while looking for her, but all her signs in the neighborhood had disappeared and she seemed to have cleared out of the area. However, it was noteworthy that she was not injured and healthy; it gave me a comfortable feeling to imagine that she would raise a new family very soon.

My interest in the itinerant tigers was incessant. I had already told the villagers that I expected greater co-operation from them and whoever brought the first news of any tiger sighting or its kill in a crop-field will get a proper reward in cash. This kept them motivated and enthusiastic. One day, I learnt that a tiger had killed a cow at a hamlet called Budka the previous evening. I decided to check. On reaching the shed where the carcass lay I discovered that it had been killed by a leopard. It had come out from the side of Suheli River and had gone further on after being disturbed. Ordinarily, a high density of tigers by definition means fewer leopards. But here the tiger density in the cane area was one for every ten square kilometers and yet the spotted-pards were frequently encountered. Now as elephants were unprocurable, and no other way of getting the animal could be found, I organized a massive drive to send it back in Salukapur jungles, in which a mob of considerable size participated.

The length of the beat extended for some eight hundred yards. The villagers were beating through the cover when I saw a male tiger galloping across my front in some very heavy crop. Almost at once I heard the eminent sawing of the leopard under the trees ahead of me; next moment it broke into a full gallop and made to pass my Jeep diagonally as to break out between me and the tiger on my right. The tiger was in bad temper, the moment it spotted the leopard he made an ugly face, and came with a terrific speed.

What happened next took no more than a split second. The leopard ran for his life and sprang over the *Nala* in vigorous confusion, taking a complete toss while the tiger also took a prodigious leap and landed across in a high *Narkul,* and then went on following him. It took me some time to cross the *Nala* and when I got there I could find none of the adversaries. Interestingly nearby, there was a nonchalant jungle cook roosting on the bough of a *Khair* tree.

Such bits of sport as they came my way during my research were always welcome for there was a freshness about them, much like harking back of my soul to the thrills of that era of guns and shooting that I had witnessed in my family as a growing child.

The night before I was to leave, a driving storm came up; lightning flashed all night, playing with its livid glare upon surroundings and in that atmosphere I heard a lively communication of tigers. It was the experience of a life time. It started from the vast expanse of sugar forests as I call these farms; where at least two range holders set out to communicating with each other. Their roars seemed to split the air. I could recognize them to be males from the deep drawn quality of sounds. They must have been some half a mile from our tent. Perhaps one amongst these was the same robust male, which having chased the leopard the other day, had reverted to the crops.

Roar is mainly a long distance communicatory signal and is mainly used by male tigers to assert their own territorial right. This performance has greater intensity and regularity when the resident tiger invites another tiger to a possible conflict or discourages him to leave his territory. Tigresses also respond to these calls and roars but do not vocalize with extraordinary volume and frequency as the males do.

Like lions, tigers do not vocalize without specific reasons. Their calls vary in intensity and volume according to the message they carry, and obviously like human beings, one tiger's voice differs from that of the other. It seemed that tigers living in this area recognized each other's calls and responded selectively, depending on the individual who was rendering it.

For longish hours the croon to challenging continued. Lying on the bed and feeling a great air of whisky, we enjoyed hearing the booming calls, drowned in peculiar, awful reverberations of clouds. Now and then a peal awakened us and made us conscious of the electric battle that was raging outside between felines and the muttering thunder. There was a surge of excitement and anticipation in hearing that memorable sound once again.

Next morning the clouds hung sluggishly overhead but there was no rain. The country was bathed in a dramatic storm lightening so that the trees and the grasses glowed viridian, when one of the striped musicians of the night appeared not far away from my tent. It was a sub-adult tiger, seated on the road and looking at us with curiosity. But he was smallish and petite, perhaps no more than three years old, and not large enough to have generated the mighty roar we had heard last night. As he perceived Om Bir's rifle leveled at him he turned and raced off across the fields in gigantic bounds.

By the time my two months of field work ended in mid-January, I had seen three tigers, five tigresses and eight cubs, each of which had left their distinct impression upon me. I thanked Raja Sahib for all his kindness; and the manner in which he had carried out everything for my comfort and the success of my expedition.

I came back to Lucknow and mulled over the facts. The worst-hit area comprised some 1,000 square miles, it lay mainly along the Sharda river which flowed south-east wards through Pilibhit and Kheri districts. The whole extent and both the banks of the river (north and south), only as recently as three decades ago, was an area of *ratwa* and *narkul* reeds. The great savannah belt was an age-old range of tigers, teeming with its food. However, once the land was taken over by humans; and its prey species drastically poached out for entertainment and luxury consumption, the tiger's old home was gone for good, but still all the tiger movements, for the most part were focused towards the south of their old haunts, the embankments of the Sharda river.

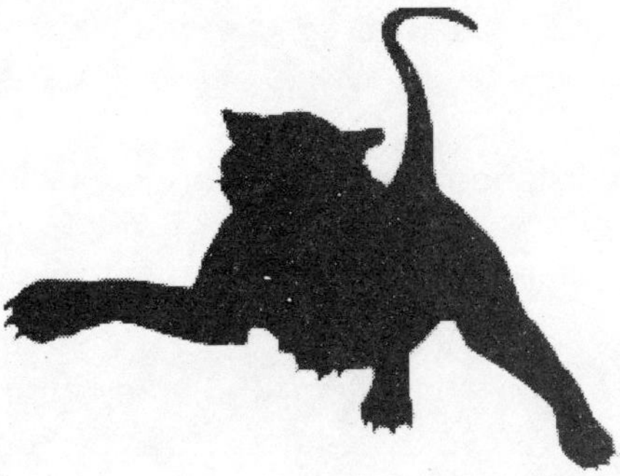

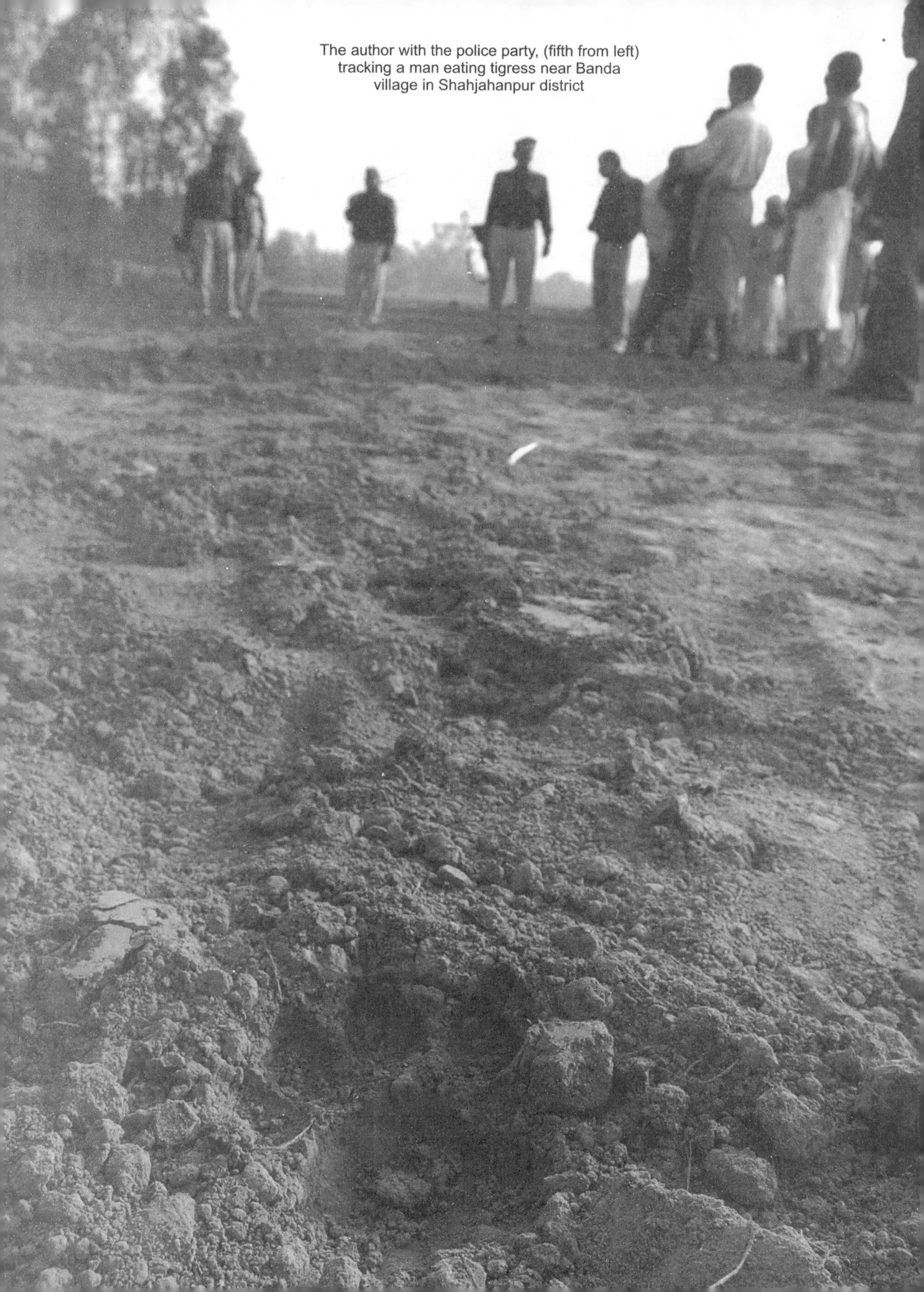

The author with the police party, (fifth from left) tracking a man eating tigress near Banda village in Shahjahanpur district

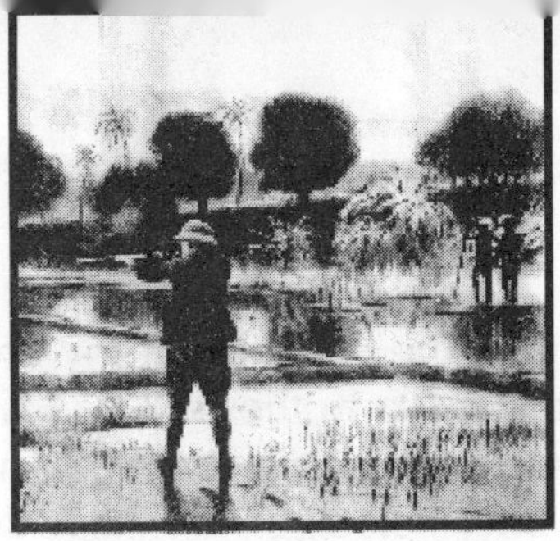

11

The Morphology of the Tiger's Paw

All truths are easy to understand once they are discovered; the point is to discover them

- Galileo Galilee

The unending phenomenon of Sugar tigers had opened a pleasing field for intelligent speculation. It was as if nature was staging some odd show for the people to fret and wonder upon. Some experts suggested that with the recent human modifications of original forestlands, tigers had been forced to adapt drastically to altered vegetations. In some parts of their range where they occur in six distinct bioregions overlapping 13 countries, they are known to have taken to plantations of timber trees, rubber, coffee and oil palm and cardamom, so the sugar phenomenon was just an extension of this tendency.

However, to my mind it was different. The sugarcane crops, adjacent to moist tropical forests of Tarai were not a small fraction of land. It outrivaled all the aforementioned plantations in their gargantuan length and width and excelled in terms of 'prey biomass and biological corridors' that offered an ideal ecosystem to its habitants. It was not only gratifying to tigers, but, with plenty of water and ubiquitous prey, it also served as competitive breeding ranges for females.

Time and again, this greatest event of nature, made me return to Tarai with never-failing interest and the hours of pursuit, time, space, danger and distance meant nothing to me. I followed them unabated through monsoon and winters and season after season. Like the finest hunters of the past who hunted alone, I never felt compelled to have company. I was an individualist and a lone ranger, who worked alone. If it seems disadvantage to some, it is a recommendation to others.

It was very tedious to travel on a motorcycle in a rugged country. There were no proper roads for several kilometers, except for the degraded unmaintained tracks, deeply rutted by the passage of cart wheels and often filled with puddles of rain water. In the core Tarai, where a flat horizon stretched for miles and every tree and crop patterns looked bewilderingly familiar and unfamiliar at the same time, I headed towards some isolated village, which had been the scene of most recent human kill and which was evidently a spot favored by tiger.

In the contest of survival, sugar tigers were the players of a different game board and it was a formidable challenge to reveal some new information on them.

I daresay if I had to advance in the direction of my dreams, I had to have some solid foundations in support of my hypothesis, I had worked single-mindedly and rationally with empirical data, having built a mass of fundamental knowledge about sugar tigers, about which no one, including the wildlife department, had the vaguest idea. Much of my data about these tigers was location specific and could be of potential value in the management of animals throughout the greater Tarai.

At this stage, it was essential to determine the current status of tigers in sugarcane. Up to now, there were only 'guesstimates' about tiger populations in the farms. Scant effort had been made to corroborate these beliefs with on-ground scientific assessment because these animals were not only difficult to come across but huge effort and material resources were needed to confirm the presence of even a single tiger.

During 1981, Dr. R.L. Singh was administering Dudhwa National Park as Field Director. A tall and suave person, deeply bronzed by the field sun, he sported a French beard that made him resemble George Adamson; a hardcore white African conservationist of the 'Bawana Game' fame and husband of Joy Adamson known for her legendary lioness Elsa.

Singh is a knowledgeable individual and an ebullient writer of many books on wildlife. I met him in his office, and found him most co-operative in my ventures. I shared my close observations with him and provided him the information of various locations where these beasts were stationed outside the park. He was highly pleased at this favour, for like me he too had been pondering over the situation of sugarcane tigers. "I am already aware of some of them, and I am working on the same line. It seems you have done your work with abundant good intent. An oft forgotten part of any enumeration is the all important pre-census work". As we discussed the matter further we got convinced with the idea that the problem needed to be properly identified and a thorough census in the farmlands was the need of the hour. Previously, there had never been any such exercise in this sphere that could have provided with a baseline data of methodology to map the distribution of tigers in farmlands and so far he knew, no rangers had yet visited the areas in question. "The obstruction is they depend too much on livestock, I have seen wild prey dropping but not too many"

Singh's response was gratifyingly swift. He briefed me about the technical aspects of a tiger census. "The census units are chosen only after surveying animal movements; then on the used paths of animals ten to twenty Pugmark Impression Pads (PIPs) are laid out and continuously monitored by the field staff. They are checked at least once in three days during the census period. We will have to orient villagers in this context to not to disturb the pads. Anyway, in this respect you have already done a good home work and you may now expect some results," he said.

I was delighted at the prospect. We shook hands in mutual agreement, glad that we had started well in the first place. I felt strongly that now the things would be much easy for me if our ideas might quite crystallize into a firm statement about the position of this animal. "You must submit your findings at the earliest. I will see how they can be incorporated into routine management programmes." he paused and then said, "I am going for a round, would you like to come along".

Huge colorful field maps adorned the walls of his office and tucked between them were the pictures of three tigers that Singh had taken in the sugarcanes. "I keep my camera ready", he said, as he hung the gadget on his shoulders and together we went out to make a fresh appraisal of things. We had too much work to do. We were to span the sugar fields and probe the estimated locations of tigers from village to village and farm to farm. This was by no means an easy matter.

The forest guards appeared with guns. Two qualified faculty from the Wildlife Institute of Dehradun also accompanied us. We roamed about the fields, almost the entire day, and I was particularly satisfied to discover no less than seven spoors of different tigers. The faculties examined the marks and interpreted them in scrupulous detail. After a thorough examination of all possible situations, they concluded that these were four juveniles and three full adults. Their measured, calculated and tempered ways reminded me of native hunters at Larti with whom I had attained my boyhood training of jungle craft. Here was similar knowledge, offered in a scientific package with more meticulous detail that I once again enjoyed to learn on my own initiative, adding new terms to my lexicon.

The equipment known as 'Tiger Tracer' was employed to get accurate tracing of the tiger pugmarks. It may be mentioned that the Late Saroj Raj Chaudhary had established the technique of tracing tiger pugmarks on glass in which only the right rear pugmark was to be used and a meticulous record be maintained, which included the date, time and soil type for proper analysis. But the controversy about the accuracy of this census method and the new capture and recapture method had already come up. Lack of standardization of methodology and the training of the enumerators lay at the root of the problem. Using pugmarks in conjunction with other techniques is probably the best method.

It takes a great deal to understand the morphology of the tiger paw. Theoretically it is simple. The front limbs of the predator are the primary means of assault on a prey. The fore arms of the front limb are used in gripping and pulling down the prey and are therefore built particularly massive in both sexes. The toes, claws and pads are also correspondingly stout. Hence the fore paw is significantly bigger than the rear one in both the sexes and if a tracing of the pugmark is enclosed in a linear frame, such a frame tends to be squarish in shape; However if the tracing of the pug mark of the hind paws are compared, those of a male fit in prominently in a square frame whereas those of a female fit in a rectangular frame. Thus it is that from the tracings of the rear pugmarks, it is possible to determine the sex of an individual tiger. It is primarily for this important reason that the rear pugmarks are used in tiger census work.

The paw is the base organ of the body, which bends itself according to the ground available for resting it. It can splay out and turn up larger on a slushy ground and look neat and compact on a hard sub-surface with thin cover of dust or sand. It will be useful at this stage to understand that even in such situations, the characteristics of each pugmark remain unchanged and the difference, mainly in size, can always be valued with reference to the habitat. On the other hand a small gravel or small hole can cause the pugmark to twist or get splayed on one side. As far as possible, therefore, a perfectly normal rear pugmark should be selected for preparing the tracing. If no single pugmark is seen in perfect condition, the tracing should be made from the best one and this should be corrected in the field by placing the plate on one or two other pugmarks having those segments in good condition which were found distorted in first one.

Only four of the toes get an imprint along with the pad in the pugmark. The fifth toe in the rear is well above the pad and does not touch the ground when the tiger walks. The retractile claws also do not come out at the time of walk, and therefore no imprints come out, except sometimes, when the tiger is walking on slushy ground. The pad is broader at the base and narrows down at the top but retains a near flat edge at the top. Of the four toes that get imprinted, two lie above the flat top edge of the pad and the remaining two lie alongside the two tapering sides, a little lower than the middle toes. In the imprint the upper edge of the pad leaves a straight line or a near straight line below the two middle toes. The tapering sides of the pad in the upper portion cave in a little near the extreme left and extreme right toes.

Unless the pug has some abnormality or deformity, it is not normally possible to distinguish between different animals of the same sexes and size. Similarly it is hard to tell the pugs of a young tiger from those of a full grown leopard. Only a man who is constantly refurbished by his field experiences knows that tiger cubs' toes are thicker in relation to its pad than those of leopard.

The lower side of pad has large lobes on both sides. A third much smaller lobe lies in the middle part of the lower edge of the pad. The joints of these two side lobes with the small middle lobe are in the form of conically tapering valleys that leave the mark of two conical ridges with well defined tips at the bottom line of the pugmark. While tracing the pugmark it is very important to correctly trace the flat edge at the top of the pad, the shape of the lobe and the two conical tips. It is important to correctly visualize the direction in which the two conical tips point. If the tracing incorporating these features is correctly made, no matter what the texture of the ground is -- from rocky terrain through wet sands, slushy banks to hard earth, soft earth and mud -- the tracking can be equated with fingerprints. Different tracings of the same tiger walking on different soil will still remain conducive to identifying the individual.

It is true that a great deal of information about tiger behaviour can be picked up from the study of pugmarks, but it is not easy. Long experience is needed to interpret whatever marks the beast has made and only those foresters who are persistently in touch with these animals are qualified to point out such dissimilarities truthfully -

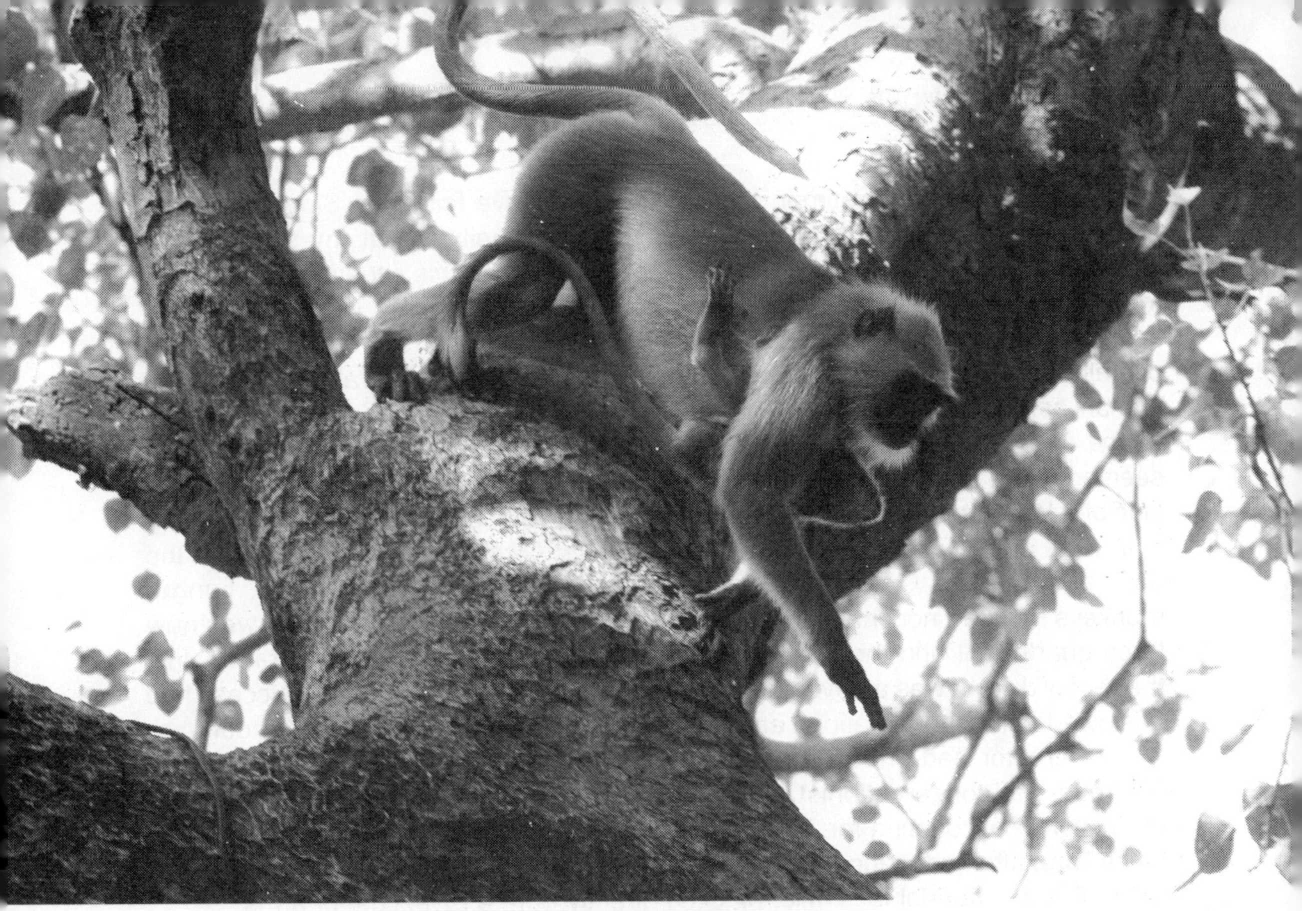

Gray Langoor monkey with her baby coming down a tree

and even they can gaffe on occasions.

At the end of the annual census, after proper processing of location-specific data, the number of tigers declared within the park boundaries was 62 and in the sugar cane fields it was 43, excluding cubs. To my surprise and delight, this figure was confined to North Kheri only. Fifteen tigers were found within ten kilometers of Dudhwa buffer zone while 26 were found over a distance of ten to twenty kilometers from the buffer zone and four were found still beyond that limit. The data was not complete - there was still no proper assessment of the total number of tigers in agricultural fields. There was a hint of danger from half a dozen other animals that were reported from still more distant places of Maigalganj and Dhaurara cane fields, in the extreme west of the district, and which our count did not include. Moreover, as natural mortality is very high in young cubs so the teams had tried to avoid counting them to not to make the census too invasive.

The count certainly showed us the monstrous extent of the problem and furthered our interest in it, but before the staff could be sent to locate them, an exceptionally violent rainstorm broke out, and the farms and their approach roads were flooded with muddy water. For a week the clouds gave no sign of lifting and the dawn seemed to break dark and murky, which brought our efforts to naught.

Until now the tiger numbers in sugarcane were only subjective speculation but here was an objective testimony that called us to have faith in it. Singh had done his job admirably and I too had availed the opportunity to put my scheme into practice, happily with most excellent results. No wonder this situation, which gave forth a peculiar challenge to conservation strategies for big cats, was unfortunately never acknowledged in the race to expand protected area net work; because, the overall conservation effort in the country was still one that separated wildlife from human dominated landscape.

The evening was like a dream. The office room was dark; the polished table seemed like a pool with only the glimmer of lantern reflected in it. We sat by the side of a large open window and raised a toast to celebrate the occasion. The dark blue vault of sky was ablaze with glittering stars. Cicadas seemed to drill into the darkness. Fireflies signaled to each other in miniscule bursts of light. Langur monkeys lounged nonchalantly on the roof of tourist canteen. The moon was now three quarter full and their demonical figures loomed black and spectral against the yellow disc. It was an evening of luxurious quiet after toil. Ultimate success had bestowed self congratulations and the sense of achievement was paramount.

The director had shot a tigress named Tara, a pet of Billy Arjan Singh, the controversial conservationist who lived close by. This tigress had a notorious distinction of accounting for 22 human kills which is a record set by any man-eater in the Tarai after independence. Her stuffed body was kept to a side in the drawing room, like an imperial facsimile, plucked directly from a royal coat of arms.

"You see it Rahul," Singh said in the vein of a jaded, blasé sportsman from the yore, "This is the most prized specimen that I have successfully obtained from all my man-eater hunts. It was a pet then, and it is still a pet. From the moment I have shot it, I made it my pet. I have treated it with respect and loving care," Singh continued settling his cowboy cap. "I wished to restore this dead creature as near to life as could be possible and it has been done well by the old taxidermists of Bangalore." I took a look at the mounted Tara, standing in the circle of light thrown by the lantern. Everything was as black as pit around her but her glass eyes gleamed in the velvet light. She looked alert and frowning, as if she were alive in her full natural splendor. The tiger arouses awe, and in deference to the might of the king of the jungle even the stuffed man-eater can send a chill down the spine. Once she was a pet to Billy and now she was the same to Singh, but no longer a fearful man-eater, no more demanding and aberrant.

Risking repetition I would say that approximate 800-km plus square kilometers of Dudhwa Park is surrounded by about 5,000 square kilometers of sugarcane fields and exactly when the landscape animals like sugar tigers cross the real ecological line is not known. The contention that the adjustment of tiger population would be contained by constriction of available habitat, does not seem to hold much meaning in the unlimited habitat of sugar forests; for in spite of everything, tigers have a tendency of transgressing their eco-systems and ranging beyond protected areas.

This report indicated a paradigm shift in the perception of the forest department that had looked at these tigers as someone else's burden. The pertinent question was that with this kind of development, whether the Project Tiger in Tarai was heading for a sustainable and sensible future, conducive to uphold and control the growth of sugarcane tiger through some scientific management? The inevitable reality is that if wildlife has got to survive it must learn to adjust itself with the tremendously spiraling integer of human beings. Population explosion of mankind is an inevitable future of this earth which must destroy and eat out everything that stands in its way. There are about four times as many people on the globe as there were at the beginning of the last century. An example can be sited from India's population which only in last hundred years, from 1910 to 2010, has registered an increase of no less than 333 percent while the gross national product has gone up about seven folds in same space of time.

Thus presently most preliminary research of the environment has to be focused on fresh threats of human-induced climate change and the issues whether wildlife can co-exist with man-kind; especially whether a landscape for large predators like tigers, can be carved out within the human landscape, isolated from human endeavors.

Complete reorientations of management principles needed to be devised at the earliest and as the tiger is the key species for controlling the environment, the fiasco of the sugar tigers offered a window to the tigers' future with mankind. In the interest of the longer rubric of conservation in altering landscapes, it presented a functional laboratory to experiment, where the integrated conservation and developmental projects could be applied as a potential harbinger of opportunity to understand the forthcoming matrix of man-wildlife adjustment. This would help us to reinvent the strategies that may augur well for their future conservation.

Scientists have long held that despite the availability of voluminous information about the present state of ecological systems it is not easy to create a model that would predict the future of the species; such predictive models fail because of the human style of functioning. Dr. Karanth believes that human reactions create stable influences and massively overhaul the system and in the case of complex systems of tigers, humans are more likely to topple the scales in their bid to correct imbalances. So the future depends not only on what is happening presently but how meticulously we respond to the existing conditions.

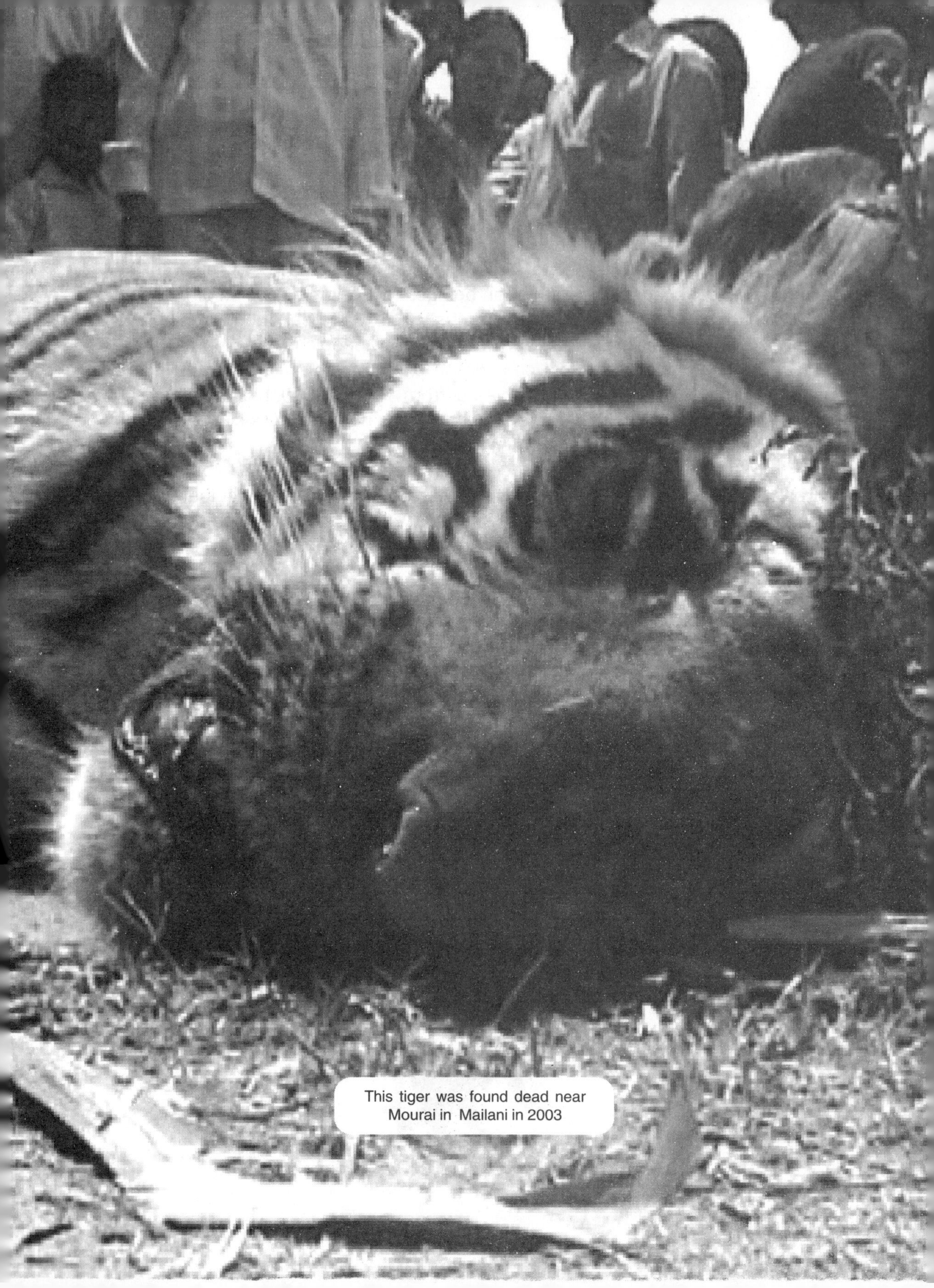

This tiger was found dead near Mourai in Mailani in 2003

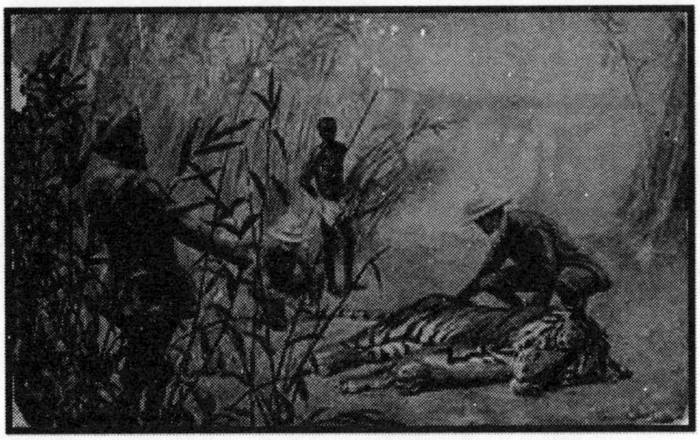

12

Man-tiger Conflict – The Max Out

We generate our own environment. We get exactly what we deserve. How can we resent a life we've created ourselves? Who's to blame, who's to credit but us?

- Richard Bach

Paraspur is my favorite tiger–turf in North Kheri. It is virtually a facsimile of my ancestral village Larti and a camp of unending interest, where inspection of wildlife is essentially combined with a comfortable home and social amenities. Now, when my outings are based on my natural need for action and I want to get away from the mundane life of urbanity, I go to this piece of land where the sugar farms are pitted with tiger pugs and the surge of tracking wildlife comes more spontaneously. One can take a Jeep and go roaming about at any hour of the day. The possibility of being able to spot deer herds or pigs on a good scale within an hour's drive is more like routine business than a regular expedition based on a settled plan.

I liked this lovely country and Mintoo Mama's sons, Om Bir and Shyamu were my constant companions. Their enthusiasm for the big cats was as much a legacy of their ancestors as it was with me and we worked as a close-knit team, I knew that without their selfless and effective assistance, I would never be able to accomplish my research.

Tiger are high profile animals. They always remains in the limelight and perhaps for this reason, the deaths caused by man-tiger conflict are always reported in the press. I was always on the lookout for such 'real-news', which verily announced the presence of some tiger in an unfamiliar area, which was not the usual haunt of the species. Every week having collected the clippings of newspapers, I would take out the Survey of India maps of Kheri Division, spread them on a table and jot down important data on the map. I would mark the place with a small cross with the date against it, signifying the place and time of each incident of man killing. In the case of a sighting, I marked the place with a black pencil, in the case of an attack, I made a green cross and in case of a human death, an orange cross served the purpose. I also tried to obtain all the possible information about the beast, the localities where

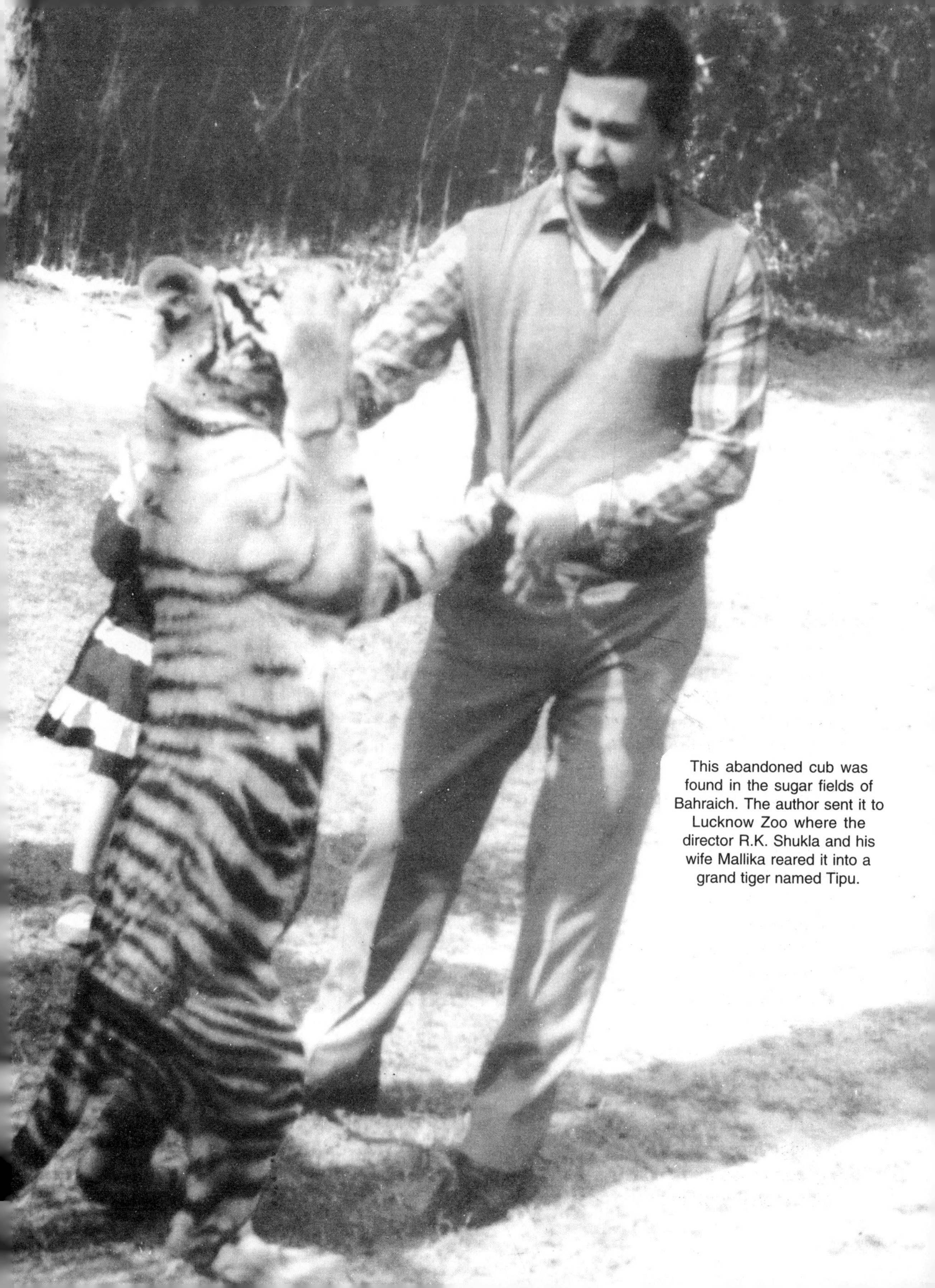

This abandoned cub was found in the sugar fields of Bahraich. The author sent it to Lucknow Zoo where the director R.K. Shukla and his wife Mallika reared it into a grand tiger named Tipu.

Till now, I had thought that killing of humans by tigers was more often than not a co-existential hazard. Human death on account of the tiger was an occupational risk ever since woodcutters and grazers entered its territory. But, here the situation was different. The habitat sharing with human and the constant competetion had seemingly altered the lifestyle of tigers and it was against this radical background — the hungry tiger and solitary villager — that the problem had to be viewed.

One day in my free time, I studied the map quite comprehensively and was surprised to see that in just one year I had made 182 crosses on the North Kheri map and 96 on the South Kheri map. Fifty of them were black, 141 were green, and 65 were orange and the rest were in red indicating the violent death of a human in the jaws of the super predators. A large encircled red cross was indicative of a tigress making a triple kill of a woodcutter and his children at a place called Kumsi in Nighasan sub-division.

To trace the history of this jinx briefly, I recall that the first outburst of man-eating tigers in Dudhwa was over by 1980. The five serious man-eaters including the tigress of Baraucha Nala and Tara, the pet tigress of Billy Arjan Singh, had been shot dead by the forest managers. After that a sudden peace seemed to have reigned over the country.

From 1981 to 1984, nine tigers on rampage were recognized as man-eaters and taken into account; thus raising the number to 14. All of them had been officially shot yet the problem persisted, assuming prodigious proportions. My mission to protect cane tigers seemed pretty hopeless at this stage; because the phenomenon had undesirably transformed into that of the so-called man-eating tigers, and this had brought the man-tiger conflict into sharp focus. My efforts to buy favour for these tigers from villagers were somewhat muddled by fright of tiger attacks creating a confusing asymmetry.

The frequency with which the kills were being reported pointed to the fact that many tigers were taking part in the slaughter. Perhaps some new collaborators had emerged to join the ranks of their ancestors and the sugar fields of Kheri were nurturing a new chain of man-eaters which was to spell a notorious phase of terror once again in the region, It was clearly 'man versus tiger' and all this unremitting turmoil was bound to make Kheri internationally notorious for its killer but doomed tigers.

It was only a week after a man-eating tigress was killed in Madhopurva of South Kheri, that a new aggressive tiger was noticed in the vicinity of a village called Rehta in the same area. News came that three persons had been killed by this recent entrant, besides four others that were lying in a critical condition in the hospital.

This had happened only ten miles away from Gurha farm where I had been staying at Sardar Mukhtar Singh's house and I quickly went over to investigate. I drove to the village and got the first-hand report from the Gram Pradhan who had himself been a victim of the beast's wrath, but had been lucky enough to escape with a few claw scratches on his back and shoulder.

The tiger had killed a cow in broad daylight when an old woman was working in a sugar field. She heard her cow bellowing in distress. She walked up to it and found the killer standing near the dead cow. She had approached the spot from the only open side. The tiger leaped, bit through her shoulder blade, crushing the bones of her chest and back and the women fell down on the ground unconscious. He then ate the cow and disappeared into the sugar thicket.

"The news reached the village by afternoon", said the Pradhan. "We led a rescue party to the place and saw the pugmarks out of a crop plot. It was not a very big thicket, only some hundred square yards but was rather thick and low and covered a wide ditch. There was a small tunnel like entrance into the bush. We concluded that the tiger had entered leaving its footprints which were clear and fresh."

The party created a great noise to flush out the tiger. They yelled and pelted stones beat the bushes with their sticks and even threw a couple of crackers into the crop. Nothing came out and the rescuers concluded that the tiger was not there.

Meanwhile, two policemen arrived. They went round the plot to find out in which direction the tiger had gone but there were no pugmarks on the other side although the ground was freshly ploughed. One of the men, who had a gun, came back to the entrance of the thicket and tried to peep into it. He got down in the ditch to have a better view and crawled inside the tunnel half way up to his waist, while his legs were still in the open.

There was a terrific growl that made the throng run for dear life. After a long sprint they attained a little rise from where the police stalwarts opened up with their service rifle and fired a volley of rapid fire.

The villagers were exasperated about the fate of their fellowman. They requested the policemen to help them in bringing him back. The request was turned down. The villagers wanted to borrow a gun but were refused, instead the policemen promised to keep the thicket covered with their guns in case of an attack so the unarmed men went back to the place where they had left their partner waist deep in the grass.

They found him in the same prone position, stretched out on the ground. His legs were still in the open, while the rest of his body lay thrust in the bush tunnel. He was dead. There was a patch of blood on his back and his head was crushed as if with a hammer blow. The tiger launched its second attack with devastating fury as the crowd tried to retrieve his body. He came out of a depression and in an instinctive death grip went for the throat of the leading man, killing him then and there. He then caught two others and pulled their entrails out in a split second, seized another and with a mighty heave of its shoulders twisted his neck breaking it; and then chased the fleeing crowd almost boxing in most of them. Hitherto furious, he caught a young boy and without pausing to kill him clamped him in his jaws and pulled him for a short distance. But then left him unconscious on the parapet and bolted inside the crop.

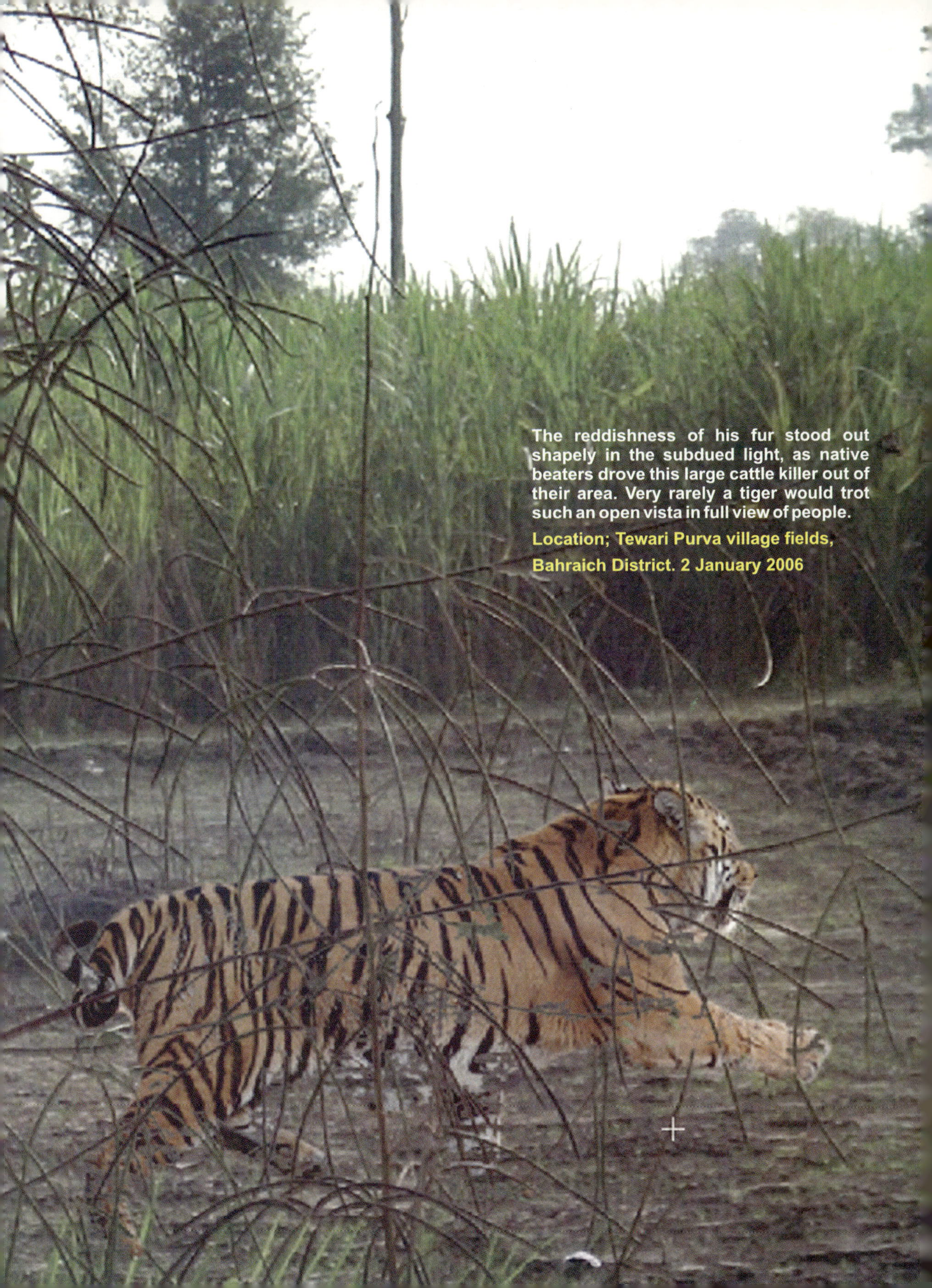

The reddishness of his fur stood out shapely in the subdued light, as native beaters drove this large cattle killer out of their area. Very rarely a tiger would trot such an open vista in full view of people.

Location; Tewari Purva village fields, Bahraich District. 2 January 2006

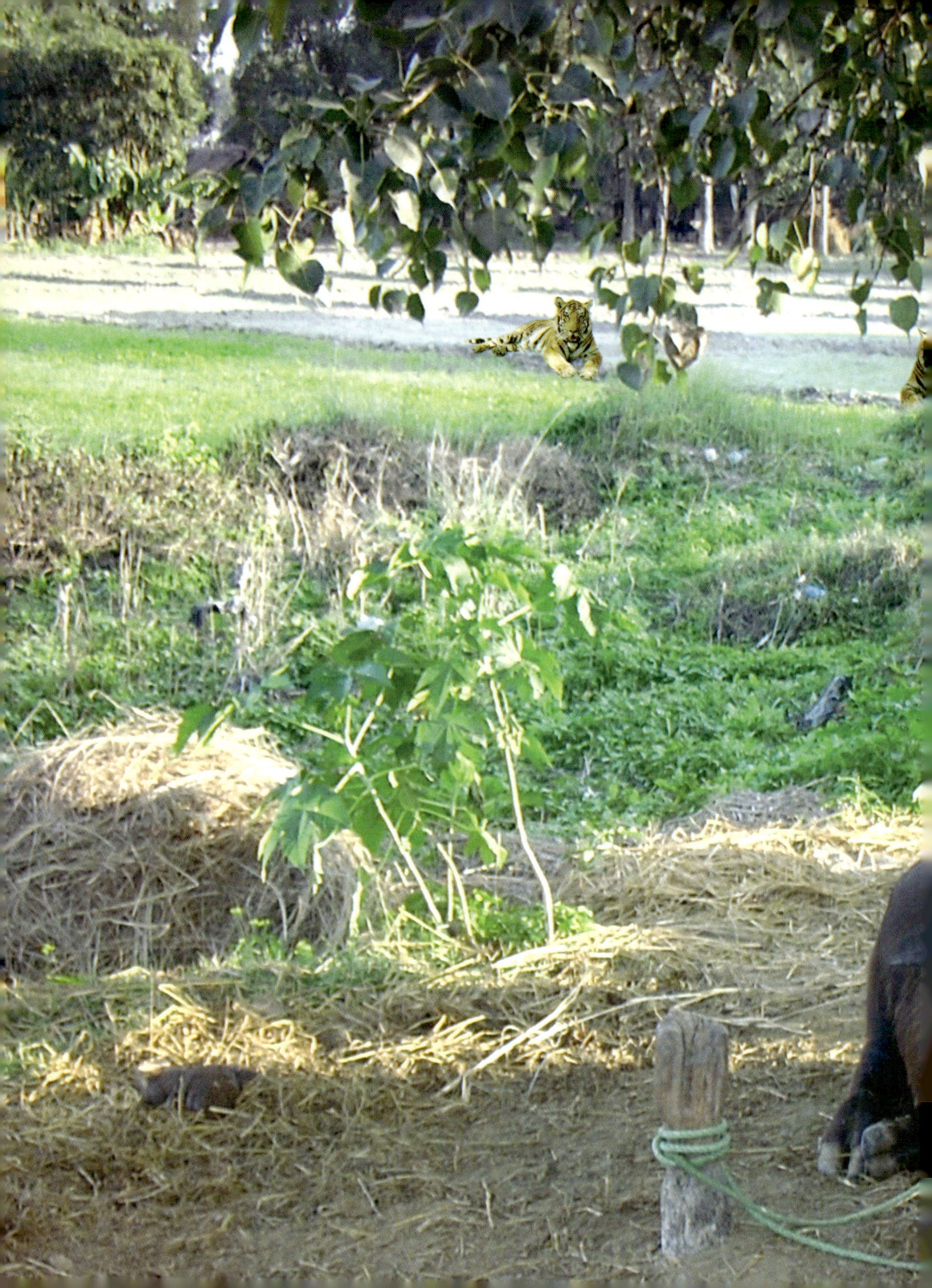

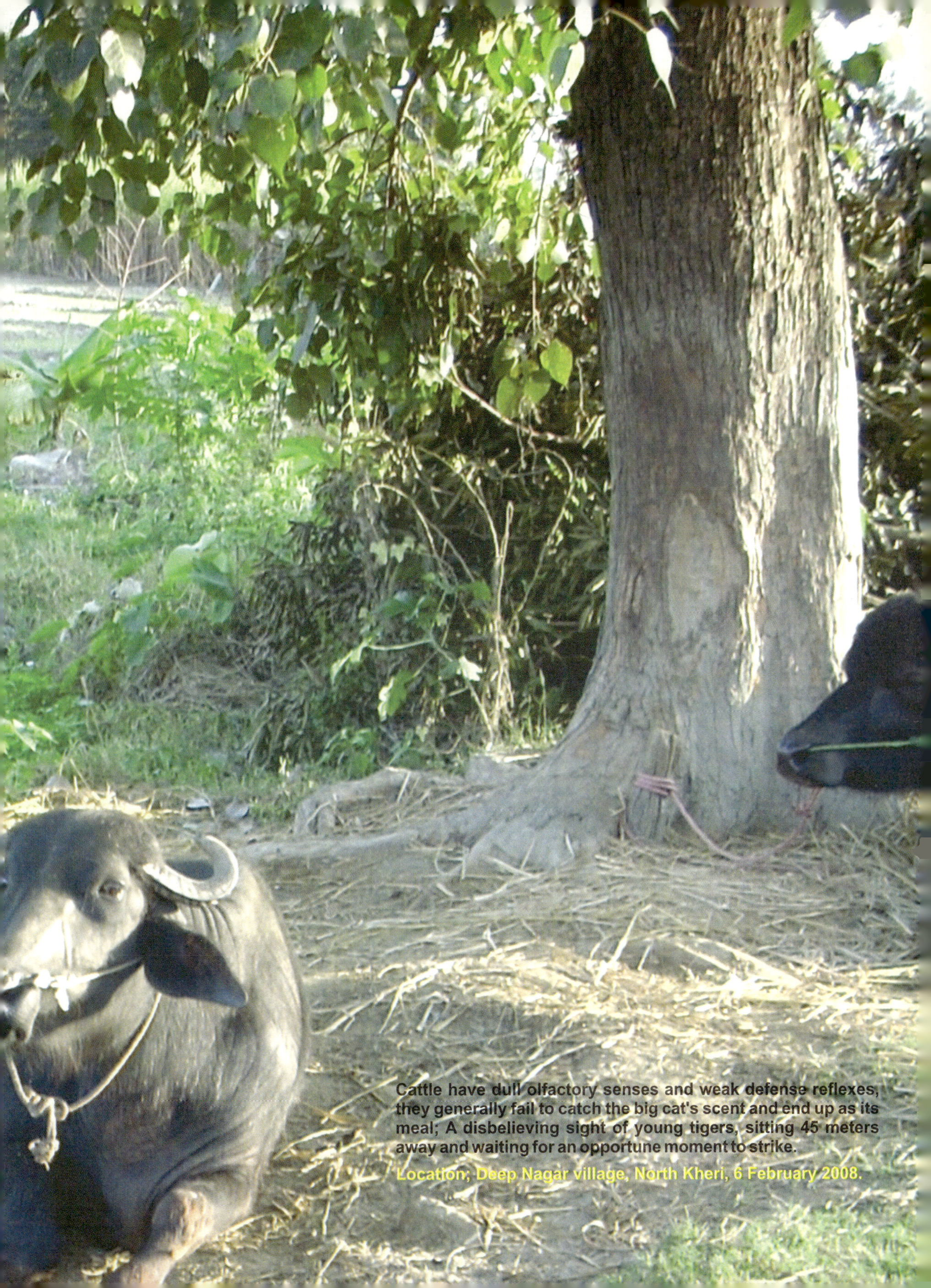

Cattle have dull olfactory senses and weak defense reflexes, they generally fail to catch the big cat's scent and end up as its meal; A disbelieving sight of young tigers, sitting 45 meters away and waiting for an opportune moment to strike.

Location; Deep Nagar village, North Kheri, 6 February 2008.

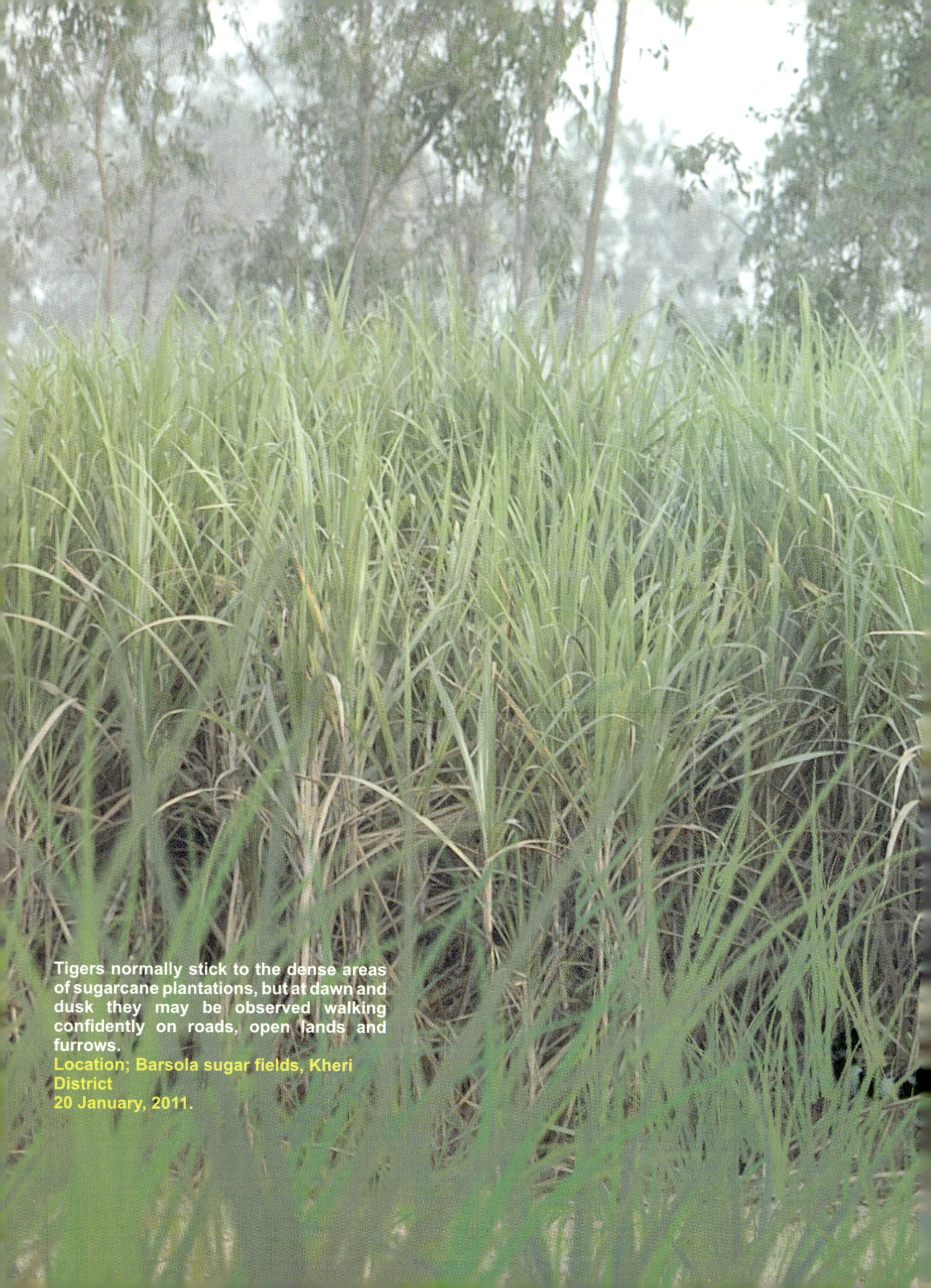

Tigers normally stick to the dense areas of sugarcane plantations, but at dawn and dusk they may be observed walking confidently on roads, open lands and furrows.
Location; Barsola sugar fields, Kheri District
20 January, 2011.

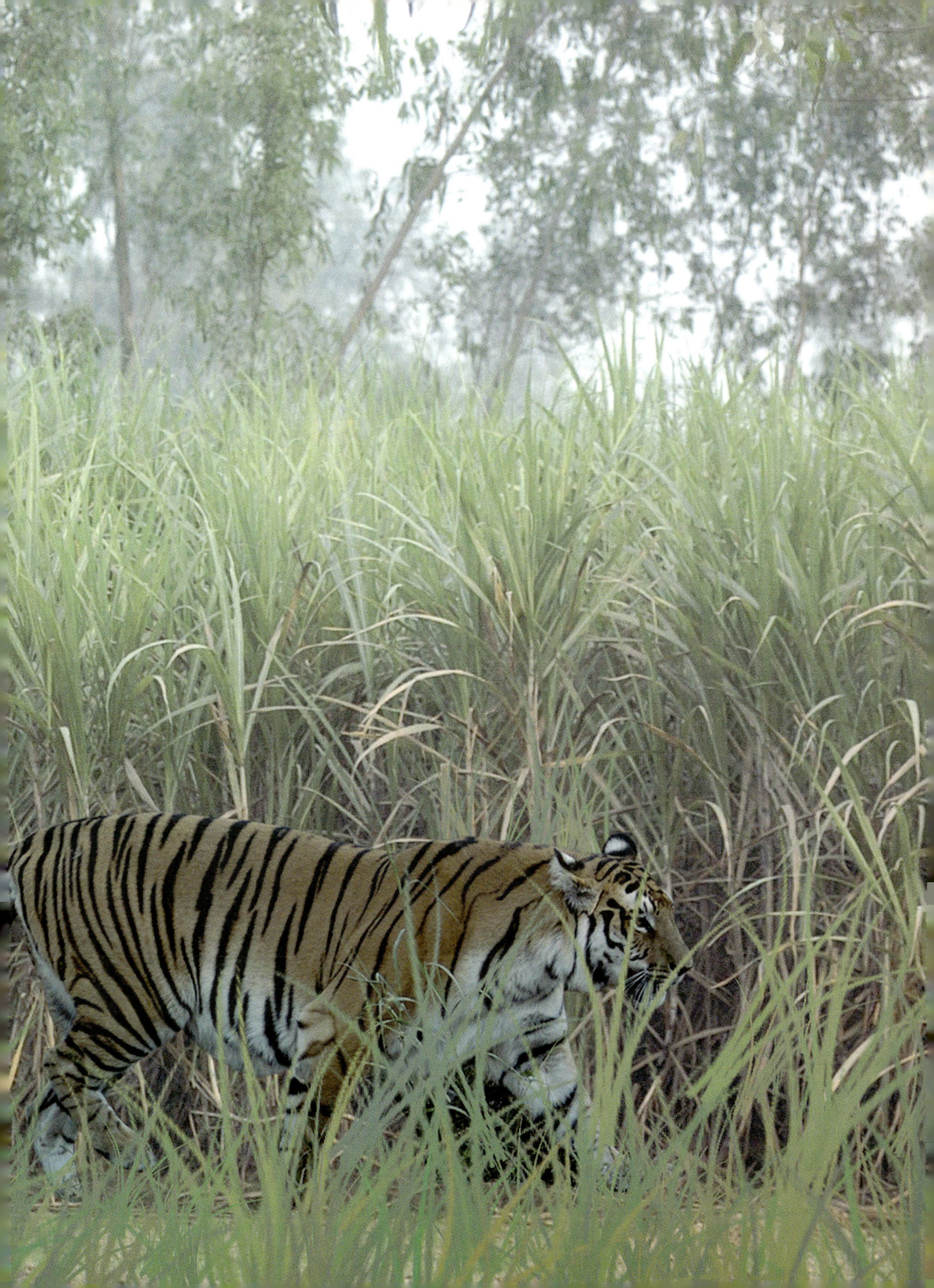

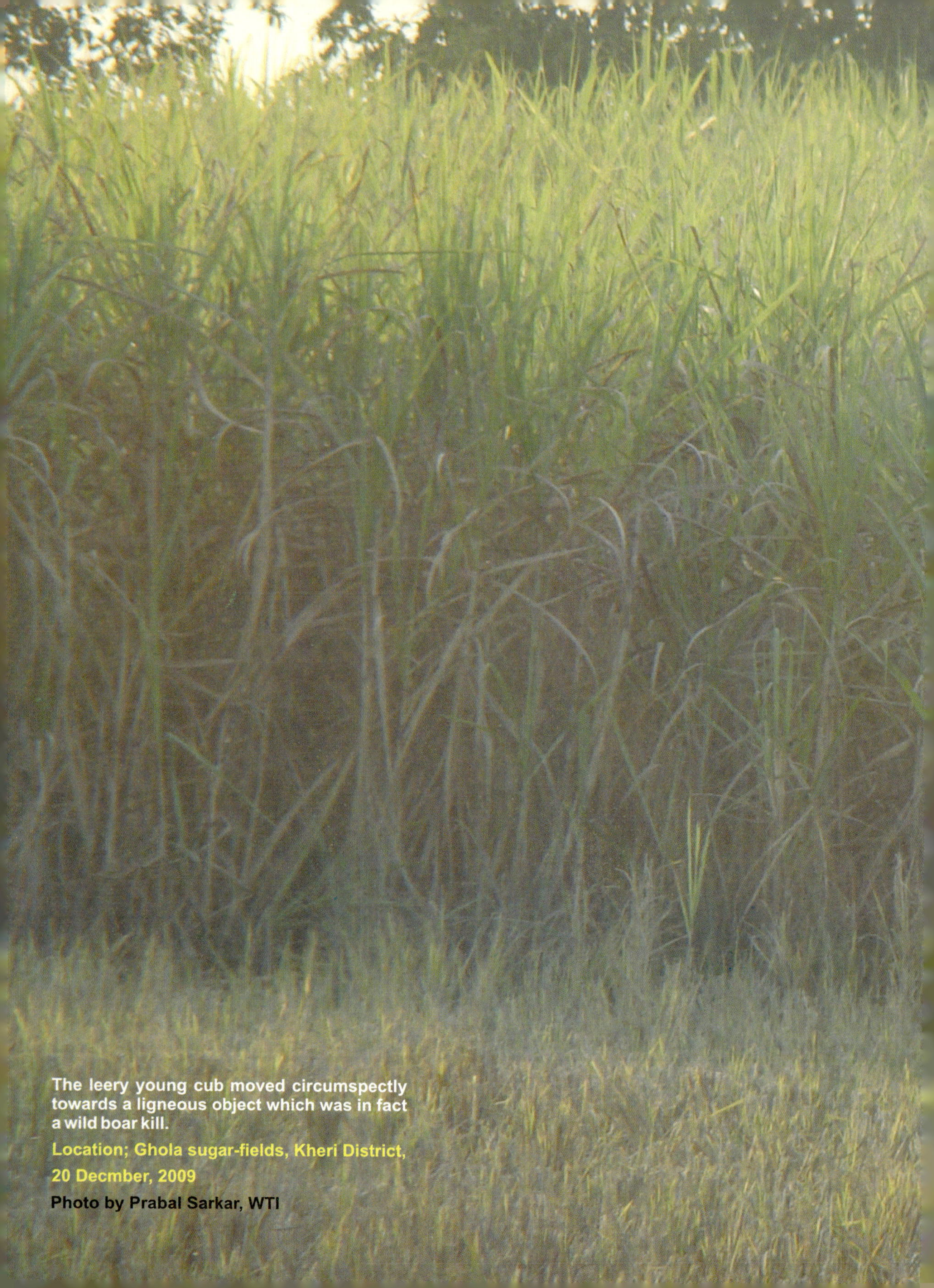

The leery young cub moved circumspectly towards a ligneous object which was in fact a wild boar kill.

Location; Ghola sugar-fields, Kheri District, 20 Decmber, 2009

Photo by Prabal Sarkar, WTI

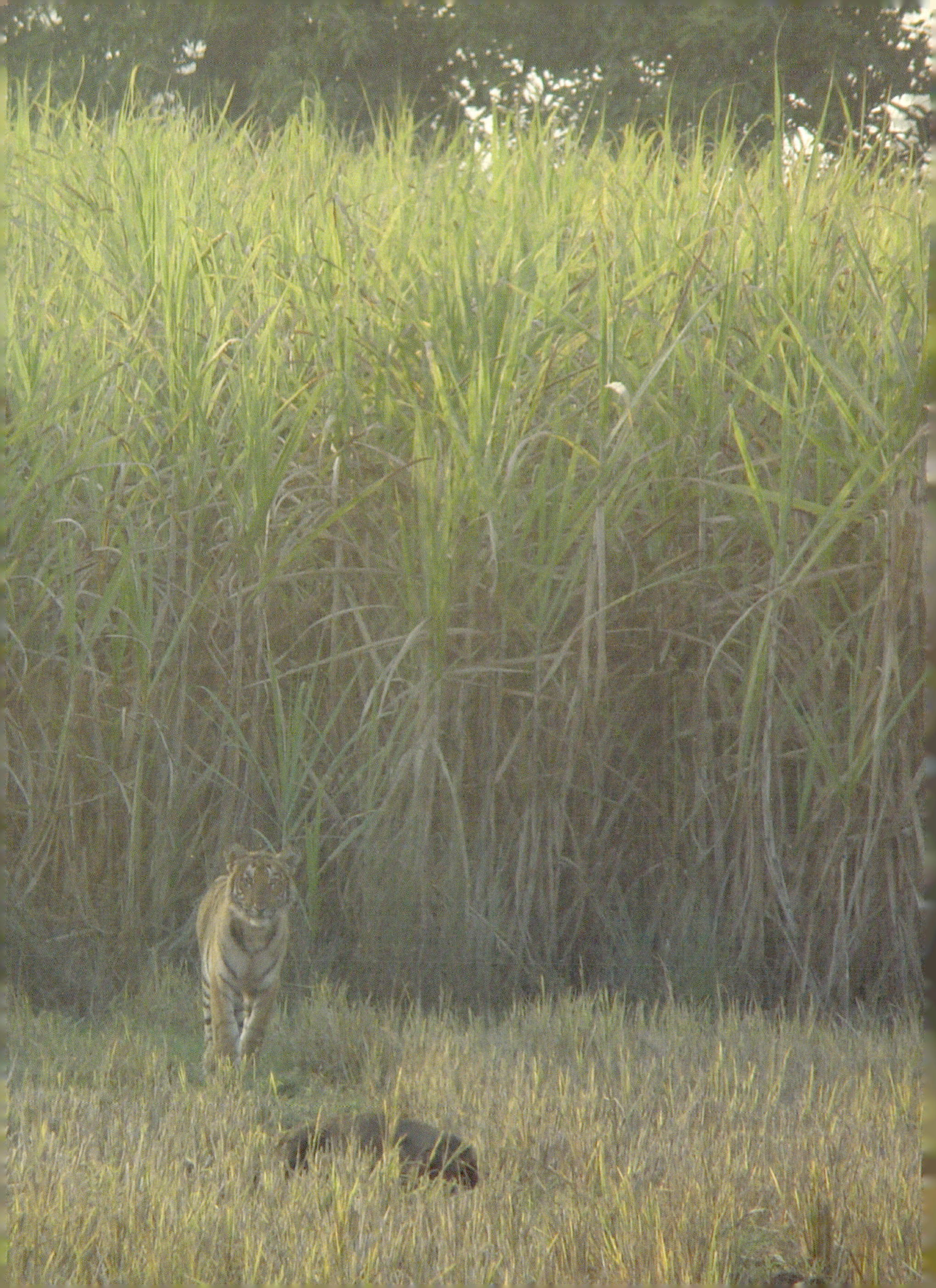

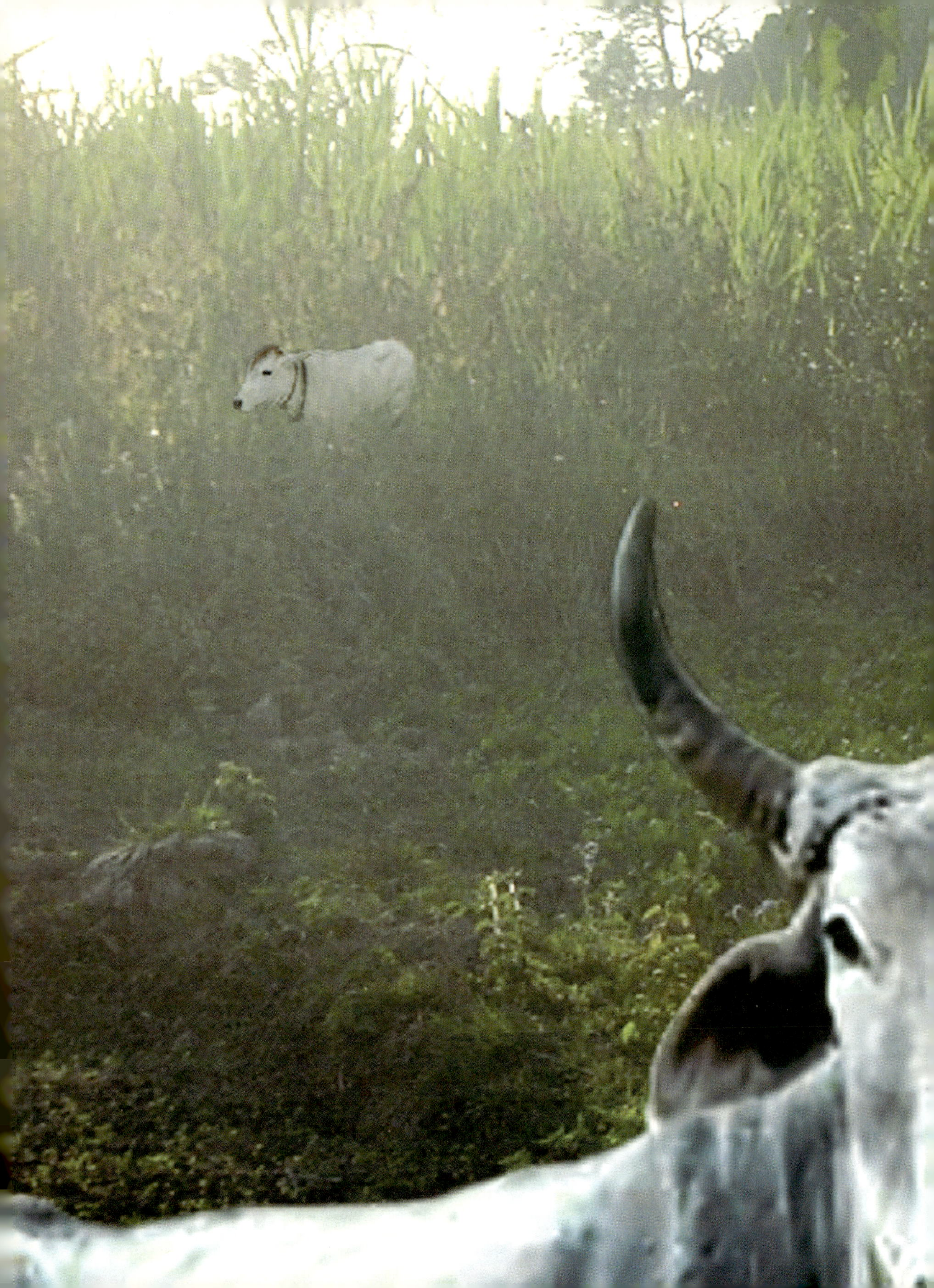

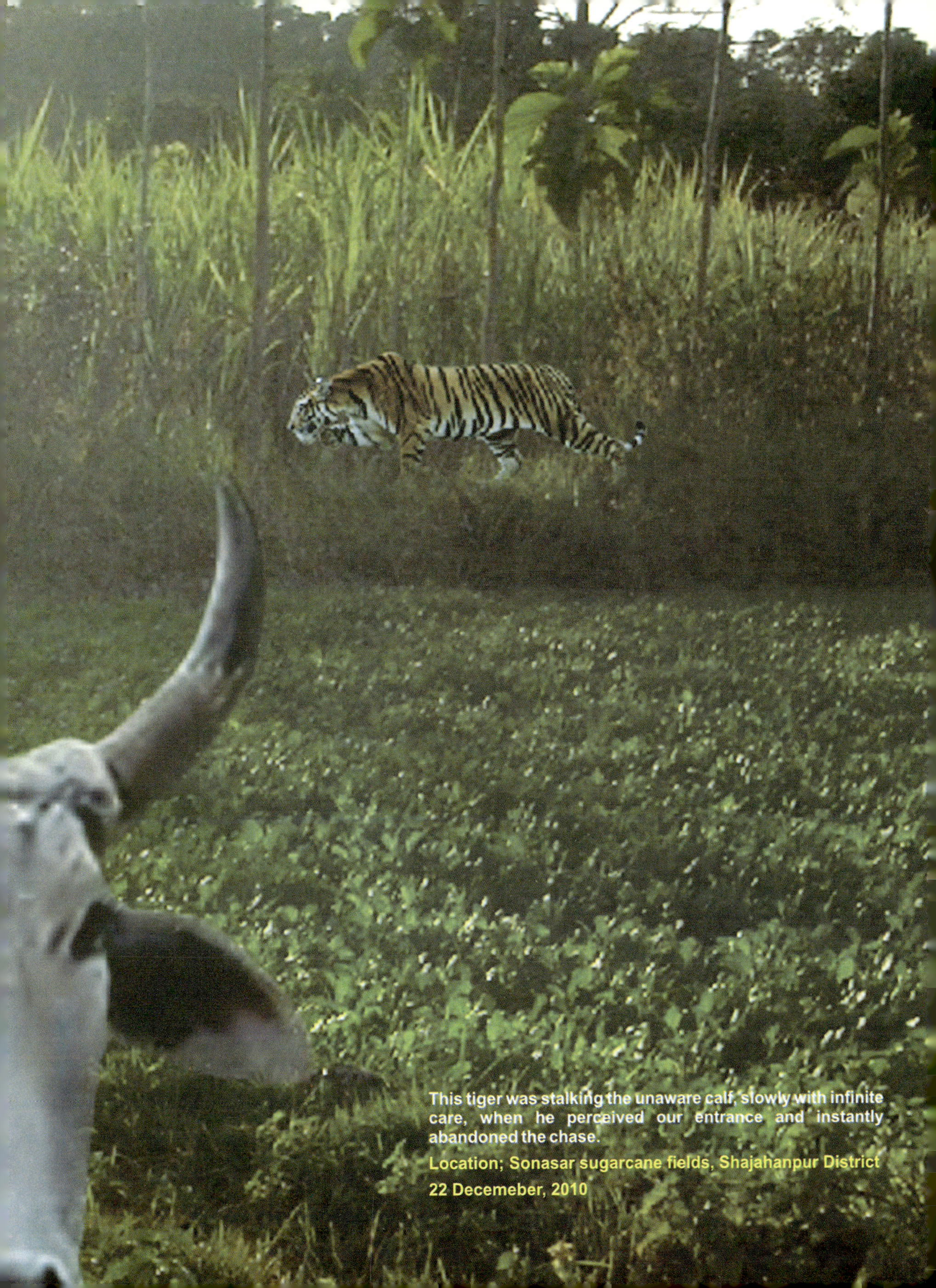

This tiger was stalking the unaware calf, slowly with infinite care, when he perceived our entrance and instantly abandoned the chase.

Location; Sonasar sugarcane fields, Shajahanpur District

22 Decemeber, 2010

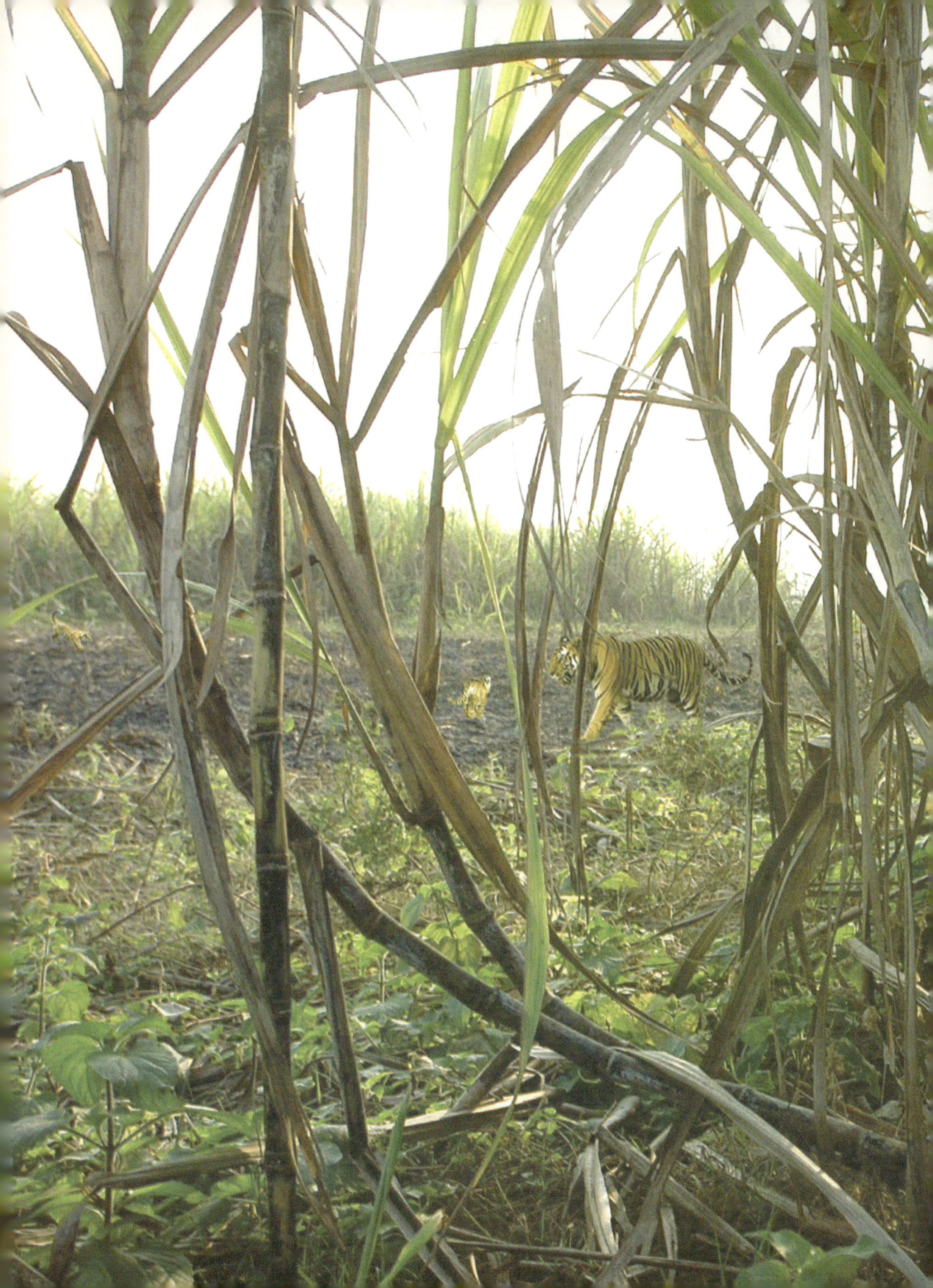

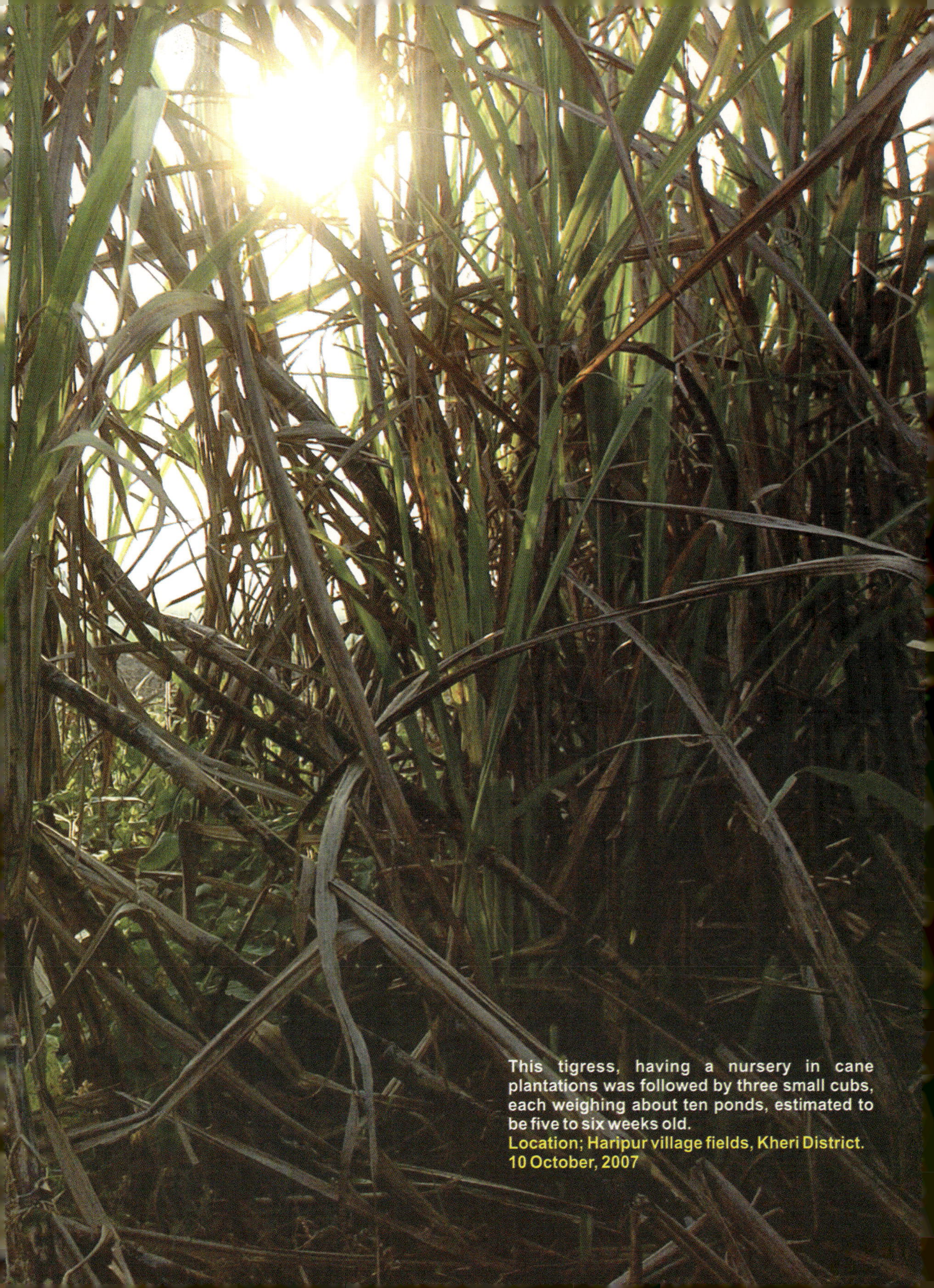

This tigress, having a nursery in cane plantations was followed by three small cubs, each weighing about ten ponds, estimated to be five to six weeks old.
Location; Haripur village fields, Kheri District.
10 October, 2007

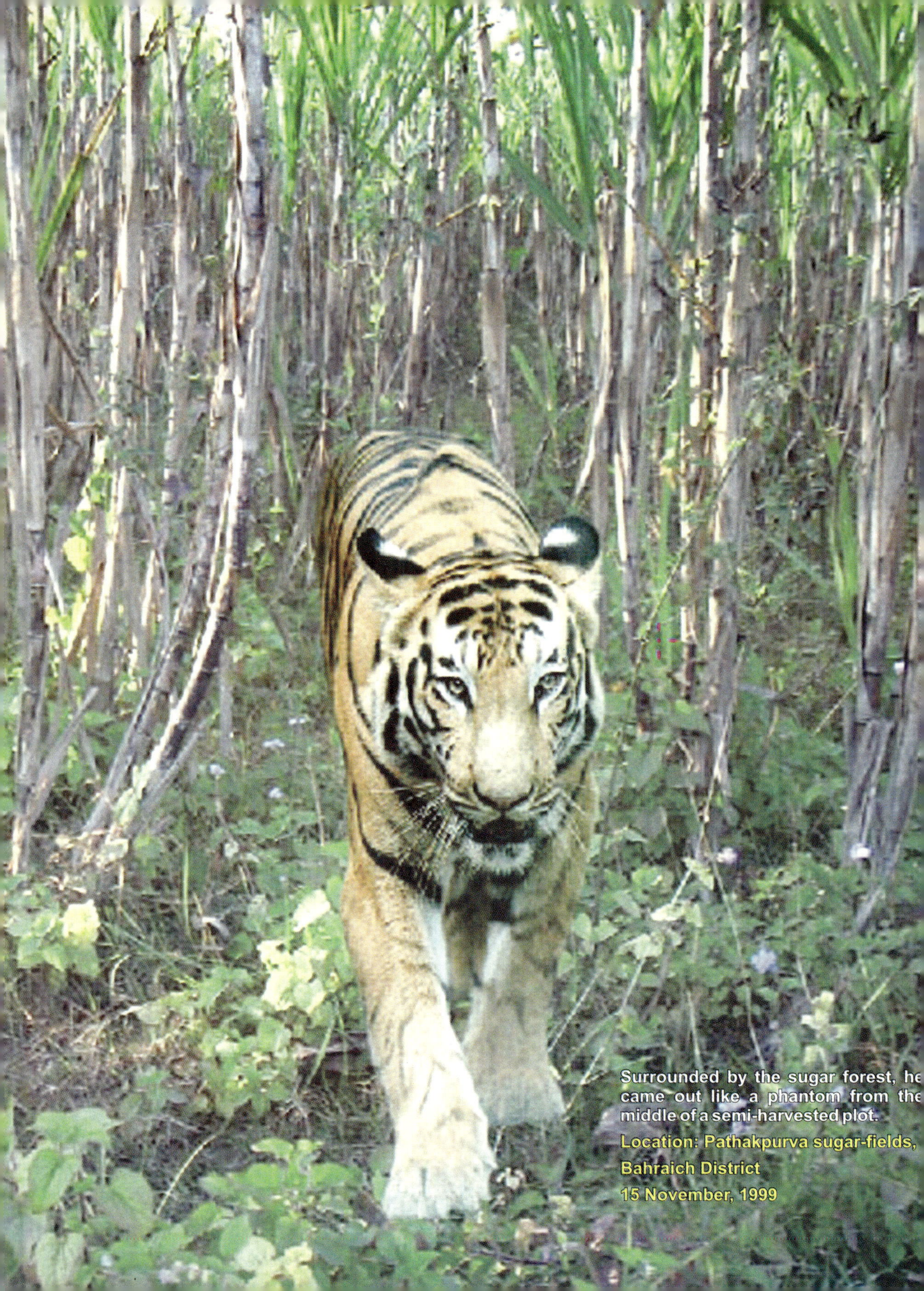

Surrounded by the sugar forest, he came out like a phantom from the middle of a semi-harvested plot.

Location: Pathakpurva sugar-fields, Bahraich District

15 November, 1999

"The human mind cannot form an idea of such a terrifying scene *sahib*. It turned our soul within. I never felt so helpless in my life," said Pradhan as he finished the narrative.

All this had happened within seconds. This can give readers some impression about a tiger's overwhelming powers of destruction. No beast of prey is so exceedingly well equipped and so specialized as tigers are for this particular role in life. It is quite ironical that all the body weaponry of the tiger, meant to subdue and tear apart hard and rough wild prey is almost wasted when he attacks and kills a man, for only a small percent of killing force is put into use. On the other hand, it is also surprising that despite so much of torment, they have still not reacted with even one percent of their total capacity to destroy.

The new development set the policemen on routine work. Bodies of the dead were taken into custody for autopsy, a *Panchnama* was done and the tiger was included in the wanted list of the government.

The Gram Pradhan's father was deeply sore at the fiasco. The old man refurbished me with his interesting theory, "*Sahib* I had asked the men to go and chase the tiger away, but to be sure not to abuse him but they made the mistake. Tigers are very intelligent animals, aware of their invincible position in the jungle. They have a great self-respect which should not be reduced. You abuse them and they know they are being disgraced. They will attack you. But these fools used the most horrible language concerning the tiger's ancestry and its female relatives... now you see what he has done?"

I liked the old man's conviction. This was not just the awe of the tiger imbedded in human psyche, but perhaps the truth that had given the great predator the status of being worshipped as a deity in animistic cultures of the Tarai. Paradoxically, it is this incredible halo of reverence that pervades the minds of these poor people regarding the supernatural powers of the beast that makes them feel quite satisfied to co-exist with it.

As the sun slipped down from the cloudless sky, a pack of jackals wailed and howled from a thickset cane beside a swamp. Customarily, when settlers had cleared the forest for farming, they had left some original trees to mark the memories. While returning, I was shown a withered historical tree, from which many tigers were shot when the area was a unspoiled jungle. Many types of bait had been tied up in the same spot, kills had taken place, and the tiger on each occasion had been driven past the historical tree. Now over forty years of deforestation, when the original forest was some six kilometers away, the tree still seemed to hold some deep-rooted attraction for transiting predators. I remember seeing some semi-fresh scratch marks upon its trunk, which were powerfully raked to the height of seven to eight feet. The animal had evidently stood up on his hind legs and pulled his claws down, making deep incisions in the bark. I was told by the Pradhan that they belonged to the tiger which had caused the debacle.

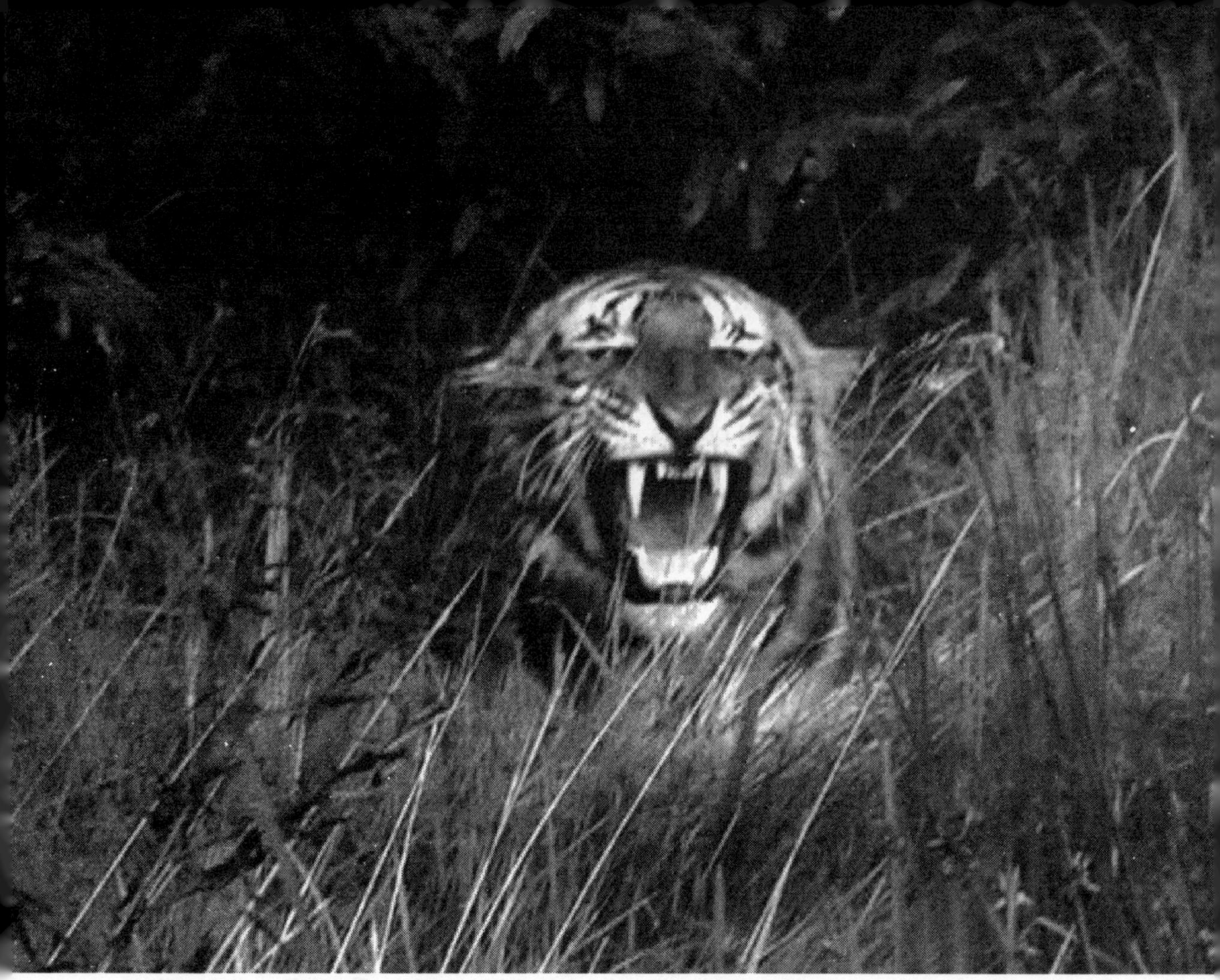

This tiger, hurt by a truck on the Khutar-Gola road, lay starving and suffering from the considerable stress of automobiles speeding past and blowing their horns at full blast. He was sufficiently upset to launch demonstrations on the team, which the author led to rescue it.

After this incident, peace was abruptly restored. What happened to this tiger is a mystery. Did he revert to normal behaviour? Or went back into the jungle or fell to the revenge for the killing of someone? Nothing is known.

In the next instance, I learnt of a new tiger that had entered a cattle pen in Makanpur village and killed six cows, he later attacked a yoked bull and when its owner tried to save it he seized him by the shoulder and took him into the canes alive. He was heard shouting for help, by his fellow-workers and by the time rescuers reached the place the man was dead. The next morning the tiger struck again, seizing an old lady outside her hut, a furlong away from the scene of the previous evening. She too was dead by the time her body was recovered. The villagers felt it was necessary to destroy the tiger, as by all reports it was a confirmed cattle killer that was now getting obstinately aggressive.

A week later, a lame cub jumped over the boundary wall of a railway pointsman's house and killed three goats tethered inside. Another juvenile took away a dog from Tikonia railway platform in the full view of passengers. There were many tigers like this and many stories of similar flavor. They created a terrible reign of havoc for some time, and then either moved to other areas or just disappeared for good. It was largely surmised that the official hunters had failed to identify the man eaters properly, and condemned scores of innocent animals to death. The real ones were still there.

R. L. Singh was sensitive about the whole issue. He told me "Only recently the tiger was a living entity to these people, almost a part of their life. When they talked about it, the reference was never in inimical terms. But now, things have taken a twist. The tiger is still a hard reality in their life but they now rebel against it."

An intense resentment was brewing in the area. Some hot-heads were obviously primed for an open revolt and perhaps a few tigers known to villagers by pet names had suddenly vanished. The revengeful lot had started eliminating them secretly and burying the carcasses in the fields.

It was a tragic situation, as human killings are invariably liable to counter retaliation. I wondered that when at least 100 people die from snake bites in the same Tarai for each one killed by a tiger, or even infinitely more numbers die by traffic accidents in undisciplined and overcrowded cities of India, then no such popular reaction is ever recorded. Why, then, such an uproar over killings by the tiger?

In far-off areas some more tigers were being heard of. Some of them had earned an undeserved reputation for being man-eaters which in fact they were not. To my mind besides normal tigers, there are two categories of recluse animals. One is the raven 'aberrant' and the other is the genuine 'potential man-eater', though both of these tigers are disoriented in their depredated habitat but there is a large degree of variance in their attitudes that can better be described as intransigent and confused. There is a very fine line between the two but that is a very important difference nonetheless.

It is similar to how a common man, who does not know about the great school of thoughts, does not know how Hobbs differs from Russo. While discussing giant thinkers one unconsciously crosses the diaphanous border and enters into the realm of the other and goes on unabated in the name of the first. Here, the situation was quite similar, there were many foresters whose walls were covered with wildlife diplomas but who had somehow managed to remain ignorant the difference between aberrant tiger and man eaters. Instead of intellectually rationalizing the nuances of the incorrigible man-eaters and aberrants, they talked about all nonconforming tigers as man-eaters, whereas there is no enigma about these two types.

They did not realize the trauma of their competitive existences, where hunger played a big role throwing such tigers away from natural controls. Until this unique incongruity was properly understood, the man-eating problem was liable to be mixed up inextricably with that of innocent beasts. The dichotomy was the thin edge of the wedge which increasingly justified the thoughtless elimination of the predator.

Most of the man-killer tigers come into the category of aberrant, each of them

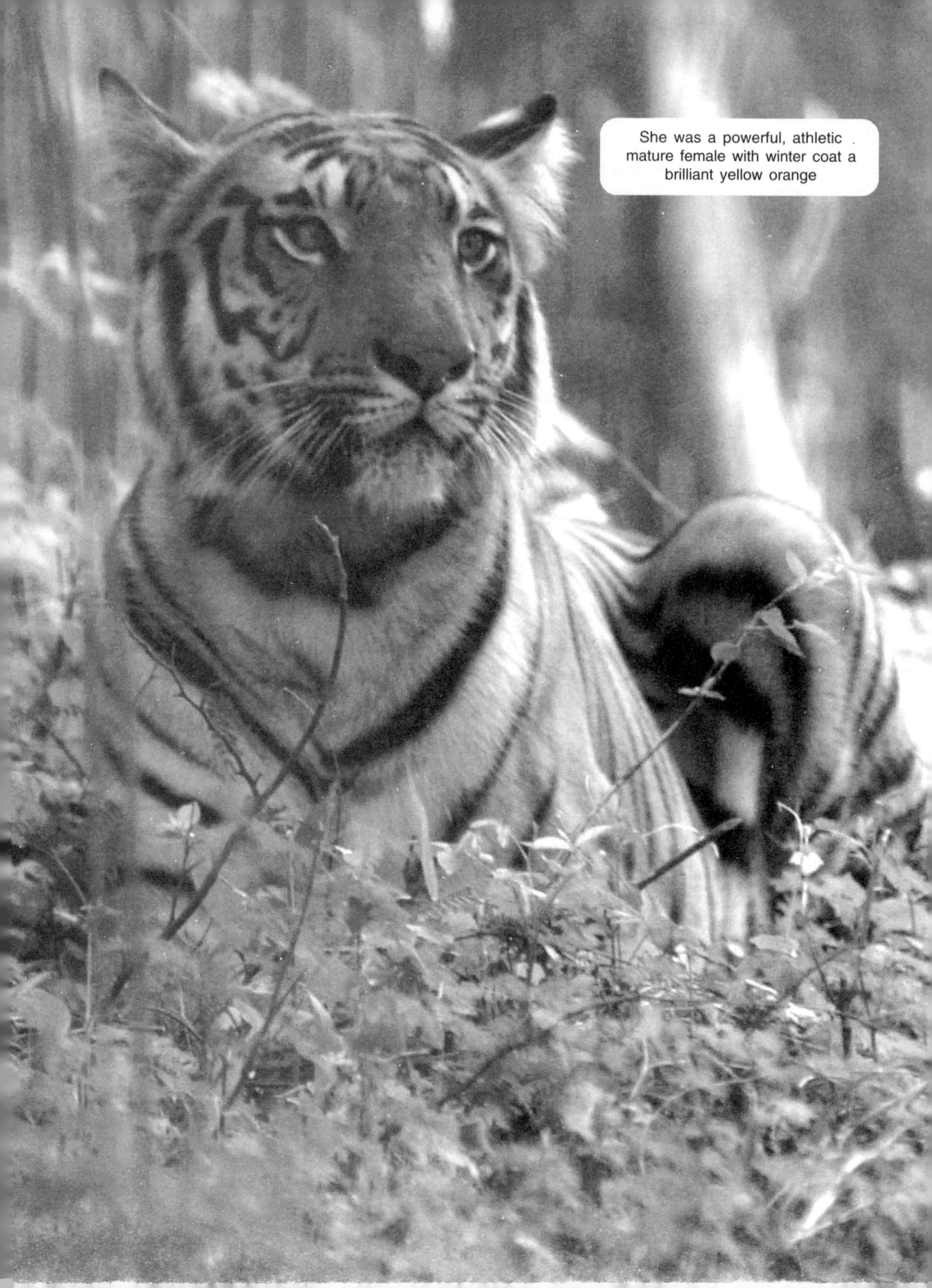

She was a powerful, athletic mature female with winter coat a brilliant yellow orange

claiming no more than one or two victims, such beasts usually attack someone who accidentally stumbles on the animal while it is on its prey, or if it is a female, with cubs. Man-eaters on the other hand, systematically seek human flesh and terrorize the district, where sometimes entire villages are deserted.

It is very much in the framework to mention Locke's observations that there are some tigers that will hardly ever come back to the dead animal which they have left uneaten of their own accord. He writes, "It is hard to account for these apparently aimless kills when the tiger goes to a great deal of trouble to secure them, but the fact remains that such instances do occur. There is no apparent reason why the kill is left?"

When tigers are known to lose all interest even in the often selected natural kills and abandon them uneaten, the normal tigers will invariably prefer to leave their unnatural kill — the accidental human kill — without protest.

I do not think other tigers are attracted to such human kills at all, though in one case, I have known pariah dogs to have eaten a human corpse for a change of taste, before it was recovered. It is surprising that the most ancient friend of mankind, dogs grow in human association yet they often refuge to acknowledge the established bond and are disposed to feed on human corpses whereas obligate carnivores like tigers, on realizing their mistake immediately abandon them and never return. Again it is a display of distaste and tigerine sanctity rather than the murderous blood thirst; they are so often accused of vehemently.

Aberrant tigers are those who having killed a man usually leave the body or at the most break their fast on its genitals. I have seen some 14 accidental human kills by tigers out of which 6 corpses had their genitals missing. Incidentally most of these had sustained deep canine injuries on the rear skull and nape and also some claw scratches on the back.

Tigers normally begin to eat from the rump of prey. It appears that the contour of human body is unfamiliar to tigers and therefore they are not sure where to begin eating it from. The normal attire of a village man, *dhoti* or *lungi* is loosely wound round the waist, it often falls out in the drag that follows the kill and the genitals are exposed. Even if there is no sufficient inducement for feeding but out of curiosity, a small bite is usually taken at the protruding soft parts of the body, which is genital in man and breast in women. This reticence may apply only to the first or at the most to the second kill and despite their having made a small meal of a human part, these tigers are certainly not man-eaters.

As the argument was in progress, I wondered if humans really constituted an exclusive diet for even one fourth of these tigers. On an average 2000 individuals would have been killed each year by only 25 tigers. The average body weight of a mal-nourished Indian villager is 40 kilograms and generally a tiger requires about ten kg of meat every day, but this was never the case. On an average 30 persons fell victim to the tiger every year and more than half of them were left uneaten, which only formed 0.1 percent of total diet need of these tigers.

Despite the large population of tigers in sugarcane, confirmed man-eaters appeared very rare and this was proof enough that man is not the normal prey species for tigers, even where the tigers are accustomed to human presence.

At Ghola, I met a man named Shiv Shanker. By an amazing coincidence, he had been seized by a tiger twice within a month. One night he was guarding his crops when a tiger walked up to him and seized him through his quilt, under which he was sheltering from the cold. Fortunately, the man's lantern overturned and set fire to the straw and the tiger decamped. Some three weeks later, the same man was stripping the cane and telling the story of his encounter to another man, when the same tiger materialized on the scene and pounced upon the man he had missed the last time. Shiv Shankar had a large piece of cloth wound round his head. The tiger caught him by the head and began to drag him. The man suffered a severe scalp wound but was not fatally injured. Meanwhile, the other cane workers began to wield sickle and axes and raised a yell. At this the tiger left his victim and ran away.

"I survived because I bear the name of Lord Shiva. He is "*Mahamrityunjaya*" the conqueror of death", said Shiv Shankar. The man had possibly created a world record of having escaped twice from the jaws of a stubborn man-eater. This seems to have impressed him with the idea that he was not destined to be killed by a tiger. Last I met him in 1999; he was happily stripping cane, and the very area was again harboring a tiger.

A week after this incident another man was killed. He along with his wife and daughter was going to meet someone when he squatted on the wayside by the edge of a sugarcane field to piddle. It was late afternoon and suddenly the tiger seized him and dragged him into the crops. His friend who was just returning after leaving him set fire to the cane to scare off the tiger, while a tractor was also driven in the half burnt field but by the time they found his body, the man was already dead.

From 1976 to 1985 over 200 human deaths by tigers were confirmed officially in seven districts of the Tarai, and the toll seemed to be spiralling unavoidably upwards. I had been watching the developments for years. In 1978, 26 people were killed by tigers for the record. In 1979, some 30 people were killed, that also included 22 human kills by Billy Arjan Singh's Tara. In 1980, the toll demitted to 18, in 1981 it was 39, in 1982 it dropped to 16, in 1983 it rose to the highest of 41, in 1984 it was 28, in 1985 it was 25 and in 1986 some 35 human deaths by tigers were recorded; twelve of them were laborers, eighteen were travelers and the remaining five were grazers. This count included the people who were left wounded by tigers and died later but not those who survived the attacks.

It may be admitted that deaths attributed to this cause had been sometimes due to foul means, because in the villages, the distance from a police or forest station being long, a body was often cremated before the officials were able to reach the spot to determine the cause of death. But the unofficial number of deaths was naturally much higher. Though 90 per cent of human corpses were left uneaten, with only genitals missing in some of them, every single human death was a tragedy that posed a severe threat to the future of the tiger, when officially it was still in the danger of extinction.

It was not easy to ascertain the reason for this chaos. For example, there were sugar areas outside principal forest formations in Pilibhit and Udham Singh Nagar that recorded the maximum concentration of the tigers; with 40% availability of tiger pugmarks, the account for human causality was nearly zero while fields around Katarnia Ghat area recorded only 10% of tiger population of the sanctuary in sugar fields, yet it was a hot spot of man-tiger conflict. In 1985, it contributed quite a significant percentage of human causalities that amounted to nearly 30%.

The very year, I was invited by the Chief Secretary of the state, Girish Mehra, to investigate the causes of problem and suggest the remedy. The baseline investigation revealed that though a tiger's position in the crops is often known to the villagers and they do exercise precautions but the most immediate threat to farmers were tigresses that were rearing cubs. It is time when tigresses are sharply alert to any danger and do not keep their young ones for too long at any one place. Their habit of shifting their cubs as a routine safety measure renders farm labors particularly vulnerable to their attacks anywhere in the terrain.

Moreover, there were non-irrigated patches of sugar crops, which when dry during the frost, were almost certain to hold a tiger. During the sharp bouts of frost towards January, tigers lived here because these were the warm spots.

There seemed no immediate remedy to this tricky situation. Anti-tiger forces were active and the villagers had automatically ganged up with them. The attitude of the forest department caused a greater dissatisfaction. They were blamed for not taking serious action to eliminate the subsequent contagion of man-eaters; and because of the lack of the procedures to isolate and identify notorious individuals; most of the anger was vent upon innocents. Many tigers who had never harmed anybody and who had no track record of man-eating were shot down by foresters. The second crack-down against man-eaters was an ensuing confusion, in which some 10 more animals were accounted for.

Government files are maintained meticulously. One tiger who had scrounged on hen and dogs in sugar fields was notified as the notorious Sarkhana man-eater and another mangy juvenile who had traversed miles of flooded lands to reach Barar farms in Pilibhit was noted as Banbasa man-killer, and a famished cub who had entered a settlement in search of food and was killed by a heavy blow of a lathi on its head was declared the man-killer of Katanga in Udham Singh Nagar district. And a tiger shot dead at old Jalpaniya swamp, near Sitarganj was also declared a suspected man-eater, without proper evidence or evaluation after it was killed.

A former student of LCC who was a DFO in Bahraich district once told me, "Sir, great felines do rouse predatory instincts in us. At the time of their destruction an intense but surprising excitement seems to take possession over my team and we justify all action. This feeling is strong enough to wipe out all twinges of consciences and pity".

Yes, he was right. This atavistic trait, concealed deeply by layers of civilization may seem non-existent in some educated people but it is like a hidden claw of ultimate killer, wrapped in a velvet glove of tutored intelligence that suddenly comes out when the murderous instinct is stirred up.

The police are often blamed for fabricating encounters while the real criminals elope; consequently, the errant cops are not only reprimanded but punished also. In the same manner, the feat of shooting teams, often singularly unqualified to deal with the situation, must also be investigated thoroughly and its pseudo heroes be penalized for slaughtering a National Animal, without establishing its proper identity as a man-eater. Fake human killings are always liable to snowball for the police but unfortunately dead tigers don't tell tales, so these image-building criminals remain immune to punishment for inflicting wanton abuse on innocent animals. This is the tragedy of wildlife.

Till now, there had been occasional discoveries of tiger carcasses in the cane fields of Tarai, most of whom had died of poisoning. Now the genocide seemed to have been accelerated. Three dead tigers were found floating down the Sharda canal. It seemed that after being poisoned and overcome by raging thirst they had collapsed as they drank, or perhaps poachers were ferrying the booty, when their boat capsized and the carcasses were washed away. No wonder a local politician analyzed the situation as uncompromising where tigers of Kheri, disgruntled with their managers, were committing egoistical-suicide by jumping into the river.

In March 1984 some Tharu tribals set fire to a patch of crop near their village known to contain a tigress and her cubs. The mother escaped but the next day, the charred bodies of five tiny cubs were found lying in the ashes. While they were being removed the tigress arrived back on the scene and followed the men, demonstrating vigorously. I also learnt of three cubs and their mother escaping the same fate narrowly in another fire, set near a village called Mahola on the Pilibhit border. Two tigers had been run over by railway engines in Dudhwa and over half a dozen knocked down on metalled roads by speeding trucks that move all through the day. Five poisoned tigers were found lying next to cattle surrounded by dead vultures and jackals, which too had paid with their life for eating a poisoned carcass. They were shot, trapped in nets and Jin traps, electrocuted by stretching live wires along the boundaries of fields. A forest guard was found burning a carcass of a tiger in Kishanpur area. A tigress was found dead in a sugar plot near the bustling township of Khutar with a compact bunch of LG pellets in her head.

A curious scene of reckoning was witnessed by hundreds of passengers from a train. It was early morning; the train had left the Tikonia railway station and was passing through cultivation fields. The passengers saw a man shooting a fleeing tiger from the driving seat of a tractor. He was firing as rapidly as he could work the lever of his rifle. Bullets rained around the animal, kicking up dust in the harvested fields and ricocheting off into space, like angry bees. The breathtaking scene lasted for some five seconds and finally the quarry disappeared, seemingly unmolested, crashing down through thick canes, in long, heavy bounds.

In 1986, the situation turned even grimmer as 14 tiger carcasses were found in the fields around Dudhwa. Three of them were killed by the use of sulphos and presented a dreadful sight. Their stiff petrified bodies, whose graceful silhouettes had once adorned the horizons of evening, lay gouged out, disemboweled and awkward in their rancid exposure. This poisoning generates toxic gas, which gives blue black color to complete lining of digestive system and the stomach blots. All of these were healthy, able bodied animals, with no physical infirmities; their coats glowed in the sheer flow of their youth.

It was greatly distressing to find that 11 out of these were young tigresses in excellent physical condition. The loss of a tiger is little, but the loss of a young tigress is invariably the potential loss of ten to twelve tigers -for optimally, a young tigress produces two to three cubs every alternate year, between her fourth and fourteenth year, and raises at least one cub to maturity.

In my enduring fascination for tigers I may add that the machismo of a tiger's head, enormous neck and heavy fulvous forearms can only be appreciated by those who have seen one dead; some four hundred pounds of muscle fused with the dynamite of power and defiance and much as one feels a pang of remorse for so handsome a beast being laid low by petty rascals. If the tiger must die, then surely the weapon of his death should be of the highest caliber, but here was the anti-climax, the feat had now been debased to the dirty trick of chemical poisoning.

Journalists had gathered like hyenas, to feed on the news of tiger-corpses, felled by the natives in historic battle for survival. The liquid notes of a cuckoo suffused melancholy in the surroundings as she cried her heart out at this misfortune. So far as I knew the feats of daring that had once captured the imagination of heroics, fostering an image of masculinity for claiming the dangerous animal, had never been so dishonored as now. Many of these animals were not even culpable in human terms. It was difficult to restrain the pangs of remorse at their ignoble passing.

During this time, my crusade of 'saving men from tigers' was in its nascent stage, now almost two years old and hugely successful. It visualized, that the cultivation of 'Conservation Will' results in increased levels of forbearance towards carnivores by local people, thus promoting a viable path towards coexistence. The actual fulcrum of my intervention was to provide a safer heaven to big cats. But instead of addressing this line of approach, news bulletins were flooded with the reports about the end of the tyranny of the animals. It was lauded as the success of natives, who were strained to check the growth of a menace to keep the tigers down to a reasonable number, while for the politicians, this killing of valued wildlife was the native way to demand justice and a resounding way of 'being heard', after years of grievances. Conservation groups were losing hope. Doomsayers were making self-fulfilling prophesy and the experts, having lost the clarity of mind, looked at the reports of disaster as unique.

This was a harsh, callused piece of evidence glowering in the cane fields of Kheri with an overwhelming force. The situation warranted a warning signal to guard against future ecological disasters, but the authorities in New Delhi were arguing on logical lines: "With all the noise and activity in farm lands it seems beyond reason that any wild animal would risk its life in such surroundings."

It was after much ruckus created by the conservationist lobby that a bureaucrat from the capital came to make an appraisal of the problem. He stayed in the Dudhwa rest house and the next morning when he went out to have tea at the outer canteen, he found imprints of a tiger on the dust road, superimposed on human foot prints, that he considered his own. "Wow, is it not the cane tiger?" he asked the people around.

"No sir, cane tigers do not occur in the jungles, they live in sugar fields only, this is a sugar-free tiger." replied Naseem, a fêted wildlife guide of the Park.

One chief wildlife warden, at a loss as to what to do, decided to outsource the solution. He issued an order that all the free ranging tigers outside the National Park should be captured and be trans-located or be incarcerated into zoos. It was a clear instance of wrong human intervention but unfortunately the imperative solution to the problem of carnivores has always been a call for their removal. I felt sorry at the decision. Conventional zoos are in reality animal prisons and as tigers cannot change their basic biological traits -they have to live on flesh- it is the final disgrace for a predator of infinite freedom to be locked up, in segregated surroundings. Schetini de Azevedo and Cipreste's studies on captive wild carnivores' show, that shifting animals -even those that have been in captivity- into another new enclosure significantly increases their stress level. A prolonged heightened stress brings about hormonal changes which not only augments their aggression resulting in injury against steel bars but also brings about stress related deaths. The ghetto of a zoo makes the caricature of a noble beast, as the powers of those enormous limbs and claws waste away and a gaunt and listless form assumes a bored expression of collapsed beast.

Consequently one problem individual and his six innocent kens were caught and incarcerated into the zoos. These mislead people into the belief that they all had been saved whereas in reality four of the beasts died within a month of their capture. The lack of guidelines to managers on pre and post capture of the conflict management was responsible for this unprofessional conduct. Without a manual containing inputs from scientists, experienced managers and veterinarians, they did not know how to take care of the animal. However, as a fanatical response to the popular doomsday prophecies about tigers, the unnecessary intervention of 'Capture-Tiger' continued but surprisingly even this did not cause any substantial dent in the problem.

(II)

Out of a dozen mammalian predators operating in the farmlands of the Tarai, sugarcane tigers were now the most conspicuous predators in the neighborhood of villages. I noticed that the man-tiger conflict was of three types -- killing domesticated cattle, accidental attack on human beings which may destroy or incapacitate the victim, and eventually the deliberate hunt of a man as prey. This last and ultimate factor of man-eating is much accentuated by a combination of circumstances and I was quite doubtful about it. For this pattern of man-eating was being wrongly equated with the compulsive and selective preying of humans as described by Jim Corbett or by John Patterson of '*Man-eaters of Tsavo*' fame or in more recent accounts given by George Adamson and Norman Carr. Kenneth Anderson also describes two cases of such types but the author is more accused

The crop protectionists were generally armed with unlicensed shotguns and hesitated to shoot tigers, but accidents did take place in the nights when the identity of animal ensnared in nets was mistaken.

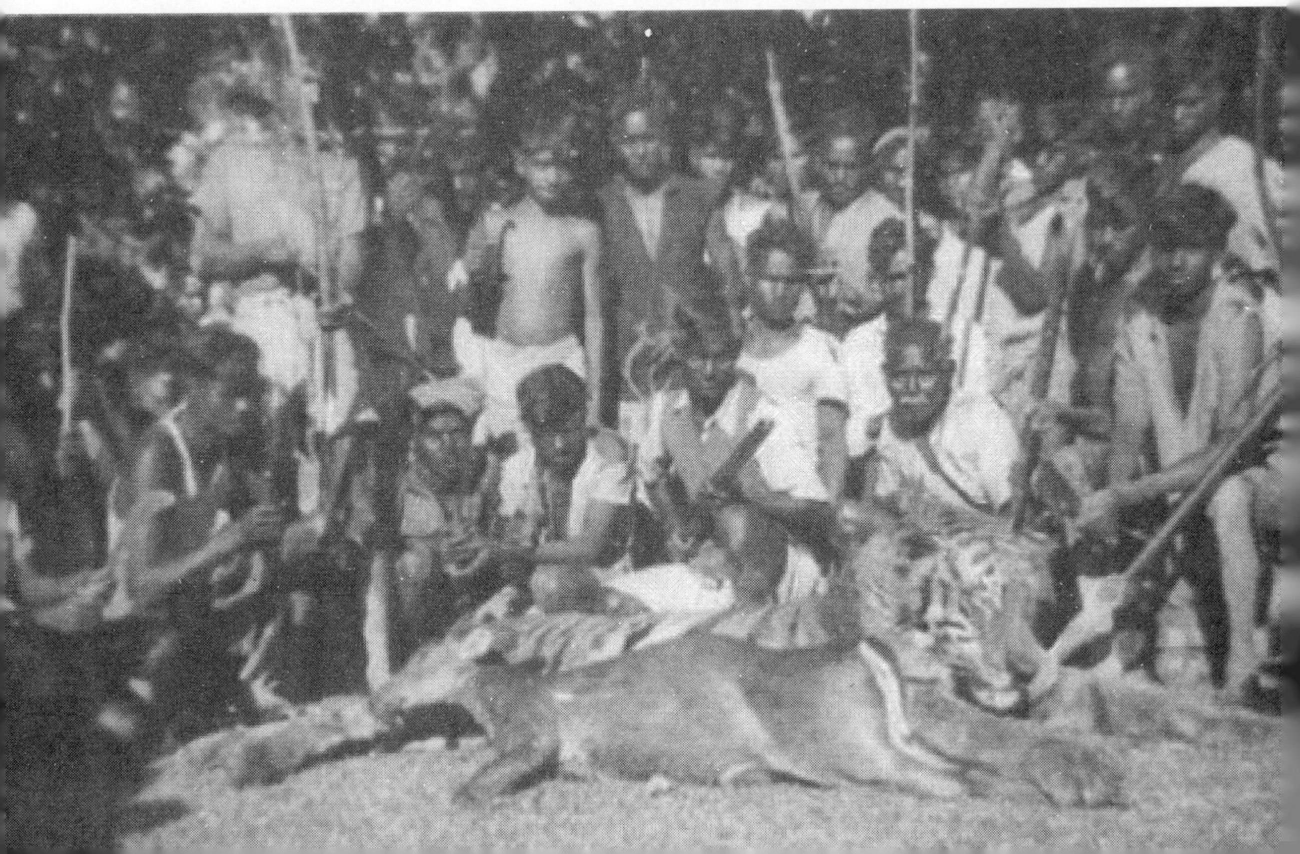

for producing reams of fiction, and his writing is taken lightly by experts because of its dubious veracity. To my mind the local problem of man-eating was an animal deviation only in the classified sense of human values; indeed, the fall out of socio-ecological incompatibility and its resultant confusion.

If the foodstuff for the carnivore is scarce in a landscape then their response is to traverse across a wider area in search of food, thus the tiger's continuous presence in the croplands implied the existence of enough cattle, dogs and goat as food to support it and also the increasing latency for conflict with man. There was a serious lack of information on the livestock-carnivore conflict aspect of the phenomenon and I needed to understand as how this contributed to the creation of problem individuals.

Livestock husbandry is a part of culture in the Tarai. Consequently a vast number of domestic animals which are undernourished, unproductive and diseased are not done away with but are allowed to exist on religious grounds. They graze without restrictions in virtually all the forests and sanctuary areas and cause serious damage to the ground vegetation, culminating in the widespread erosion that is particularly common in fragmented forests.

Interestingly the scourge of abandoned cattle compensates for the shortage of food for cane tigers. Statistics by Schaller and MacDougal suggest that out of twenty attempts made by tigers, only one succeeds in getting it a slain prey. In comparison to the hard work of game killing, a cattle killing is no challenge at all for a big cat. Success is absolutely assured.

My investigations found that the tigresses of the area were potentially inclined to have a meal set upon cattle. Some of them had even made cattle their staple diet. Perhaps they were raising cubs and during this period the mothers are most insecure. If humans intrude in their area, they show a promise of violence in defense of their cubs and remain an imminent danger for several months. This is the time when they also look for easy food, and cattle both feral and domestic, give them a real edge in sustaining the family. In areas with a large cattle population and the wildlife having driven away, the tigresses in trying to get at the cattle sometimes accidentally killed several herdsmen, as they will knock down any obstruction that stands in their way. If for some reason the cattle escape, the tigress returns to the first knocked down victim and begins feeding. This combination of circumstances is rare but when it happens, the tiger invariably becomes a man-eater as such accidental killing, often forever, puts an end to the instinctive dread of man and prompts its sudden acceptance as food.

Scientists believe that an intense compulsion is required before a tiger embarks upon the alien diet of human flesh. My experience proves that it is more aggravated by high rate of accidental-confrontations of tiger and man than the essential scarcity of prey species. However, nature has made tigers the predators of the highest degree and the great Homo, primarily being an animal was their natural food for long, before it became Sapiens and moved out of their prey list.

It seems unlikely that only a small percentage of tigers should come into conflict with man when there was a substantial number sharing the same living conditions. To understand this unique variance we must examine the ethological traits of tigers. Though it is difficult to put down inflexible rules in this regard but right from the nineteenth century some experts appeared inclined to assign certain reactions to the tigers in their encounter with humans and they termed it as personality. In the context of sugarcane tigers this model seems relevantly applicable.

In dealing with the animal kingdom, it is dangerous to try to establish an intellectual hierarchy. Anthropomorphism often leads us astray. Nonetheless my own experience suggests that the tigers living in the biotically disturbed complexes are in fact clever beasts. Their constant and extraordinary association with man has tutored them with time serving manners. A few tigers react against the ravages of their eco-systems when the cane is harvested while others just avoid the harvesters. A few take it casually and a fewer still react timidly and run away into other fields. They display a great variety of personality and approach towards man and their characters vary as much as those of humans.

It bears remembering that in that period about forty percent of the land area in the Indian peninsula consisted of forests and tigers had a verdant habitat to operate in. Their prime homes always remained undisturbed and inaccessible. Between the jungles and pockets of cultivation there existed naturally huge buffer areas of scrub and grass lands. Thus both the species, viz humans and tigers, had ample room to avoid each other. It will not be an exaggeration to say that in those days, despite hunting being prevalent, many tigers still lived in peace and died a natural death, without ever setting an eye on a human being in their life.

Now the situation had reversed and there was nothing bizarre about the present outburst of man-tiger conflict; the reason was the advancement of human settlements into tiger habitat and its negative consequences. In some particular areas farm tigers came across much larger human settlements, where the prey animals had been obviously reduced by crop protection guns, which in absolute terms were substantial and the cane had been planted right to the boundary of the village and attack on livestock indicated that wild prey is not present in sufficient numbers; thus virtually almost all the ingredients towards coexistence were missing.

The influence of the environment on animal behaviour needs to be understood. For in day-to-day life animals interact with the environment on a one-to-one basis. Different environments condition behavior in many ways. Some tigers, bamboozled by this turbulence often come into direct conflict with humans and create problems. The familiarity with man develops a strong sense of courage in them. Quite a few individuals, who have accumulated experience about mans' limitations and helplessness and their success in escaping from any probable harm from man, even exaggerate their reactions against the species. Their hunting instinct guides them to approach man as he is the easiest prey. The weaker or the smaller the prey is, the less reason for the nicety of a clean kill, one preying lizard can easily hold down a struggling fly or one bird of prey a sparrow, whilst the meal is begun. Such tigers often begin to feed on their catch immediately and do not bother to kill them.

All these factors reinforced by my field surveys' prove that the causes of man-tiger conflict are simple. The sugar tigers at the first opportunity exploit the resources of food supply raised by humans-and occasionally even humans as food supply. Their curiosity and basic fear of man is considerably diluted, they disregard human presence and are not much effected by lights, sounds, and movements of the mechanical gadgets used in cultivation. The act invariably lands them in competition with man. Unprovoked demonstrations are occasionally heard of. Excessive slaughter of cattle often occurs. On opportunity, they kill more than needed and are bold enough not to relinquish their kills when challenged.

The predatory inclination of a tiger is triggered off by instinct. His solid armory, ultra fast reflexes and habitat of restricted vision dictates its natural impulse to attack abruptly on moving targets, and an unexpected meeting with man is liable to produce disastrous consequences for the latter. We must remember three things; first the tiger's large upstanding ears are highly attuned to catch air borne sounds. Like other cats, they can register sounds in the frequency range of 100-200 KHz as opposed to the maximum 20 KHz or so that the humans can hear and in respect to these sounds its sense of direction is extraordinarily accurate. Secondly their forward facing eyes, like humans, register a considerable overlap in the images which results in binocular vision allowing the assessment of distances on a very fine scale. And thirdly, a tiger's muffled tread and sinuous gliding movement combines to affect his stealthy approach to his prey. They are marvelously fit for striking the prey, holding and killing it immediately. From these facts flow certain consequences that can lead to an instantaneous death of fragile species like humans.

Tigers are also exempted from the complications of dentition. They have scissors like teeth and four long straight canines set in a short muzzle. There are gaps in the jaws just behind the canines to permit these teeth to submerge fully into the body of the prey. Lateral motion is absent in the jaws of a tiger. Their broad condyle bone is set so perfectly into its socket, that a prey's departure from up and down scissors like action is impossible and so is escape from its claws. They remain sheathed in its talons and are kept sharp and safe by this peculiar arrangement. While catching the prey, they suddenly project out, hold and demobilize the animal. Precisely all these arrangements ensure the greatest power of destruction and the simplest mechanism for producing it.

Man is so feeble an animal that tigers do not require any special method to kill him. Given this propensity, even if it catches a human being haphazardly, his claws and teeth strive to retain the hold on the struggling and moving body with two massive paws encircling each shoulder. The jaws exert a pressure of 500 kilograms per square inch. Thus the injuries inflected within a span of few seconds are mostly fatal and man, the paragon of animals, instantly reverts two million years back to a defenseless prey, crumpled to earth with colossal weight upon him. By the time the big cat realizes its mistake of having caught something it does not require and leaves the victim, it is all over for the poor chap.

The accidental killing of a man helps the tiger overcome his generation bred reluctance to attack man and it may at times induce an individual member of the tribe to include humans in the list of its prey, or may even convert him into a habitual man-eater.

The tiger's attack is extremely dreadful. They are predators of huge dimensions. It is difficult to escape their formidable armor. I personally know over a dozen men who have been mauled by tigers. In every case they have been partially or more than half crippled. Some have lost arms or legs and others might as well have had them amputated for they are of little use to them. Apropos their strength, Brander mentions an incident in which a "man-eating tiger had driven in a man's skull into the torso, simply with a blow from its paw delivered on the top of his head."

I endorse it, for I have personally examined the corpses of three cane strippers, Dubar, Ram Adhin and Tauley, all killed by Katna man-eating tigress near the bustling township of Gola and Sarju Jatav of Sitarganj, whose necks were completely broken by the stroke of tiger's arm. I believe that tiger's forepaw is a real engine of destruction and the weight of the limb is the valid cause of the mischief. Thomas Williamson, (1807) in his book *Oriental Field Sports* tells that the operation of a tigers forepaw is "Similar to that of a hammer, the tiger raising his paw and bringing it down with such a force as not only to stun the common size buffalo but often crushing the bones of the skull."

To my mind, even the attack of inexperienced tiger cubs that are over six months old, are hazardous, for their phylo-genetic inheritance commands them the procedures of killing and they instinctively aim for the neck of their victim.

The result of this build-up was essentially an unprecedented increase in the number of man-killers. The Dudhwa tigers seemed to have dwarfed the intemperate man-killers of Sunderbans. It was an extraordinary situation. I had witnessed the whole gamut closely, from its commencement to accentuation, and also the changing paradigms of man-tiger conflict. One of the key components to this disaster was the attitude of natives who had developed increasingly hardened feelings towards wildlife. The ongoing onslaught of retaliations had left many a normal beasts injured and incapacitated and thus qualifying them to agree to or decide on aberrant behaviour. The vacant territory of such animals when captured or removed was filled by younger animals, which potentially proved more dangerous in their normal, inexperienced and disoriented state of mind, than the previous, 'partially invalid' but experienced occupants.

It was a clear cut case of mismanaging carnivores' population in populous country

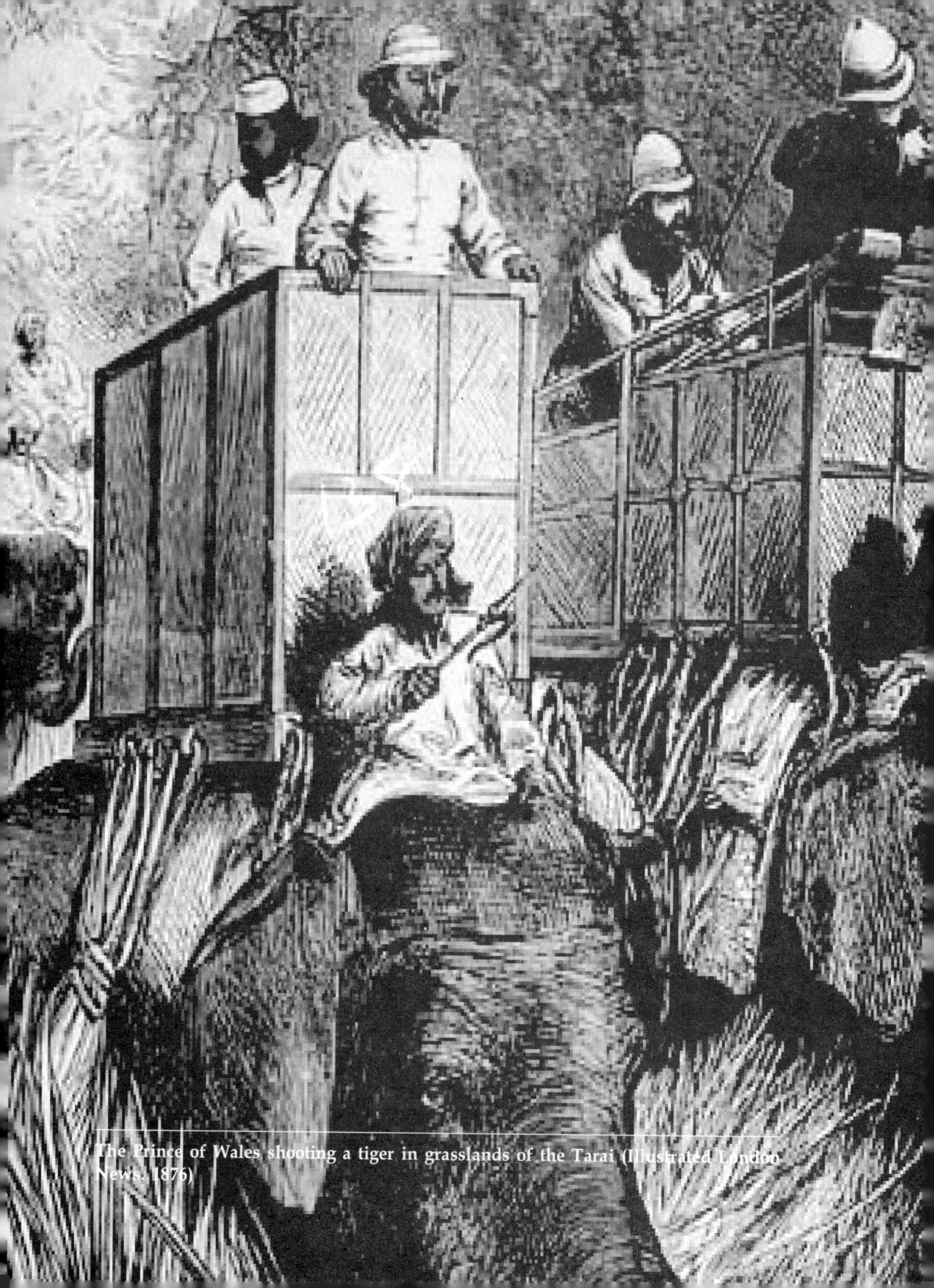

The Prince of Wales shooting a tiger in grasslands of the Tarai (Illustrated London News. 1876)

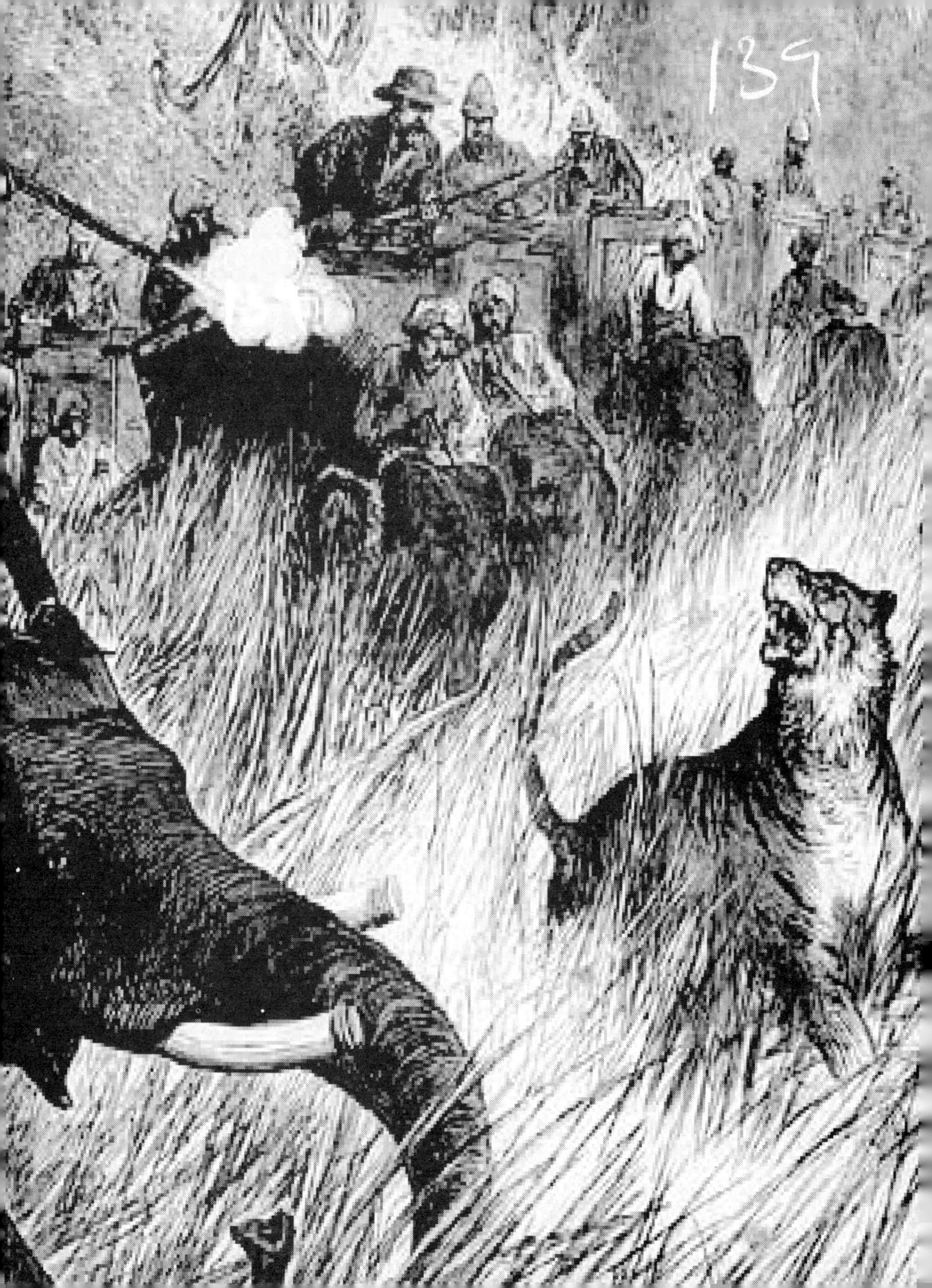

like India, which had lead to an increase in their potential for danger. Small hamlets, consisting of small farmer families had since become the hot spots of conflict. With both feline and villagers sensing the threat from each other, the vulnerability of both had increased manifold.

A closer look at the data indicated that purposeful attacks by tigers were isolated either temporarily or spatially. Premeditated attacks were anomalies, some of which had elusive inconclusiveness - a way of dropping the victim and fading away- needed to be examined on a scientific scale. Poets and dreamers might see such actions as compassionate but it is just an aspect of the unending temperament of big cats. In fact, no one knew why tigers behaved like this. It seemed like a wonderful combination of romance and frosty inescapable truth about their changing state of mind but there was no meticulous underpinning to this behavior.

It was obvious that a good enough understanding of tigers modes had gone astray and experts were unable to give a rational answer for it. So I maintained that at this stage of confusion, my idea of sugarcane tiger is at least better than none. Carnivores have wide ranging habits and the only possible conclusion is that the conflict, which was earlier made of 'stress of circumstances', wounds or old age, now is the direct result of adaptability of tigers to human dominated terrains. Different Environments condition animal behavior in different ways; hence a scientific understanding of landscape ecology and its connection to tiger biology was the desperate need of hour.

I was disappointed and worried. I wrote letters to the Forest Department, but they being too pre-occupied about schemes of revenue generation failed to respond. The Project Tiger bureaucrats seemed singularly unqualified to deal with the problem. They failed to figure out the fundamentals of this conundrum and grasp my side of the picture. Perhaps, because of data scarcity, the outdated notion was still heavy on the minds of authorities; much like the 10th century Christians, who considered an earthquake to be a display of God's will, rather than like the 20th century westerners who understand the upheaval in terms of geological shifts.

Interestingly, in the treatise of science, one important aspect of paradigms is that they are incommensurable, which means that two paradigms cannot be reconciled with each other because they cannot be subjected to the same measure or common standard of comparison. That is, no meaningful comparison between them is possible without fundamental modifications in the concepts which are part of the paradigms being compared. It is not knowledge opposed to knowledge, but this was a different knowledge altogether. I wanted the experts to think outside 'the box', for it more meaningfully defined an explanatory model of a new tiger crisis. It was not the equation of man being in the jungle like in the Sunderbans and getting eaten there but this was of some tigers moving in the human zone and then taking to inveterate depredations.

The appalling surprise was that when all the obdurate man-eaters had been destroyed, why were humans still being attacked by tigers? Were the farmlands of Tarai destined to be ruled by born man-eaters? Or all this gory extravaganza of 'tooth and claws' was just accidental; simply because a necessary change was wanted at several different levels in the human approach towards tigers, such as that of farmers, rural labors and small traders who moved in sugar crops and whose current methods of dealing with the dangerous animals only resulted in an increased aggression. It was apparent that many people, public representatives, managers, telecasters and media anchors were not aware of the biology of the animal and its relation to the problem.

Perhaps the cane tiger phenomenon still did not fit into the conceptual framework of the managers. Besides, as an attitudinal change among local people is generally difficult to achieve at such a large scale; various sections of rural community also needed to be educated on this line.

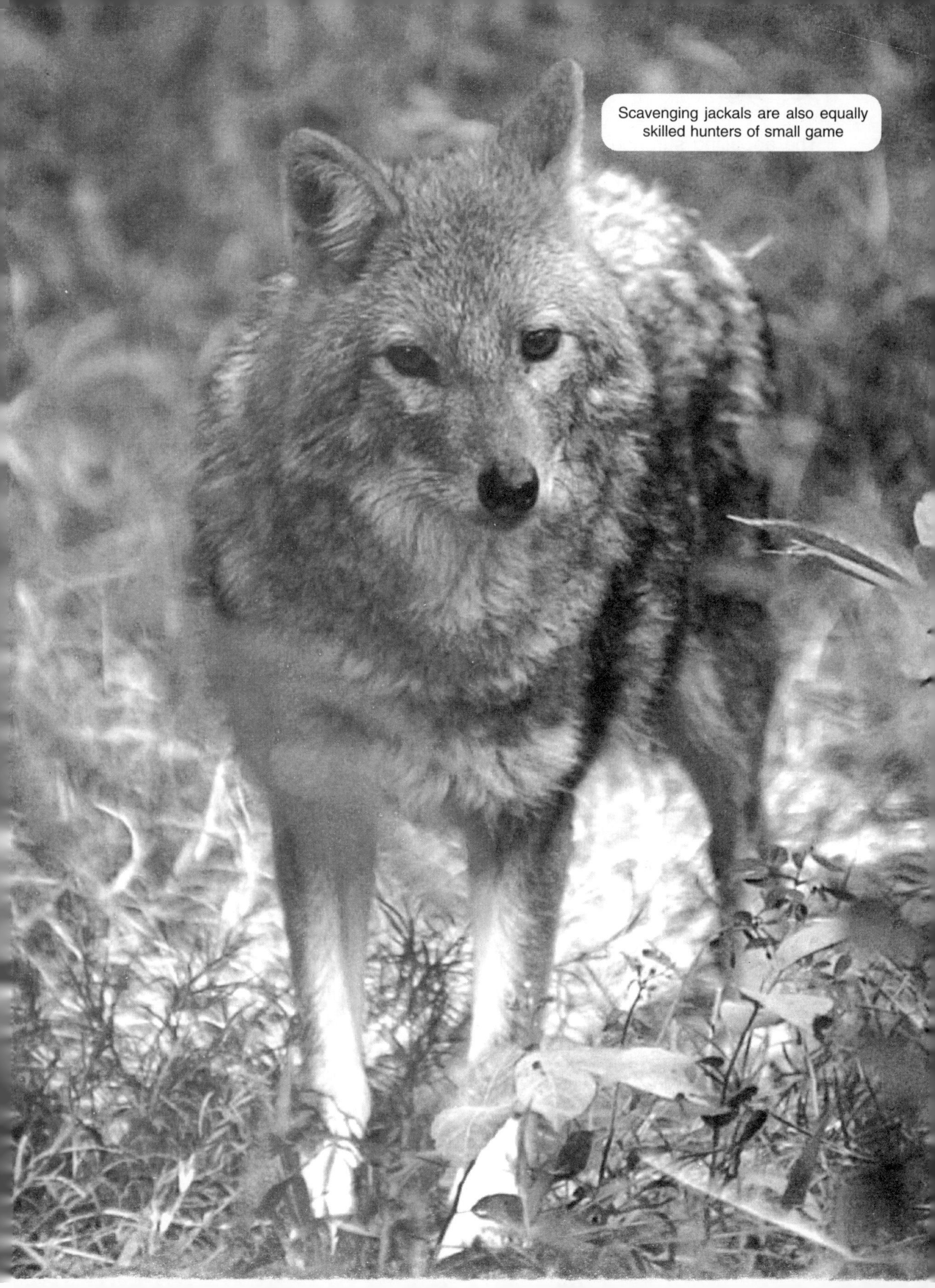

Scavenging jackals are also equally skilled hunters of small game

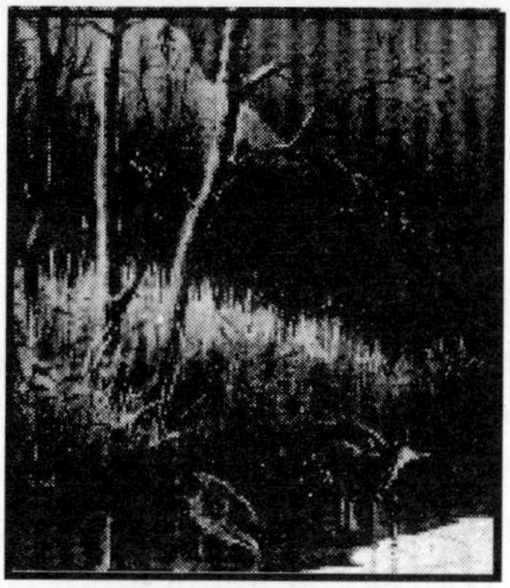

13

The Barotha Tigers

"Cats are a mysterious kind of folk. There is more passing in their minds than we are aware of."

- Sir Walter Scott

I am one of those for whom the call of wild is irresistible, however reassuring the amenities of civilization may be. In the middle of October 1987, I had the tiger itch overcoming me. The monsoon was over and the oppressive heat of summer had gone by when I eagerly planned my trip to Himalayan Tarai, just like the old childish trick of reaching after the moon. Only in this case the moon was an emotion; the thrilling adventure of chasing tigers in the freedom of humungous farmlands by whose charm I was entirely captivated.

Even if wild animals are expected to be confined to an existence inside forests, some species like jackals, wolves, hyenas, civets and leopards including cobras, easily thrive outside the forests in human dominated landscapes and in the case of Tarai, even tigers are no exception. I had heard of a particular village called Barotha in the Nighasan tehsil of Kheri district, around which a scattered population of tigers was flourishing for quite some time. My piece of information, based on local intelligence revealed that they lived in a matrilineal colony, which included a mother cat, her duo of daughters and a granddaughter. This temporary overcrowding pointedly implied the existence of justifiable food to sustain them in the area, and since no clashes had taken place in the region, it also signified that tigers had been living in the crops without menacing with people.

As I gained the opportunity to observe these tigers in earnest, I came out with some challenging documentations that created a new stock of knowledge. It was in terms of shifting prey base for long term sustainability that yielded a tremendous landmark breakthrough for my project. It was quite different from the basic concept of tiger's predatory patterns. As far as I know, before my personal probe into the ways of Barotha tigers; the sugar-tiger's flexibility to modify the rules of their predatory behavior-based on changing local environments and circumstances in face of biophysical conditions and anthropogenic disturbances- had never been taken into account. No expert had ever sought to explore the question as to what lifestyle large carnivores might adopt to eventually share living space with man without being at odds.

It is a mind-boggling fact that India with an average population of 345 people per sq km still retains 57 out of 58 predatory species (the Cheetah being lost in the last century) of which 14 weigh more than 10 kilos and are formidably dangerous to humans. Yet many of these exist in human landscapes on friendly terms with man, at least on their part, and never fall prey to serious human extravaganza of large scale exterminations. This corroborates that there is some entrenched reason to this continued survival of carnivores in human landscape, which includes some deep-rooted stratagem, some rudimentary caution, inherent environmental awareness and eventually the orientation through stressful experiences, that affects their attitude towards man in their day-to-day living. We have yet to understand the aforementioned factors on scientific scales but we can casually acknowledge the tolerance of some wild animals that deliberately avoid competing with humans, and thus are better able to adjust in human landscapes. My experience with Barotha tigers was something on this line.

One early afternoon, having had enough of city life, I reached the old township of Nighasan and almost immediately after a luncheon left for Barotha. A local transporter named Sardar Ram Singh Dhillo and his two mechanic boys accompanied me on this venture. In my enthusiasm to drive a truck, I took on the steering of the new vehicle and drove it through the narrow streets of shabby township that were full of goats and cattle. We could take the pleasure of fresh air only when we came out in the wide open countryside. The road was probably one of the most beautiful twenty five mile stretches in the district. We went through the rustling green country of sugarcane and past mud-walled villages basking under the Kodachrome blue of the sky. A cool westerly blew and the prattle of birds mixed incongruously with the groan of the truck.

The region was grossly underdeveloped with all the signs of backwardness. There were no infrastructural facilities like schools and dispensaries and even people seemed to live at the leisurely pace of a forgotten era. The land was bathed in a benison of light. I lit a cigarette and tilting my hat to shield my eyes from the glare of the late sun, drove with a Sunday driver attitude. I was skirting a low lying area called 'Dhuria-wala-khalla', when we were confronted by a large herd of *Nilgai* racing in the open with astonishing speed. They frantically crossed our path from north to south and then suddenly, for some nameless reason, about turned and crossed the path again, making a furtive retreat. Before I could perceive all this happening, the truck had travelled into their middle, and when, in the hysterical melee a luckless female bumped violently into left door of the truck and fell badly hurt, with its head cocked on one side.

"My gosh! This creature must have lost its mind entirely", exclaimed Sardar, lurking out of the window as I stopped the vehicle screeching on the tracks.

Soon after this, the injured doe got up and even in the painful crisis of the instant, made a prodigious leap in the air. She went across the entire height of the truck sideways, and landed smoothly on the other side. The magnificent spectacle of power displayed by an injured *Nilgai* was a lifetime sight. The way she carried herself across the truck with an effortless ease left us in disbelief.

Nilgai is a tremendous animal and the largest antelope of India. I never knew that the burly, slate grey brutes with their sloping withers and rolls of fat are such a great jumpers; four hundred pounds of muscles fused with the dynamite of power. The experience left us aghast as we watched the doe melt into the herd that was fleeing away, raising clouds of dust.

It needed no soothsayer to suggest that the antelopes were running scared of some predator. I switched off the engine and looked around for the cause of turmoil, when a mechanic lightly touched my shoulder and extending his other hand pointed out in the distance what he had spotted towards the other side of the road. To our immense delight, some two hundred yards from the road, in the green lintel fields was another fine sight waiting for us; a stupendous tiger crouched in possession of a dying *Nilgai* bull it had just caught. The hind portion of the bull convulsed in the gasps of death. Evidently this charge had triggered the rush of herd. *Ahr-r-r-uf...* He growled in a low menacing snarl and begun to drag off the carcass towards the shade of a *Pipal* tree where he intended to eat at leisure. The tiger would straddle the bull, lift it by the neck, and walk clumsily a few paces. Then he would stop to rest, panting like a huge dog, as the mega-herbivore must have weighed nearly a thousand pounds. I was greatly impressed by the strength the old fellow displayed. He was lithe yet powerful and muscular with profusely grown 'Dundreary whiskers' that made a big ruff round his face and even hid his ears.

From the distance, I could clearly see the puncture marks in the bull's neck. I was in the process of taking out my fixed focus camera out of the bag when Ram Singh, also too energetic in his quest for adventure, jumped down the truck in excitement and the tiger's attention was distracted. He first slunk behind the body of the bull and then in an instant bounded off at a great rate and entered into the plot of golden crop. The maze was tallish and the great yellow beast went bounding through in great leaps. Although the tiger is absolutely noiseless when stalking, he makes a surprising amount of noise when he runs, his big pads thumping distinctly as he leaps along the ground.

This new experience left deep impression on us. Ram Singh and his boys were delighted with this unusual entertainment while it seemed to me that Tarai had so magnanimously bestowed her supreme gift upon us just for free.... Exhilarated by this successful culmination of a happy afternoon, I set on the road again, now at a leisurely pace and reached Barotha in an hour's journey. The village stood out on a slightly high ground against the gold sky where we were welcomed by a Sikh chief named Sher Singh and a crowed of his henchmen.

Sher Singh had a luxurious beard; rarely wore a turban, and usually kept his shoulder length hair loose which gave him a swashbuckling look of a Robin Hood kind of bandit. His deep voice with its Punjabi tilt was a remarkably powerful facet of his personality. I conversed with him about tigers and he briefed me with some fantastic tales and personal knowledge about these animals. I had brought along an old map of the Survey of India on which I had divided the area into four approximate compartments and marked the ballpark locations of two tigers. The man declared that they were very accurate as he had perceived the occasional glimpses of tigers around these settlements. He told me that there were not two, but four tigers here -- three females and one male -- and perhaps there was another tiger about twelve miles away in the Gauria and Bangawa fields. This news was amazing, somewhat difficult to digest. At length even if a standard discount is given to village versions, there must at least be two, I guessed.

However, it was mid-eighties, and considering the success of Project Tiger, the number of the wild tigers in India had more than doubled and the standard count in the state of Uttar Pradesh had already crossed to over 700, thus this information was most likely to be right. Conservationists were worried about what would happen to all the surplus animals. As principal forests could not accommodate this large number, tigers will have to settle down outside into agricultural expanses.

When I asked the grazers if these tigers were cattle killers they vehemently denied it. "Yes, they are no doubt tempted by the presence of hundreds of cattle that graze around the village," said a local man. "They often stalk them but they fear grazers; when challenged, they run away. These tigers do kill *ban-gaili gaiya* (feral cattle) and *Nilgai* but there are packs of aggressive jackals, which attack our stray calves or lift lambs and goats." They showed me a buffalo calf that had been severely lacerated by jackals only last day. To me, this appeared a wearied situation that here the poor rural people were affected predominately by jackals rather than tigers.

The people in this part of the Tarai were lucky that the tigers near their settlements were still hunters of natural game. To my mind, the configuration of the country and natural features did not support the existence of large hunting animals and since nearly 80 per cent of the land area was arable, natural wildlife was scarce. The place did not seem to carry enough food to sustain potentially deadly predators. Although I knew that there are many cases where animal population resources are affected in terrestrial ecosystems, but the factors that determine the long stay of predators in such systems remain poorly understood. However, while on the way to this village, I remembered seeing numerous strings of native bullock carts; the patient bell tinkling cattle crawling unguided along the road with their drivers muffled up fast asleep behind them. In such enticing conditions, I wondered for how long these tigers would wear the tag of inoffensive game killers, invariably restrained in their interactions with humans and still having their home alongside their home.

Livestock losses to predators are higher where natural prey is scarce but almost everywhere in the Tarai farms, feral cattle top the list of natural prey for tigers for they are unwanted and not actively protected by people. They also work as a cushion against the predation of livestock. Moreover there were dogs in every village, and predators avoid the area where guarding dogs are patrolling or barking loudly.

The young men of the village were eager to help me. A haphazard beginning to look for tigers somewhere from the middle would be unsystematic and depended too much on chance, so if I hoped to be able to locate at least one tiger during my stay I should begin operations from one end of the area and work forward towards Bangawa, rather than the other way round.

As the evening fell, the stars begun to glimmer, the sky sworn as thick with glowing gems as a field with seeds. Even though full darkness was yet to descend; an intense caterwauling of jackals started from across the fields. We saw a jackal family, a male female and two cubs, moving restlessly. They turned their heads to watch us, ears pricked and muzzles narrow. Just then, in the distance, I heard a tiger roar. At length, there came a mighty resonant *H-O-W-N* thrice at high pitch. The whole atmosphere suddenly appeared energized with an electric current; the jackals ran away, urinating freely while the outlying packs instantly stopped calling each other. This celebrated thunderous holler of tigers is produced by taking lungful of air and then expelling it vehemently against the crown of the mouth, the lower jaw being slowly closed at the same time. The terrific call resonated and reverberated in the air for a short stretch and then gradually subsided into deep sighs and finally ceased altogether as the night was left to the hours of darkness.

Researchers believe that sounds produced by individual tigers do carry an acoustic fingerprint. I could make out from the heavy gruffness in the sound that it was a male, perhaps the same, I had seen in the morning pulling the *Nilgai*.

Intending to obtain more information on the frequency of roaring, I asked Sher Singh whether the tiger calls regularly. He said he had never verified it, "but natives tell it occasionally does so, only after he has killed an animal."

I felt a surge of excitement because tigers do not vocalize without specific reasons. It meant that this tiger had an immediate partner; most likely a female and was calling her for a sumptuous dinner. F.W. Champion (1927) noted in a few cases that roaring is quite prevalent when tigers have killed a large animal such as a buffalo or a cow. In the dead stillness of nights, this loudest and most stirring sound echoes through the cultivation fields for over three to four miles. In such a situation the tiger is believed to be giving an impression of trying to draw attention to its ample food supply.

Scientists believe that by understanding the selective pressures behind the evolution of behaviour that at first appears altruistic in animals, we learn that there is a natural and necessary element of self interest in such behaviour.

A part of the answer can probably be found in the socio-biological theory of kin selection. Fitness in the term 'survival of the fittest' does not refer to how physically strong the individual is, but rather to its capacity for survival and the number of genes that the individual passes to future generations. The animal can increase its genetic fitness in two ways -- directly by producing offspring that carry one-half of its genes; and indirectly, by enhancing the survival of its more distant relatives such as cousins, nephews, nieces who carry a smaller proportion of its genes.

Of course it is not altruistic behaviour but natural investment, which some of the predators who possess the helping gene make, to perpetuate their own lineage, and tigers are no exception.

The fire died down to red coals, and the moon peered over the canopy of trees, flooding the fields with a silvery light. I could hear the rumble of a tractor and see the sweep of its bright headlights back and forth across the countryside. Some hardy farmer was busy plowing his fields at the zero-hour. The jackals were beginning to caterwaul, their quivering howls adding tension and menace to the landscape, when we finally slid into our beds and slept.

(II)

The next morning I awoke to the shrieking flights of parakeets. The first glimmerings of dawn were beginning to seep against a goldening landscape and the Tarai air, distilled through immense jungles and earth, was like fine rare wine - heady and intoxicating. When the sun had fully risen, I took a quick breakfast and set out to meet the local communities and take an appraisal of the area. Save for two moderate stretches of thorny wilderness, this area was almost completely devoid of jungle and was more than fifteen kilometers away from the principal forests of North Kheri. Most of the fertile land had been cultivated and a continuous strip of cultivation had already eradicated many a fragments of grass and shrub lands that usually border the Tarai villages.

Of the natural wild fauna, the prey base was very scarce here. We drove for miles and saw practically nothing of importance, but for some troupes of rhesus monkeys and a small herd of blue bull, having some twenty animals, mostly females and calves with only one handsome jet black male. I never came across any other stock of wild animal worthy of prey for a tiger. The nonappearance of game even gained me the impression, that, perhaps due to too many tigers, the predator pressure on the game species was excessive.

Jackals were incredibly numerous in this part of the country. They came out from the safety of burrows and bushes nearing sunset and gathered in the open fields in great numbers with the onset of darkness. They lived on ground-roosting birds, rodents and reptiles, and also fed on fallen fruits and raided sugarcane, maize and corn fields in the villages. Towards midnight, a horrible discord of low mournful wailing arose from the fields and mingled with the ferocious howls from the distant packs this continued incessantly for several hours.

Barotha was a sub-optimal habitat with many ecological constraints for tigers. With diminished prey resources, and with cattle killing reduced to negligible, I was unable to understand the puzzle of the large predator's survival. The question as to what they ate and how much their ranges expanded was intriguing. It is said that tigers never rely on chance. They are essentially able to calculate, far in advance where and when they will be able to find prey. So I was quite sure that the band settled here for the duration of over two winters was quiet naturalized and their hunting ranges carved out in different directions were their preferred dietary niches, where their mechanism for survival was by some means normal.

Two days later, I was investigating a distant terrain between Barotha and Bangava villages. It was a large patch of grass and trees with a hefty banyan in its centre, the roots of which stretched like the ribs of a Paleolithic skeleton. I was near a canebrake, when I described a magpie robin, chucking softly and warningly. It leapt out of the leaves of a *shisham* tree and dived as neatly as an arrow into the *nala*. Suddenly, the magpie uttered three brief, harsh chucks that sounded rather muffled as though its beak was full of food. The bird's attention was riveted on something in the centre of *nala* and she was calling with some purpose. I hurriedly reached the *nala*. It was some six feet deep and ten feet broad, which was dry in the winter but a raging torrent in the rains. It consisted of detritus wash down from surroundings. Such places are chosen spots for tigers to retire in the afternoons; and it is usually by such routes that tigers travel during the day time when there is a lack of cover.

I walked along the *nala* curious as to why the bird was calling when I happened to find a pile of animal bones lying at a place. This was a dump for remains of cattle that die a natural death. Such places lie at the outskirts of villages and serve as a restaurant for scavengers, where given a favorable wind, the pestilential odor broadcasts a mouth-watering invitation to crows, kits, vultures, caucal, jackals, foxes, monitors, mongoose, rodents and many lesser lights of lives who survive on it. Even a hungry tiger finds dead cattle as acceptable as the kill he obtains himself.

I felt curious and descended the mud encrusted bed to examine the bones. The bones, picked clean and chalk white, lay scattered over a vast area of roughly some forty feet. The spot was also marked by the gorgeous plumage of a male peacock, scattered about in hundreds of resplendent fragments.

I proceeded further inside the *nala*. At a cool point shaded by creeper clad undergrowth, I got the shock of my life for there in front of me lay a large number of bushy tails. Tigers normally pluck and spit out the tail before commencing to eat from the rump. The odoriferous plucked relics, not less than fifty in number lay scattered all over the dry bed of the *nala,* and were unmistakably of jackals. There was also a blood smeared and partly chewed off head of a freshly killed jackal whose entire body had been devastated without any scrap left. The severed head of the carrion had been tossed to one side where blue bottle flies were buzzing over it forming a black halo. The bird that had guided me here was feeding on some innards, as she saw me coming towards her she screeched in a frenzied alarm and flew off hurriedly.

The discovery of another bone pile signified that it was the dining room of a tiger, perhaps the den of the Barotha tigress. None of the bones were large enough to suggest that they belonged to cattle. Sizeable measures of them seemed to be of moderate size animals, seemingly of goats and dogs but in fact were of jackals. I was bewildered at the evidence of such a large scale killing of scavengers. Never

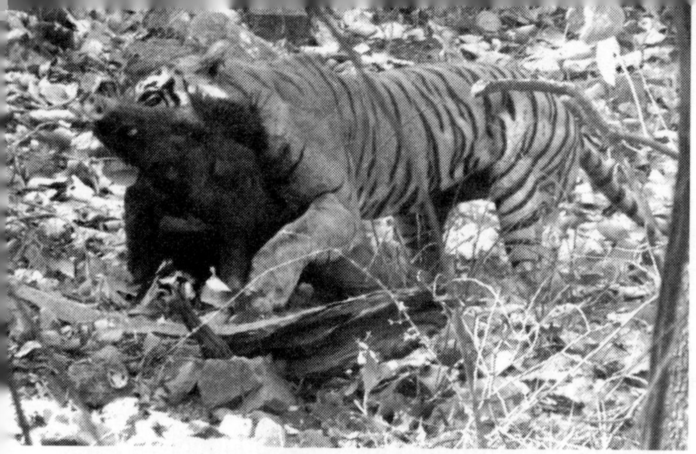

The tiger cuts the juglar vein and carries the wild boar away

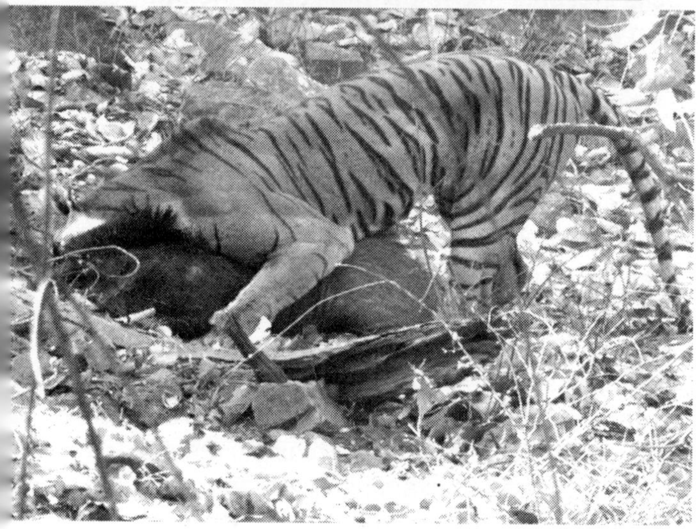

before I had heard or read of such a demeanor of tigers in old accounts. Could this be an act of needless slaughter, a transitory aberration of a predator? Or I was witnessing some new predatory conduct of a tigress, whose life maintenance strategies had undergone some definite change.

A fully grown jackal stands about 15 to 17 inches in height; the length of its body from head to the base of tail is from 2 feet to 2 feet 6 inches and weighs up to 15 kilograms. Some bigger and heavier animals may exceed up to 18 kilograms. If one includes the energy requirement of a predator, the undersized species is of little food value to a tiger that has evolved as a killer of large animals.

An American biologist Melvin Sunquist made some calculations on the amount of live prey eaten annually by the Tarai tigers. In his study conducted at Royal Chitwan National Park of Nepal, he estimated daily food requirements of a female to be 11-13 lbs and of a male 13-15 lbs. Presupposing that 30 percent of each carcass is inedible, and that some meat is lost to scavengers, and through disturbance, he estimated annual requirements to be 5,700-7,200 lbs for a female and 6,800-8,100 lbs for a male. Seeing the gargantuan food requirement of wild tigers, it is wrong to assume that the puny jackal would form their staple diet and even if it does then the killing and consumption rates are expected to be very high, which in long term will certainly remove a high percent of standing crop biomass of that very species.

A trail of the tigress' pugmarks was clearly visible on the bed of the *nala.* It showed that she had visited the place only the night before with the jackal kill. It was for the first time I had gained knowledge of a big cat that was an obsessive jackal eater, with a developed taste for their flesh. Though the farm dogs were disappearing and people were aware of it but nobody had even the slightest hunch that she mainly existed upon carrion meat and had gradually become adapted to this compulsive selection of prey, which otherwise comes low on their list of priorities. The pile of tails, numbering over 50, substantiated that the tigress was successfully preying on jackals and her killing rate was no less than one achievement in two to three attempts.

It is realistic to understand that on one hand, there are complex energies and alternative paths of existence in all ecological and biological systems that enable a living organism to sustain itself, whether big or small. On the other, the organism also sometimes adopts an innovative technique to trap a quantity of energy, which helps to ease its path of survival. The key to the guiding principle of an animal's survival character is to be found through its sensory system. Survival senses are intuitive intelligence and develop before any other instinct and reason. The character and actions revolve round this dominant sense. It is through this sense that the brain chiefly acts and it also determines the main character of the animal.

This produced a revelation to my mind. She was truly a sugarcane tigress in her natural state, whose only area of operation were sugar farms by naturalization and whose dietary habits were governed by the clear-cut guiding principles. It is open to doubt whether any such case had ever been pointedly verified by responsible scientists in the past, across the penumbra of the tiger's conventional prey. This important breakthrough was to mark a major turning point in my project.

There are numerous past records of sportsmen/naturalists regarding the killing of jackals by tigers but rarely has anyone witnessed them devouring the mangy beasts. Statistically, tigers account for less than one percent of the jackal death rate in the wilds, which leads to the conclusion that tigers do not eat jackals. But my continuous experiences in the predation pattern of Barotha tigers made a zilch of these statements. It was years later that I found accounts of two sportsmen of the nineteenth century who differed from the prevailing view and mentioned that tigers ate jackals occasionally, which raise their caterwauling at the killer's sight. "It is like an excited wail of self-pity from a lost soul in purgatory, yet it seems to serve the same purpose as the anxiety of birds at the sight of a predatory snake," wrote Stein & Wood in *India Sporting Review of 1882.*

My every fiber tingled with curiosity at the great cat's behaviour. It was a secret unseen by anyone but me that opened up spaces for engagement of biologists. Out of a snooping desire to interpret the event, my thoughts went back to the old stories of the jackal and tiger associations, romanticized by authors. Even I had been nursed on such stories by native hunters in Larti, some of which I have also written in my previous books that jackals don't mind living in close proximity of tigers and go in search of food with them. Even Brander writes, "The jackal is a cheeky, adaptable and insignificant animal, in no danger from the tiger, but to whom it is quite conceivable that he might be useful… he is the only animal which has anything in the nature of friendly relations with the tiger". This may be partially correct but the scavenger also knows how vulnerable he is to fall prey to the great predator. Perhaps the unearthly tremulous pheall cry, *P-i-a-a-o-o, P-i-a-a-a-o-o-o* given by the jackals at the sight of tigers, which is entirely different from their normal cry, is generated under the influence of the fear of death. It is interpreted as a general warning as well, issued to communicate the danger to other jackals.

The lifestyle of every creature is designed in such a way that it leaves its next generation in a more secure habitat; and the species that step out of line, die. The presence of tigers in the sugarcane fields showed that even amid such an apparent confusion of place, objects and events, there was definitely some kind of order that had held the species firmly there, whatever its prey base may be.

The level of population of available prey in a particular habitat shapes and determines the nature of that biological system. The school of chaos believes that there is orderliness, sequence and rhythm in everything, for the intelligence of nature finally generates a pulse of life from it. Nature may be taken as rude and incomprehensible at first but the sum total of such events tells us that the basic ecological rules are never overruled or nullified. These tigers had adapted themselves efficiently and fast to changed circumstances. Their system tuned itself to fit their behaviour according to changes in the environment or in parts of the system itself. Tigers are able to exist as scavengers for long periods and are equally able to live on scavengers too. Had these tigers hit upon the selected clues that made the future of their progeny safe.

I wondered as how this innovative diet of jackals representing a shift in the delicately balanced food pyramid of tigers could be a new clue to their improved ecological resilience. Though in addition to eating frequently the instinctual creatures like tigers can go for days without eating anything, yet the reason for this was instinctual to keep their digestive system in optimal condition. It was an essential break-open type of approach in a world where remorseless ecological cycles regulate and control the lives of the creatures that live in it?

My discovery had been immensely rewarding. I was able to establish some reason for the unexpected prey selection of this tigress. It was possible that other tigers in the vicinity might also be practicing this similar trait, feeding on a primary product of the environment as infallible means of survival. It may be said that energy is used to maintain chemical dis-equilibrium, which is a criterion of life, and qualities like the type of energy, type of nutrients and physio-chemical living conditions determine the survival of a species in a specific environment, where the biological equilibrium is often subject to laws that are apparently contradictory and even anti-natural. Marginal habitat means, less cover, less prey and closer to humans. Was this an alternative to switching over to any other novel diet, a supplement against human livestock; certainly these tigers' had evolved to realize that if they kill cows people would kill them and the application of this solution based knowledge on their part was a potent way for nature to avoid offense against the formidably dangerous human agency?

In life sciences, the term adaptability is used variously. At one end of the spectrum, the ordinary meaning of the word suffices for understanding. At the other end, there is the term as introduced by Conrad, referring to a particular information entropy measure of the biota of an ecosystem, or of any subsystem of the biota, such as a population of a single species, a single individual, cell, protein or gene. It was also reasonable to suppose that some teensy genetic component had made these tigers adopt this odd area as their basic home where they were managing admirably with changed hunting habits, without competing with human outfits. Thus, they steered clear of being harmed by them.

William Baze says "if a tiger discovers an area which is rich in the kind of food he enjoys he will plan his life to get the best out of it for as long as it lasts and move off only when its stores are running low." It seemed that the environmental factors had taken over these tigers so completely that they were effusively naturalized with the system and satisfied with their queer diet card of candies.

Here, I may rationalize that due to post independence human-led extermination of large predators in the area, the lesser lights of life had seemingly forgotten their anti-predatory patterns. Now, when the tigers had re-emerged in an area where they have been absent for long periods, their prey had not yet salvaged its former anti-predatory behaviour. Thus, typically the hunting success of re-colonizing predator was initially high, but it was bound to decrease over time as the prey would re-adapt to the constant presence of its destroyer agency and learn to evade. The re-adaptation of anti predatory behaviour in a prey species may occur in as short a time as one generation, which in case of jackals is hardly a couple of years.

From October onwards I frequented Barotha periodically for over six months. Nothing else out of the ordinary occurred save for I saw all the three tigers quite repeatedly' Twenty times at least' but I admit that I never learnt to recognize them individually. Most of the time when I saw them, it was dusk or dark and the sighting was never for more than half a minute. And it was not possible to scrutinize their faces closely or distinguish the individual marking by which experts recognize them. Once, a dark type of object sitting some seventy yards away in a maze field, watched me with curious interest. Its head was perfectly still and gazed steadily at me but owing to the bad light conditions I could not identify the animal, when its great mouth opened in a yawn, and a deep long-drawn sigh followed, I could know that it was a tiger.

It sometimes happened that I heard a tiger coughing a warning roar when I inadvertently closed in on him on my walks and when I endeavored to detect the beast; it slipped away unseen, too quickly for detection. On occasions the setting light of sun revealed just a flickering flame of colors in the grass or a disappearing tail was all that I could see, then not wanting to disturb the cats I knowingly avoided following them.

(III)

A few miles due north from Barotha was a farm called Grant Number 12 where a young tigress was nursing her singleton progeny, a six-month-old cub. She was most probably the daughter of Barotha tigress who had successfully mated with her father, the big male and raised a family. I assert this information because my observations suggested that this meta-population of three females and one male, occupying the territory around Barotha and Bangava (the male was the resident of both the areas) was in fact a matri-linear family group. Looking at the possibility of home range inheritance by female progeny, I was sure that all of these females sharing the same home range were related.

The favorite residential terrain of this tigress was an open type of country consisting of a series of *Nalas,* where sugarcane and reed grasses grew. One late February evening while traveling alone by motorcycle, I confronted this tigress on a sodden road, leading to *Sonatar Baghar*. Rain had fallen the previous night and she was on her usual perambulation. I stopped the motorcycle, and sat silently, getting an unusual opportunity to observe her through my binoculars for nearly half an hour. There was a raw red wound on her shoulders, apparently inflicted by the ripping action of the assailant's claw. Though a covering layer of fat had partially healed it but the seepage of sanguinary fluid was still continuing and a ten inch piece of skin quite unconnected with flesh hung loosely. It seemed that the tigress had landed in a soup with a powerful antagonist while on a kill or trying to save her cub from probable fatality.

It may be useful to mention here that the common fighting method of tigers is rough boxing where the claws hook deeply into the hide, peel off the skin and inflict such wounds. In the case of an acute fight, biting of the shoulder or back is often registered which causes a paralyzing effect. And in case of cubs being killed by adults, a bite through the skull is commonly executed.

A week later while I was in Barotha again, the ranger of Majhgai contacted me with a message from the headquarters that the deputy director of Rajaji National Park Uma Shankar Singh was in Dudhwa for some official work and was coming to my area of the study to take an assessment of the situation; it would be better if I appraise him and guide him in the area. Uma is couple of years junior to me in age with experience and a fine knowledge of wildlife. He arrived the next day, a tall polished man, full of bonhomie and vigor. We talked about two natives mauled by a tiger in North Kheri, about their recovery and traumatic. Uma told me that at present, the count of Dudhwa tigers, excluding Kishanpur and South Kheri was 121 out of which 79 were contained by the jungle and 42 were living outside the park in the sugar fields. The animal concentration map of the region also included the count of 5 tigers operating in my area of study.

In wildlife affairs, the element of luck is too powerful a factor. After a brief conversation towards the evening, we set out on a field survey in an open Jeep and by an amazing coincidence, met this tigress again at the same place. It was her favorite ground of operation. The sun had gone down but a green twilight hovered in the sugar-fields when we heard of several jackals calling in the frenzy of frustration. We reached the point hurriedly and I was surprised to see a pack of half a dozen jackals surrounding a crop plot and behaving agitatedly. They yapped hysterically and we could not realize what they were up to. It was as if they wanted to attack something but were unable to muster up courage.

This was an extraordinary conduct of mangy creatures. We stopped the Jeep and watched them silently for some ten minutes thinking what on earth had induced the old fools to indulge in such reckless behaviour when the rapid twilight closed in and it became darker. Suddenly the appalling stench of the predator accentuated in the air and the young tigress emerged out of the crop. It was deathly still but I could smell the tiger distinctly, and we understood thereby that the air was settling gently in our direction. A mangled half-eaten carcass of a jackal dangled in her mouth. She walked nonchalantly on a narrow path, like an indolent queen with the jackal's hind legs trailing on the ground. There was a curious fascination for me in her solemn movements as she walked under the stars that trembled against the dying sunset glow.

I could immediately recognize her from the large blot on her shoulders, as the Grant No. 12 tigress. She appeared weak and famished. Her wound seemed to have subsided reasonably but there was enough swelling around shoulders. Her face and neck were already covered with blood, perhaps she was in the process of dining on the fresh kill that bubbled of hot blood. The scavengers immediately distanced themselves from her. Some trotted in confused circles while some of them whined loudly as the alpha predator swaggered along the border of sugar plantations. Even though the occupants of the jeep were overflowing the sides of small vehicle in their excitement to see her, she never hastened her pace.

The surroundings had grown perceptibly blurred and only the tips of sugarcanes were outlined against a faintly luminous background. In the subdued light, the white spots on the back of her ears stood out brightly. I was sure that her cub was somewhere nearby and she was carrying the kill to him, when responding to some undistinguishable signal from her, a small shadow like object emerged on the *Kuccha* road at about twenty-five paces. It was her lone cub, looking really starved and weak, may be for the reason of some disease or insufficient meals. His hip-bones stuck out on either side of his backbone. He followed her greedily at the sight of meat. A big owl fluttered out of darkness, sending its weird quivering cry in the hushed evening. It circled over the duo and settled on a tree nearby. The mother and son watched the owl for a while and then strode into the canes. From there the sounds of their eating commenced soon — the crunch of bones, the grating of incisors cutting skin, the occasional snarl or cough of minor dispute between the duo.

I glanced at Uma and the forest staff. Like me they were fascinated and at full alert. It was a poignant and also a historic moment for all of us. We had witnessed an astonishing accomplishment, a successful hunt of a tigress that was adapted to an entirely different prey base.

It was quite late in the night when Uma left for his camp and I flipped through my notes pondering over changing prey base of tigers.

Self-defense is more a matter of mindset than a matter of techniques. Different animals react in different ways, if the predation becomes heavy on them. No doubt the tigers had accepted the jackals as their food and the courageous jackals were constantly challenging them. Perhaps this impractical and energy inefficient communal maneuver was being done in a false hope of releasing their kin from the grip of a superior predator, whose solitary hunting strategy, like one gorilla operating alone, had beaten the group vigilance of pack hunters, showing a high degree of evolutionary modification. The experience also proved that as a consequence of local predator extinction, prey may lose the knowledge about its natural predators and fall an easy victim at preliminary stage but usually express swift behavioural adjustments after return of predators. That is why predation is recognized as a major selective force in the evolution of behavioural characteristics of animals.

In any habitat, tigers customarily have the first claim over the best prey base in comparison to other predators. It was intriguing how they had deliberately opted for a second order prey biomass. Could it be due to some ecological reasons or due to some innovative stratagem, or probably due in part to the fact that tiger and jackals are both nocturnal in habits, who move and feed mainly in the safety of darkness? Although, in summers another reason for coming out at night is to avoid the midday heat. However, a jackal being a nimble opportunist searches for food in every nook and corner and comes in contact with almost every living organism of his environment, thus it is normal for him to cross the tiger's path.

This bizarre situation raises many questions, the answers to which can provide viable alternative hypotheses for long-standing patterns of habitat selection of large predators as well as their prey species, and their coexistence therein. The preference for such non-customary prey also establishes the fact that given the relative paucity of protein available to carnivores, tigers can and do take to opportunism and live successfully. The experienced opportunists literally live by their wits with no special adaptations. But in context of larger predators, some particular type of food is often chosen as ideal after a careful consideration. Such food being the primary product of the area and being abundant in the area, where the source of a predators next meal is almost certain in the same prey species, regardless of its size, may often develop into 'singular-feeding-adaptations'.

Thus, such singular 'feeding-adaptations' of predators generated by an eco-system approach for survival, often facilitate them to cope with the crisis of a degraded habitat. This is despite the fact that the greater mass of larger prey outweighs the greater numerical representation of smaller prey species in a predator's diet. This approach, positively advantageous to village communities even helps a predator to contradict the potentially formidable onslaught of human agency and thus helps him to survive longer in the human zone. An animal's brain is wired up according to what is important for its survival. Tigers that rely largely on instinct or highly context-specific learning, only quickly learn things related to the environment it evolves to live.

The farm tigers of Tarai have a good understanding of the daily routine of the village folk and they know as what kind of actions on their part attract human attention and might throw them into a conflict. They tend to avoid such complications and their selection of prey is also a part of this strategy. We know very little or practically nothing of what passes in the minds of animals but we are prone to ascribe human modes of thought to account for their actions. We only judge intelligence by comparing other creatures to ourselves, and in the present case if my assessment was correct, then I was really looking into an exceedingly thoughtful mind of the tiger, as though she was a mentally defective human rather than a specialized carnivore. To keep pace with this new mind was a challange which surpassed all my previous challenges in the study of sugar tigers.

Cats also have "ecologically surplus ability" that is the capacity to crack problems outside of its specific adaptations to its environmental niche. Ecologically, surplus abilities permit animals to cope with rapid or unexpected change in the environment, which are often hard to measure. When food is scarce, cub-rearing tigresses are the first to suffer, since their movements are limited around the nursery and they are unable to hunt for long hours. Under such constraints the mother tigresses often turn to cattle lifting or even man-eating. It was more likely that during such a desperate situation, some blundering jackal might have approached too close to her den in search of food and provided her with a hearty meal. Jackals are enterprising animals. Their exploratory and inquisitive behavior, ready to make use of what they find, invariably makes them poke into every niche including that of tigers. Mother tigresses are constantly watchful of scavengers who pounce on their helpless cubs. They kill the attackers in a flash and often also consume them in anger. This readily-available buffer of alternate prey must have supported her for a long time and later turned into her routine diet.

The flesh of the larger animal is tougher and a family rearing tigress often has to eat it where it lies, and later in the night bring her family on the spot, whereas a jackal carcass can be easily carried into nursery and is particularly tender. She must have essentially féd her dependent cubs on the scavenger's tender flesh, so they too had grown up accepting it as normal, potential food, which was a salient biomass of their environment.

Tiger behavior is governed by its immediate environment. By the same principle, the frequent hunting of jackals had made the juveniles' specialized hunters and opportunists par excellence. Tigers are handicapped all the time by an exceptionally voracious appetite so I was sure that the mother had passed on this fiendish apparatus of 'eco-system approach' to her progeny — 'take protein whenever you can get it'. Young cats seem to learn far quicker from their mothers about correct solution to "proper food object discrimination" problem rather than from examples set by unrelated cats and they relish that learning as gospel of truth. They had adapted themselves so well to the surroundings that the dislikable flesh was their first preference. Mammalian neuroscientists believe that such early feedings in some cases even become an addiction.

It can be partly accounted for by the fact that jackals are habitually more prone to go singly or in couples, and are less inclined to forming packs unless hunting. Though every single animal is more or less law unto itself, each one is wary and shy, invariably alert, using its facilities of sight, hearing and smell to detect and avoid predators yet their 'on their own' venture makes them vulnerable to predation. Tigers exploit this vulnerability to their great advantage.

It is said that the dilution effect as an anti-predation behaviour is the main theoretical reason for grouping in animals. It is believed that all individuals in a group have an equal risk of being predated upon, if equally spaced from each other and the predator. This apparently does not apply here as jackals group to hunt and not for the purpose of their defense.

I never witnessed this tiger family in action but the grass cutters and herders and a forest ranger named R.D. Bathom who had watched these cats, stalking, hunting and killing jackals in the field told me that the senior tigress increased her chances of attack success by preferentially targeting single or in case of group, non-vigilant individuals. She seemed to want to get in much closer for an attempted kill and used to take the quarry from 5 to 10 meters, often killing more than one animal in a single chase. A jackal's most common response to predator is flight. Bursting open from cover, she would chase the prey for a short distance and execute a mighty sweep of forearms to topple the balance of fleeing animal. The jackal often went flying up to five meters from the blow of paw and lay severely crippled with its neck or back broken. She would hold on the trachea and slay by preventing breathing and then returning to the other crippled beast, slay it too.

The behaviour pattern of her daughters differed sharply from their mother. Inclined to take more chances, they used to charge from greater distances and were seemingly more confident about their strategy. This unique method of making game of game, devised by them was an extraordinary and quiet exceptional form of predation, which besides ambushing, which is a true tiger trait, had now materialized well in her daughters.

It is supposed that the tigers never allow their hunting expertise – on which their survival depends – to become atrophied on tame animals. They often bypass even tethered bait and go on looking for a wild prey. I believe some tigers indeed nurture this useful tendency because they look for the game element in hunting, and jackals do offer that in plenty when persistently hunted as an easiest alternative form of prey. The Barotha tiger family clearly demonstrated this relevant aspect of predation in their way of life.

The character of this tigress was unique. I discovered quite late that she was using an incredibly big area; the different localities falling within it contained the farm fields of nearly sixteen villages, in a liner beat of some twenty miles. My experience led me to surmise that a high-quality prey density is not necessarily a pre-requisite for some big cats because establishing a large territory and making an effective use of it adequately compensates for all the paucity of prey and this strategy is obviously successful. "The larger carnivores are commonly assumed to be density dependent on the numbers of possible prey," writes Brown, who then comments; "it is doubtful if this is really so." He notes that by virtue of territorial behavior the predator may maintain a larger home area than it actually needs, so that the likelihood of a population crash on the part of the predator is remote even if calamity suddenly reduces the number of prey. It seemed true here.

(IV)

With the advent of vernal equinox the harvested fields stood barren and there were no further reports of tiger sighting in the area and the same was true for the jackals. It seemed that tigers had to make at least one kill every day or so, and this had perhaps increased the pressure on jackals; and if all the three tigers were hunting daily then it was safe to assume that it had forced a bulk of scavengers to move away from the area or they had gone back in hiding, increasing their vigilance to such a degree that any kill was harder to pull off. It was also possible that the tigers were still frequenting the range clandestinely in search of their favorite prey and that their predation had a strong depressing effect on the demography of jackals.

Jackals breed throughout the year, producing from four to six young in a litter, after a gestation period of two months. The population of prolific breeders was greater than every nuisance in the area. Sources of nourishment are found everywhere in varying degrees of availability, and given the relative paucity of protein available to carnivores, the major diet of the particular species was an exclusive advantage of the area. The tigers were doing a job which man could not do well – controlling a vermin population that had disrupted the fragile balance of nature. Its predator pressure on any prey species within the area must have been unduly excessive.

Predator-prey history is an important factor in shaping the behavioral ecology and interaction of current prey species and their predators. I do not know for how long this prey and predator correlation had been developing around Barotha sugar farms. I only happened to witness its concluding phase of last six months from October 1987 to March 1988, when its graph had just crossed the peak and its limiting effect of prey population had also started in earnest.

To the best of my knowledge, during this time the territories of no less than three tigers -all of which were seemingly fervent killers of jackals- overlapped around the particular terrain of around 10 sq. kilometers. (It was evident that they were also intricately involved in the maintenance of rights to an area). A rough assessment suggests that besides feral cattle and *Nilgai*, and in some measure rhesus monkeys, the prey base of jackals contributed nearly 50 to 60 percent of the tigers' total prey. The rate of predation upon the prey could be assumed to be proportional to the rate at which the predators and the prey met at close range. Thus, it was nature's mechanism to profitably exploit the breeding potential of jackals and also justify the presence of a superior, opportunistic predation agency in the existing system as a regulator of its own equilibrium.

Predators may increase the biodiversity of communities by preventing a single species from becoming dominant. Such predators are known as keystone species and may have a profound influence on the balance of organisms in a particular ecosystem. These tigers, like conditional keystone species -the condition being as long as the prey is available- had not only managed to use scavenger population to their advantage but were an extreme example of specialization in cropping an initial resource of the environment.

The impact of predation on the number of prey can never be expected to be constant. It changes seasonally from year to year and also from species to species. It is reasonable to accept that if this so-called 'temporary-aberration' of singular feeding adaptations becomes a regular feature in a predator's life, then this is in fact an eco-system approach of a predator, which presents an extraordinary model of 'Prudent Predation' where it temporarily plays a temporal keystone species. This apparent intelligence, flexibility and ability to adapt new situations and often an interim role of keystone species are born out of the need to survive in extraneous environs.

Many years later in the capacity of Honorary Wildlife Warden, I once raided a Kanjar camp and recovered a big pile of jackal bones and skins. "Where is the flesh?" I asked. "We have eaten it all," was the reply. The nomads told me that jackal flesh is exactly like that of a dog and is very tasty. Until then, I had regarded the animal as an abhorring and ill-chosen prey but that day my knowledge was carried a step further on this point and I could connect it to Barotha tiger's passion for jackals as food rather than any in-built hostility towards the creature.

A Russian scientist, Vladimir Tronin records that 'tigers don't like dogs but they prefer fresh dog meat to any other food. It is not a matter of flavour; it is a matter of utterly incompatible natures'. Dogs and jackals belong to the same family of *Canidae-canis*. Uneasy, noisy jackals like dogs irritate the quiet, peaceful cats with their eerie yelping and caterwauling. They are effective predators, who stick their noses into tiger kills and compete for food with them, causing anxiety and panic amongst tiger's normal prey, especially when helpless creatures are parturient and fawns are too weak to stand. On the line of this logic, thus when a tiger destroys a jackal, it not only gets a scrumptious food but also begets order to its home range.

On one hand, this model of 'prudent predation', leads to suggest the behavioral limitation of a predator which has evolved on group selection and on the other it exists in nature because some prey species are capable of tolerating increased predation, at least temporarily, without their rate of reproduction being seriously hampered. Predation only becomes a significant threatening factor when it occurs at a high rate and is more severe over the long term when predators take a constant proportion of the prey base, and when predation is across all age classes. It needs be remembered that the relationship between predator and prey is one which is typically beneficial to the predator, and detrimental to the prey species. But sometimes, predation also has indirect benefits to the prey species, such as when the old and weak are eliminated, the younger lot gets an opportunity to contribute its healthier genes and the population of species abruptly increases.

This model also demonstrates that the tiger does not consciously make a decision to live on its prey capital but such equilibrium flanked by the densities of predator and prey species is the product of the forces of natural selection that function on an evolutionary time scale. Hence, the reasons for such prudent-predations cannot be directly related to scarcity of proper prey base; much more research is needed before we can draw any firm conclusions about them.

After March 1988, I could never visit Barotha again but the reports trickling in confirmed that the jackal population had drastically thinned down. A year later, the senior tigress was once seen near Barotha but there was no information about her two daughters. It was not certain whether they had died a natural death, had been poached or shifted their range elsewhere; and in the want of jackals their predation pressure had shifted on which species.

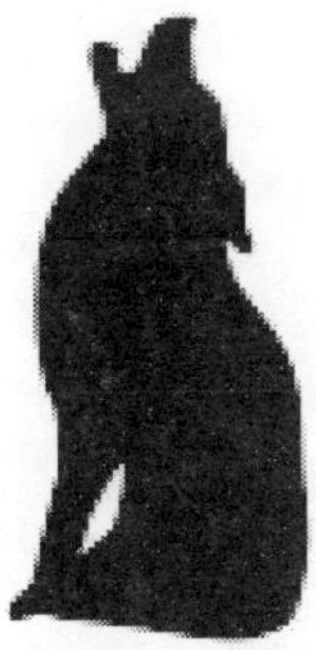

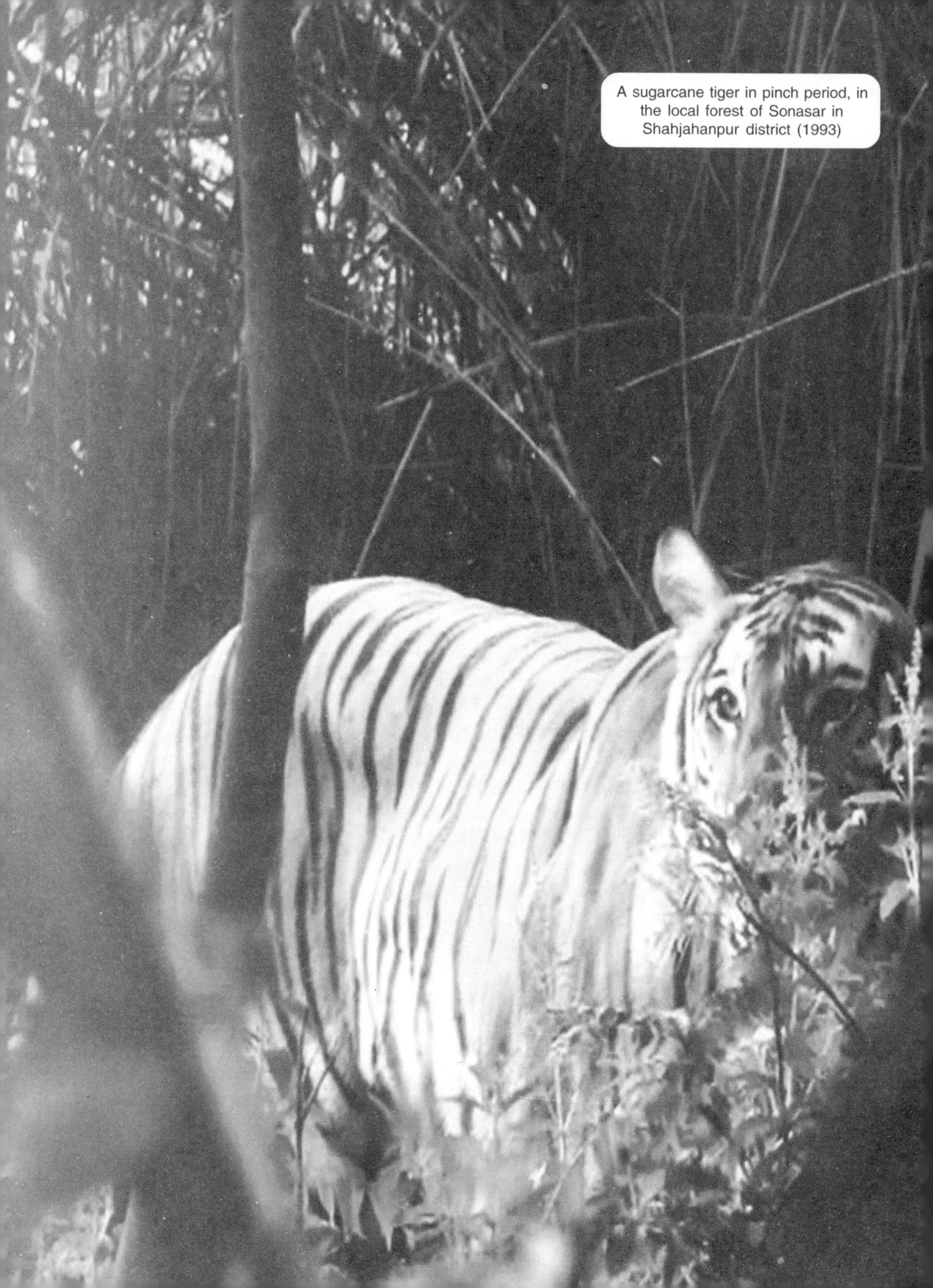

A sugarcane tiger in pinch period, in the local forest of Sonasar in Shahjahanpur district (1993)

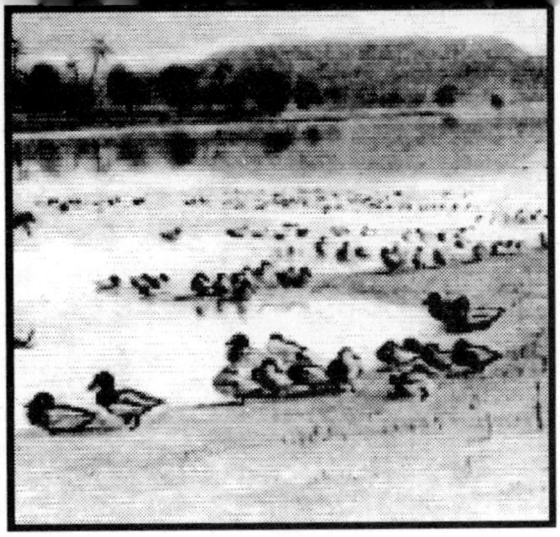

14

Pinch Period and Return to Fragmented Wild

Environments are not just containers, but are processes that change the content totally.

- Marshall Mc Luhan

The hard summers set in by the month of April. The awesome energy of the sun radiates its devastating power. The blisters pant over the dusty fields as the most potent god of Hindu scriptures, so inextricably linked with life on earth as a life force, burns the earth. The temperature soars tremendously, the water dries up and the blistering heat simmers, as the soul of the universe, the sun controls the animate as well as the inanimate patterns of life.

This is the pinch period. By this time the sugarcane crop is entirely harvested and the fields lie bare, where the dust devils dance. It is a tough time for the sugarcane tigers, which display great intolerance to heat. When the sun burns and the temperature soars to 45-48 degree centigrade; the big cats feel exhausted, they sit panting like a dog, their tongues lolling and saliva dripping from their chin whiskers. Their metabolic rate increases – meaning a faster burning body furnace— and they turn listless and lethargic. It is partly because supplementary energy is lost in the form of heat, from their surface areas. The normal luster of their coat diminishes gradually and their hair thins out. It is perhaps nature's way of shedding the excessive temperature. The transition is so complete that in summers the animal looks a totally different beast than when he appears in his full winter dress. They move about sluggishly and the area of their beat gradually shifts to around some water body.

The splendid sugar fields that were once a comfortable forest of fresh stems now stands destroyed. Missing too are the cool spots where tigers could spend long hours, no longer does the thick wall of vegetation offer them a prized habitat and no longer do they find the prey animals which they ambushed secretly.

This phase also accentuates food shortage; wild animals vanish almost as completely as the original landscape, so the tiger matrix of the area also undergoes a drastic change. The complete harvesting of habitat - deforestation from the animal point of view- renders the prey animals less vulnerable to attack while the stalking predators are put at a further disadvantage by loss of cover, so vital for a close approach to prey. Unable to support their family, tigresses often desert their subnormal cubs to die of starvation. Sometimes, the entire litter of healthy cubs is abandoned to its fate and sometimes even killed. For a mother in these circumstances of inevitable hunger and tension, this is the only way to end the misery of cubs. It also enables tigers to maintain some balance, especially when there is a shortage of prey*.

As the weather gets warmer, the deserted fields seem silent and almost featureless. Some un-harvested crops may be still standing but the water supply to them has been stopped. Most of these are infected by pests -red rot and boring beetle- which reduce the sucrose in juice and make it as dry as a bone. These are now marked for burning. Since it is too hot inside the canes for the tigers to hide during the day, it is time to bid adieu to the place and pack up for a different pasture.

It is at this time that traveling several miles, this new contingent of farm tigers arrives in the jungle. The favorable niches are already occupied by powerful residents and the residual slots are not big enough to accommodate the displaced outsiders. The time is burdened with tension and inter-species fights. Conflicts erupt as the new entrants try to adjust with their kin. The water level in the ponds and rivers depletes. Many predators center on such places. Their beat will run along river beds and *nalas*. They seek water, drinking many times a day. Even in the night their beats are limited for they do not want to leave the place so easily till they are challenged and chased away by some more powerful antagonists.

Occasional fires also trigger hazards. These not only destroy the jungle but reduce the amount of good ambush cover, and force the tigers to move uncomfortably close together, producing a temporary overcrowding.

This is crucial time for the jungle and is fraught with problems for tigers as balance of power is tested by a number of means other than force. Consequently, many immigrants prefer to stay on the sidelines and do not penetrate the main jungles. They adjust to the ragged frontier of the forest belts or to take to the areas of the eco-tonal lines, where the environment is relatively safe and sound. There are bands

---

* I have documented one instance in particular, which impressed me deeply. In the dry season of 1988 three orphaned cubs were reported to be sheltering in a crop plot at a village called Pipal Purva in south Kheri. A small one among them was weak and sickly and was barely able to keep up with its siblings, which were quite healthy. But for some unaccountable reason the tigress had left the whole bunch behind. It was later surrounded and tormented by a pack of jackals that killed and ate them. Nothing was left of them, save one small skull, which was later collected by the villagers from the spot and submitted as gory evidence to the foresters.

Along the lengthening border between field and forest there must be multiplication of other similar incidents which are known to locals but go unreported and therefore do not see the light of the day.

of rapid gradation from trees in the forest to that of grass at the periphery. The edge is usually a band of richness, fast growth and diversity and offers a high degree of attraction to species endemic to both sides of the edge, where these tigers stabilize for the time being, dwelling in a state of limbo.

The eco-tone areas have medium-prey-density and because of their firm occupation by either the past prime adults, recently thrown out from the natal area, or the pre-prime adults, preparing to find a foothold there, the new contingent remains in trouble. The crisis of such tigers is no different from the problems that the wildlife managers complain about the translocation of a captured tiger from one territory to a different territory, where a relocated predator may not be acceptable to the local residents.

While the ecological crisis perpetrates in the jungle, there is a section of tigers that chooses to establish itself more securely at the exterior of it. It settles down in local fragmented grass and bush lands for a summer sojourn. This is the pure cane category. This motley group is the master of its new environment. It lives an incognito life in utterly desolate places and uses every bit of terrain to its advantage. They live un-noticed and secretly, waiting for the crops to grow up so that they may return to them soon.

It is noteworthy that much of the remnant tall grasslands of Kheri are located in the plains of the district. During my course of investigation, I was surprised to discover numerous fragmented verdures of wilderness surviving, unharmed by mankind, outside the demarcated forests. It was a kind of unused land, comprising sloughs and marshes, lush and damp with *ratwa* and *narkul* grasses, with big mud wallows for wild animals. These were ideal homes for sugarcane tigers to spend their crucial time in the pinch period. One of such noted places were the Nighasan glens. Created over a millennium ago by the instability of waterways, this grassland was the centre of common avian species of the district and was ecologically important. I got the opportunity to visit the place in December 1985 and came to know this local jungle well, while searching for a group of tigers that lived there.

I was staying in the house of Dr Pramod Kumar Singh, in charge of Nighasan government dispensary when I briefly happened to meet a party of villagers who complained about an assemblage of tigers that lived in the desolate marshes. It was a bowl like shallow area forming a rough circle of about six kilometers in diameter upon which a chain of pools lay scattered like huge pearls. Here the deposition of rain water had created a sort of exasperating swamp where it was impossible to reach. With many awed gestures they told us that there were quite a few tigers in the swamp and the leader of the group was a tigress with two half-grown cubs. I was not in the least alarmed at this somewhat startling announcement but also I knew from past experience that nearly all native stories of this kind are widely exaggerated-not deliberately but simply because there is a natural desire to inspire a quality of enthusiasm in the listener who has touched upon the thrilling subject of tigers.

The swamp patch was about one and a-half a mile long and one mile wide, tapering to a point at the far end, with an open area all around for a distance of more than hundred yards. The doctor was so much overpowered by this fascinating information that he thought it was worth investigating. Finally on the clear and sunny day of December 20, a group of diehard naturalists, Chhotey, Phagunia, Doctor and I started for the swamp. We took a twenty mile drive through lush fields and finally entered a wasted land which had no road at all but for a cattle track. It took us a couple of miles through bush land, when the swamp began in earnest and all of a sudden the track disappeared into it.

From here onwards the area was dense and inaccessible and there was no way for the jeep. It was mid afternoon; the time was around 3 pm. We got down from the vehicle and proceeded on foot. In the way, we met a grass cutter and a cyclist who warned us to not to go ahead as they had heard tigers snarling deep inside in the bog. At all events it was cheering news. 'That means luck' whispered Chhotey, bursting with the excitement.

The afternoon was quite bright. Countless game ducks waded in the small water shallows. Way out in the distance a pair of *Sarus* cranes flew over glens with their newly-fledged chick, relishing its loud, sonorous and bugling call in the air. There were dabchicks, painted storks and black storks, pecking around the small water bodies. A pink blotch in the distance proved to be a block of Greater Flamingos.

The tigers could be anywhere, hiding in the ocean of tall grass. It was not easy to find them but Chhotey and Phagunia, the sagacious natives with unnumbered generations of jungle ancestors behind them, had an instinct in this lore. They were hunters at heart and no naturalist is as ardent as a hunter in the pursuit of his query. Their eyes were as keen as of an eagle and they crept along with the air of a tiger about to spring on its prey.

It was imperative to proceed noiselessly and never speak above a whisper. A light drizzle in the morning had made the ground wet and therefore it was possible to move over the wet grass without making much noise. Though often the sounds of the soft crunch of my rubber soled boots and the occasional crackle of twigs when pressed hard under my body weight could not be avoided.

The swamp was throbbing with life. A large water deposit towards the west was a kaleidoscope of migratory birds, where pintails, shovelers, and coots swam between water lilies and lotus flowers. A *Nilgai* strolled around the pond with an egret contentedly riding on its back. Birds twittered all around and there was a general vibration of insect vociferation filling the air. Chhotey kept his eyes glued to the surroundings, and his ears, all alert and strained for any sound or movement. It is very difficult to discover the safe resting places selected by animals but the old man had had a knack of finding animals like a needle in a haystack, so he was sure that he could spot them at any moment, if any of the animal showed as much as the tip of its ear.

Some 200 meters away a pair of crows was cawing. Their frustrated calls indicated the presence of meat which was in sight but out of reach. These birds provide excellent indication of a tiger's presence. Chhotey proceeded in that direction through the long reeds and as he broke out into an open place he immediately drew back into the reeds again. He caught hold of my shoulder and asked me to sit down. I got my binoculars set and pushed through the reeds. And there in front of me was a young tiger, perhaps two years old, looking at the crows with its head raised and sleepy eyes half-opened. It was lying on a grassy parapet and was so well concealed in the grass that except its head hardly any part of it was visible.

Close to him was a tigress, sitting near a *Jamun* tree contentedly recumbent amidst her twin cubs. The scene before my eyes offered a most fascinating sight as if it was straight out of a movie. Both the cubs some six months old, sat at a distance of five meters on either side of their mother. The cub on the left seemed weak and thin while the second cub was in a grass thicket and I could faintly see his stripes.

A little higher up the escarpment was her mate, not very impressively handsome but certainly the lord and the star of the show. He prowled to and fro wagging its tail in some obvious mood swing but seemingly in an undisputed control of the situation.

Now by this time, having met tigers at many anomalous places, I had almost got beyond the surprise state where they were concerned in sugar fields, yet I must admit that the sight that met my eyes fairly took my breath away. I was thoroughly startled by seeing no less than four stripes assembled in the covert.

I was equally bewitched by the restless walk and wagging tail of the male. The tigers living in captivity do saunter in the limited space of zoos, turning about when the bars hinder but they do not wag their tail. This was for the first time I had seen a free-ranging tiger doing so in his normal home. The psycho-experimental studies on feline suggest that tail wagging in cats has the opposite meaning to a dog wagging his tail.

However, despite his conflict, the reason for which I didn't know, the male was a grand sight indeed. The declining sun created a familiar jigsaw of light and dark over the mound as his striped beauty was restlessly silhouetted against a golden sky.

The area had quite a few raised mounds and our vantage point was approximately three meters high. All four of us remained fixed to our respective places, I half lay on the reed bed focusing my field-glasses. The slightest relaxation in caution might have pushed one or all of us into dire disaster. The jungle concealed us perfectly from the watching eyes of the tigers.

The tiger is slow to distinguish a stationary object, but quick to see the slightest movement. The tigress had not perceived us but she had raised her neck a bit, she was constantly gazing in our direction with fixed stares. A few seconds later her cubs also did the same, as if trying to listen for a prolonged moment. Every muscle taut with apprehension, they sniffed the air as their ears scanned for the leery sounds of unwelcome visitors. I felt that the big cats had become suspicious of our presence. For a second or two I held my breath but none of them looked unduly alarmed, they were rather poised, and things seemed relatively unfussy. I thought that perhaps they were familiar to humans violating their habitat and that this was an infrequent part of their existence but I could not be sure.

Then a male tiger appeared unexpectedly on the further bank. He had heard the signals of disturbance and had come to see if everything was all right. Next couple of minutes was quiet exciting. I heard the fresher growl, to which the bigger one answered with a louder and an even more convincing roar. He then instantly plunged into the water. The pond seemed to erupt in an explosion of spray as he went bounding after him and soon both were lost in a thick cover. Through my binoculars, I watched the wonderful chase with absolute clarity. I could scarcely believe my fortune. Nature was in one of her most charismatic moods! It was predators going about their lawful business. It was like a glimpse of an incredible and historical Tarai, of a lost epoch, of a world frozen in time.

The honing sounds of tigers were so intense that the flock of flamingoes took off from the swamp. It wheeled about in perfect synchrony, adding a weaving splash of pink to the natural tapestry. The moment was pure magic. I knew that the entire setting was far too complicated to capture in a camera, but I relished the flavor of rare event, and regretted not having a camera in my hands.

The tigress was in a passive mood, she remained perfectly comfortable with the sub-adult male's presence, half lying and resting, spending her time in the ritual of grooming. Her rough tongue worked over her claws, shoulder, chest and whatever part of the body it could reach. Pretty sure that it would not move till dusk we spent one fascinating hour watching the unsuspecting tiger family.

The sun rays grew more slanting and the shadows lengthened. The blood red ball of fire was declining in the west when the sky suddenly darkened. The dusk came with hovering fat clouds which threatened to rain. Towers of white, brown and dark clouds boiled up and intermingled ponderously above the glen. Finally the storm broke. A blinding flash ran zigzag in the sky and a terrific crash of thunder boomed. The tigress stood up facing the dead leaves that were blown about noisily by the wind. She sniffed the rapidly cooling air, whirled round and then moved into a thicket. The cubs raced after her scattering the dry leaves; and as though suddenly responsive to their recklessness, they stopped and stared towards us for the last time, which seemingly demonstrated that they were aware of our concealed location. I let the caution go by; I stood up enchanted and waved my cap in air as a farewell gesture. At this they looked a bit surprised and in the twinkling of an eye, vanished into the blackness of the swamp.

As the rare drama was over, we lost no time in tracing back our steps. The sharp blue light of lightening illuminated the surroundings in blinding flashes. The wind tore at the tree branches and a driving rain lashed out the swamp. We backed off at a fast pace, stumbling along through the downpour for the best part of half a mile before we risked slowing down our pace and walking properly. I was not unduly nervous about getting out of the vicinity of the tigers but with the growing darkness and a lashing rain storm, it was also not advisable to take the swampy glen casually. These glens are fed by all sources of nature, ground water, local water bodies and of course rainwater. The sheer violence of the rapid flooding of such places is spectacular and can cause severe disasters.

Clearly, it was a place for the tigers to smile about, where nature could safeguard the balance and maintain the safety valve between man and tiger but how it worked was not clear to me. Especially in context of these tigers' compulsive adaptation to sugarcane plantations; these basic questions needed a detailed research. This re-kindled my curiosity and I wanted to know more answers.

(II)

This glen was some 20 miles away from the regular jungle and a very small place for the tigers. In Chhotey's opinion they were the original dwellers of sugarcane who had provisionally gathered at this point to avoid the hustle of human commotion and the bustle of machine sounds. Human intrusions like plowing the field, product collection, excessive movement, irrigation management, cane stripping, burning fires, livestock grazing and even occasional hunting of ungulate prey disturbs the equilibrium of a predator's life. It was natural to assume that traumatized by the shock operations, they found capital covert here and shifted during the day time and then as dusk fell, they again left the place for the night ramblings through the canes.

Sometimes, knowledge is gathered in strange ways. An interesting paradox is that whereas the pressures from farming, animal husbandry and forest product collection, including the huge developmental projects, degrade the physical quality of many tiger habitats, sugarcane plantations stand as a contradiction. Until harvested, they remain in a first-rate condition for months and there is no physical degradation of the reed-like crop, in fact there is a constant improvement in the quality of habitat.

By October, the monsoons transform the landscape into a verdant paradise. The steady irrigation of sugar farms also continues to make it an even better habitat; the sunshades formed by the fronds give the plantations a character of canopy forests that appears welcoming to the tigers. As the feel of the closed environment becomes much stronger and more overwhelming, there is a marked increase in the density of prey animals. They are scattered everywhere, wandering at their will, without restraint as to water or sufficient cover. Many more arrive here to bear their young, followed by some more tigers from the jungle. That is why sugarcanes have many tigers while there are a lot of jungle areas which have no tigers.

We have already seen earlier that sugarcane plantations, like perennial grasslands are extremely productive habitats for tigers. In the jungle, the geology, topography, rainfall, evaporation, regular grazing, and controlled fire by the foresters are factors that control or limit the form of vegetation. In agriculture fields, crop harvesting creates a similar effect and manages the continuation of this extremely productive habitat.

Tall coarse grasses have little food value once they have grown past the young palatable stage. By the time they have flowered and die, most of the food has been transferred to their roots for storage- an evolutionary adaptation designed to cope with the oncoming dry season. The controlled fire is judiciously employed in phases so that the wildlife is not harmed, and it later creates a more suitable habitat for the ungulates that rapidly move into recently burned patches to feed on succulent and nutritious new shoots.

Similar to the disproportionate annual grasses in the jungle, the sugarcane attains full growth in nine months. Once the maximum protein/fiber, glucose and cellulose ratio is achieved, the crop sustains it for a couple of months and then starts declining and its edible value gets reduced significantly. The skin becomes thicker and harder, and the small stomas in the nodes, called eyes, sprout out petite green root like shoots that indicate that the ageing of sugarcane has begun.

This is the season when the harvesting starts in phases. From a tiger's point of view, the main importance of a dead or dying sugar crop is apparently to afford cover and shelter; but sugarcane grows perennially from the root system known as ratoon rhizomes that remain in the ground and re-sprout from each stalk. Ratoon crops grow faster than the primary crop plants because the cutting blade is placed at a height of three inches to prevent the loss of roots. This speedy regeneration restores the habitat within months. Moreover, the entire crop is not harvested simultaneously – it is taken in installments, thus the wildlife gets ample time to seek refuge in other patches which are often of considerable size.

It has been established that grasslands produce a greater animal biomass than the monotypic forests. Harvesting temporarily retards the habitat and also works as a check on the population of farm tigers as well as of ungulates. This significant feature indicates that exclusive harvesting of sugarcane crop, like the spring season grass burning in the open plain after frost has made it inflammable, is a natural and ecologically sound exercise. It later improves the habitat and allows it to meet the food shelter requirements of most of the ungulates.

It may be noted that grass fire doesn't add to the number of nutrients in the soil – it just releases them from dry grass making them available for the nutrition of the plants. Similarly the stripped-off sugarcane leaves left as mountainous loads in the fields are later disposed of by burning, leaving plenty of nitric compounds and organic matter to enrich the soil. The opportunistic grasses and lentil seeds also germinate simultaneously within all type of crop plots and the natural young growth easily attracts grazers. The function that the annual grasses perform for the wildlife in the jungle is achieved to some extent by the sugarcane in the fields.

In 1973, C. S. Holling introduced the word *resilience* into the ecological literature as a way of helping to understand the non-linear dynamics observed in ecosystems and in its actors. Ecological resilience, functional on both biotic and non-biotic components of environment, is defined as the amount of disturbance that an ecosystem, as well as its living organisms, can withstand without changing self-organized processes and structures. Other authors consider resilience as a time of return to a stable state following a perturbation. A new term, adaptive cycles, is introduced to describe the process that modifies the resilience in life systems.

Differences in perception arise from different viewpoints. Funny as it may seem, the impact of harvesting is not very tangible on the mainstream tigers, for it is just a part of their adaptive cycle that goes with the crop rotation patterns. Yet as the impact of habitat degradation is exceedingly subtle and consequently more lethal in its consummation, the animal might come into head-on conflict with the livelihood requirements of people and the cases of man-tiger conflict and even man-eating might increase at such times. As the farmers start harvesting cane crops the frequent visibility of tigers' increases in areas and the tigers are left with no other option but to come out in the open till they seek a safe hideout in local forests including the gulches of Sharda, Ghaghra, Ull, Katna and Barauchha nala and other such water bodies. This illustrates that inanimate patterns determine the animate patterns we encounter in the environment. Such interaction between flora and fauna, and people living next to them, keeps the sequence of the environment in motion and triggers a new resilience in life systems. And finally these ecological parameters coupled with interesting animal communities shape the unique animal that is known as 'The Sugarcane Tiger'.

Naturally I could not expect people to view this phenomenon from my point of view, but at least now I could look at the theory of 'sugarcane tiger' as a brainchild of mine, brought up through considerable exposure to danger, stress and troubles of all kinds. Study of sugarcane tiger required being deeply rooted in physical reality. An ordinary naturalist of course knows nothing about such prevailing conditions in the Tarai and his first response is always of a great disbelief, and those who are a bit aware of wildlife matters doubtlessly think it as a common problem of displaced tigers, which is sometimes very insignificant indeed.

(III)

It was the dead of the night, when we eventually reached the shelter of home. The warmth and the comfort of a fire were never as welcome as on that day. Listening to the wind and terrific thunderbolts crackling outside, we enjoyed a hearty supper and congratulated ourselves on being safe under a roof on a night as wild as this. There blazed out constant violet coruscations, vividly illuminating the somber earth but as the lightening passed, it left a sensation of stygian darkness. We retired to rest, discussing the events of the day over a cup of hot tea, and a sociable chillum. The rain thundered on the tiles of the house roof. And there was a pleasing reflection, within our light hearts, that we had found out yet one more answer to the convoluted riddle of the sugarcane tiger.

The next morning the storm had passed and the fields stood in soggy silence. The incessant rain of the night had given way to an early dawn and we were taken aback by the light and freshness of the morning. We set to the task again and resumed our search for the tiger group. The stony silence provided a perfect setting for a fresh effort. Nature seemed to be holding its breath while drinking the life giving moisture. The rain had washed out every vestige of last evening's drama, yet we squelched our way through sopping and bedraggled clay and combed all the sections of the glen carefully. To our astonishment, it was completely deserted, and wore that appearance, unmistakable to an accustomed eye, of utter desolation and absence of animal life.

This was extraordinary; so my men repeated the search through the grassy hollows that only 14 hours ago had teemed with tigers and birds. It was as if yesterday we had beheld some fairy vision, some illusory caprice of the brain.

Again and again we explored every nook of that isolated patch; but to no purpose. After three hours' diligent search we finally returned home; unaware of the reason of the solitude which had so swiftly fallen on this favored spot. The villagers told us that the tigers were living at the place for some months. Sometimes they were seen together and then suddenly they separated. Perhaps due to the tensions caused by the tigress that periodically came into estrus or some conflict over food, they dispersed and moved away but had a tendency to join up again. Perhaps, the last day's incident was a typical example of such a situation.

It is noted that when the cubs grow large the tigress often keeps them with her while she is in association of a male. Such groups consisting of a tiger, a tigress, and two-third grown cubs have been periodically recorded by naturalists. But this group was different, a mother with two dependent cubs -as large as matured leopard-one extra female and two males. The second female was elusive. Though we never saw her but Chhotey competently read the tell-tale signs that provided the evidence of her existence. Perhaps she was establishing her rights to the area.

Old wildlife literature records make contradictory observations in this context. A large section of authors observed tigers as a solitary animal. Ingles (1892) wrote for example "in their habits they are very unsociable and are only seen together during amatory season. When it is over, the male betakes himself to his solitary predatory life."

But Forsyth (1889) stated "I have twice known five, and once, seven tigers to be driven out of one cover." Brander (1923) and Sanderson (1912) wrote about seeing two males and even three females with a male on a kill. Hewitt (1938) noted "a family will be met of a father, mother and two or three cubs sometimes nearly as large as the mother before they leave her." Berg (1936) also seems to agree that "The tigers do socialize if the conditions are convenient."

A perusal of old writings shows that there have been observations of a similar type of adult group and non-family associations in the past. Edward B. Baker (1886) in his book *Sport in Bengal* writes, "This animal is not an unsociable creature as it is commonly understood to be. On the contrary, it is fond of consorting with others, and not seldom three or four may be found together; a mother and nearly full grown cubs; both parents and half grown ones, or a charming party of young males, and females living and hunting together for a considerable length of time."

A. A. Dunbar Brander in his book *Wild Animals in Central India* states, "The largest party I have ever seen together, consisted of six animals; one large male and two fully grown females accompanied by three young animals almost as big as the tigers."

There were six tigers often congregating in this small area living in a sort of cordial relationship. It was a 'non family group'. They had probably established a rank order but it was not at all a social group, for tigers cannot form a social group. Either way, it is positive attraction of animals to one another which maintains the social group. A group of vultures on a dead cow is not strictly speaking a social unit, since the group is formed by individuals attracted not to each other, but to an external stimulus.

Schaller points out that the social interaction of adult tigers can best be understood when considered separately in the context of hunting, mating and feeding on a kill. In areas of plentiful prey, tigers are tolerant familial groups and tigresses with common blood line often associate with each other while Valmik Thapar's observation of nine tigers at a single kill in Ranthambhore, makes the same conclusion that "tigers might sustain kin links throughout their lives and many tigers can feed off the same carcass without unpleasantness". The juniors are safe until they do not transgress the protocol.

The nature of the species food resource determines, in general, the form of its conditional or enduring social organization. The result is a relatively tranquil order in social groups, which ensures less energy is used in bickering and more in surviving.

An abundant food supply means that the tigers can afford to be more social and live in transitory groups. A rare and sparsely distributed food supply would soon be depleted by a group. Thus, at the least social end of the social continuum, the solitary tiger will again figure out, which because of the exigencies of prey consumption would show no tendencies towards socialization.

This group of tigers, howsoever temporarily formed, raised a serious question; do the tigers in sugarcane reflect a curious blend of the semi-social and the solitary beasts at the same time? Whether this behavior is due to the changeable nature of the land over which they roam? Or it was due to stressful conditions, generated by human pressure all around that they sought refuge in the glen and recurrently spent a disproportionate time together.

A host of questions that had plagued my mind came flooding back. Is this independent scrap of forest a world in itself, like many others in the Tarai, actually a special one, a micro-habitat, a sort of core zone for farm tigers, where 'come together social groups' were formed under certain compulsions? Prater has suggested that the congregation of species depends on the supply of food. It was a small six sq km area, where three prey species of wild boars, *Nilgai* and an occasional hog deer were certainly the staple food for these tigers and they were making effective use of the area not only as day-time cover but also as a hunting ground.

I was especially curious about how the behaviour of these groups changed in response to diminished prey resources and other ecological constraints. Would a serious scientific study reveal some new obscure aspects of tigers that move here in summers after their sugar habitat is harvested? And why these tigers, instead of going to the jungle, preferred to shift to swamps and fragmented forests, to spend their interim period of summers; precisely the four months of April, May, June and July.

It may be paradoxical to argue that perhaps these tigers were unable to meet the harsh compulsive demands of the forest. Partly because the constant pressure of the resident tiger's generated fear in them and their adjustment with local population was difficult to achieve and partly because their skills to survive in the jungle were constantly put to test against the depletion of prey. It was also possible that in some tigers, these skills were drastically diluted and unable to meet the acute competition in the jungle, they preferred the sugar crops. Here too they lived under optimum conditions where at least there was some easy food and water.

Interestingly when Project Tiger was committed to the philosophy of total environmental preservation, with its management limited to eliminating or at least minimizing human disturbance and to repairing the damage already done by man in prime tiger pockets, the queer creed of cane tiger was flourishing in human proximity. The untamed wild animals had taken to tamed human environments where their life-style was so compulsively altered that they had acquired a series of skills to compete with man and the factors that were of big economic consideration for villagers such as crop harvesting and animal husbandry.

Though rain hampered my further observations but I had ascertained that from this very base these tigers took to their nocturnal forays in the agricultural fields. They avoided those parts of the sugar savannah where the cover was deficient, and moved to wherever it was thick enough to offer some protection, and then, as the cane stems grew to an adequate height, they finally returned into them, adapting to the fluctuating heights of fronds and occupying their discriminating niches of existence. For such tigers it is a 'return to the long grasses.'

My query about the pinch period immigration of sugar tigers had lead to this interesting discovery. The presence of natural game along with feral cattle gave little reason for the tigers to take to domestic cattle and with an abundance of food available just for the taking, there seemed to be no cause for the tiger to ever turn man-eater. Tiger mobility is affected by seasonal changes, prey movement and availability of water. It is observed that over the short term local tiger densities tend to be fairly stable, but in the long run they may go up or down in response to significant ecological changes. What exactly is the effect of acute summers when the water levels recede? Where do the tigers go then? Do they seek a further resettlement? I wanted to solve even this last question.

I visited the place again in summers. The dry season had crept in and the whole glen was sweltering under the burning sun. Water sources had dried up. Just a few birds stood sleepily around the muddy remnants of the pond with their beaks wide open in the vain effort to lessen the dryness of their throats. The stifling heat beat down on their heads and the dry westerly hot wind called *Pachhiyaon ki loo* ruffled their feathers. This wind blows daily in May to ensure the ultimate drought of pre-monsoon up the Gangetic plains. The villagers, to my inexpressible joy, told us that two tigers were still living at the place. The two males and the young tigress had moved away, the weakling cub had died but the other was still at heel of his mother. In the process of becoming independent, he was often seen wandering further a field at an earlier age.

It was interesting to note that from the selective occupancy of principal forest formations, the tiger had been forced into baleful and concomitant existence with man. I could not help thinking that a small family crowded into limbo, where its chances of direct competition with man were evidently high, was still living comfortably. The glen was an approximate centre of the tigresses hunting range, which included some 20 sq. kilometers of area.

"The glen is drying, do they get enough water?" I asked the accompanying villager.

"Sahib, they come out in the night and drink freshwater in our sugar-fields" he answered.

It needs to be understood that even in this pinch period the rhizomes of sugarcane are constantly irrigated. Though the small fronds don't offer enough cover for the tigers to move in, but as water is obtainable, they keep visiting the old haunts periodically, in nocturnal perambulations, to wallow and quench their thirst like erstwhile tenants coming back home, which is once again 'under-formation'. Throughout summers, as the fierce sun exhausts all moisture, this irrigation remains a substantial resource of water to the wildlife of farmlands and in their nightly rounds tiger's inspect most parts of their range periodically. Although their movements are related to searching and killing prey, yet in a way they sustain their rights to the area.

During the wet season when the crops rapidly gain height, they thinly disperse throughout all suitable areas, feeding on wild boars and a generalist's range of

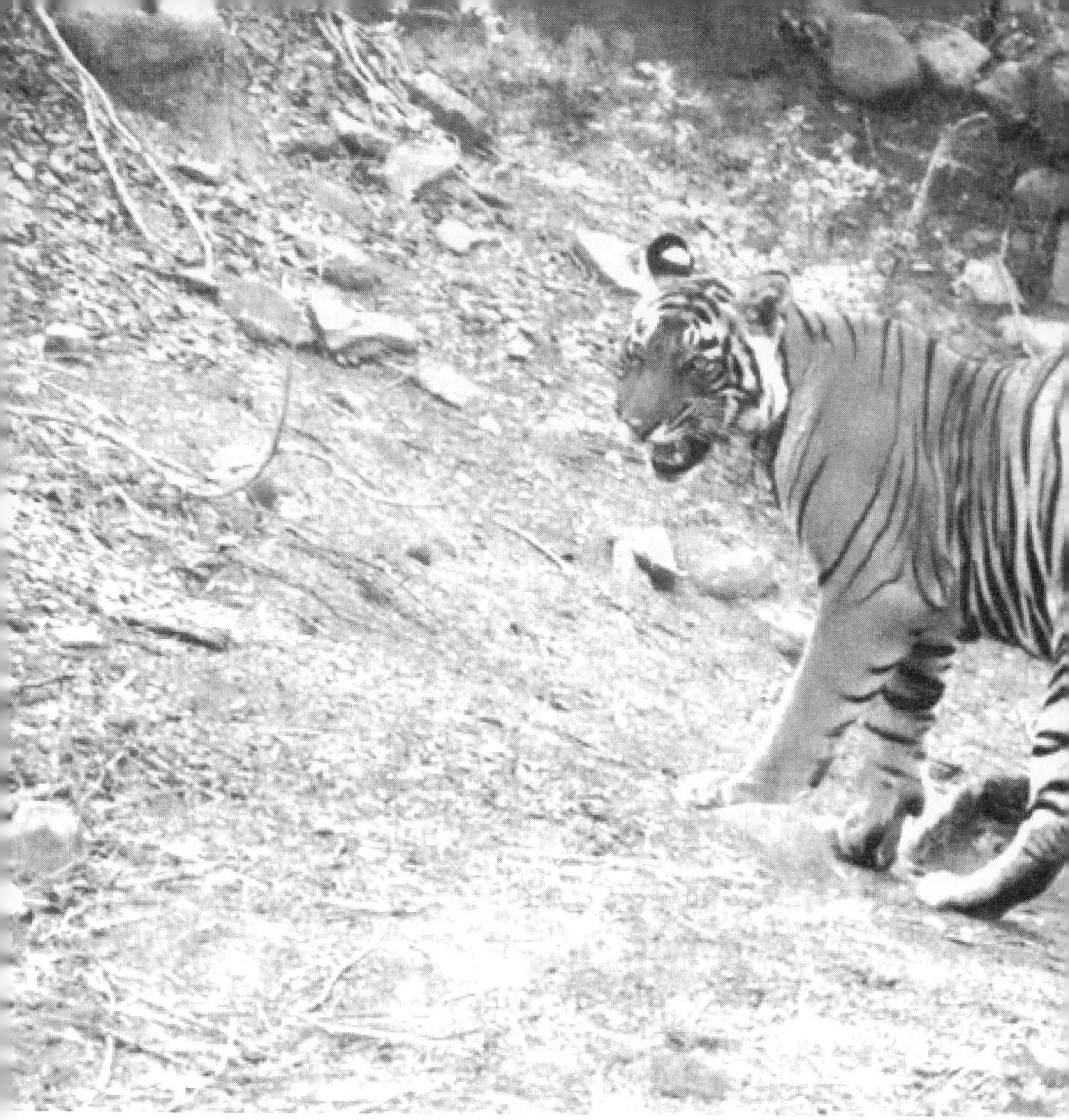

animals who roam about eating juicy sugarcane and in turn themselves become juicy food for the tigers.

Nighasan glens were indeed a beautiful place; an isolated verdure of initial jungle, settled in the middle of agricultural landscape. It abounded in wildlife, perennial grasses and short vegetation. During 1994 the Tarai was still in the throes of expansion. The population was moving up and agriculture demanded more land. The populist policies of the state government allowed the *Gram Sabhas* to lease out their extra land to landless people for the purpose of small farming. Politicians

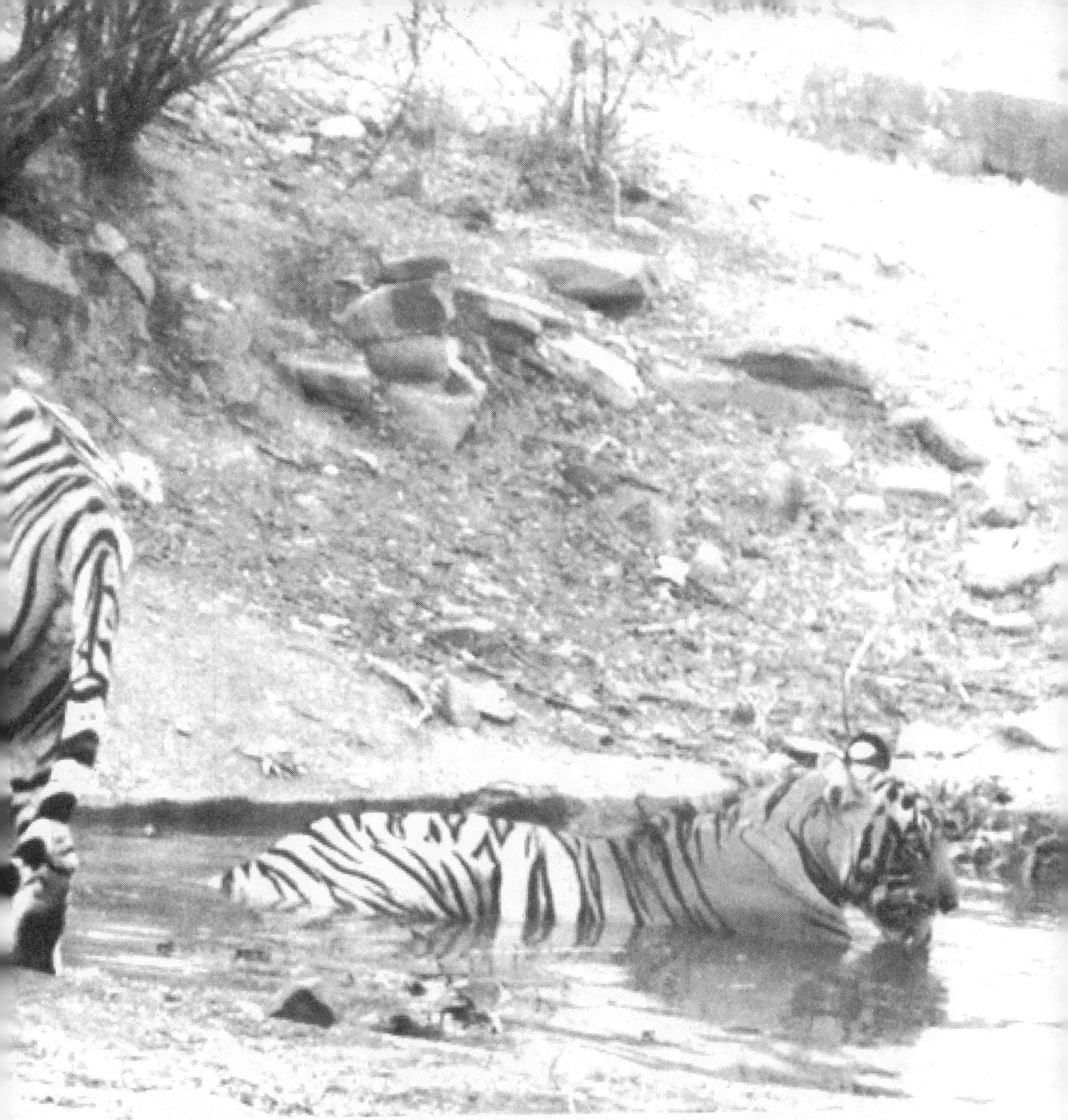

and land sharks exploited these glens in the name of helping the poor communities who were actually victims themselves. Many tractors were brought. Hundreds of hectares of fragmented forest land, with ten feet high *ikra (Erianthus ravennae), nal (Arundo Donex),* and *Jhau (Tamarix dioca)* grasses, were cleared and put to the plough. The whole cycle of events repeated itself without any protest. And with that the once prized glens -a timeless world since the inception of the Tarai itself- ceased to exist.

Like in many other cases the mystery about the sudden disappearance of the tigress and her cub remained unsolved.

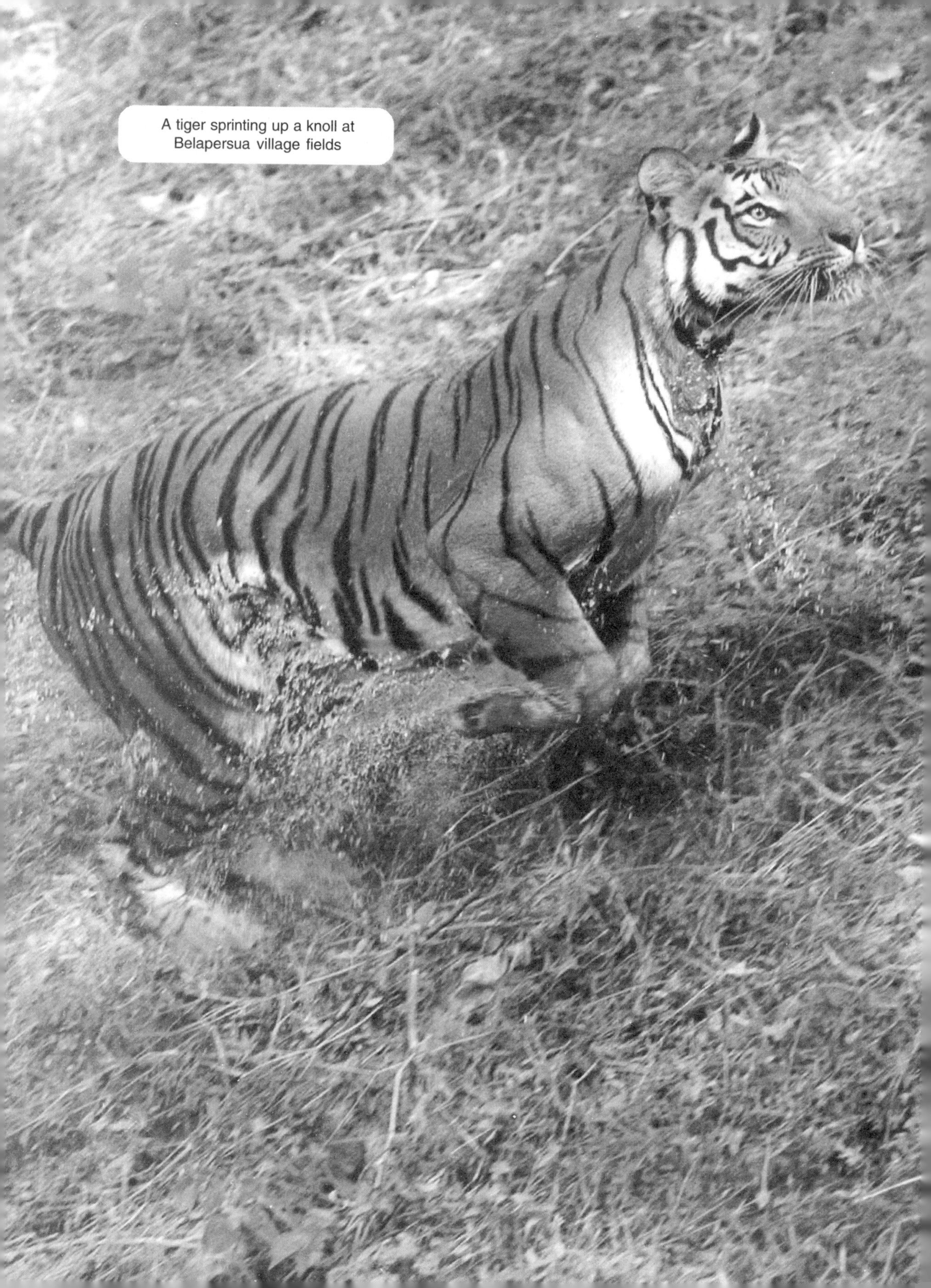

A tiger sprinting up a knoll at Belapersua village fields

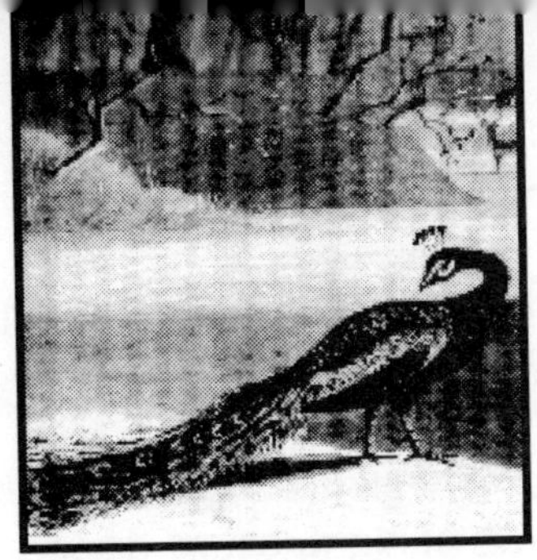

15

Tiger's Den!

The world was made for tigers to suit their way of operating.

- Billy Arjan Singh

I consider myself supremely fortunate to work as a teacher. I continue to be fascinated by my chosen field of endeavour, which makes me much better off than many men, who are chained to jobs they hate. My job never interferes with my life. It fact it has always helped me to achieve my ends, where I could get two months' vacation in summer, one month in winter and a fortnight's sick leave every year, all with pay. It is a soft-berth which has sustained my outdoor ventures very well.

In intermittent years, I had done several short-term surveys in the sugar-fields of the Tarai. The feat had resulted in the generation of a systematic hypothesis about the farmland tigers that I had vaguely started calling the cane tigers. It was certainly an exception to the normal conjectures on large carnivores and bound to contradict the opinions of many known cat group experts from all over India. The phenomenon was being witnessed by hundreds of people every day and my experience, attained at a much wider level, was slowly gaining acceptance. It was a hard, practical, academic piece of evidence achieved from innumerable hours of fieldwork and an acute analysis of empirical data. The fresh facts coming to my knowledge were necessarily fitting themselves into the scheme and as a result my temporary hypothesis, once put forward for argument's sake, was well on its way of becoming a theory.

In the Tarai farms, the continuous strain of human presence results in much shifting and adjustment among these tigers. Sometimes they are there for asking and at other times it is extremely difficult to locate them. Wherever I stayed on farmlands to investigate tiger ranges, I made it a custom to take a walk each morning for some distance in order to get familiar with the terrain. Farmlands were my laboratory and it was necessary to get a rough estimate about the type of wildlife that lived in it, in order to understand the template that favors large carnivores.

The pugmark tracings in the jungle reveal that tigers use roads, trails and game paths to move swiftly between areas where they actually attempt to hunt. They follow the same habit in the canes. They travel great distances by night in search of prey. They may be tracked along the edges of crop plots and adjacent open areas. Their chief desideratum is to use any vista along which they can proceed silently, which is free from obstructions and along which they are afforded a fair vision. More rarely they wait along paths, likely to be taken by animals in anticipation of ambushing them.

Cats normally do not prefer to walk through the path on which the bushes and grasses, often wet with the dews of night, cause discomfort by brushing their sides. However sugar crops are planted in such a demarcated manner that enough space is left in between each plot, forming an elevated boundary around it. Labor gangs and as well as tigers move on the edges of these parapets, which function as walkways.

It often took me a considerable time to search for fresh signs of a tiger; and once I concluded that they were worth following, I would easily sneak into the carnivores' realm. It was most interesting and exciting work to advance through unending plantations of sugar grass, which a master predator had chosen to coexist with his competitors. There would be scrapes in the soil and scent markings on the paths and the trees and often signs of a dust bath taken by the tiger. I followed the trail with confidence, convinced that at any rate it would take me to the place where the animal has taken cover.

The ways wound through the plantations for several furlongs without a break and it was quite confusing to move unaccompanied through a closed environment. The exercise was nightmarish, for there were characteristic places, flanked by tall shading fronds where tigers liked to hide themselves along paths, waiting for an opportune moment to ambush prey animals. They possess hair-trigger hearing capacities. They could hear me walk and breathe and even hear me take out a cigarette from my pocket. It was madness to move on foot alone and expose myself to an accidental ambush, yet it was the only method possible.

I am not a man of great courage but I personally believe after a few days of this sort of constant practice, if one had an aptitude for wildlife, the senses sharpen again. Instinct buried for eons under the rut of civilization, reawaken. The ear strains to reach the million different sounds each of which tell a different story. The nose quickly perceives anything unfamiliar in the smell. Nothing is overlooked by the casual eye. The eye learns to stretch its range of vision-to note the soundless message of the field. And all this comes automatically but with time.

With a rifle slung on my shoulders, I moved on the narrow paths with great care. It was not unusual to get further and further into the depths of this claustrophobic world, an immense greenhouse, where I consciously missed the usual clamor of wildlife; the lingua franca of the jungle that ensues at the sight of a tiger in the wilds. This language of alarm of those hunted by the tiger is a great guiding factor to a naturalist but here the sugarcane crops hung back exceedingly quite, as if their recesses were lifeless. One might think that then there was no one to raise the alarm if I got into trouble, but I was absolutely positive that I won't run into anything that I cannot deal on my own.

On the way, my eyes searched for stripes in the crop. Scanning to right and left to make out an odd shape or a shadow that is not familiar in the consistency of land, I kept a sharp lookout all around, expecting to come across -a pungent whiff of wind, a slight movement or a short growl of admonition- and a tigers face to pop out at any moment. Once I found the tracks of two tiny cubs that were some three months old. They had walked through the puddles made of cart wheel marks and then pushed their way through cane. But ordinarily, I came across nothing much, save here and there a few partridges or peafowl, a hair or a monkey, a jackal or a wild sow accompanied by her train of shaggy piglets. She would scuttle away to safety with much grunting, evidently very annoyed at my intrusion of her domain.

Once while negotiating half way round a plot, I came across fine leopard lying on the middle of the parapet and basking in the morning sun. I had approached the place quiet noiselessly but he got up quickly and made off before I could take out my old fashioned camera and try a shot. Perhaps a leopard is too circumspect a beast to be caught napping.

I liked to follow the nightly course of tigers on the muddy paths that crossed between the crop plots. The track led through fairly unexpected plots where the traces of wild boar and hog deer would be numerous. It was a cumbersome exercise, for the big cats, on their reconnaissance trip, walk five to eight kilometers every night, and over and over again move off from the path, making zigzag sweeps through the crops trying to flush some deer or a wild boar. Thus their own imprints keep appearing and disappearing on the same path.

My guide in the area was a one eyed tracker named Ram Prasad. He knew his way about and everything about wild game, a dirty looking but likable fellow, fitting admirably into the wild surroundings; he was employed by the forest department. His job was to survey waterholes and other possible slots of tigers in sugar fields. He was a hunter and no doubt a poacher and we soon became friends. He once told me that there was a particular tiger in Salimabad fields that patrolled his beat in the night. The tracks of this tiger, supposedly a pre-prime adult, did not actually go very far. Just padding along the dusty path that registered the impression of his wanderings with unfailing certainty, he took a round of four to six kilometers, and then with interesting regularity returned to the point from where he had initially started.

My experience in Larti jungles had taught me that tigers have definite and individually distinctive patterns of movement, and in the years past, I had been familiar with the movements of no fewer than twenty tigers in different parts of the Tarai but this behaviour was strange, and most unlike of a tiger. Since it was a male it couldn't have the liability of the cubs to nourish but there was some irresistible compulsion that always drew him back. It actually raised a question in my mind of whether this tiger was occupying some kind of permanent home. The tigers inside the forest are naturally better off, for plenty of cover provides them enough concealment to practice their traits and keep themselves safe from strong opponents. They indulge in hunts all through the night and in the morning, terminate

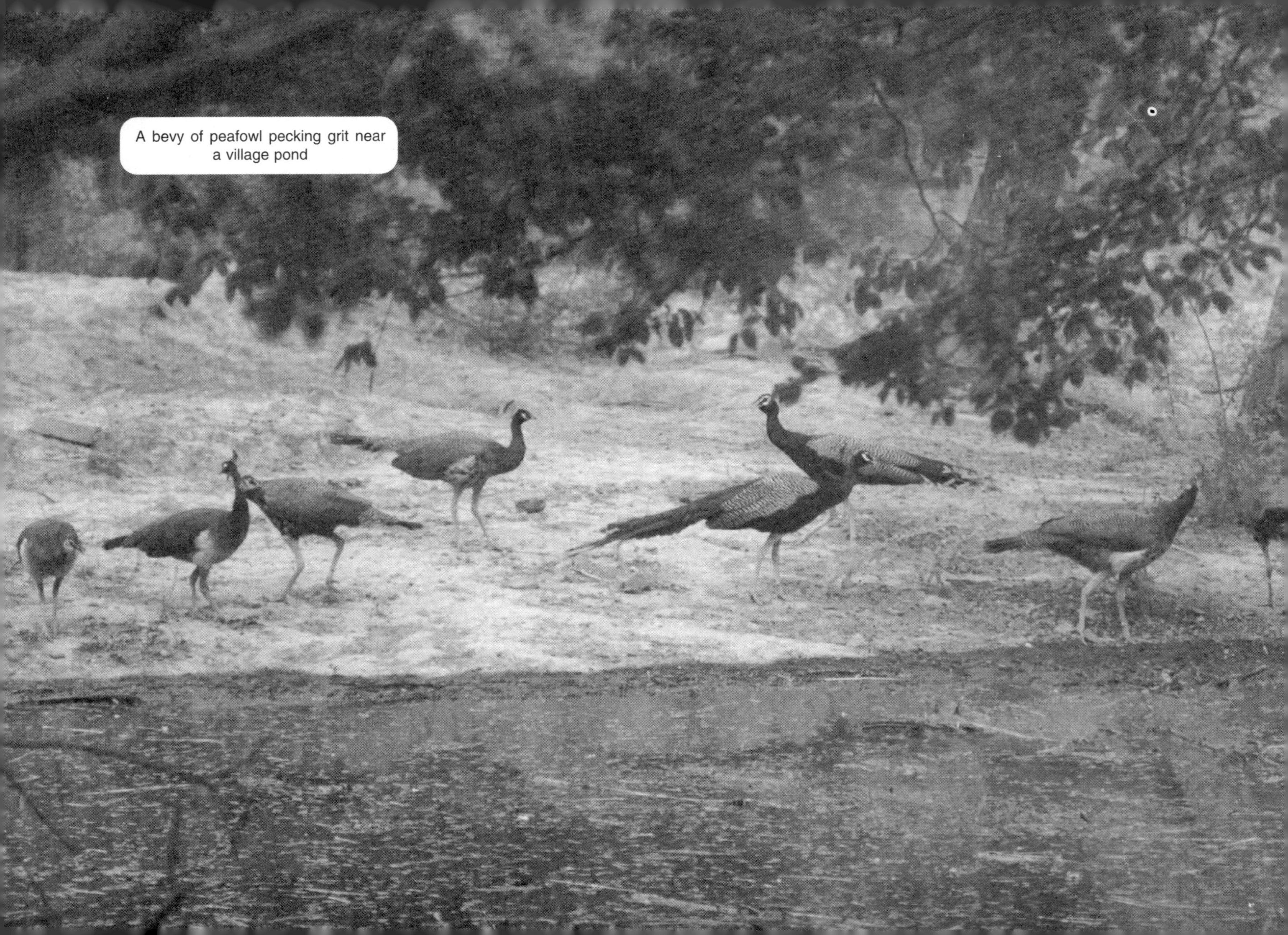

A bevy of peafowl pecking grit near a village pond

their search and stop off at one of the halting stations within their territory. They do not have a permanent residence and are rarely to be found at one place for more than a day. Actually, these marked stations only provide them with temporary resting places from where they can go out hunting the next day.

The tracks of this male juvenile were so exclusive that the entire pattern of his activities could be traced by them alone. This point was of curious interest. I decided to take up this case as a test for my cane tiger theory and see how far I could take it. Long back I had independently chosen this research question to build my thesis of cane tiger. This was a major part of my study agenda and here was a prospective opening that could provide me with the right answer and help me establish fresh benchmarks for evaluating the presence of tigers in the canes. Moreover years of focused study had taught me that no finding is worthless in the field research. There are innumerable examples where seemingly irrelevant knowledge later turned out to be extremely valuable for the management of the animal.

The following three days, the tracker I made a determined search; after a great physical exertion and with great expenditure of thought, skill and guile we picked up several clues to the hideout of this tiger. The place laid in an 'odd area' quite far from the sugar fields. Odd areas are sites not well adapted for cultivation, such as seeps, bogs and ditches, that grow to provide habitat to a variety of animals, and where permanent trees, shrubs and grasses protect areas of shallow water near or within crop fields. Generally, exclusion of livestock from some areas provides the best vegetation diversity and structure for wildlife habitat.

The place was a mile away across a *Kuchcha* road harboring a big belt of reed grass. Beyond this was much swampy ground, where this animal lived. It was a damp ditch, ideally located in a *sarpat* patch, well shaded and cool and under the dark shade of a cluster of *Jamun* trees that were loaded with hundreds of the nest of weaver birds. The irregular pinnacles of termite mounds surrounded it in three directions, rising to a height of 6 to 8 feet. The place was rarely visited by villagers and remained relatively undisturbed.

I entered the den from the moor side. A number of snakes' swam off in shallow water to get out of my way. The den was quite secure and impregnable. It reeked of big cat with awful smelly urination. Here, I found the heads of two recently eaten dogs whose cranium had been cracked open to chomp at the brains. I had heard about this fussy leaning of tigers from native hunters but had never seen it in life. Some tigers often practice this 'nonstandard trait' with the heads of small prey animals whose flesh they find tender and tastier. And the urge is, to enjoy every scrap of the small carcass; hence even the brain is scooped out.

Delighted at my luck, I rummaged around, looking down at the ground and came across some sopping wet substance. It seemed the tiger had vomited quite a few times. The vomited material consisted not of food but largely of ping pong-sized hairballs, a couple of which lay near the base of the *Pipal.* Vomiting may be related to disorders of the stomach but cats vomit quite readily and such occasional vomiting does not indicate any abnormality. Hairballs occur because cats groom themselves extensively and often also lick their prey lustily before commencing a meal. Their tongues are equipped with backward-pointing spikes which aid in their grooming and also scoop up loose hair. The disadvantage of this is that cats end up swallowing a considerable proportion of the hair they lick off their own coats or their prey, thus retaining a large amount of hair in their stomach.

Hair is not digestible and usually it doesn't get bunched together. It may pass through the cat's stool, while at other times it accumulates near the throat or in the upper digestive tract of the stomach and is vomited periodically as hairballs. There are times though, when the hairball becomes too big, and it can't be expelled. In such cases, it could be dangerous for the cat.

At such times tigers eat grass to aid the removal of hairballs through vomiting before they become unmanageable. They may subsequently swallow the froth that they cough up but the hairballs are not re-eaten.

A closer examination of the den revealed a few more dirty looking balls, dry and half-dry and certainly harder than the first lot. The expulsion of nearly half a dozen hairballs could not have taken place just in one bout of vomiting because the lots lay scattered here and there at odd places. Only couple of these were fresh and the rest were older. Moreover, expulsion of hairballs is a periodical feature, which happens with a gap of one to two months in a cat. I wondered if the zoo felines reflect this tendency at a normal rate in their life, reason being they are given the properly chopped and washed pieces of hairless meat; therefore their regurgitation rate is low and the matter contains the hair of their bodies only, while in a wild tiger, that swallows a lot of hair of its prey in his each meal, besides his own that he licks the regurgitation rate is much higher. The stockpile of so many hairballs clearly signified that the tiger had been living here, at least for few months.

Tigers cough up such hairballs only when they are at ease and purr. The sound triggers the brain to release a hormone which helps it to relax and acts as a pain or stress killer. Done with "specific intent" the purring creates vibrations in the stomach which potentially helps the tiger to dislodge hairballs from the pyloric valve. The stock of so many hairballs clearly signified that the tiger had been living here at least for few months. This was like the den having a nameplate of "tiger-in-residence."

I collected the hoard and sent to the Director Lucknow Zoo, Rashmi Kant Shukla. The laboratory examination done by Dr. A.C. Das, revealed that the largest hairball, about the size of a cricket ball was made of pheasant feathers, mostly of peafowl and brown partridges, besides some of tiger's own hair.

This was valuable information for me. I could see the break coming. For until now, like the Project Tiger mandarin, the existence of a pure sugar-brand tiger had been seemingly an 'incomprehensible-probability' to me, which had held my conjecture in reserve. I had often thought that farms could not be a normal habitat for a tiger, for unlike jungles there is no way for the tigers to relieve the pressures imposed by human intrusion into cane crops. But here was the evidence, which inveterately substantiated my contention that the tigers had discovered the deep layers of utterly desolated tracts to attain tranquility. They may be away from the jungles, but they were stress-free and favorably contented at strategic slots.

Locke suggests that "Contrary to popular belief, tigers do not have lairs, although they will occasionally carry off their prey to the same spot when no alternative feeding place is available" Jim Corbett described the life of one tiger which had its home base in a hollow tree and William Baze found that a tiger "is strongly attached to its permanent quarters and uses them as his base for his foraging expeditions." Jerdon noted that the tiger returns to the same lair at dawn. To my mind under conceivable circumstances, any temporary lair is abandoned as soon as the corpse is all eaten, which may take several days, but if a tiger repeatedly brings its kills to a certain place then the place is but his lasting lair.

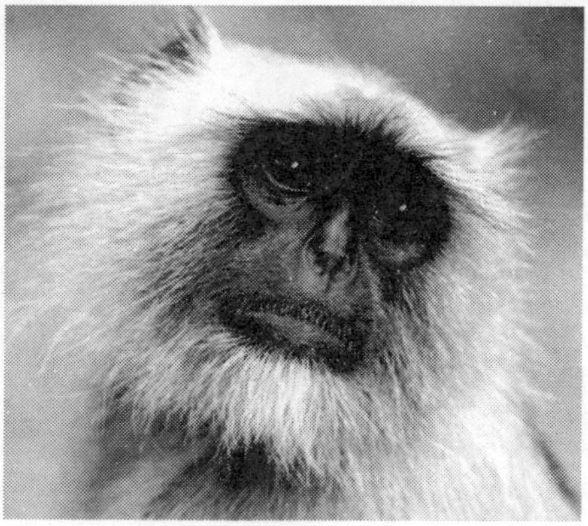

A Langoor Monkey

These and other observations indicate that in some areas, a tiger appears to have a more or less a permanent abode to which he returns each day. In forests with scanty undergrowth, localized water supplies, and heavy disturbances by man and livestock it seems probable that the tiger retreats daily into one of several pieces of preferred cover.

In the Tarai cane fields, however, the shade, water and other requirements are widespread, yet the tigers have a predilection for certain lairs. Once the great cat has made the transition to the completely different surroundings from the jungle, nurturing the instinctive avoidance of man, it inevitably seeks isolated corners where it feels secure to retire for the day. When such habitat is a selective possession of a tiger -a core zone of its territory that fulfills its biological and ecological necessities- it shows a strong disinclination to move out. It endeavors to stay in residence as long as possible.

Perhaps such soothing places that keep the nocturnal predators away from adversarial contact with man have been a major factor, underlying the continued survival of sugar tigers in the farmlands of the Tarai.

As I stood on the crucial spot with a revolver in my hands, the sun was setting, turning the close by moor into a wonderful autumnal panorama, over which a folk of spot bill ducks was leisurely sailing and I knew I had found what I had expected. I was in high spirits and content with a sense of achievement that I had discovered an incredible and at the same time a ground-breaking secret.

"Good heavens" I cried, "It is marvelous".

******

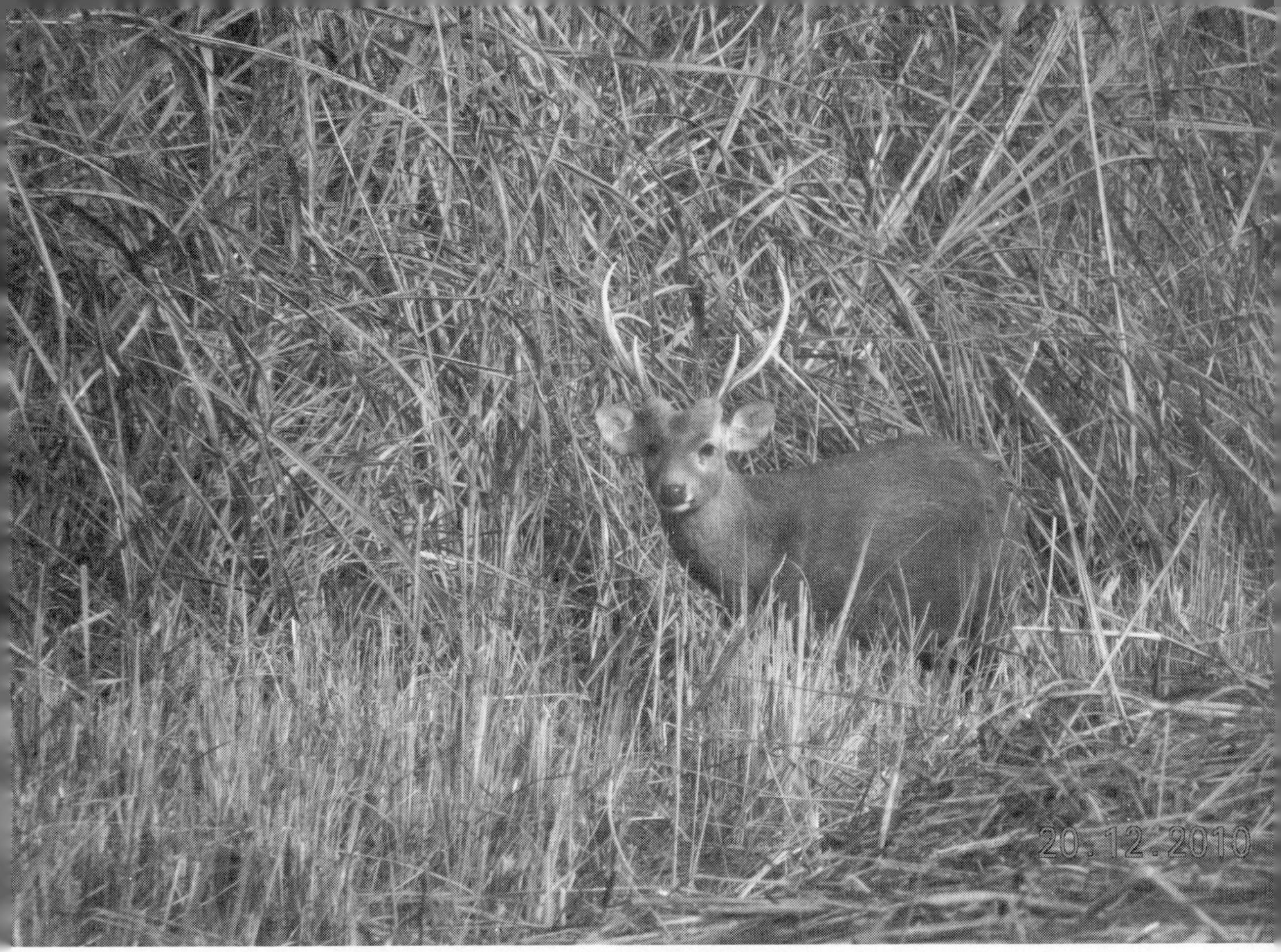

A Hog deer

Evolution is often thought of as something which happened ages ago, an event which has reached its end since all possible creation has been made. But truly, evolution is a constant process and life forms essentially keep changing in response to the demands of an ever-changing environment. Modification of behaviour will go on as long as there is life. The contemporary dynamism of evolution in the *Tarai* was most apparent in these tigers.

Sugarcanes are sub-optimal habitats, yet these beasts, having accepted farmlands as their new and complete environment; do not return to the jungles again, they do not take even to the eco-tonal belt of their previous ecosystem. In the event of interspecies or intra-species tension, they rather penetrate deeper into the cane country, in which they are seemingly integrated and take to local jungles and marshes.

Lifestyle changes of this magnitude suggest that distinct from the general macrocosm they are a microcosm of an evolving putative creed; the hard cores of compulsive sugar tiger, who know the coagulated codes for continual existence in the farms. Philosophers of an earlier age had held that facts exist independently, and that truth is born when human beings discover these facts. Often truth is also conceived as something created - not discovered, but created - by man. How does truth change from something discovered by the mind to a thing created by it? I was cautious, if unintentionally, I had not become responsible for so momentous a transformation in tiger studies. But the answer was a big 'No', for my school was everyday experience in the field, where my roots went deep into the lessons learned from on-ground initiatives and where each day with something new, something never seen before, good or bad was teaching me distinctly.

No matter how different it was from the rigid view of science.

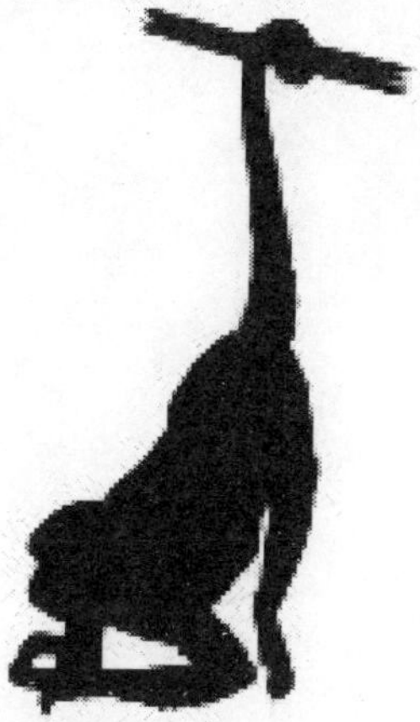

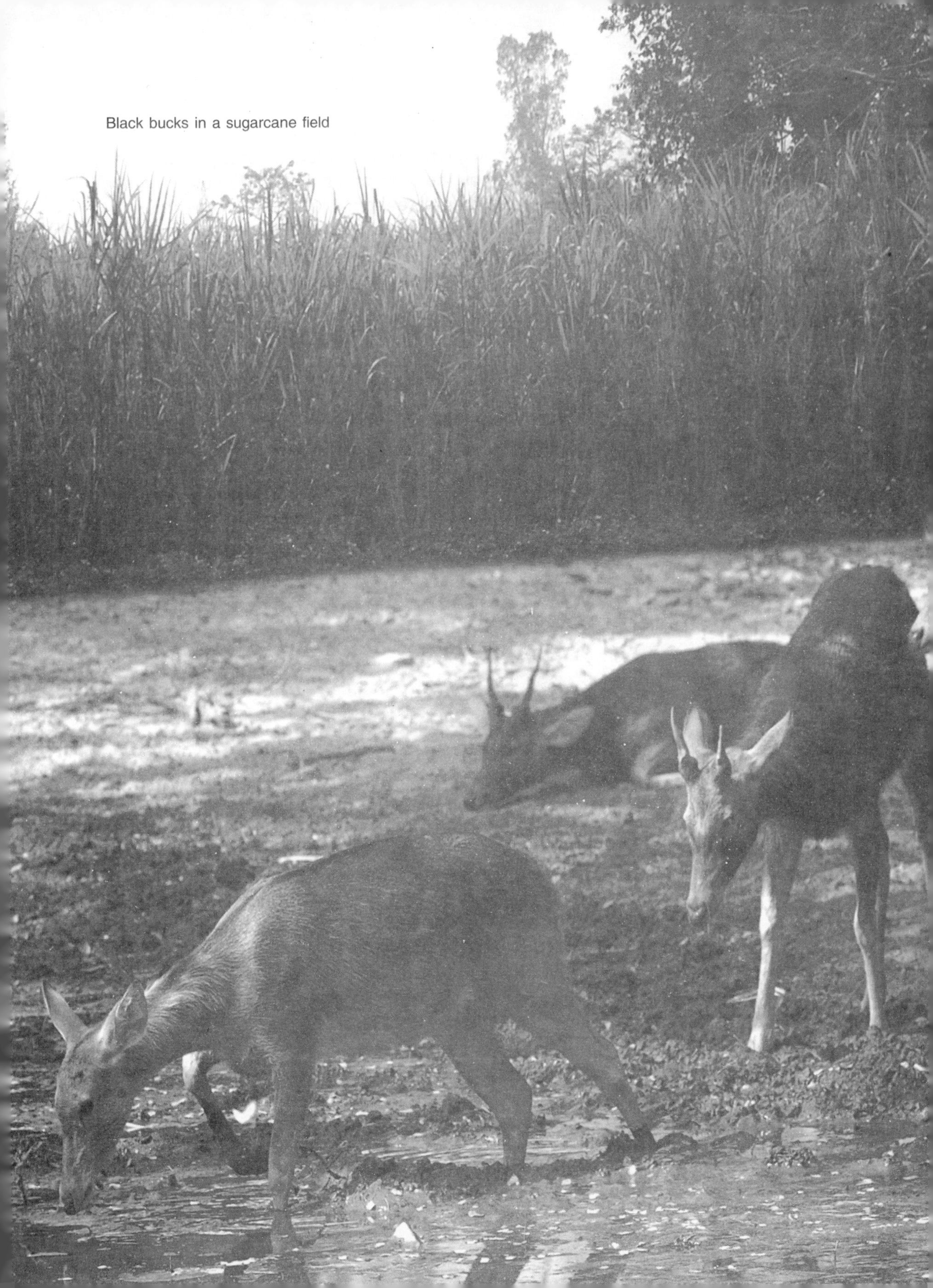

Black bucks in a sugarcane field

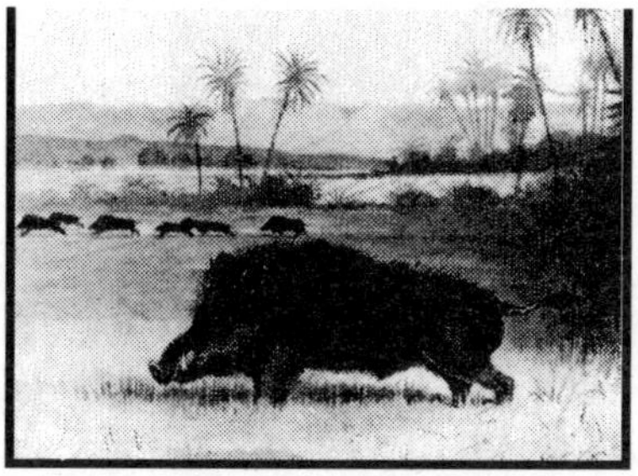

16

Prey Base

Livestock has assumed an important role in providing the cat with prey in many areas.

- George B. Schaller

The existence of large carnivores in farmlands is a subject generally and signally ignored in books of sport and natural history. As indeed might be expected of popular authors' to have a tendency to ignore farmland wild life in relationship to jungle life or follow one another even in perpetuating errors of facts and views about large carnivores by unjust stigmatizations and unscientific generalizations. My object in writing this treatise is to present a comprehensive view on the ecological dilemma of cane field tigers to better understand their characteristics and temperament. Thus this treatise is certainly the ultimate word on the controversial subject of sugarcane tiger. I say this on the basis of my singular qualifications of intermittent field work and the conclusions gathered from original observations.

The nature of an animal's food supply dictates its whole lifestyle, limits its absolute abundance and regulates its numbers. The second law of thermodynamics states that the weight of carnivores in a stable ecosystem will invariably be much less than the weight of herbivores because the carnivores keeps the herbivorous population in check. This is true but the most general case is that the herbivores control the carnivores' number. A curious turnabout when the fate of the fearsome cat is dictated by the population dynamics of timorous prey.

The prey base has far-reaching effect on the consumer for it is the ultimate determinant of the morphology of the predator. The vigor of a predator is reflected in the vitality of its prey. To understand the matrix of food source in a tiger's life we must first know as how do they exploit the prey base within their habitat and what are the patterns of their prey selectivity? Only then we can understand the anomaly of their survival in sugarcanes.

Different tigers have different food habits. Those who kill and eat a buffalo calf slowly in installments of ten to fifteen pounds a day often demolish a 100 pound chital just in two days may be because it has a better taste. In my experience, cane tigers are not selective predators and being crepuscular in habit, they constantly make contact with domestic species and naturally feel more tempted to kill them.

In a revealing study on Chitwan National Park in Nepal made by the American biologist M. Sanquist in 1981, it was found that the daily food requirement of a tigress was 5 to 7 kg and that of a tiger was 7 to 9 kg. Discounting the inedible part of the carcass and the loss of some meat to scavengers, it was estimated that the annual requirement of a female was 2,800 kg to 3,600 kg and that for the male was 3,300 kg to 4,000 kg. On the basis of this and using certain established estimates, it was calculated that the crude biomass (or live weight of prey) available to a tiger was between 3,500 kg and 5,600 kg per square mile.

This pertains to the availability of natural prey as the studies were conducted in the forests where there are no cattle available to tigers. Ullas Karanth says that "Through the massive overkill of their prey base, hunters have depressed carrying capacities and even eliminated tigers over most of Asia. A simple rule of thumb can assess this deadly impact; for every 50 deer hunted in a year, there is room for one less tiger on this earth."

Charles McDougal also endorses the same point but in a little different way, "In addition to wild species on which a tiger depends primarily for food, it supplements its diet with domestic cattle and buffalos when the opportunity presents itself... Nonetheless the tiger cannot exist without natural prey, and where this has been eliminated from forest areas, the tiger does not survive, even though there may be plenty of cattle and buffalos to prey upon."

The question may be raised as how the generations of captive tigers in zoos breed and survive on rationed meat of cattle and buffalos and live their full cycle of life. Tigers of Chinese farms are not fed on wild prey, yet they are healthy and show a gargantuan increase in population. Even wild tigers of Vladivostok are known to gather round small townships to live their snowy winter on stray dogs. This means tigers can survive on any kind of animal protein provided it quantifies to fulfill their nutritional requirement.

As regards McDougal's point, it is responsive to understand that wild tigers are sometimes unable to absorb the sudden pressures of prey depletion and perish but when it comes to farm tigers, we presume that they inhabit the retreat by the process of naturalization, thus their prey composition, its availability, as well as requirements are certainly different and this is where that they biologically differ and must differ from the jungle tigers. This behavioral adaptability to new prey and a new habitat is that specialized qualification, which finally brands them as the sugarcane tiger.

Terms like threatened fauna and flora, prey depletion, endangered ecologies and exacerbated terrains normally used to explain nit-picking aspects of tiger conservation landscapes do not apply here. Jungles may stand entirely denuded of prey but farmlands are never devoid of it, in fact farmlands are bottom-heavy with exploded prey numbers and with no top-level predator to nosh on them, thus the prey base of a sugarcane tiger figures as a critical question. I have already said that different tigers have different food preferences thus they do preferentially kill certain prey types. The prey offered to farm tigers is not the customary prey; more often it is a mixture of both wild and human livestock. The percent of their customary, primary prey that comes out of the jungle vis-à-vis the percentage of non conventional, secondary prey in the form of pets is mostly lower. And when we analyze the crude biomass available to tigers within their range; it also includes human beings living per sq km. And that alone surpasses all the density of fauna obtainable in the area.

This makes the food situation diametrically opposite to that in the jungle. And in juxtaposition to this difference, the percentage of such farm tigers, turning into ardent cattle lifters and subsequently man-eaters should also be higher. Tigers may not go for alien food easily but it is undeniable that its attainability for them, with such increased access, remains optimal.

But all this is mere conjecture, as no exhaustive study has ever been conducted of such mundane a thing as the variation in the prey list of a jungle tiger and a farm tiger. The impact of co-existence with humans on wildlife is also not known but there is enough reason to conclude that wildlife gets seriously endangered as a result of loss of fodder, food and habitat.

Interestingly, farm lands falling within ten kilometers of the jungle function as eco-fragile zones, and contain small wildlife of their own. Wheat, pulses, *channa*, and barley etc. grow here simultaneously with the cane. Herbivores of all kinds are attracted by the crops. Wild boars, porcupines, chital, hog deer, swamp deer and monitor lizard visit these fields in the night and also breed there some times. Thus, the tigers here select their prime preys.

Sugarcane is the perpetual pleasure for wild boars. They move in it as soon it is sown. They would dig up the sets which are planted and covered with earth. After the sets have germinated they take shelter in the crop itself, and as the crop matures, they build shelters against rain and squally weather by piling cane leaves in huge loads, and getting under the pile of trash, they finally elevate it to form a kind of igloo. They would dig into fresh earth to form breeding shelters, and breed outrageously large families. They live in their larder and eat at all hours. Given that most ungulates produce one or two fawns per year, the wild boars do not have any fixed cycle for breeding. These prolific breeders are supposed to compensate for all the lapses in the production of prey species. Their tribe grows in geometrical proportions and produces an annual surplus of nearly 30 per cent. A sow delivers thrice a year and each litter carries 15 to 20 piglets which easily survive till maturity, increasingly competing with mankind for livelihood. They constitute the principal prey for tigers in the jungle as well as in the farmlands.

I have seen the remains of 32 wild animals killed by tigers in the cane fields. They represented eight species — four of chital, nine hog deer, twelve wild boar, one monitor lizard, one python, one swamp deer doe, one peacock and a porcupine. I have discovered a pile of over fifty detached tails of jackals, devoured by Barotha tigress which I have already described. (I have also witnessed one monkey's predations but never found its remains). A friend of mine once gathered some quantitative data by collecting rumen samples from some kills. It showed that sugar cane was the primary diet of ungulates, especially of wild boars.

Amongst farm dwelling herbivores the resource of sugarcane seems to be shared in a mutually beneficial way. Because of its coarse structure, a mature strand of sugarcane is physically unavailable to the small deer, and even unpalatable until broken by the heavy feeders like the herds of *nilgai*. Wild boars uproot it and munch it like carrots. Even jackals pull down the cane by breaking its base to suck its sap. Once the stem is broken the deer family and monkeys move in and take up coarse feeding, with a moderately low leaf to stem ratio. They may be followed by some more animals like monitor lizards who hunt for bird eggs, frogs and chameleons in the canes and also suck the succulent juice from busted stems.

Sugarcane is a highly nourishing plant and serves as a wholesome food for many. It contains a number of nutrients, including sucrose and exquisite minerals and salts, high calcium content, carbohydrates from sugars helping later in development of fat, finally turn into protein, and a large quantum of roughage. Hence it is far more nourishing than common grasses and if there is a craving for some specific mineral hunger, boars briefly move elsewhere and satisfy it by eating cereals and herbs and uprooting saplings for tubers and then again come back into the canes.

I do not know if the wild ungulates ever become diabetic by eating so much of sugar but monkeys are certainly susceptible to it. I have observed that monkey troops eating excessive sugarcane turn considerably thin due to high glucose in their blood but when the cane is harvested they turn to other foods, their diabetes level wanes and they start gaining weight.

The boundaries of ecological tolerance for various species are abrupt. As the distance of farms increases from the jungles, the feature of the environment changes and the capricious species like deer thin out yet a few basic wild preys remain. *Nilgai* and wild boar in ungulates, rhesus and *langur* monkeys in primates, pea fowls in birds and finally some lesser lights like porcupines, hare, mongoose and cats, might possibly still serve as humble prey base to a tiger. This list of fauna apparently represents the second order prey, which occurs in most of the pockets where cane tigers have been often reported. The place can be as far as 15 to 20 miles from the jungle. This *carte du jour* also supports straying tigers.

(It is interesting to note that in 2009 a tigress straying from Pilibhit to Faizabad via Lucknow district had covered more than 500 kilometers between November and March. She had unintentionally killed 5 human beings and eaten none of them. Its kills recovered by tracking forest guards, included 3 chital, 6 *nilgai*, 22 goats, 4 buffalos, 13 dogs, 4 wild boar and 11 feral cows. Once located it was constantly pursued by natives and foresters beyond reasonable limits. Under the widespread pressure of the native crowd, hurling abuses and baying for its blood, most of the kills were left uneaten or half eaten, pressurizing the hungry tiger to kill even more. At many points, it had also scavenged on the putrescent carcasses of cattle that had been thrown away by the villagers.

However, this medley of prey cannot be used as a decent predictive model of a farm tiger's prey, as a great deal of it was knocked down under excessive hunger generated by harassed conditions, where the consumption rate of a carcass of slain prey was almost as good as zero in comparison to the exceptionally high killing rate. Moreover, the tigress did not defend its kill nor did it return to the site. It was not in the propitious conditions in which the sugar tigers seek their existence. I am sure that in terms of prey size, the effective utilization of such kills invariably lowers the killing rate of a tiger.)

The ungulates of the open plains are much more prolific breeders than solitary animals. It is due to the induced communal activity, where one female brings another into season, and the male has the ability to serve several females. Nowhere is this factor, scientifically described, as 'synchronous breeding dynamics' is more applicable on *nilgai* in the Tarai. As the cane zone recedes further away from the jungle, the wildlife drastically thins out but the *nilgai* herds invariably stay on. I have seen the huge deposits of their droppings nearly everywhere in the Tarai as these ungulates have a habit of regularly using the same spot to defecate and also as rendezvous point. There may be a few black bucks at some places but they usually frequent arid terrains.

Thus, sugar plantation is a perfect combination of prey and cover for a tiger, for here they naturally run into a larger variety of ungulates in contrast to their jungle counterparts. And in reality, there is nothing like legal or illegal prey for a hungry tiger. Necessity knows no law. The biological traits of tigers enable them to prey upon innumerable species that share their home and being, in the apex position, they can prey on even the calves of elephant or rhino. So in the sugar, where an opportunistic lifestyle is called for, tigers have a little cause to worry for food.

The tiger is a product of wisdom that nature has selectively evolved. The only problem is that man reprimands this wisdom for his own purpose, as a greater quantum of it does not fit into the scale of human values. A tiger, whatever it kills, never reprobates against natural laws, but it always sins against human laws.

My experience leads me to believe that real cane tigers feed on primary production of the environment from varanus lizard to monkeys and partially on feral livestock. I have counted at least eleven species of livestock, which they often kill, ranging from buffalo, cow, horse, mare, donkey, goat, sheep, domestic pig, dog, cats, ducks and hens, out of which cows and goats are more vulnerable, whereas amongst wild prey a monkey's predation is extremely rare. It may be accredited that the sugarcane tiger's area of expertise is its aptitude to use a wide range of food resources; it is a strategy for dealing with the seasonal changes that dominate the cycle of their year.

I reckon that they kill randomly, thereby taking different types of prey, not only certain types, roughly in proportions that occur in their habitat. They do not preferentially kill certain prey types. Ullas Karanth explains this in a complementary, scientific manner, "If tigers are indeed selective predators, they kill their prey animals based on species, body size or some other factor that renders the prey vulnerable to predation."

Thus, vulnerability is the first factor in prey selection and cattle are the first to fall in this category. They are ever exposed to predation, because of their dulled senses of self defense and also because of their relative abundance. The only deterrent is the human factor, which is a deterrent in every way. Even if a tiger kills a wild boar or a hog deer, the human factor often steps in and its kill is often plundered for a village party. I have witnessed this paradox many times. If a farm tiger kills natural game, he starves and if it is feral cattle, he can at least gobble it in contentment.

Tarai is overcrowded with feral cattle. Cows being sacred to Hindus are never traded with butchers. As a result, hundreds and thousands of emaciated cattle which, when left of no use, are cast off by their owners to fend for themselves. Such a gaunt lot, sans an owner gradually adopts wild ways and becomes feral cattle. They collect in groups of tens and twenties and voraciously devastate the crops ready to be harvested.

The farmers have no permanent solution for this problem, so they keep driving the herds away from their territories. They are chased across numerous villages and blocks, sometimes south and sometimes north, from where they are again chased east or west. They are chased from corner to corner and the process is constantly repeated, bringing a temporary relief to farmers. For such large herbivores substantially exceeding 400 kg in adult body mass, predation is a negligible cause of mortality until a tiger arrives.

In ecology, predation is a simplest mechanism of population control. This menace, of feral cattle, falls an easy prey to the sugarcane tigers. So the big cat is not without a 'functional-response' in a humble villager's economy.

Then there are still more cattle moving in herds. They are a part of animal husbandry, manned by grazers. Sugarcane tigers competently distinguish the essential difference between the two segments, as feral and domestic cattle they do not forage together. Thus tigers don't turn their attention to herds despite the effective target area being large, and the greater being the chance of a hit. They rather instinctively go for wild cattle.

Tigers take their prey base in a sustained comportment. They do not overkill nor do they exhaust the capital but much like human beings they moderately try to live on its interest. To my mind, a tiger in sugarcane survives by cropping just one to five percent of its prey base, whereas in empty jungles, with wild prey base radically reduced due to poaching, the same animal might crop somewhat thirty to fifty percent of interest or even come down to the eating of capital; it is not to be forgotten that this also includes a relentless input in the chase.

A tiger, living near Palnapur village in South Kheri, once presented a classic example of this accomplished hunting. In a period of 18 months, from March 1985 to September 1986, he killed around 66 feral cattle and was never harmed by villagers, because he was actually helping them. He used to kill his prey with a rare technique of biting it on its nose so that the animal was asphyxiated to death. Though feral cattle were the most important prey species of this tiger yet he was never branded as a cattle-lifter. He was rather considered a prudent benefactor and a regulator of natural equilibrium in the environment. I remember seeing his pugmarks along the banks of Ull River and the whitening bones of many cattle in the grass around and also the gleaming crops that had clearly come to life that winter.

Now, when the farms have pushed back forests everywhere, such beasts with apt 'feeding compositions' are more cunning, more individualistic and are better able to escape the threat of extermination because the advantages they provide, in the long run, outweigh the disadvantages.

(II)

Tigers are obligate carnivores, meaning that they have a diet strictly of meat. They have evolved as a specialized predator of large herbivores. Full-grown tigers prefer to hunt larger prey. Investigations prove that large tigers show a definite preference for semi-mega herbivorous species such as cows and buffalos that weigh more than 300 pounds, than over medium sized and smaller prey. In some areas the killing of cattle —wild, semi-wild, abandoned and domestic— contributed to over 70 per cent of the meat eaten by tigers in cane zones. In some cases it was even 95 per cent. I believe that the tigers that were exclusively living on such predation were either old or incapable beasts, cub rearing tigresses or last but not the least, to advocate my point, the able-bodied but hardened cane tigers. Unfortunately, some false claims for compensation on wild cattle devoured by tigers projected as domestic cattle, led the officials to brand them as aberrant.

Normal tigers hunt mainly at night. They are not often too exposed to the temptations of domestic stock which are usually herded back into enclosures at dusk. In some areas they do take to domestic cattle. As domestic cattle are only available during day time, the tigers in such areas also display diurnal habits; their biological clock works according to the habits of prey.

We have already seen that such tigers, who gradually switch over from wild game to abandoned cattle, have improved opportunity of surviving in sugar fields. Cattle meat is effectively available in different measures in different places and its anti predatory responses are also poorer. This factor makes the prey composition of a sugar tiger diametrically opposite to that of a jungle tiger, bringing a radical change in their diet, which is widely divergent. I also sometimes doubt if tigers have any developed taste glands at all, their incredible versatility in feeding habits, that even includes grasshoppers, locust, centipedes, maggots and many other creepy-crawlies, proves that they must be and should be indifferent to taste. However, this complex subject too remains an under-researched area.

To repeat the point, this transformation seems a pre-requisite for living in the sugarcane for it essentially gives these tigers the real edge in terms of food over others who live in canes but look for wild prey. R. L. Singh says, "A tiger can survive in the sugarcanes if he behaves properly." This means he has a lot to learn by seeking to live near man. The key word 'behaves properly' denotes being dexterous enough to survive a direct impact of multiple ecological influences as well as of the human excesses imposed on the environment. Until this proper behaviour does not change direction against both natural and man-made laws, where energy is used with tranquility, the tiger can live as a strategist; significantly it also includes the process of learning how to avoid its only predator — man.

Predators are the strategists of the highest order. Multiplicity of selective pressures –as all the animals seek to minimize the risk of being killed and eaten-results in any one final form of behaviour for a carnivore. In the light of these facts, cattle-eating is an acquired taste and its hunting is an indispensable part of a sugarcane tiger's life, because they are both vulnerable and large in terms of prey size. Cows, fat, slow and clumsy, must seem the ideal prey to a tiger. One can hypothesize a number of advantages as well as some disadvantages to such a predation. Imagine a tiger wandering about, looking for something to eat. If there are 500 cattle in his range, there are 500 possible targets he can encounter. Cows are large animals, more conspicuous and easier to detect. Thus, tigers selectively exploit their increased vulnerability. No normal tiger, even an ardent selective game killer, will leave an easy food that comes to him asking to be killed.

It is in such paradoxical ways that the search of knowledge sometimes takes a step forward. With the slaughter of a cow, the tiger gets detected and the inevitable human factor steps in. Domestic cows are human possessions and as the man tries to save it, the tiger lands up in a conflict. Some miscreants loudly proclaim themselves to be the owner of abandoned cattle, devoured by tiger and demand compensation from the government. All they need is a suitable pretext and the presence of a tiger in the area. This gimmick inspires impecunious characters to find old piles of bones and skeleton somewhere and lay claim upon it. The officials know this but as wildlife schemes are perennially short of funds, so their investigations are very tough before even a paltry sum is released. The confusion creates problems and more often than not the big cat eventually pays a heavy price for it.

The argument that cow meat is inferior and tigers don't readily go for it is utterly spurious; the misleading notion has no scientific background. From a large carnivore's point of view, a cow contains a substantial volume of meat, which if not wasted, can definitely sustain it for days. Hungry tigers are sometimes reduced to eating humble foodstuff such as fish, frogs, crabs and bird eggs. Brander declares that once he was shown a heap of cow dung "part of which had been eaten, of which he was assured was the work of a sick tiger". My observations lead me to conclusion that when Barotha tigers devoured jackals and berries as their staple victuals, then any meat of phlegmatic cattle is indubitably a lofty cuisine, which also includes carrion in an advanced state of decomposition.

Schaller endorses this point. He says, "Taking India as whole, domestic cattle and buffalo are the most important items in the tiger's diet. With the wildlife in many forests is decimated or eliminated, the tiger has taken partly or wholly to living on livestock, which is easy to kill and readily available. At least ten percent of the cattle grazing in Kanha Park and on its fringes are killed by tigers each year."

Cattle essentially serve as staple food to wild tigers. Brander states that "The great mass of tigers is partly cattle killers and partly game eaters, but some animals living in forests... hardly ever kill cattle. On the other hand, in many parts of the province tiger lives on nothing but cattle and follows the herd about as these are shifted for water and grazing".

The purpose of evolution is to take active practical measures and solve problems of life to make it easier for survival. The sugar-cane tiger reaches a completely unexploited food niche of hoofed animals and exploits the solid food source in feral cattle. These surplus animals which otherwise create problems and die of malnutrition or starvation greatly help, particularly at the time of stress, in taking off some of the pressure from the wild prey. This source of food is simply unavailable to most other tigers inside the principal jungle. Thus a forest dweller may starve but a devious tiger of farmland will not.

However, because the prey communities are different, the diets of two populations of tigers are quite dissimilar. Forest tigers feed mostly on wild game; Phlegmatic cattle are included on availability while sugarcane tigers, are juxtaposed to such situation.

The diversity of fauna in a sugarcane field is a measure of its richness. There is a complex community of ungulate prey, about fifteen species for taking, both wild and domestic. With so many foodstuffs available in the sugar farms a wide spectrum of mammalian predators can live an easy life, so why to question a tigers existence only. It is correct that a large carnivore's home is in the jungle but at his very doorstep extends a rich belt of sugarcane which supplies him with best food and best cover. To my understanding, this is an extraordinary condition where a tiger's access to an overwhelming profusion of prey might and must prevent him from revisiting his prey reduced jungles, and in process must precipitate the progression of his naturalization in the sugarcane plantations. Considering their killing qualifications, their armament, power and size, these food resources stand under-utilized by them even during the leanest period.

Arthur Locke says, "Tigers will eat almost anything they can kill or which they find lying dead." Thus the problem is not food; the problem is of a socio-ecological nature, and that is a monstrous problem since any attempt of survival is brought to a naught by man, the paragon of the artificial world, who cannot share space with alpha predators for a long length of time, as the familiarity will eventually evolve in its recognition as a prey species, and nature's protection device will become fractured. Arjan Singh states, “If this transpires then it will really be a precarious situation for not even a great quantity of other prey will put a stop to human casualty”.

The message was clear; the sugar tigers were seemingly straightening into an eco-type strain, with a number packing a 'big punch'. They should either be effectively saved for the future by some imaginative strategic conservation or be left disregarded to die of poisoning, poaching and 'shoot-at-sight' predator policies of some local Surds'. A rethinking was essential in this context and we had to rummage around for some viable solutions before man-tiger conflict assumes menacing proportions and becomes the cause for revengeful elimination of the entire farm-tiger population by the villagers. An American international conservation body believes that a certain amount of predator control is necessary to regulate nature's balance. It advocates quotas on the commercial hunting of predators that are menace to livestock.

Out of many hit and try methods, this predator control philosophy might be translated into an active programme to manage sugar tigers. Instead of maintaining a blanket ban on game shooting and allowing poachers to have a blast of time why the legal hunter should not come back on the scene once again to manage tiger conservation issues. The way forward in conservation is always to develop an economic mechanism around the species that will pay for the animal's own conservation. At the crux of this argument is the notion that conservationists should exploit the fact that the tiger is a valuable and renewable economic resource to generate the funds to save it, rather than denying the animal's economic value and focusing solely on law enforcement as a tool of conservation, where as trophy hunting can as well be used as a vital tool for conservation.

The presence of a confirmed man-eater in a sugarcane tract is a dreadful scourge to people who have to pass through those areas daily and no man on leaving his house can be sure of returning. At least the hunting of deviant tigers, the so called man-eaters could be started as marketable business to earn foreign exchange. The speedy removal of a 'proven aberrant', would mellow down the native spree of revenge, appease their anger and fear and put a halt to the wholesale demolition of innocent tigers and eve discourage poachers.

It is also argued that hunters by harvesting unwanted animals perform a most important function in conserving and managing the wildlife. So when the species is close to extinction in the wild, this 'quota killing' may mean the difference between survival and oblivion for the same in its chosen habitat. The revenue realized from this provision should be used for the remaining lot of tigers which may save them from inevitable and nearly universal destruction; because the men who struggle for existence against these tigers, depending on their crops to sustain their families, care nothing for laws aimed at saving these valuable cats.

In short, predatory animals, injurious to mankind and those damaging property are controlled when necessary, making use of most selective and human techniques. This approach may seem logical to managers and locals --but until quite recently the tiger was the ultimate big game trophy, thus this would push the animal once again into those days, and was bound to invite considerable opposition from millions of wildlife conservationists. It is for sure that the presence of trophy hunting operators, as demonstrated by African game management techniques in Zambia and Tanzania, can reduce illegal hunting. Lease agreements in these countries require assistance in anti-poaching from operators in hunting concessions and they often conduct anti-poaching to protect the wildlife resource on which they depend. Moreover trophy hunting generates high revenue from a low volume of hunters which is often much more than the income generated from hundred bus loads of echo-tourists. It is also a self regulating discipline because low-take off is required to ensure a high trophy quality and marketability of the area in future seasons. It is important to reinvest revenue from hunting into conservation and to share it with local communities. This will create a financial incentive for the villagers and the benefited will surely favour the protection of this tiger.

The important point is that the animal damage control must be practiced with good reason and judgment. Therefore the reduction or suppression of their numbers should be done only as a means of accomplishing specific management objectives.

It was time to evolve new and more efficient managing techniques to cope with the changing needs of our wilds and shed the orthodox conservation philosophy. As each area's needs are different, and management ideas and plans must therefore base themselves on amalgamated needs of local communities and wildlife. Experience shows that an improved assessment of conservation role of controlled hunting, diagnosis of problems and prescription of site specific-solutions are drastically needed and its market principles be recognized, than merely discussing the wildlife conservation issues on failing moral and ethical grounds.

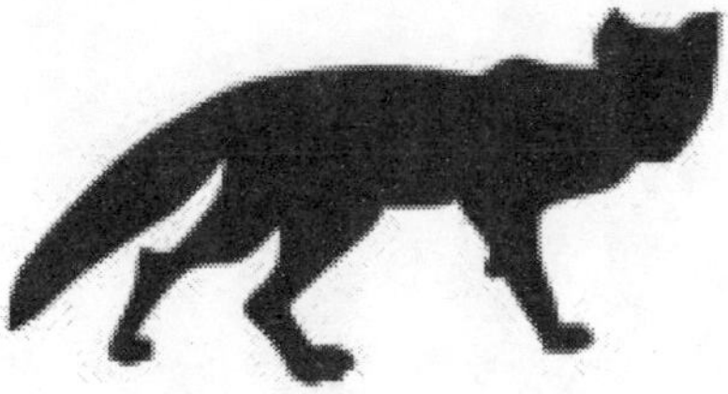

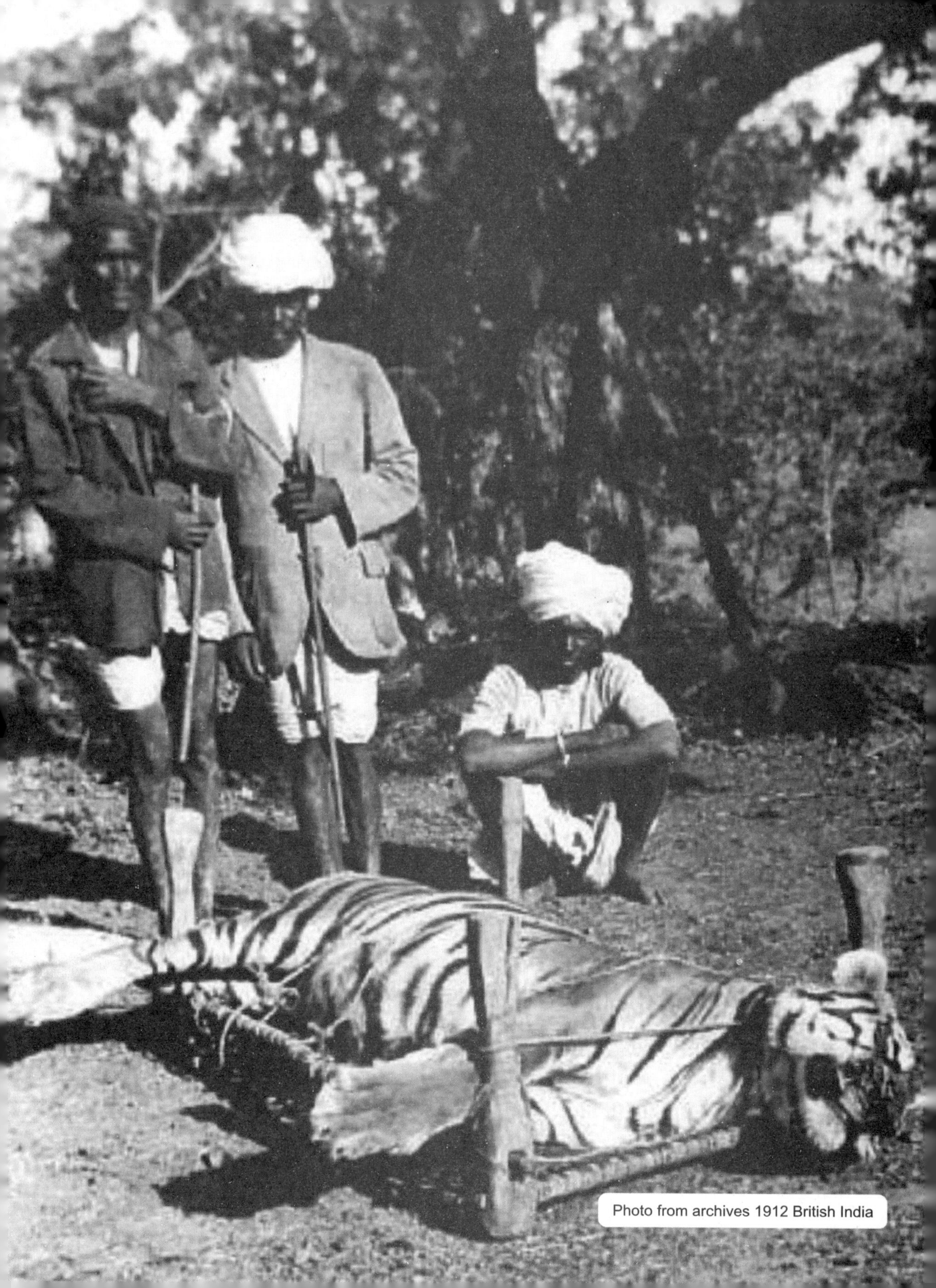
Photo from archives 1912 British India

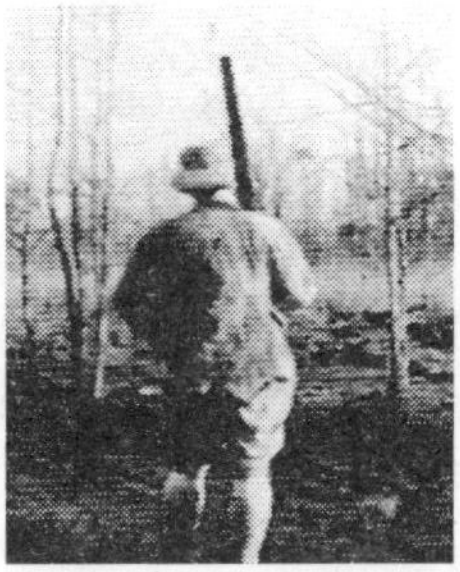

17

Night Belongs to the Carnivore

When I was twelve, I went hunting with my father and we shot a bird. He was laying there and something struck me. Why do we call this fun to kill this creature who was as happy as I was when I woke up this morning?

- Marv Levy

November is the most picturesque months to be in the countryside. This was the month in 1989 when I got back to my dreamland and camped at the house of Dr. Pramod Kumar Singh at Nighasan. The annual winter migration of birds had started. Every day assorted flocks of wild ducks crossed over the sky in a typical V formation, honking their cheery songs. The birds gifted with remarkable sagacity flew over cultivation fields, looking for a suitable wetland of their liking. The colour and the picturesqueness of all this was indescribable; it was among the loveliest pictures, I saw in the Tarai

The birds stretched out their legs and necks perfectly straight as they moved through the air with powerful beats of their wings. I watched them placing themselves in two oblique lines, forming a triangle, or a single line when the battalion was not numerous. The bird at the head of the triangle cleaved the air first. When fatigued she retired to the last rank to repose and others took her place in turn.

They flew without tumult to accomplish their journey which displayed their high degree of intelligence and a combination of their unerring instinct that is hard wired in their genetic code. There seemed an arrangement, a method and a system in place where each individual kept his rank and followed the body of the army with little or almost no fatigue.

As winter advanced, heavy fog started to hang over the fields often hiding the sun. Meanwhile, sporadic news of tiger movements poured in from various places. From a farmland called Banghatia, there were reports of a number of tigers calling around the village, and one had shown itself rather ostentatiously more than once near the village tube well. In last one week, their restless moaning and whining punctuated by roars had not only increased but had become a rather regular feature in the night.

I visited the place immediately. An examination of pugmarks indicated the presence of three females in the area. It was a case of preponderance of adult females with no male being around. All the three were in season and desperately vocalizing to get a mate. I heard the unmistakable calls of these tigresses several times but was unable to locate them accurately for any observation.

The area was live with snakes. Just outside the village was the hole where a cobra lived. This snake had been made a pet by the village womenfolk. He was believed to save the villagers against all deadly snakes, which he killed and ate. He had never harmed a villager and was often fed with cow milk. I could never see the big cats but I saw the cobra many times. After a week's futile effort I returned to Nighasan.

The range of a tigress is smaller, by nature's arrangement, chiefly because she has a distinct biological function. Whenever she has young cubs, they secure her to a moderately small area. Charles McDougal mentions his observation in the Royal Chitwan National Park where tigresses did appear to outnumber the tigers. He based his figures on the records mentioned in the old hunting literature, where the number of shot tigresses was always higher than tigers. He took an account of the gender of unborn fetuses found in dead tigresses in the wild and found them to be equally divided, and also that the figures of birth in captivity are equally balanced. He thus came to the conclusion that some process of attrition must thin out wild males before they reach maturity.

It is a real statement and not an illusion, as claimed by some experts. To my mind this is the reason why females should preponderate. The territory of a dominant male includes the area of several females and there is always a number of young males seeking entry into it; a chance to take over the range permanently from the present incumbent. This ignites violent confrontations and many a male juvenile is killed in the duels while new females are rarely killed and welcomed in the harem. Forsyth, Baker and Hicks attribute the preponderance of females in the adult population wholly or in part to the killing of male cubs by adult male tigers. Perhaps this is nature's way of shielding the female to perpetuate the species. It makes the density of tigresses high in the jungle as well as in sugarcanes. However, it is easy to hypothesize about the function of excess females, but not easy to discover the mechanism.

Although, Dudhwa had become a part of Project Tiger and elaborate rules of conservation had been established, the local poachers did not seem to bother much about them. Many of the old ungulate slots were being thoroughly exploited by them. One night some poachers of Lalpur- Dhaka, a village in North Kheri division, set a lightweight contraption for a deer and a tiger was caught in it. Once a tiger is cornered or trapped, shooting it becomes a relatively simple matter. The trappers come near the beast with a serviceable muzzle loader and fire from very close quarters. The charge of gun powder was little and damp; it took time to ignite and finally when it blew off the gun was not steady. The first shot of pellets grazed the predator's body and the second shot crossed through the stomach went into the earth. Now the pain-maddened tiger gave a mighty jerk and wrenched himself free from the Jin-trap. Blood bubbled copiously from his wounds yet he first killed both the poachers and then escaped into the canes.

Next day, as the foresters had no suitable weapon and there was also no one experienced enough to deal with the situation I was called by the DFO of North Kheri to check on the site. In those days, due to my regular forays in the fields, I had cultivated a skill for tracking tigers through their most dreadful haunts, which was probably why they had asked for my help. When I arrived, the bodies had been taken into custody by police and the trap was confiscated by foresters. A surviving poacher was regaling the officials with a vivid description of the catastrophe, explaining things with illustrative gestures.

I examined the ground of tragedy. The scene resembled a theatre of war. Three spears, a towel, a turban and several pairs of sleepers were still lying there. The large quantity of blood deposit and other signs indicated that the tiger had been wounded in the upper region of stomach and low down in a limb by the nails of contraption. A clean cut hole made by the bullet bled freely both at its entrance and exit points, but there were no signs of internal hemorrhage. The tiger did not bleed from the mouth; however he had coughed a quantity of reddish tinged foam

The hunting hawk

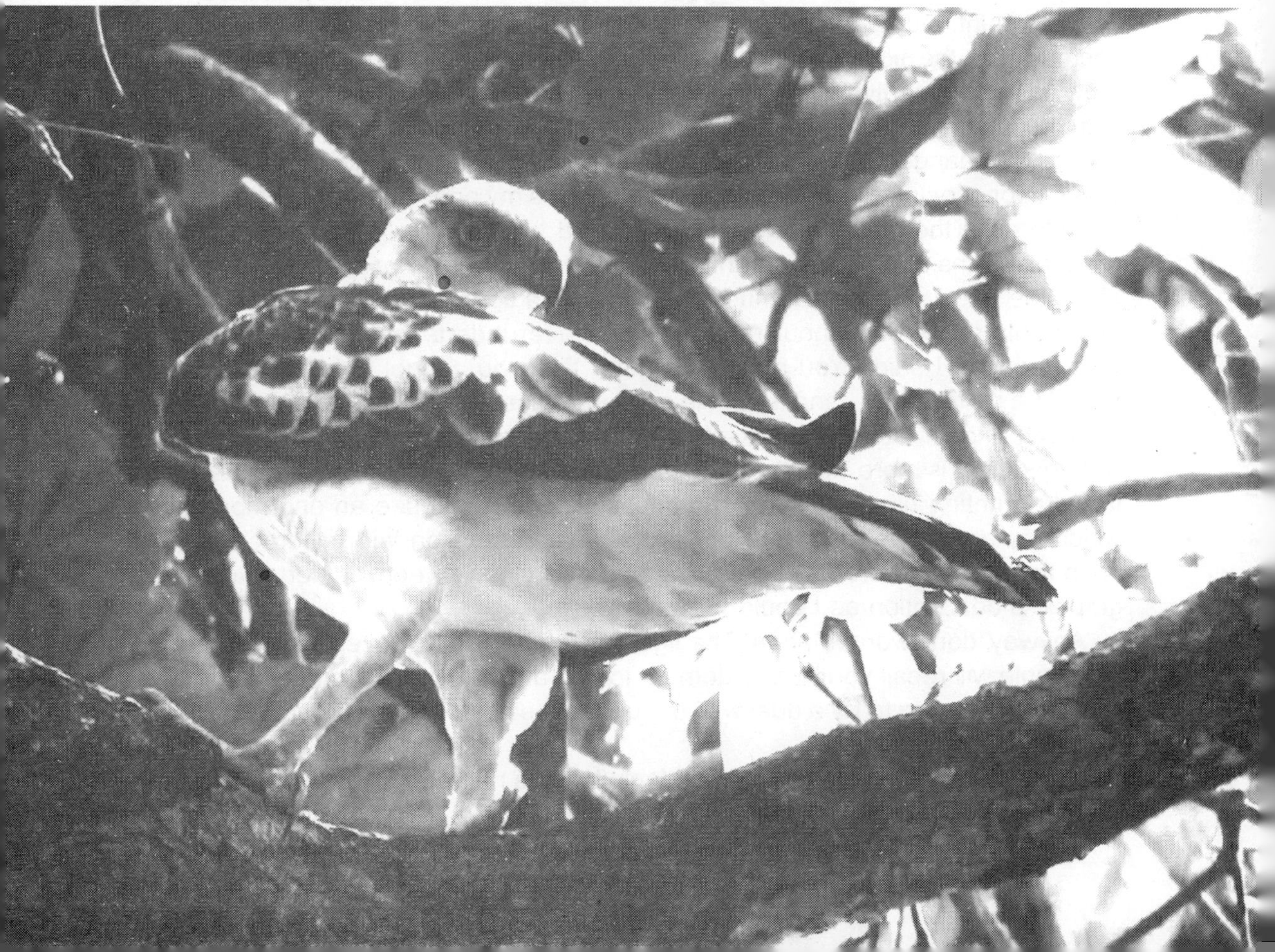

on the grass indicating the route he had taken to escape. Nobody had attended to this uneven trail because the sugarcane was very dense.

The animal when wounded appears to dash off at a great pace, but experience has shown that it does not travel any distance and if it is not followed up at once, the shock and severity of the wound will induce the animal to rest. The loss of blood creates insatiable thirst and the tendency of the wounded animal is to seek thick cover and water, if the latter is within a reasonable distance.

As a general rule a tiger is not considered to be dangerous for at least 24 hours after being injured. In the case of a light flesh wound, it usually moves away on being approached whereas with a painful bone wound it might continue to be dangerous for several days. There was a pond nearby and by guess work the tiger must be hiding there. In the light of the fact that it had just killed two persons he was likely to be highly dangerous.

Many a Sikh from the nearby villages had come on the scene and as usual they were carrying an assortment of smooth bores, including two .315s. Their tempers were running high and in a spirit of war they were adamant to follow the trail blindly, hoping to stumble upon the tiger and pump him with solid lead. I had also brought along a double-barreled .375 Magnum Holland & Holland, so they wanted me to lead the hunt. But as I sensed the foul mood I gave up the trail immediately. It seemed that the tiger could be further molested by the unruly mob, which was growing ever assertive with the arrival of new persons and more guns.

In the interim some hooligans had entered the crop and were throwing stones in it. This was dangerous because a wounded tiger cannot be moved from cover to cover, sooner or later it will charge. His safety was my principal concern so I decided to undermine the crowd's confidence. I called their leader Mahua Singh and two unsavory Sikhs and with an intention to spawn fear in their minds, I let them know about the ferocity and great muscular power of a tiger, called into play when he is thoroughly roused. "Without realizing you have undertaken a highly dangerous performance," I said. "You must remember that you cannot hold the determined dash of a pariah dog… and here it is an injured tiger. These beats are accustomed to attack and kill other animals—they have weapons of offence for doing this. A wounded tiger is more likely to charge and charge home. He usually comes straight for you grunting his purpose with ruthless violence. You see an enormous head, which rapidly grows in dimension as he would come on with a ferocious rush, bounding from a short distance taking you in a clean sweep," I tried to create as graphic a description as I could.

"Anyway, don't worry Mahua. The tiger is a humane killer; even if you depart this life people will recall your martyrdom for long. Take my rifle and make history. This is the best weapon to try a dual with the beast," I said as I handed over my .375 DB to him.

At this, the man hesitated and suddenly lost his nerve to follow the beast. I was happy to make out a look of terror on his face.

My ploy had worked well and the rebellion was nearly over. The tiger did not seem to be in imminent danger, his disability appeared temporary and there was a fair chance of him becoming normal again, so I felt morally bound to support his leeway for survival rather than work for his nemesis. The villagers were sober and easier to handle after that, the tigers might have been indulgently viewed so they withdrew first and then to my great relief the Sikhs also returned to their farms.

I admit that I did not take up the unpleasant task of locating the tiger inside the dense sugarcane as the visibility within was almost zero; moreover the animals are of hard nature, they will endure the most frightful wounds without uttering a sound and never give any clue as to where they actually are.

Next day, a brief follow-up showed that the tiger was still going strong. Towards midnight he had come out of his hiding and crossed the river Sharda to enter into another massive sugar plantation. His tracks were unevenly indented on the ploughed mud and a grotesquely twisted mark of the forefoot showed that his wound was bad enough to make him necessarily hesitant from venturing into the open. Large heavy predators become helpless if they have lost the use of one leg but given the magnitude of the anti-synergistic forces, his wounds healed slowly and painfully and it was a miracle that this tiger survived for quite a few years in the surrounding area.

I had all appreciation for him the way he had fostered himself to recovery and salvaging his range once again. The shotgun pellets had been absorbed by his body but the suppurating scar left by the jaws of the trap was conspicuous on his right forearm; a hallmark of disaster that was to follow him throughout his life.

It is vital to empathize that the wild tiger has only to get wounded gravely, not killed outright, as a result of being hunted, Septicemia, physical invalidity, infections, malnourishment and starvation are often the agents that eventually lead to the death of the tigers who supposedly effectively break away from native contraptions; because it is difficult to get at the wound and keep it clean of flies and maggots.

Here, I must say that his recovery produced a revelation. Whereas on one hand the scientists are talking about the need to continuously monitor the impacts of human activities on tigers, their prey base and habitat, on the other hand this man made shelter of sugarcanes, with its reassuring ease of food, water, cover and space had precisely played a critical role in the survival of this tiger. It had worked as a medicine, as an elixir of life, striking home the fact that only a potential habitat -where optimum conditions exist- can produce situations conducive for the convalescence of an injured predator. All these factors point to the conditions of the habitat as key to maintaining viable, healthy populations both of wild ungulates and of predators.

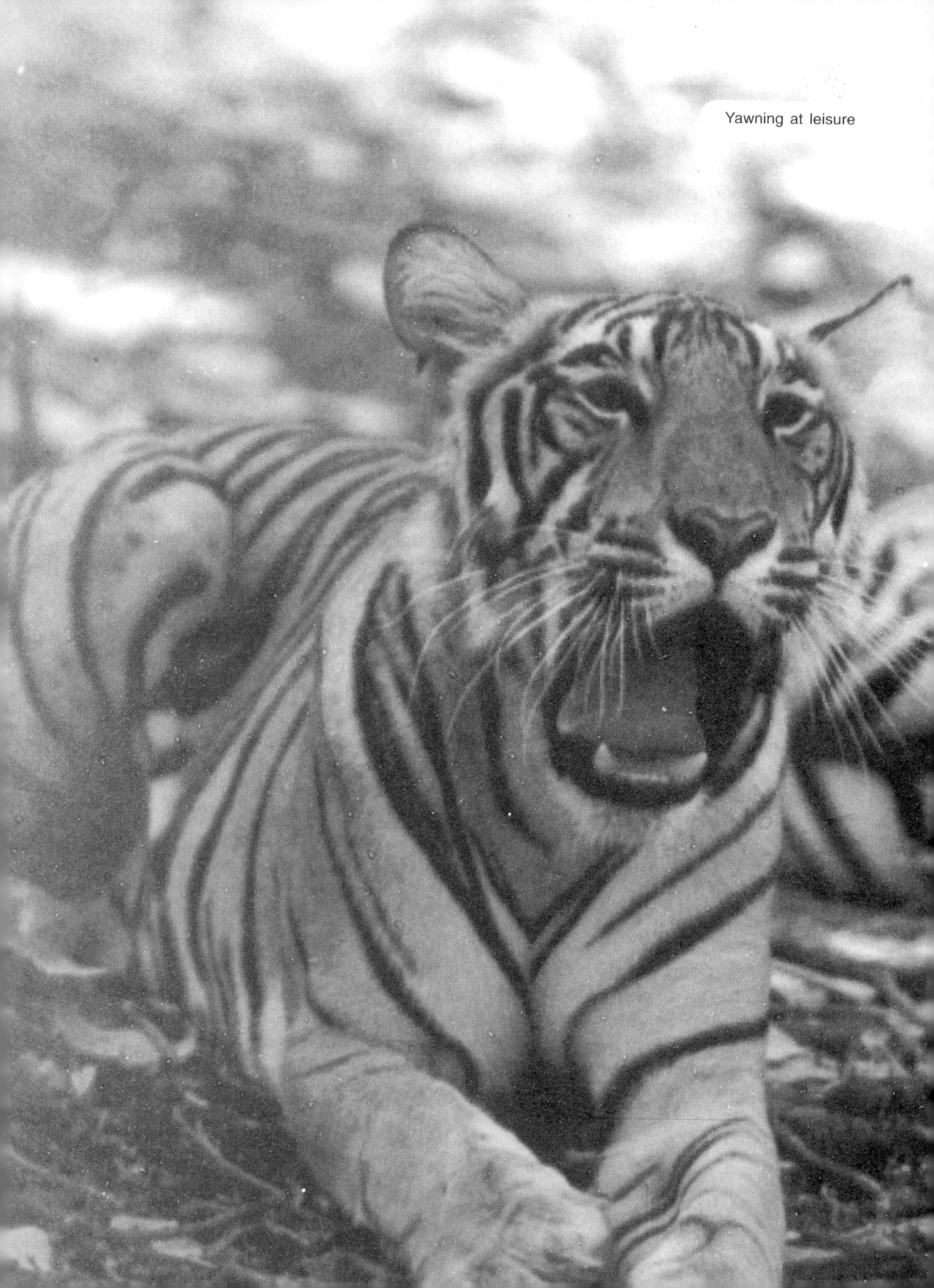

Yawning at leisure

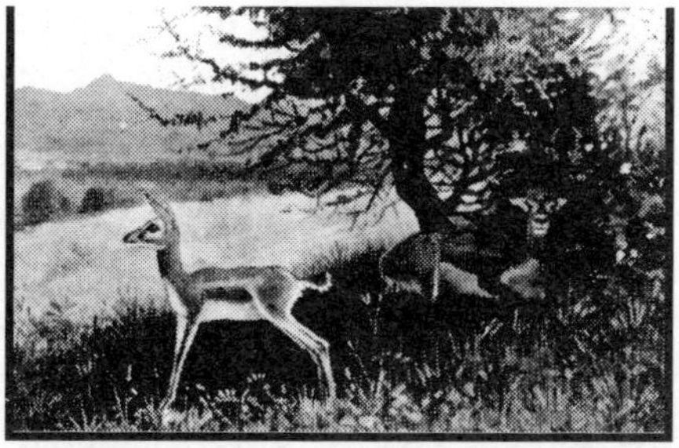

18

The Old Boy of Navrangpur

Nature is an infinite sphere of which the center is everywhere and the circumference nowhere.

- Blaise Pascal

Ranjit Bhargava became Chairman of U.P. Chapter of W.W.F. in 1988, but his much-assured project on cane tigers could never materialize. A sagacious and incorruptible man, he unfortunately failed to motivate the interest of the W.W.F. in Delhi to get financial support for this cause. The state, however, seemed partially convinced with the idea but the mandarins claimed that the budget was not enough for human needs and any expenditure for the protection of wildlife in ersatz habitat such as sugar farms would be a luxury. All this was seemingly nonsensical; for the central command of the W.W.F. sugar tiger was utterly unrealistic and its preservationist measures were unnecessary, while the state foresters, under conventional totem of being perennially short of funds, had more pressing problems than to pursue this new but hypercritical agenda.

I hardly need to say that I felt frustrated to consider the points put forward by people in positions of authority. I tried to figure out what had gone wrong on my part. It was one thing to write a proposal and quite another to get finance. I did not know how to make my proposal attractive to a potential sponsor. I had invested my life's savings, my dreams and pride in this venture, already brought it to a half-accomplished stage and I was still practically starved of funds. There was no reason to leave the project at this stage, and if I did, I had nothing to go back to.

Perhaps the major international conservation bodies were naïve regarding the essentials and the status of these tigers. They considered them as seasonal gypsies who attacked cattle and humans and then went back to the jungle. Hence, the management policy proposed to crack this conundrum was to capture or eradicate them and not to protect them, while I was trying to sell the idea that at this stage the knowledge gap of foresters was very critical and decisively going against this tiger, for the crux of the problem was yet not clear. At the bottom line, a hidden part of this population was a putative strain in the making, a cluster of lesser known animals that was behaviorally adapted to breeding in canes and needed to be understood in a different way from a jungle tiger.

I was still using my old set of maps made by Survey of India and constantly updating them with the information gathered from trustworthy sources. This was an 'only one of its kind' record which for the first time showed the tiger distribution in farmlands of Tarai, on a rather rough scale. Most of my data about tigers was obtained by plotting sight records of known individuals on a map. In Nauganwa, Kanp-Tanda and Bajpur areas, a significant change in tiger behaviour was reflected in the shift from nocturnal to diurnal activities. On reaching these places, I was greeted with the news that many Gaddi herders of the area knew these tigers as individuals. They had dubbed them as Lalli, Gudia, Bachava and Kallu. These tigers had never ever reacted aggressively and operated in the cultivated tracts without any disruptive effect. They existed on friendly terms, at least on their part and their activities went through a predictable daily cycle. Each morning, for a bit they were seen sitting on some exposed piece of ground to take a sunbath and then went away into dense sugarcane as the human activities started. The grazers recognized them perfectly well as if their names were written on their forehead and the tigers probably also recognized glaziers in turn.

This intriguing friendliness seemed to have opened up a pandora's box of possibilities of mutual tolerance and individual recognition between man and tiger, generated by sharing the same landscape. Could this be the basis of much easier co-existence between two species than has hitherto been thought possible?

Two Muslim Gaddi's, Sher Ali and Dilbahar, were seemingly familiar with their history. Lalli was considered localized. She was said to have successive litter of three cubs for last two years, at a den site that rested concealed inside the intertwined ravines of Sharda. The senior Gaddi claimed that she was herself born there some six years back. Unfortunately none of her litter had survived but her repeated appearance on the same terrain was an amazing feature. It clearly indicated the way in which tigers sustain deep-seated primitive memories, which direct them to the old hideouts for a certain purpose such as to lay litter, and that, they do assimilate functional information about genial terrains for their future use.

Mammalian neuroscientists believe that cats have a memory that can be up to 200 times more retentive than a dog's. However, they will only remember what they consider to be useful, and therefore their memory can be quite selective.

A question that plagued my mind was: Did they have a lair in the canes too? Were they born in the canes only? Had they never experienced the real jungle? They may stroll around their hunting range, using a series of different halting stations to rest by the day, yet some of them preferred the familiarity of their original den where they were born and raised and were to be found there most of the times. Were they the hardcore, unremitting cane tigers, content to stay within their prime farmland boundaries, and feeling no urge whatsoever to leave their own little chosen acreage?

Reflex action and conditioned learning are part of normal behaviour, but a different type of learning is required for more flexible behaviour, one which enables the cat to predict the consequences of its own actions — especially in their relation with human beings -- and modify its actions based on past successes and failures. I believe that such tigers know their country well. They know the spots from where they can watch the daily routine of village folk. They know the habit of their prey animals. They know when the people are occupied in their own affairs and when are likely to go poking around into their coverts. They know when it is not wise to disturb them. I maintain that the tigers that belong to the farmlands hereditarily possess the natural etiquette of living in the human environ.

Countless ancestors of such a multi-generational being have lived in these farmlands and their neuron-conditioning has evolved, predisposing them to interact with their environment in a certain way. They nurture instinctive orientation as how to live here safely or why else do they stay back in the crops for so long. However, this is not to say that they had become house cats; they were still completely wild and potentially dangerous predators, yet their conditioning hardly made them confront the villagers.

The fact about the mechanism of symbiotic existence will be topical to understand at this juncture. The co-operation is usually thought of as being a relationship which involves a more or less conscious sharing of effort to produce a single mutually beneficial effect. Symbiosis is a form of pre-conscious, unintentional co-operation. Essentially, a symbiotic relationship involves two species doing more or less what they would do in any event but tolerating the close presence of one another while they do it. The toleration is the key which costs virtually nothing in terms of energy, but increases the chances of survival.

Perhaps a brief golden age of sugarcane tigers had been temporarily achieved. This was an undreamed of golden age in the relationship between humans and tigers, where two different species were going about their lawful business. Humans as well as cats showed a degree of hard-wired behaviour. Such behaviour allowed them to go about their routine tasks on autopilot and free up more of the brain for confronting other challenges. The cases of human as well as tiger fatalities were reduced to near zero, making it a good model for conservation to build upon. It recapped Victorian hunter Fletcher's words of 1911 that "A person is safe anywhere with a walking stick."

Having gone to New Delhi as Director Project Tiger R.L. Singh had forgotten about the plight of cane tigers. His passive attitude was unfortunately a significant departure from his previous stand. He showed no desire to circumvent the normal proceedings of the department though he could have done so if he wished. I hardly need to say I didn't grudge it because the nature of such top posts is oriented more by political principles than through innovations. The occupant automatically starts playing chess (without a board) with his friends and rivals alike. So Singh had changed. For friends he excused himself from controversies and for foes he paddled very hard — to stay where he was!

After him a series of directors followed, who as usual showed very little interest in securing the future of this tiger. These departmental bureaucrats, with little knowledge of technicalities, had no dreams for Dudhwa, nor did they want to break away from the old jingoism of lucrative exploitative practices. During this time, no accurate accounts of field surveys were ever generated and no forest rangers were ever entrusted with the job of keeping an eye on these tigers. If the livestock were killed by tigers, the owners were given no compensation or were very tardily awarded with the subvention cut for corrupt officials who assessed the claim. Even though the central government had unilaterally committed the statutes for payment on domestic stock suffering annoyance of tigers, yet the foresters often claimed to have no budget for such expenditures.

Of course there were no straightforward strategies to protect these tigers and I was surprised that the stalwarts who had laid the foundations of Project Tiger and wildlife initiatives were maintaining a golden silence on this point; as if this was a 'non-subject'. There was not a single policy statement on the status of sugarcane tigers.

I had been patient, but now my patience was fast running out. Until now, I had worked unfunded and completely on my own with three interlaced strands to my struggle; study of cane tigers, working for their protection and containing the man-tiger conflict but every so often I doubted, if with this much of constrain on my part, I could really boast of a real success story. No one knew for sure if the head mounted skins, with their teeth bared in prayer to mankind to spare their race, that still went through customs were of these tigers.

Fortunately 1995, the State Wildlife Advisory Board was constituted after years of interruption, and I was appointed a member and later also the Honorary Wildlife Warden of Kishanpur Tiger Reserve of Dudhwa National Park. Once I got the position my table was bombarded with conservation reports and I was bewildered by the wide range of conservation activities taking place, many of them in places I had never heard of and most of them of complicated nature. Regardless of ideological instance, all conservation ultimately concerns ecological targets be they habitats, species, ecosystems or ecological processes but I was surprised to see that when over the years, a variety of approaches had been adopted to protect large carnivores -from strict patrolling to co-managed buffer areas and community managed forests- there was no mention of sugarcane tigers anywhere.

In the summer of that year, I added sugar tigers in the list of state government but in determining conservation action for them -as the rational for action had to be necessarily based on scientific evidence- the burden of proof of their validity also came upon my shoulders. However I felt that I could now utilize the infrastructural facilities of the department, apply my tools in context specific manner, conduct "occupancy surveys", generate a new location data and identify far more precisely the places, where my conservation interventions might be more effective.

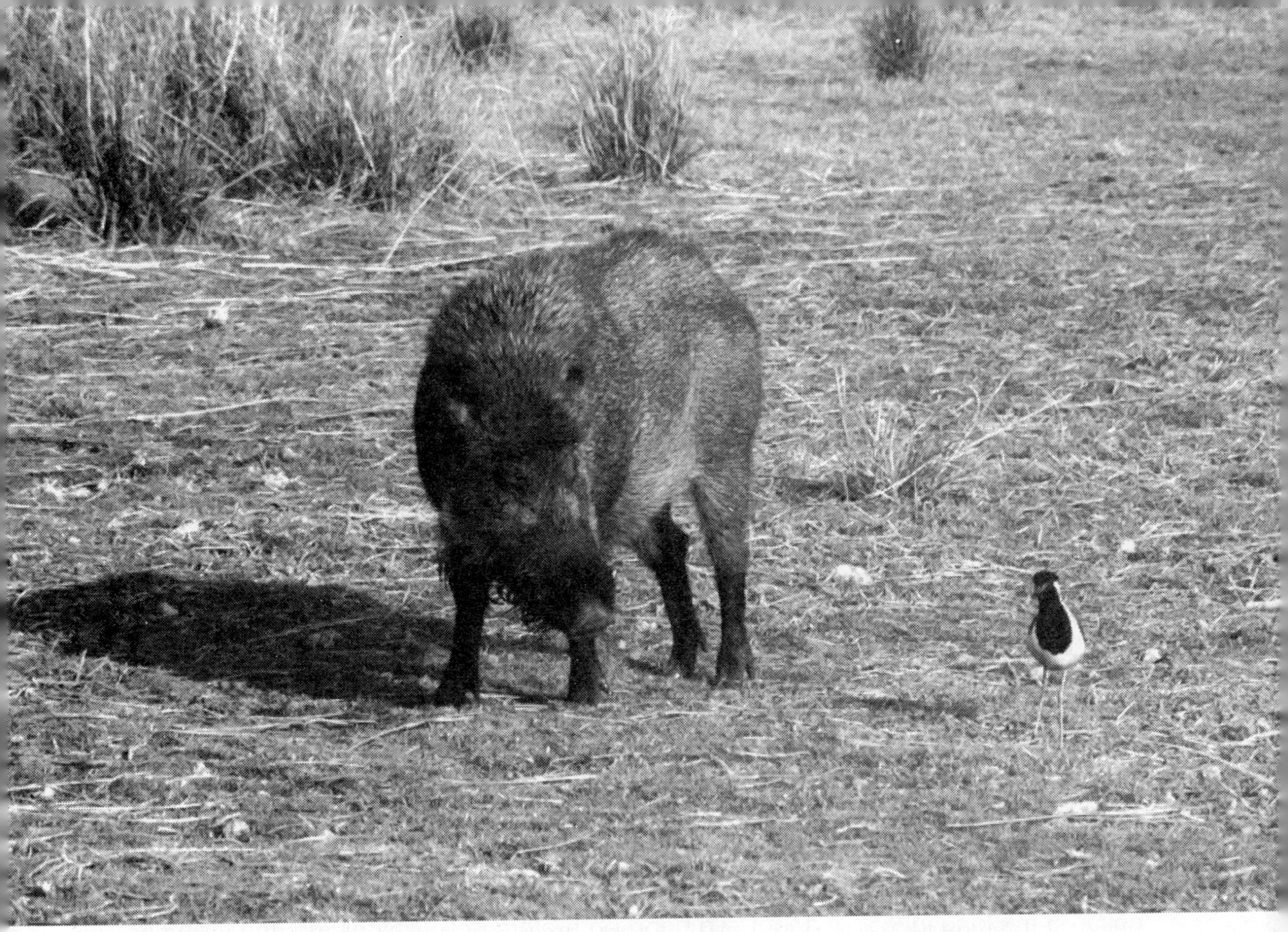

A wild boar looking at Jacana

I told this to the forest Secretary Dr. P.L. Punia, whose steady interest in wildlife was very encouraging. "Rahul," he suggested, "now all you have to do is to utilize the platform to advocate the cause of cane tigers, narrow down the conservation interests of board members for this tiger and support the measures and projects that could be of tangible long-term practical benefits to this animal."

Little I knew that political and parochial bickering had already hopelessly muddled the main concerns of wildlife conservation. The complex debates on wildlife and livelihood matters had deteriorated into emotional polls on who- whether humans or animals- should enjoy priority in a democratic country and there was no magic mantra that the board would accept without qualms?

(II)

The old settlement of Navrangpur lies on the northern banks of the Sharda River and just outside the boundary of Dudhwa Park. It is hardly five miles away from Paraspur and is connected to it by footpaths and cart tracks. It was in 1995, a happy go lucky period of my life, when I took the charge as honorary wildlife warden of the area and my quest for the tiger magic took me to Navrangpur. The ancient country, squeezed between Dudhwa and Kishanpur reserve, was said to harbor an old stripe that had lived here for years. In course of time many tales of sagacious cunning, woven around the personality of this tiger, had framed an aura of admiration around him that had gradually resulted in his being a revered animal. He was known to spend a disproportionate amount of time along the boundaries of river. Though tribal people and gypsies, who mainly hunted deer passed through that way, did pose danger but he was claimed to be guided by some uncanny intuition that guarded him form every impairment.

The day was March 11, 1995. I was with two of my friends namely W. Longwa, the Deputy Director of Dudhwa and J.V. Sharma, the D.F.O of South Kheri. We were on a patrol at the western precinct of the National Park. As Red fowls rendered their farewell calls to the day, we found ourselves encountering several coveys of Grey partridges scratching the dust on the cart roads, when some laborers returning from the fields informed us that they had just seen a tiger walking along the escarpment of Sharda River. The news was encouraging. We hurried in the direction to see if we could catch up with the animal.

Rounding a bend, the escarpment fell opposite the settlement of Navarangpur. Dusk was falling, the sun had already set but there was enough redness in the sky, when Longwa descried a moving figure on the escarpment silhouetted against the horizon. We halted our vehicle, shut off the engine and watched the figure silently. It was a tiger. He moved slowly and his gait seemed to lack the usual smartness. It covered the long length of about two hundred meters in a straight line and then sat down on a rise overlooking the sugarcane fields, to watch the tranquil evening scene that stretched before him.

The twilight was fading fast, but due to the openness of the vista the objects were still identifiable. Soon the last streak of daylight faded from the sky. The gathering darkness enshrouded the landscape and the silhouette of the tiger faded in the haze.

As our eyes grew accustomed to the gloom, I got an impression that the animal had swayed stealthily and moved down the declivity on our side of the escarpment. A lapwing called from near an irrigation channel as I switched on the jeep headlights. In the glow we saw, the brilliant emerald eyes moving at right angles to our west. He was too far to show his stripes but the eyes like spots of phosphorous told the way he followed.

We switched on the search lights and focused on him. The animal was coming down the declivity. After perhaps five minutes, I saw his head half facing me, thrust into the circle of 'halo' like beams, thrown by the search light. Then he advanced fully into the open terrain and the accompanying ranger immediately recognized him as the old boy of Navrangpur, who had returned to his favorite haunts after an absence of a couple of months. For some time he stood glaring at us and considering the source of light and then decided to move away into the gloom behind sugarcane crops.

We came back to Navrangpur. The village chief Dhani Ram offered us the hot tumblers of milk and insisted that I stay with him. After a sumptuous treat, my friends went back to the headquarters while I stayed back. I discussed about the tiger with the chief and his henchmen. He told me that this particular beast was well known to the people of the area as he had been living on the outskirts of this village for many years.

"For how many years?" I asked him.

"Since my first child was born," he pointed at the boy playing near the cot. I looked at the boy, hardly three feet in height. He seemed to be of no less than four to five years.

"What is his name?" I asked casually.

"Sahib we call him Sheru. He is named after the tiger, you just saw."

"So this tiger is called Sheru," I concluded, "Right, we will look for his whereabouts tomorrow morning."

Meanwhile, the cute little child wandered near me and shyly gave me his wooden toy; I put a five rupee coin in his hand, which his mother promptly took away.

That night after a late dinner, I lay down on the cot; the moon was almost full and on her way to zenith while the silvery light was clear and unobstructed. The time was around 11 p.m., the small black bats, swept silently across the grass in pursuit of fireflies whilst the night jars slid smoothly on their silky wings along the fence, uttering a peculiar cry that sounds like "*Chyeece*". The hour of the witches' Sabbath — a supposed midnight orgy of devils and witches — had commenced. The wind moaned in the sugarcane fields and a mournful, wild and hungry cry of a jackal incessantly broke the silence. It was deep and low like that of a baying hound, but infinitely wilder. The moonlight poured down on the fields around me and somewhere in the east the tongues of fire were flickering on the skyline as a sugar crop was being burnt.

I closed my eyes and my thoughts went to the extraordinary demeanor of the wild beast I had discovered lately. I considered myself supremely fortunate to have come upon such a tiger, whose existence was a groovy riddle. He was claimed to be a resident of this area for the last five years and this was a hell of a time for a tiger to stay at one place. I knew that the stories of this effect are prevalent in most of the jungle areas but the natives who relate them are generally truthful and accurate in matters of this nature. The tiger had perhaps occupied this slot as a middle aged animal and with the waning of his youthful agility had found it more comfortable to establish himself as a subsidized custodian of the neighboring sugar farms. These were now his longstanding home where he was living alone.

I remember, that in the last eddies of my consciousness, I was reviewing the statement of William Baze if tigers live in a particular area, then they do live there well and proper. Shifts from less suitable localities to improved ones may be made while social spacing keeps their numbers more or less steady in spite of the seasonal abundance or scarcity of prey. The mechanical sounds of an irrigating tube well,

"*Phook-phuk! Phook-phuk*!" sounded like a lullaby in my ears. I pulled up the quilt and then came the dreamless sleep of those who make their bed under the open, starry sky.

Next morning, I woke up to an early call just after dawn, a troop of *langur* monkeys had arrived. They were sitting on the string cots and chairs in the verandah and playing pranks, when we drove them away before breakfast, they shifted to some distance from the house and were soon feeding in the trees around us.

As the early sun illuminated the fields, I took Dhani Ram with me and went to the place where the old beast was said to be residing. The place was on the banks of the Sharda. Hog deer were peculiar to this region. They showed themselves frequently amid breaks in the cane fields giving impression of being ebony statues on the pedestal of gold; at times singly, sometimes in pairs and often in herds of three. They leaped and scampered to shelter as soon they saw us. On the way, I also saw tens of sick and emaciated cattle that were discarded by their owners, to fend for themselves. With so much of food around any aging tiger could live in the vein of the proverbial cat in a cream jug.

We finally arrived at a fragmented bush land called Roheni where we expected the tiger to have retired. Skeletons of cattle littered the place in scores; their bleached bones stank to high heaven. Apparently some of these must have been killed by the tiger and some having died naturally, and thrown here, must have been eaten by him. It was an isolated place and people rarely visited here. The scene and the stench of putrefaction proved that a tiger could be occupying the grim place and living in isolation. Though he moved out of the area for a week or a fortnight he invariably returned to his favorite haunt.

An accompanying villager told me that once he had seen the male loitering on the banks of the Sharda when a female arrived from a different direction, both of them rolled in a gesture of appeasement and then moved away together. A male undoubtedly mates with whatever estrous females, resident or transient, are found within his range. It is a natural sequence in the jungle that the old tigers whose powers are waning are driven away by the stronger tigers from the areas of plentiful food to the areas of less competition. A similar treatment is also mooted to the ripened tigresses by their youthful counterparts.

Perhaps this tigress was also an old timer. Her stripes were dim and some of them seemed to have disappeared altogether. Her relations with the old boy were amicable, whenever the male found any dead animal or rarely killed some prey; he was known to render calls that seemingly meant to invite her to dine with him. The sound would be subdued at a lower pitch than a roar. This was the second case of calling the mate I had seen. Skeptics may take it as an exception but this demonstrates that sometimes the practice of peaceful joint maneuvers for food is continued, even by aged tigers because of their established associations from the past.

The average age of a tiger in the jungle is 15 years, so the last three years can be taken as old age in which the fertility of a male reduces and so does the frequency of his mating. In such a case, if old male mates with a young tigress it may result in the production of cubs but with a tigress of equally old age, the possibility of conception is drastically low.

Schaller, who had also studied Serengeti lions, says that among one group of young captive lions only 38 percent of mating had been productive. Now as tigers and lions are biologically similar and breed on a similar schedule, I can vouch that when the tiger pair is past its prime, old enough to have a couple of years left in their life, their nuptial exercise will largely be sterile and the production rate will be as good as zero. The convincing signs of estrus or heat may occur on odd occasions like flank rubbing, cheek rubbing, or the female rolling on her back and making a distinctive puffing sound called *prusten*; but very few tigers can manage to breed at this age.

Mintoo Mama had observed this tiger quite a few times on the lower banks of the Sharda. He told me that the old boy was having some rather symbolic bouts of copulation with his partner rather than fully consummated ones. I think they are an essential part of courtship for young tigers, without which the volatile reactions of mating partners might lead to serious injury. Mating involves numerous copulations and a minimum number of copulations may be necessary to trigger ovulation in a tigress before conception occurs. Different from the young tigers, the old tigers' courtship displays are only a part of their sex lives that demonstrates infrequent sexual approach and mock battle withdrawals but there is rarely any actual copulation.

This tiger, like others of his kind from the sugar-brand, showed an inclination to eat both type of spoiled foods; a vulture-operated kill as well as festering meat. It is important to be *au fait* with knowledge that in the closed atmosphere of the jungle the consumption of prey is not influenced by the presence of scavengers, especially vultures. The plentiful cover, without a hole in the forest canopy, enables them to hide the prey from the preying eyes of airborne birds. And the kills bleached by vultures are customarily abandoned by the jungle tigers for they seem to dislike the musky odour of ammonia gases that their excreta emanate.

Such dislikes are generally absent in sugarcane tiger. May be because hardly does a tiger kill in sugar fields goes undetected by vultures in the blaze of daylight, or may be because the birds are essential creatures to the operation of the tropical grasslands, so sugar tigers — like lions — have to meet the terms of their functioning too.

The vultures soaring in the sky continually cast a baleful eye over the eco-system down below, watching and waiting for someone to die. Even if the carcass is tucked away under the bush and invisible from above, the scent rising on a thermal is enough to attract them. They effectively operate on most of the tiger kills, and tigers later consume them without any qualms. Over the years, I can recall at least half a dozen tigers I watched in sugarcanes that readily snatched kills from vultures and ate them. I had once watched a similar instance in the Banveerpura tigress at Katrania Ghat described in a previous chapter. She had killed a macabre bird and partly feasted on it before switching back to the normal food that lay for her – a dead cow.

This peculiar behaviour of cane tigers may appear as a riddle to a naturalist but to my mind its answer lies in the power of the environment. The transition is perhaps an answer to the strictures which the closed, deep and dark environment of forest places on orthodox predator species. Quite justifiably so, there may be some biological explanation for this retrogressive behaviour. Or could it also be the reflection of the trauma of competitive existence?

As regards eating of decomposed flesh by tigers, some eminent sportsmen of authority like Capt. Richard Hamilton, 'Hawkeye', Blyth and F. Bruce Simpson, maintain that tigers prefer putrid flesh to fresh meat, or at least are very partial to it and will readily eat animals not killed by them. A tiger is also recorded who in preference to live calf showed a proclivity for dry moldy bones of a domestic pig that were nearly two months old and were lying submerged in about one and a half feet of water in a drain. Night after night he visited that and finished without touching the heifer.

The Navarangpur tiger was certainly one of its kind, perusing his own solitary existence. And I knew that it was not a random isolated event, but I was invariably glimpsing into an indispensable part of the system, the part of a biological process that the structure generates to sustain the waning energies of a living organism; but my question was still unanswered whether a tiger can stay at a place for so long a period.

I contacted wild life institutions and asked experts if a tiger could stay at one place for so long? There was not even a single source of information that could provide satisfactory answer to my question. Foresters took it casually while many easy chair tiger activists found it hardly palatable, questioning whether this model could provide insight into the late age functioning of tigers. W. Longwa was emphatic that the villagers spread such rumors out of ignorance, which later become a good material for writers and discussion around a bonfire. "This is a contradiction to the habits of the tiger. They are constantly moving. They don't stay at a place," he remarked out of his experience. A good friend though he knows much about tigers but I knew that at this point, much of the discord arises among tiger activists because of the school of knowledge one follows. The chief argument against credence in stories of this nature is the difficulty in imagining how so formidable and massive animal as a tiger can continue to fulfill his food requirements just from one area and villagers remaining tolerant to it. So I had my doubts too.

I have been a voracious reader and after returning to Lucknow I took to hard classical literature on the subject. Evidence indicated that such animals may stay in a particular locality for several years. Sanderson writes. "when a tiger becomes old and fat, he usually settles down in some locality where beef and water are plentiful, and here he lives on amicable terms with villagers, killing cow or bullock about once in four or five days..... Nutritional needs of such tigers are usually low; they also scavenge meat of several animals that die from disease or other causes."

I checked a number of publications and used the factual material to supplement my data. Old *shikar* buffs had taken a considerable interest in such native stories. Baker (1890) noted that a male stayed for fourteen years in a locality and accounted for 500 cattle in that time. Brander stated that one tiger remained near some villages for fifteen years and Sanderson claimed that one tiger remained a cattle killer for twenty years. Although, these lengths of time may be highly exaggerated — as they are literally the full life cycle of a tiger — the reports do attest to their probable long occupation in a locality.

The most scientific answer was from Schaller that "A tiger appears to have a center of activity within its range where it spends much of its time." But even he never specified as what length of time it may be.

(II)

Navrangpur was five kilometers away from Paraspur and as usual I was shunting between the two field-stations. The later had its own distractions; first it was lovely jungle home and the other was Mama and his family's ever-warm company.

Towards middle of June the regular monsoon set in. The change of season from dry to wet happened almost overnight as the clouds rained with increasing frequency. Dark clouds massed in the afternoons and came down with thunder, lightening and high winds which did much damage to the trees. Where only yesterday dust storms blew across the sapphire sky and the land lay dry and arid, today there were pools and rivers. At length, the time had come for me to give up the delicious feeling of freedom and bid adieu to my host.

Next day, I woke up too early. I was getting ready to catch the Sanctuary train that starts from Palia at 3.30 am; I distinctly heard a leopard moving about at some little distance off behind the house and eventually heard him chase a wild pig. When my Jeep left for the railway station, the sounds of frenzied hunting had quieten down but the raucous, resounding alarm barks of *langurs'* were still renting the primordial darkness.

There was a long stint of interval, before the Dussehra vacations fell. I accordingly took the opportunity to make a short visit to Navrangpur again. The monsoon was over and the county was vividly fresh. Its overwhelming impression was of a benevolent green. The ancient tiger was still there, running in the sixth year of his stay. It seemed that nature, in its infinite wisdom had ensured its survival and recompensed by its gratis bounties, he was lingering on admirably in the range. Sometimes he disappeared for two or three weeks, eked out his life on small pickings and then reappeared in his former haunts; hungry enough to check the old cattle skeletons again for the food.

Carrion scavenging in tigers has received little notice. We need to understand that ecological niches work in a pyramid-based format, with apex predators like tigers at the very top. The higher the animal is up the pyramid, the less biomass is generally devoted to that species, and that is why the animals high on the pyramid are generally also more susceptible to extinction. But interestingly in some historic extinction's where most plant life was wiped out, the animals that survived were actually scavengers rather than dedicated herbivores or carnivores. Thus, scavenging or necrophagy is an important feeding behaviour of big predators, which keeps them nutritionally as sound as the hunted food does because the carcasses produced by "natural" death generally carries no dangerous parasites, as most such deaths result from malnutrition and old age and not any disease. Moreover, as dead prey does not possess any active defense, scavenging is much less hazardous than hunting and that is why, besides old and atrophied predators even healthy and nourished ones are partial to this easy way of life.

In the first week of October 1996, some grazers found the old boy sitting near an intact carcass of a buffalo that had been thrown at the cattle graveyard. Though tiger's teeth can cut through the toughest skin like a pair of shears but initially, inflicted with denture problem, he was unable to open the bait. It was only when vultures had poked its eyes and pressure of rumen gasses had burst the bolted stomach of buffalo, he could dine on it with comfort. He spent several days at 1000 lb carcass, gobbling the pliable flesh slowly in installments of ten to fifteen pounds a day and drinking water from a malodorous puddle covered in green slime. He often growled, hissed and spited to keep the vultures and crows away, which essentially scavenged more than half of the meat. His feast continued till the carrion become full of maggots and reached an advanced state of decomposition. He bore very emaciated looks, walked slowly and his skin hung loose in folds. His confidence seemed sapped by physical infirmities. The tiger was conscious of its waning powers. Villagers told me that now he was semi-immobile and spent most of his time in a cluster of trees. Sometimes at night, he went to a close-by mud wallow and churned the mud.

A week after in the afternoon a grazer brought the news that the Old Boy had been just sighted, lying at the banks of Sharda River. Mintoo Mama and I lost no time in reaching the escarpment. The sun beat down like a furnace. Across the Sharda river, a small heard of swamp deer had come out of forests to stand in knee deep waters under the shade of a tree. There were several old pugmarks of this tiger indented on the dusty path. They seemed a bit buckled showing that advancing years are liable to disfigure a tiger's pad. The grazer led us to the point from where the big cat had just been sighted.

On the farthest rise, almost 500 yards straight ahead, we saw a band of *langur* monkeys sitting on a large mound. It was hurling screeches and peeping curiously below it. We stopped at their sight and focused our binoculars. On cautiously scanning the adjacent escarpment where yet another small band was busy raising the alarm calls, below it I saw a tiger resting at the banks of the river. He lay solemnly in the water, half submerged and drowsy but intermittently looking at the tumult-raising monkeys. Through the glasses I could see that the monkeys were seemingly enjoying the joke of being at a high rise and out of the reach of a killer beast, who looked apparently frustrated.

We took up a strategic position and watched the tiger with a binocular. The eight power Zeiss lens magnified his expressions as well as of the rippling currents of the river. His asymmetrical eye-spots and cheek stripes were very clear. His hair had fallen out in several spots along his back, leaving circular grey spots. Scars of old wounds were slashed across his muzzle and many of his whiskers were broken. As the beast yawned, opening his cavernous mouth to the full I got just the right time to have a look into his mouth. It showed his pale gums and the condition of his denture. Its molars in the lower and the upper jaw were in sound position, right and left upper cranial were considerably worn; one incisor was missing and the upper canines were thin and smooth as small needles while the lowers were broken and at level with the gum.

The old boy was comfortable and the evening light around him was extra-luminous. He yawned repeatedly quite a few times, slowly and luxuriously, his eyes closing in rapturous expression of tigerish bliss. Evidently, he could not hunt any substantial prey but his continued existence was enough to prove that tigers are able to subsist as scavengers for long periods. A huge J-shaped callus on his shoulder also indicated that he had suffered some bad injury in a fight or perhaps from a deer horn, which had now healed.

"He must be facing long bouts of hunger," Mintoo Mama commented on his condition, "despite the fact that hungry tigers are the creatures of great determination and cunning, I have never heard of him attacking any man. Perhaps he recognizes people as old acquaintances that live in the same territory and often feed him". He said meditatively as he concluded with a punch.

Though we were in shade but the heat was stifling. The superheated surroundings were muggy with no movement in air. We observed him for good three hours, with sweat pouring down our backs in rivulets. Undoubtedly, the tiger was aware of us but it had decided to ignore us. All his attention was concentrated on the boisterous monkeys, which were mocking at it from a safe position.

An hour passed as the dusk approached. Like a giant balloon the sun seemed to hang low over the plains. A growing shadow covered the river gorge from the west. A jackal materialized out of grass and made off with a dry bone that lay abandoned at the banks of the river. At a distance a covey of brown partridge called endlessly, while I examined the tiger minutely through field-glasses. His hindquarters were very weak, his waist drawn in, wasp-like and the hip bones sticking up prominently. The physiological limits set by ageing, like supply of blood to outsized muscle masses, nutritional problems and loss of agility associated with large body were all conspicuously apparent. His brown eyes appeared sunken and lusterless. I estimated that he must be in the final months of his life and as is the way of his tribe he must be under pressure of young males converging in on him. Seemingly with no powers of retaliation left in him, he was bound to go under to a more powerful opponent, because territorial overlaps are normal amongst tigers.

The sky had turned from amber to deepest bronze. Sharda was still bathed in reddish mist or dust haze, illuminated by the afterglow of sunset. Luckily, it was one of those tropical evenings, when sunset merges imperceptibly into brilliant moonlight, and the empires of day and night meet and overlap as it were, awhile in a common duel role. Distant tinkling of bells denoted the home return of cattle some half a mile away, when suddenly a great commotion started amidst the monkeys. I registered their wired expressions as they looked down at tiger, with bared teeth, wide eyes, and wry screwed up expressions. There seemed to be more monkeys than ever on various errands, all calling hysterically. I could almost hear them making chuckling sounds when the tiger got up from the water and moved away and they too finally scampered away over the horizon into a mirage of dust.

It is said that the tigers incapacitated by old age or injury take to man-eating and this theory is immediately acceptable. These prejudices have potentially closed our minds to other aspects of tigers during their later age. The lifestyle of this very beast taught me an enormous amount, it proved that despite the powers of a predator atrophying with the old age, the acquaintance with human being does not essentially turn a normal tiger into a man-eater; if it had been so he would have been living out the last years of his life as a menace for human beings rather than a friend.

This was my last, unmistakable view of that historic beast which turned out to be of immense value. After a few more sightings by herders the older carnivore was seen no more. On November 26, 1996, his remains were found in a dry ditch along the course of Sharda river.

My old friend, Prabhas Jha, then a special secretary in the forest department of the state was on an official tour to Dudhwa. He was passionately interested in everything about big cats. We immediately went to inspect the spot. A rank smell of death pervaded the atmosphere. The carcass was already badly decomposed and a pair of Varanus lizards was feasting rapaciously upon its stomach contents. They dashed away to safety at our approach. The pungent rumen gasses assailed our senses as the forest guards turned the dead body for examination. There were several stab-like puncture wounds on the hips, infested with maggots and much of his skin had been peeled at places. There were multiple puncture marks on the abdomen region and left shoulder. All around the ditch where he laid a large amount of coagulated blood suggested that he had been terribly injured and then killed by a powerful antagonist who had passed through the area.

There were two deep wounds one on the upper side of his neck and other inside and near the anus. It seemed that the aggressor had ambushed him from back and while holding his neck had successfully scratched his rear claws that had inflected the later wound.

It was sad to behold the garbled remains of a familiar acquaintance, rotting in the stifling heat of sun. Thousands of flies and ants swarmed over the dried blood, much of which had trickled into the earth – the atoms in an eco-system must be consumed by worms, fungi, moulds and microbes who thus short circuit the classical food chain and break organic material down into inorganic substances.

No matter how ferocious the carnivore or how spectacular the herbivore, all eventually yield their material to the decomposers. This is the nature's way of feeding itself, for when the decay is complete, the elements are back in the soil again around the roots of trees that manifests them into leaves and grasses, and from there once more, they get ready to run through the system to maintain yet another class. Soon the lush grasses spring up at the place. Grazers stop by it harvesting as what they need in a mutually beneficial way. The rapid conversion of materials into edible stuff, belonging to a cadaver of a predator then moves into the bodies of prey animals to keep the cycle of natural world in motion.

Some organisms consume dung and others move seeds, some bacteria may play role in making clouds but all of them make soil richer and fertile, and eventually the nature is merciful to all these hungry kids.

The declining sun touched the surrounding fields with gold. When the foresters finished their work we got into the vehicle and proceeded for the headquarters. I had a queer satisfaction that the 'Old Boy' had not met his nemesis in a poacher's snare or by poisoning. He had packed up a gallant way, killed by a rival, which the infinite wisdom of his tribe has bestowed upon its members. The long line of gracefully posed mounds along Sharda, where his body lay stood out black and sharp against the flaming western sky, in the quiet evening air. A moment later, we swung around a bend in the road, and I took a last look at them with a sigh, realizing that the 'Old Boy' of Navarangpur was now a memory of the past.

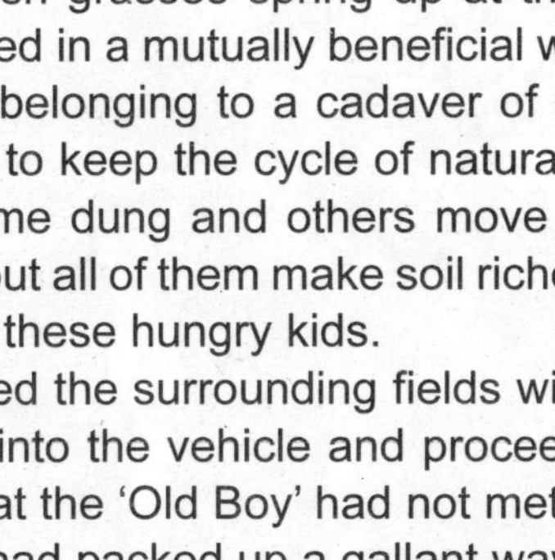

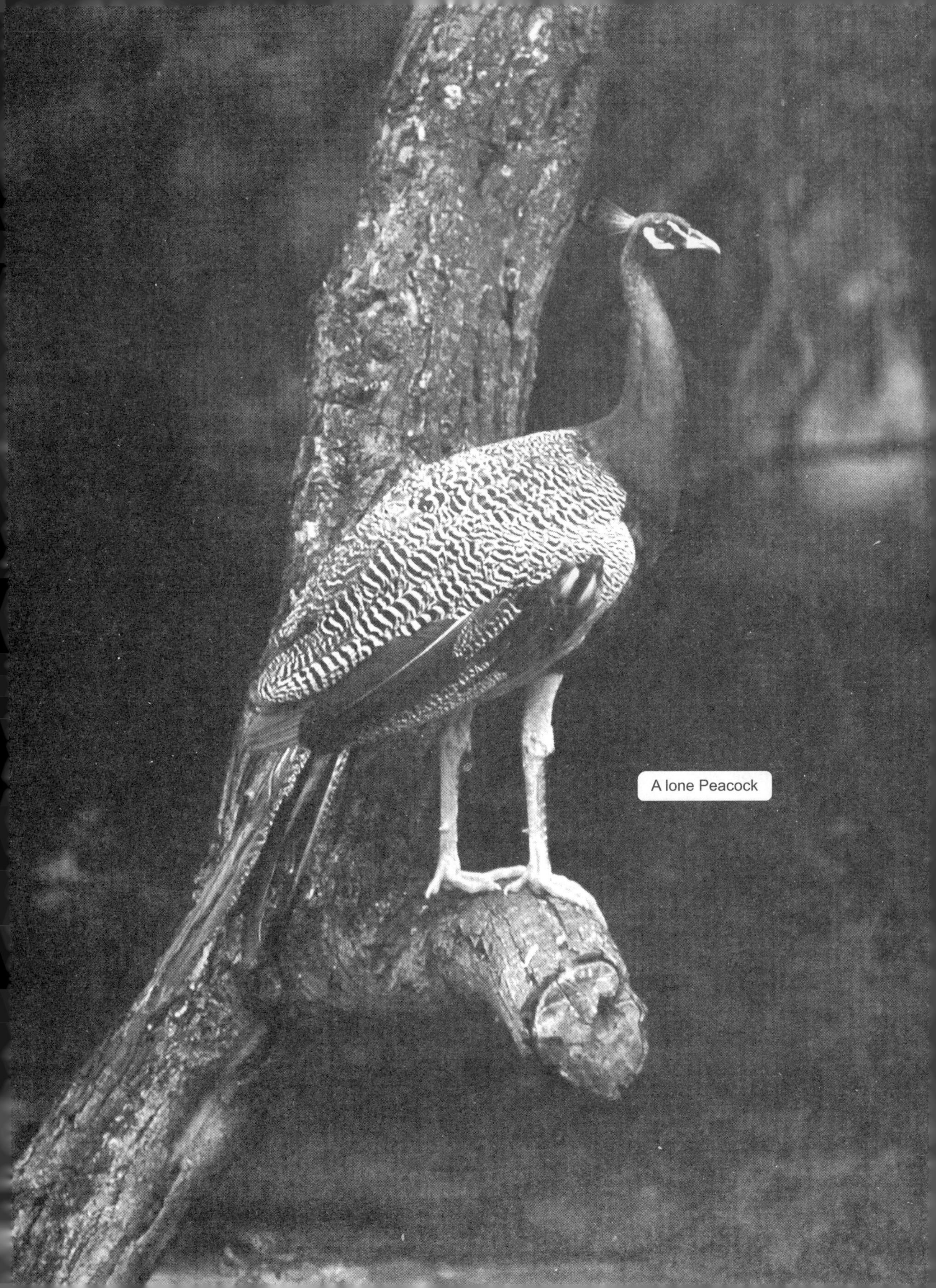

A lone Peacock

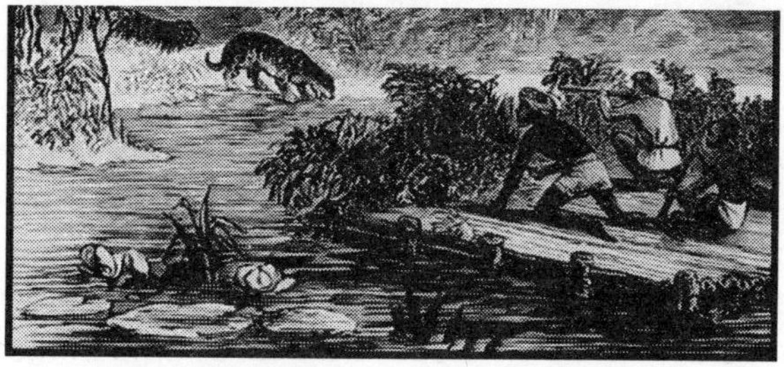

19

The Dispersal Dynamics

Nature always tends to act in the simplest way.

- Bernoulli

In the agricultural fields of the Tarai, there is a great deal of divergence in tiger activity. Tigers tend to become more mobile in winters. Their beats extend in winters and shrink in summers. The lower temperature and plentiful water helps to disperse prey species around numerous water holes which form during rainy season. The phenomenon of cane tiger increases in the winter as the population of peripheral jungle tigers spilling over to farmlands joins up with the habitual incumbents. There is also a ready generation of young cubs that is some two years old and that has reached the stage of independence. Potentially capable of killing a large and tough ungulate prey, it is all geared up to break away from their mothers and seek new postures.

At this stage the 'parent–offspring conflict' that occurs in many animal species, including humans becomes most visible. A more recent theory argues that there is time after the young are properly weaned and have become larger and more demanding, and it becomes too costly for the mother to provide food, energy for defense and manage other resources for her sub-adult young. Instinct advises her to abandon the existing progeny and devote the same effort toward the production of new off-spring. So she also encourages her young to seek independence and begin breeding.

The classic explanation for this behaviour is that the tigress is still caring for the juveniles by forcing them to become independent, which is necessary for their survival. This practice is also of genetic benefit to her because her own genes will be passed on by the young she has just alienated, as well as by herself to create a fresh order of life.

This behaviour is often difficult to observe in tigers and may not be directly perceived until closely observed, perhaps for months. My observation suggests that once the mother has trained the cubs the art of hunting efficiently and effectively, she abandons them by becoming indifferent rather than cubs leaving her at first. Though mothers withdraw and force their adult cubs to fend for themselves, they do keep in touch with their movements for a long time, through scent and occasional sounds.

This period of transition is a risky one in a juvenile's life. When the young tigers are launched on the critical process of independent living, they like to assert their presence at best spots which offer water, prey and shelter. In the jungle, such spots are normally not vacant. They are essentially in the possession of some powerful tiger, the resident male or female who spends a lot of time in marking the area and does not allow any trespasser to enter it. This results in conflict and weaker ones either leave the place or succumb to the onslaught of rival.

Last year, on the outskirts of a village called Ranipur, a grievously wounded young male tiger was found lying near a pond surrounded by cane fields; all around him the earth had been dug in a death struggle, which had raged over a vast area. His face was hideously swollen from an old infected wound. He was pounced over by an average size female, having small cubs and was mowed down. One common tactic of for such abrupt defensive attacks appears to be biting the shoulder or back that inflicts a paralyzing effect and often immobilizes the victim for practical purposes. Later a bite through the skull was also employed, crushing the heavy male down. The beaten animal was too weak from hunger and gangrenous wounds; and before he could be provided the proper medical aid, he died the next day.

Scientists having the relevant data building speculative models of tiger populations, give a crude idea of high natural attrition rate among tigers, Dr. Ullas Karanth believes that "out of 100 cubs born, only 60 may become juveniles and 54 may reach the dispersal stage and only about 20 tigers may ultimately reach the breeding age." The mortality rate for the passers-by is estimated to be as high as 35 percent per year in jungles whereas regarding farm tigers, I don't feel any such record data has been ever generated by any tiger scientist.

It is difficult to assess the home range of farm tigers. Their landscape is dotted with hostile human settlements and they live a life of different challenges in contrast to their kin in the jungle. And as it is not practically possible to go chasing them for all the 24 hours, burning up precious gasoline all over the countryside to know their areas of visit; the best thing to do is to conjecture on the basis of information available. My feeling is that the farm tigers do not have a well defined territory. I even doubt whether there is something like territory amongst these tigers; in fact they have hunting ranges which overlap with the areas or ranges of other occupants.

A territorial male is essentially preserving a part of the population food reserve — small enough to be effectively defended and large enough to attract females and nourish. The females which wander into his sphere of influence mate with him to ensure continuation of his line. The hunting ranges are by no means constant, and usually reduce and grow according to the season; for instance, contracting in monsoon period and widening in winters.

On the contrary, territories of adult tigresses are held primarily to obtain food and protect cubs, the males are much more concerned with containing and mating with as many females in condition to breed as possible. The females entering the area of other tigers are accepted but the males are not. They avoid conflict by keeping three or four miles from each other.

Usually in the jungles, the numbers of slots for the resident tigers are limited and there is no room for vagrants. New tigers became residents only as the old ones move away or die, creating vacancies; males replacing males and females replacing females. There may also be correlated shifts in land use, such as one animal moving in as the other moves out. But in the sugarcane, space is no problem, as long the crop fields extend and tigers have the advantage of cover and chemical communications. They feel safe and may carry on for larger distances.

If the regional number of tigers becomes incompatible with the food supply of the area they abruptly abandon the range and move away overnight. During winters, it is common for the villagers to come across the signs of sub-adults of both sexes in their agricultural field, moving on an exploration trip and desperately looking for a propitious niche to settle down.

Resident tigresses often make room for their daughters by yielding a portion of their ranges for them. Dispersing tigresses commonly try to establish home ranges next to their mother but the male tigers disperse over great distances away from their natal ranges. The tigers that survive through the second year of their lives disperse away from their natal ranges. They become somewhat larger and are relatively safe from threats posed by climatic conditions and predation. They try to establish their own home ranges and tend to move further in canes thus increasing the chances of passing through hostile human dominated landscape where they face higher risks.

These shy animals remain hidden and move about mostly at night. They are on no joyride as their survival needs are in head-on conflict with the livelihood requirements of people yet they manage to live in the sugarcane because the 'carrying capacity' is not restricted.

(II)

Tigers move around and patrol their area for many important reasons besides search for food. In spite of the ideal conditions of a landscape that holds everything right from water, shade to food and cover, the big cats do not patronize them for long. They frequent them for temporary periods and move on to continue their affairs. The localized stable supply of baits or natural food does confine a tiger to a limited area. It carries on with its normal pattern of activities. This is an atypical sidelight of a tiger's temperament that they are great wanderers. At times, they seem to lose themselves and get into most extraordinary places.

Intra-specific aggression is a conventional medium of population control among tigers and is an unremitting process in the areas of optimum numbers. In comparison to the finite jungles that have limited slots for predators, the boundless sugarcane offers much larger scope for a tiger to avoid such confrontations. In fact the problems of space do not exist in the canes. The contention — that in natural state the expansion of tiger population must be contained by constriction of available habitat, after which they will adjust their own populations — does not seem to apply appropriately in the sugarcane.

Here tiger movements are not complex. Instead of mooching around in the face of inter-species tension and competing predators in a given spatial area, they prefer to defuse the tension by crossing over to further lands. The land use pattern is tiger-friendly. The sugar crop anywhere is essentially a crop of similar nature, to which they are completely familiar and into which some of them are hereditarily integrated. The cane corridors allow a lot of dispersing tigers from source populations, to move to pockets where they often go off the ecological radar. Such aggressively exploring tigers may move thirty or forty miles through hostile human landscape before finally trying to settle down at some isolated place.

Males are susceptible to tremendous mobility, often without a focal point. Looking at the recent history of straying tigers, I can safely say that the vagrants who traveled

A sambher stag disinterring a muddy wallow at the edge of Jhadi Tal. This practice is typical of a rutting stag.

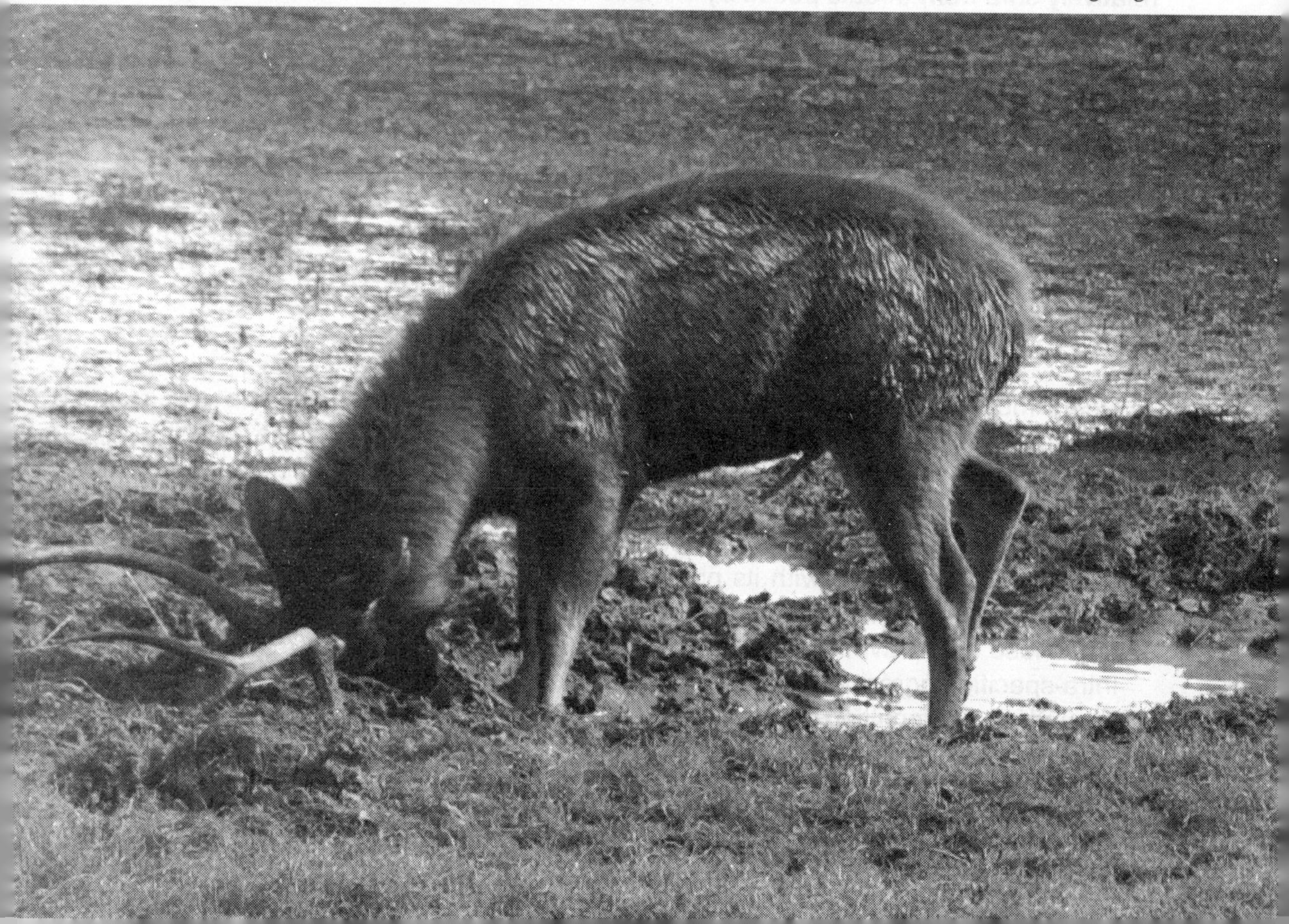

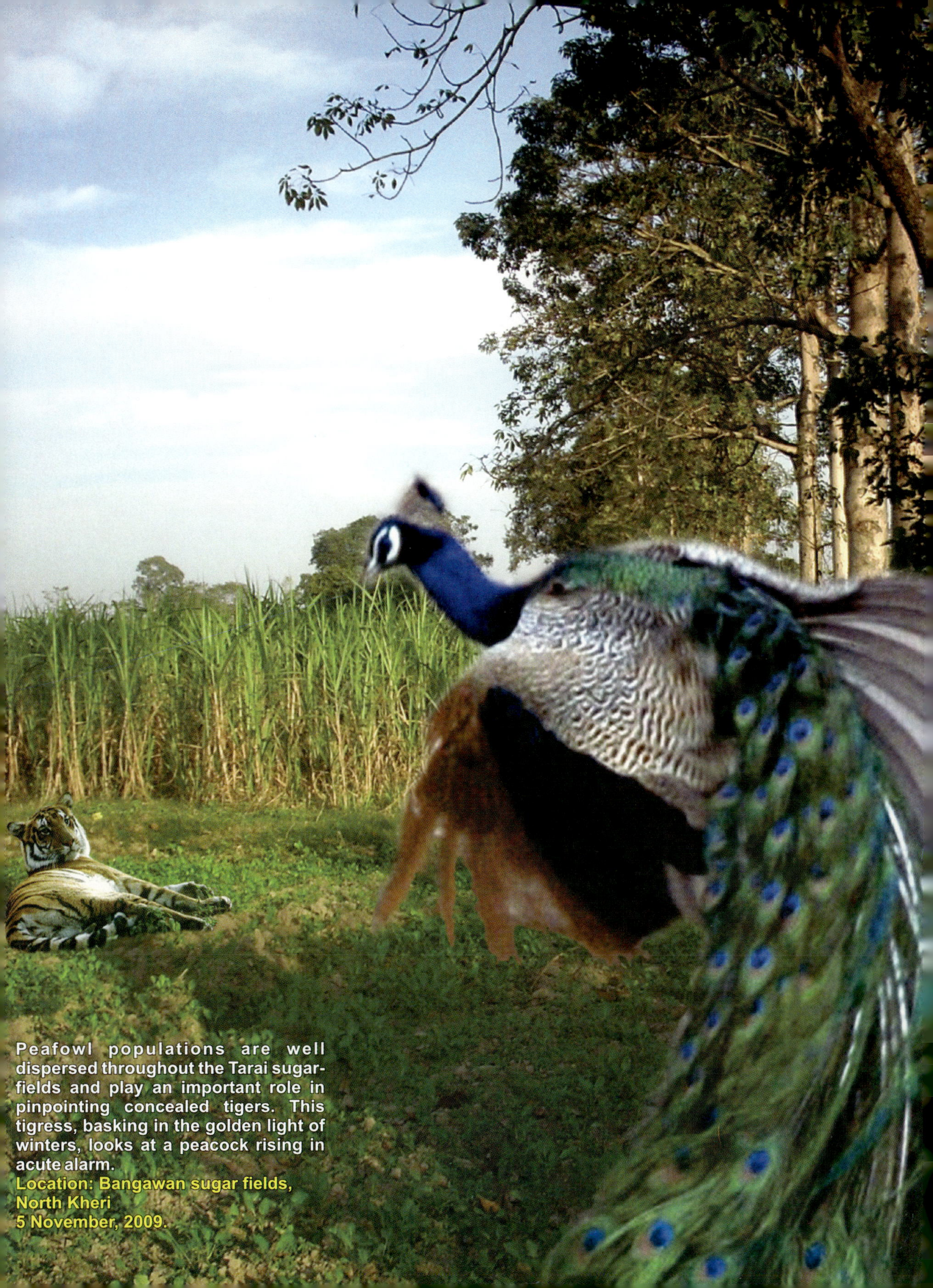

Peafowl populations are well dispersed throughout the Tarai sugar-fields and play an important role in pinpointing concealed tigers. This tigress, basking in the golden light of winters, looks at a peacock rising in acute alarm.
Location: Bangawan sugar fields, North Kheri
5 November, 2009.

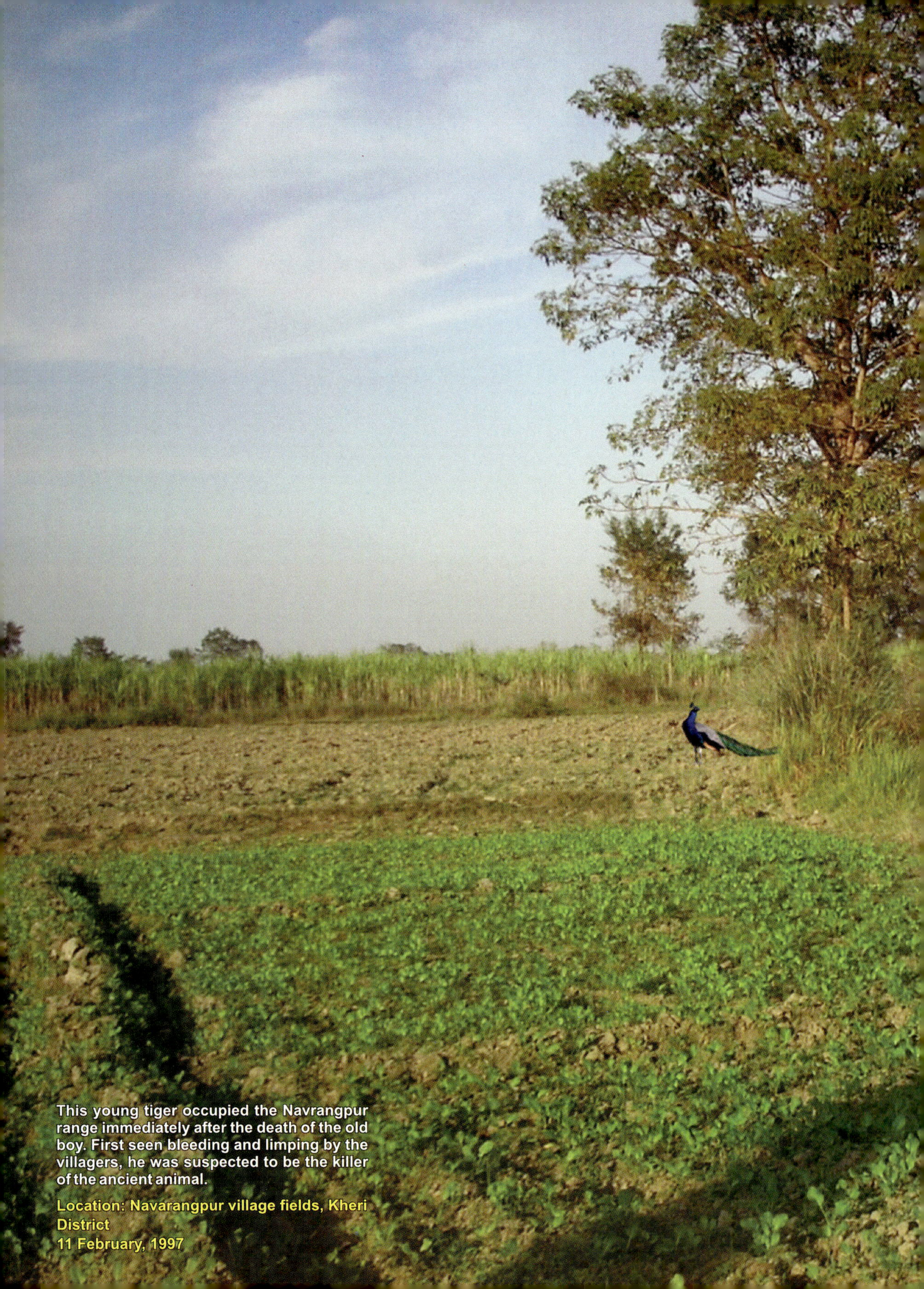

This young tiger occupied the Navrangpur range immediately after the death of the old boy. First seen bleeding and limping by the villagers, he was suspected to be the killer of the ancient animal.

Location: Navarangpur village fields, Kheri District
11 February, 1997

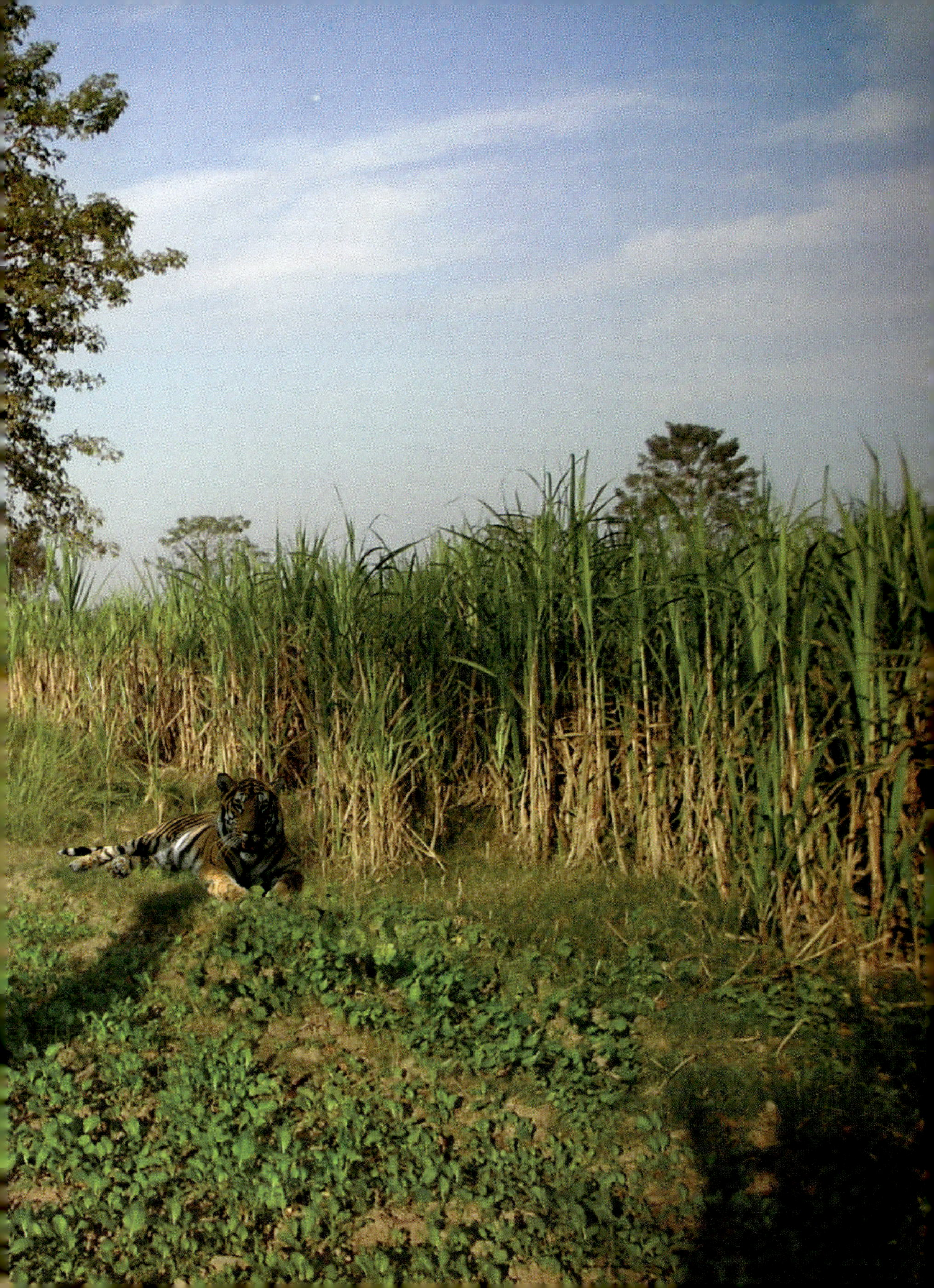

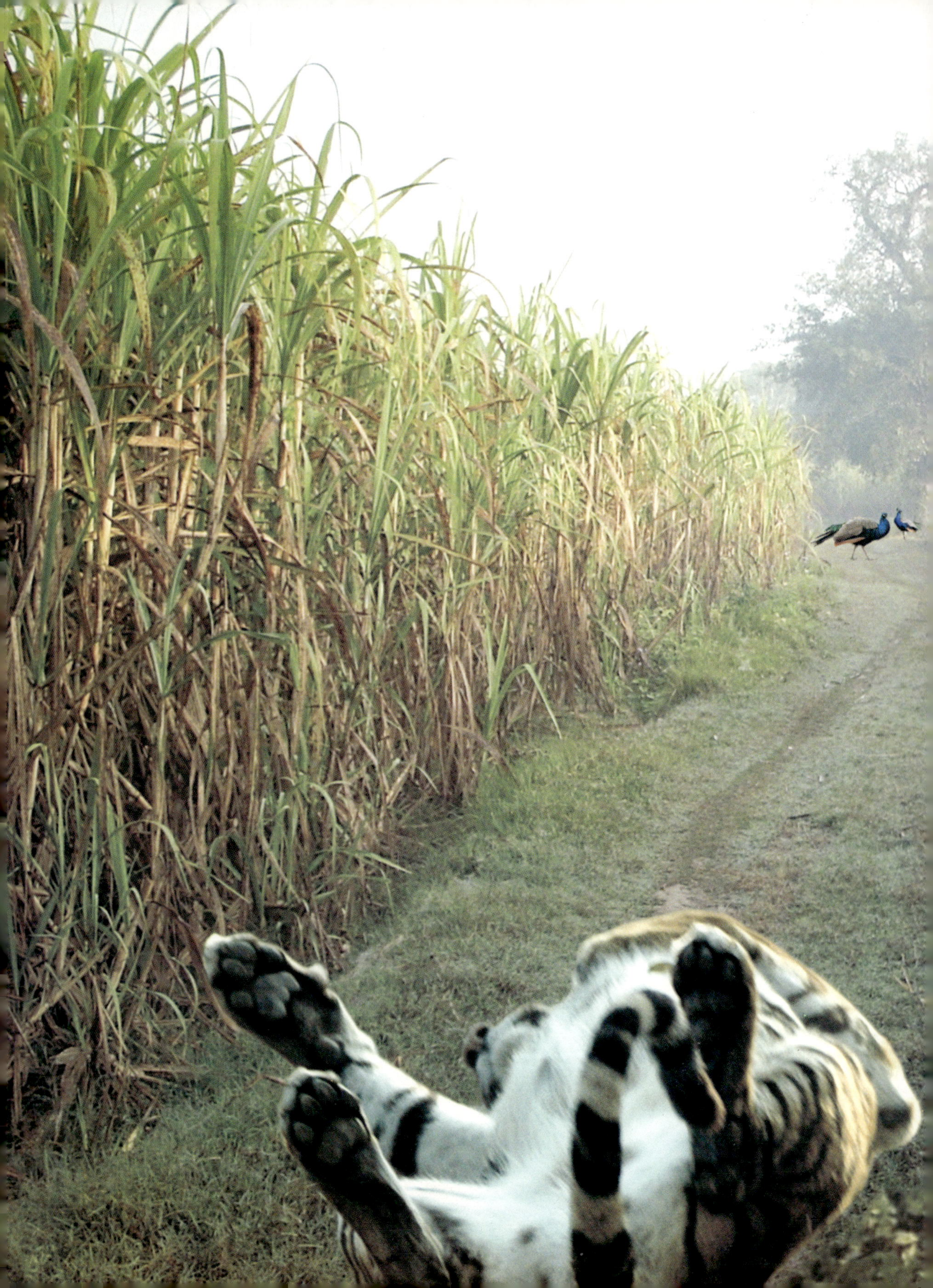

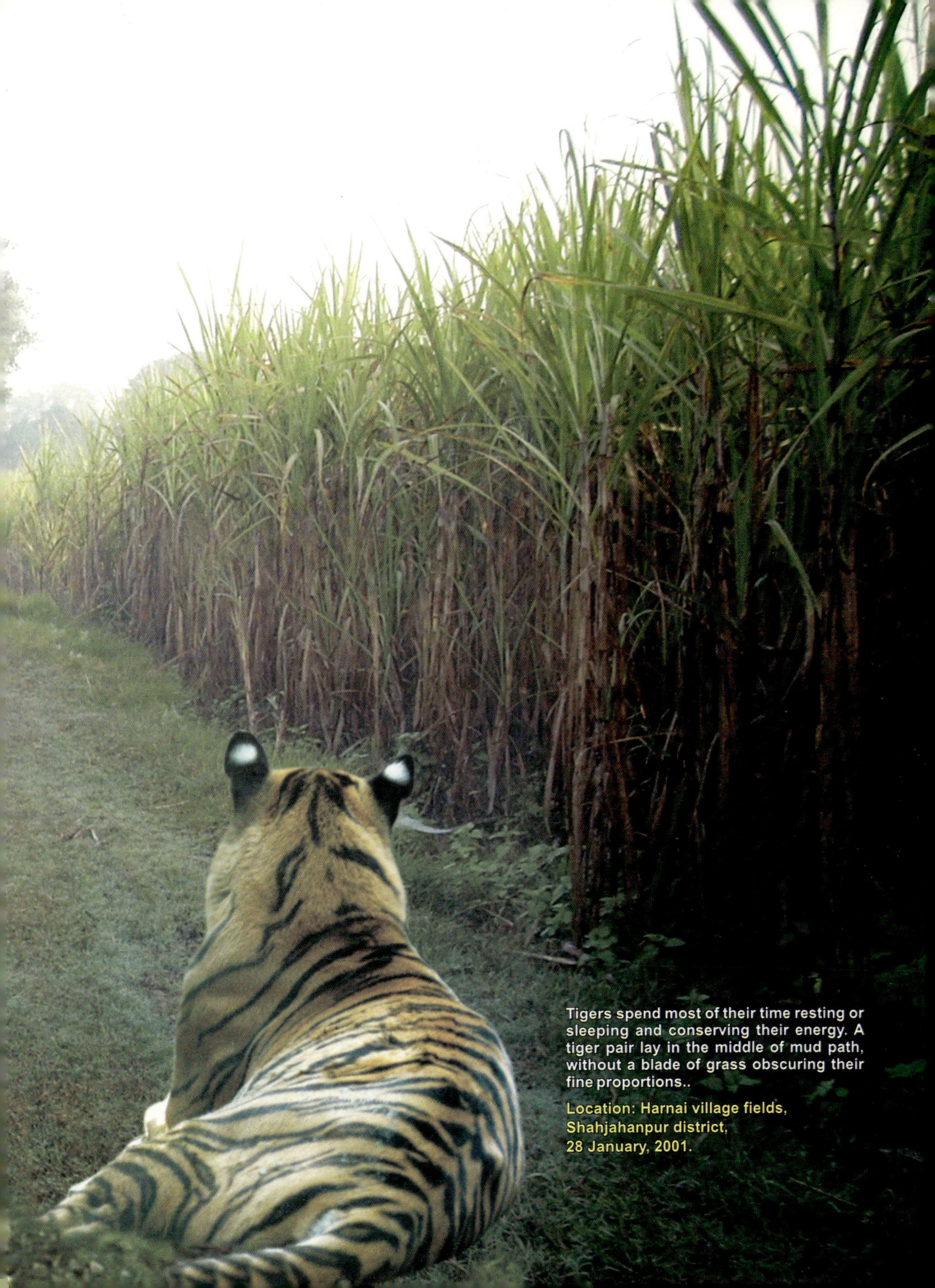

Tigers spend most of their time resting or sleeping and conserving their energy. A tiger pair lay in the middle of mud path, without a blade of grass obscuring their fine proportions..

Location: Harnai village fields, Shahjahanpur district, 28 January, 2001.

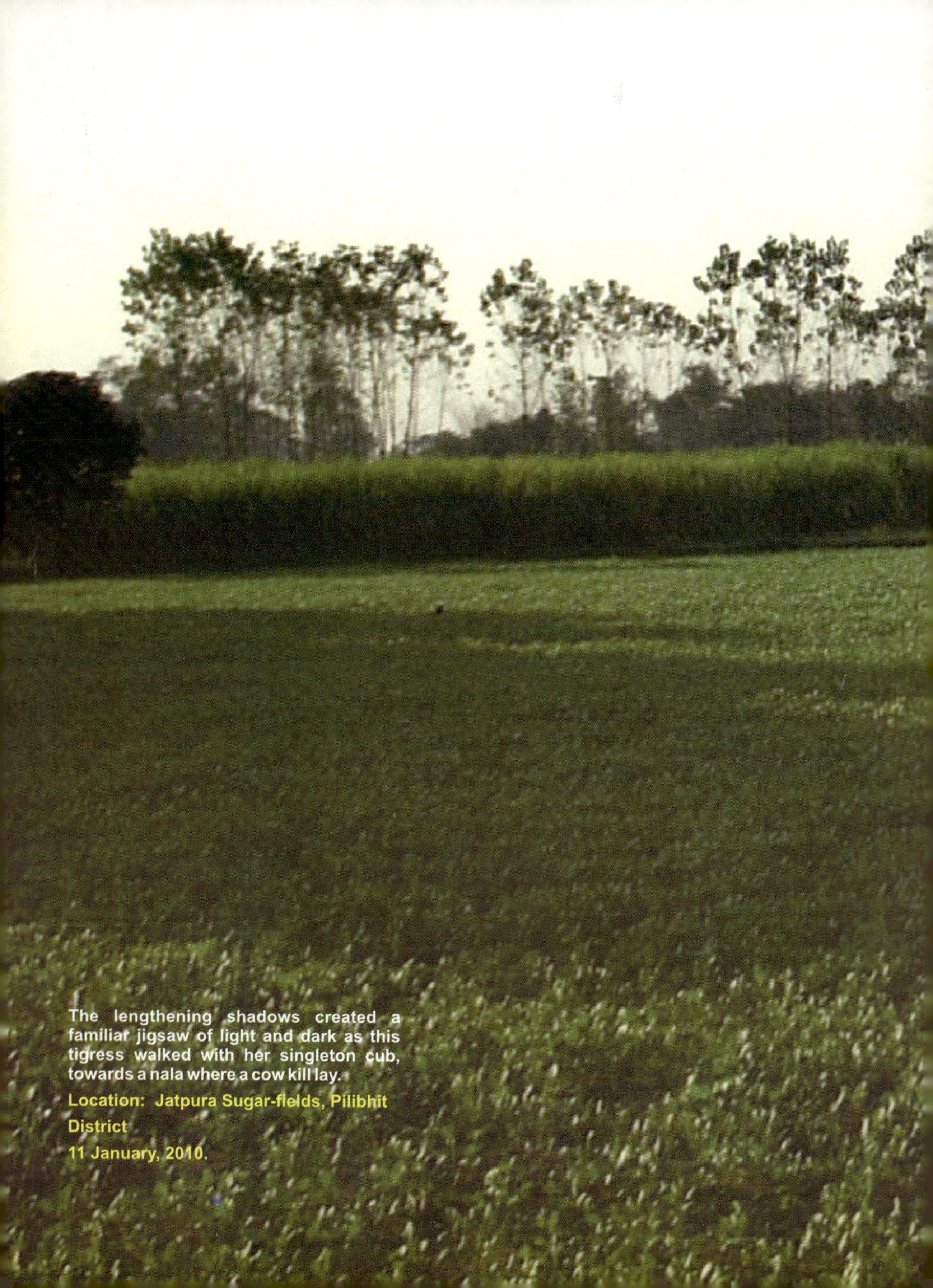

The lengthening shadows created a familiar jigsaw of light and dark as this tigress walked with her singleton cub, towards a nala where a cow kill lay.

Location: Jatpura Sugar-fields, Pilibhit District

11 January, 2010.

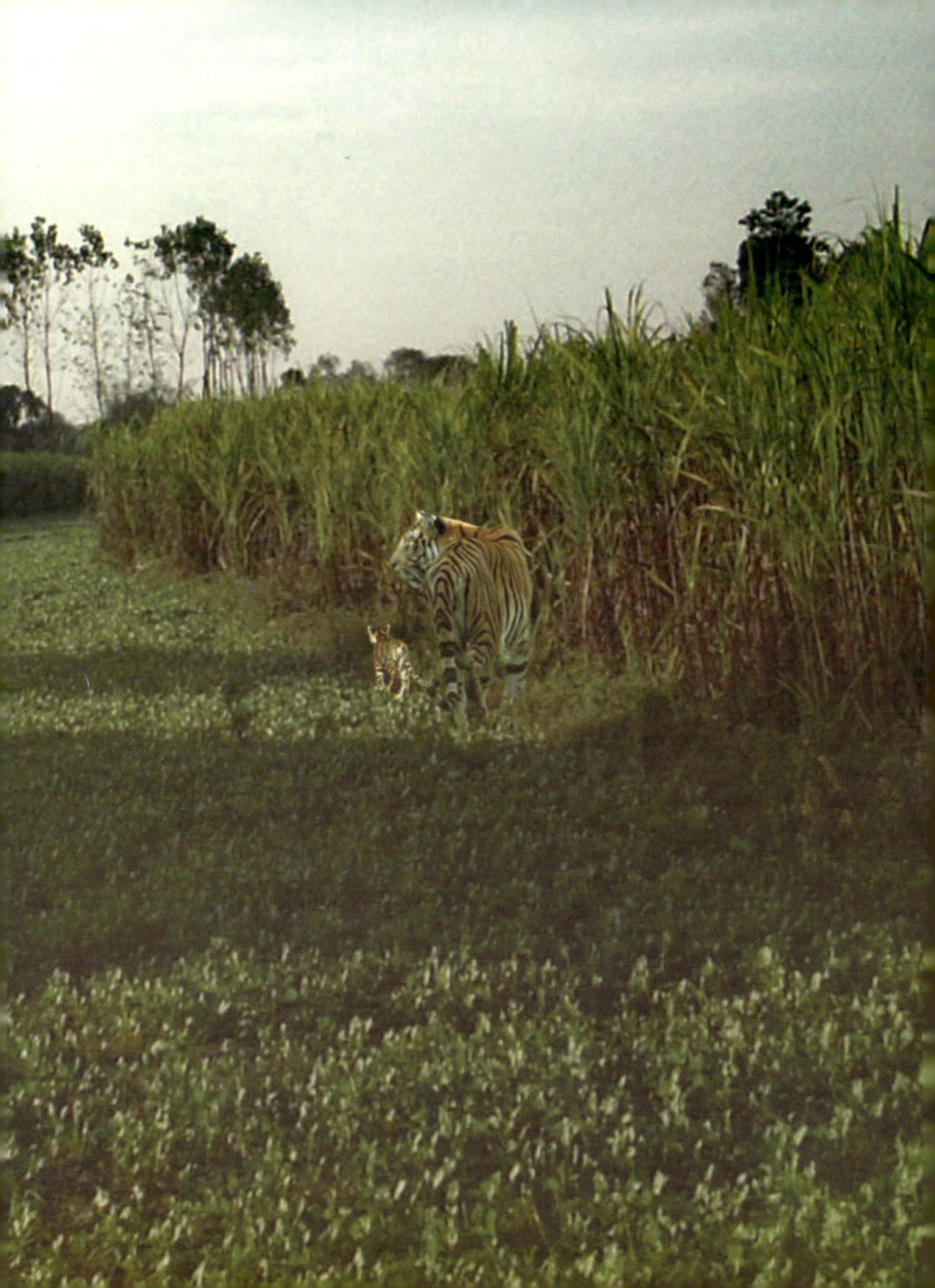

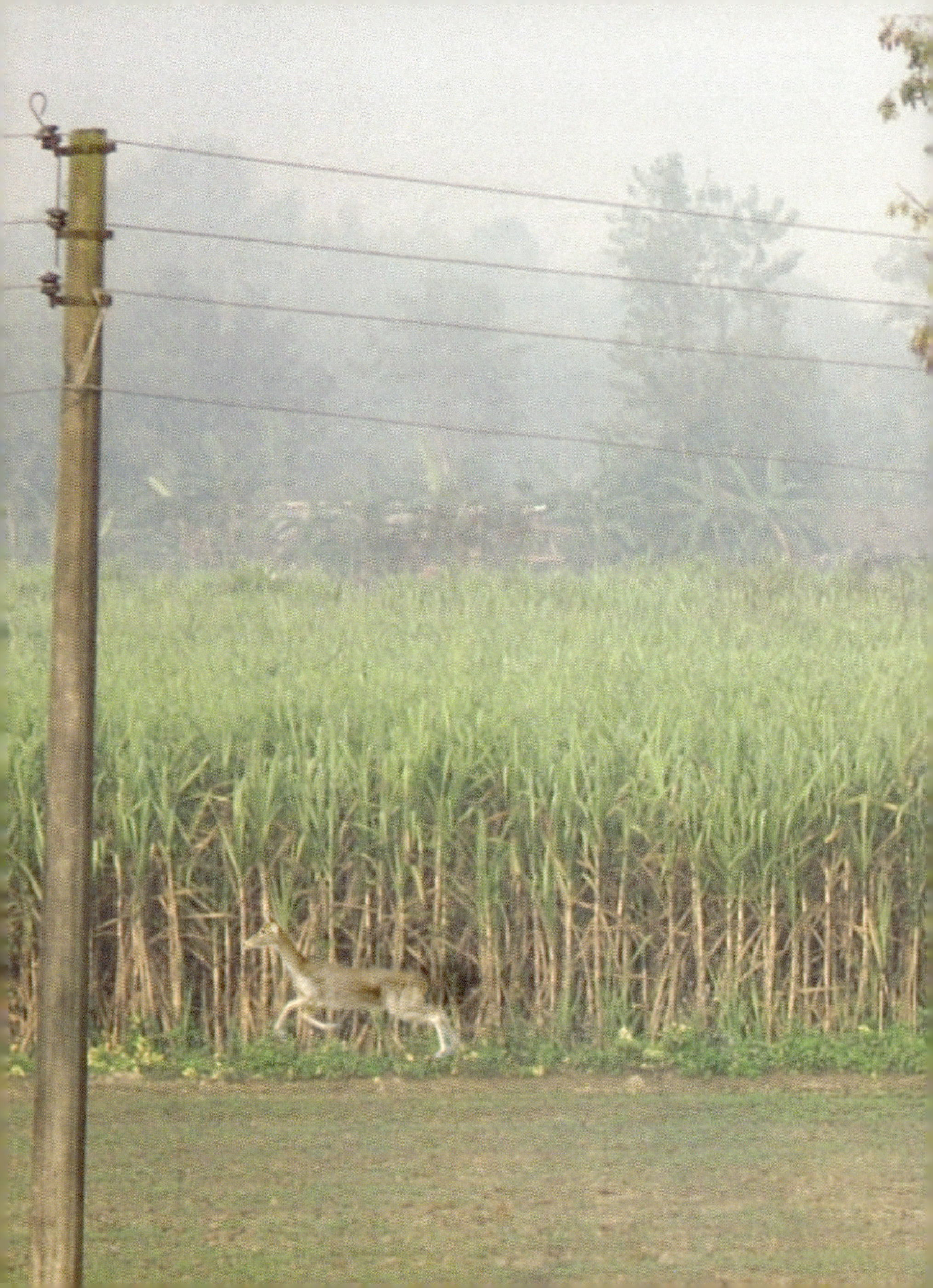

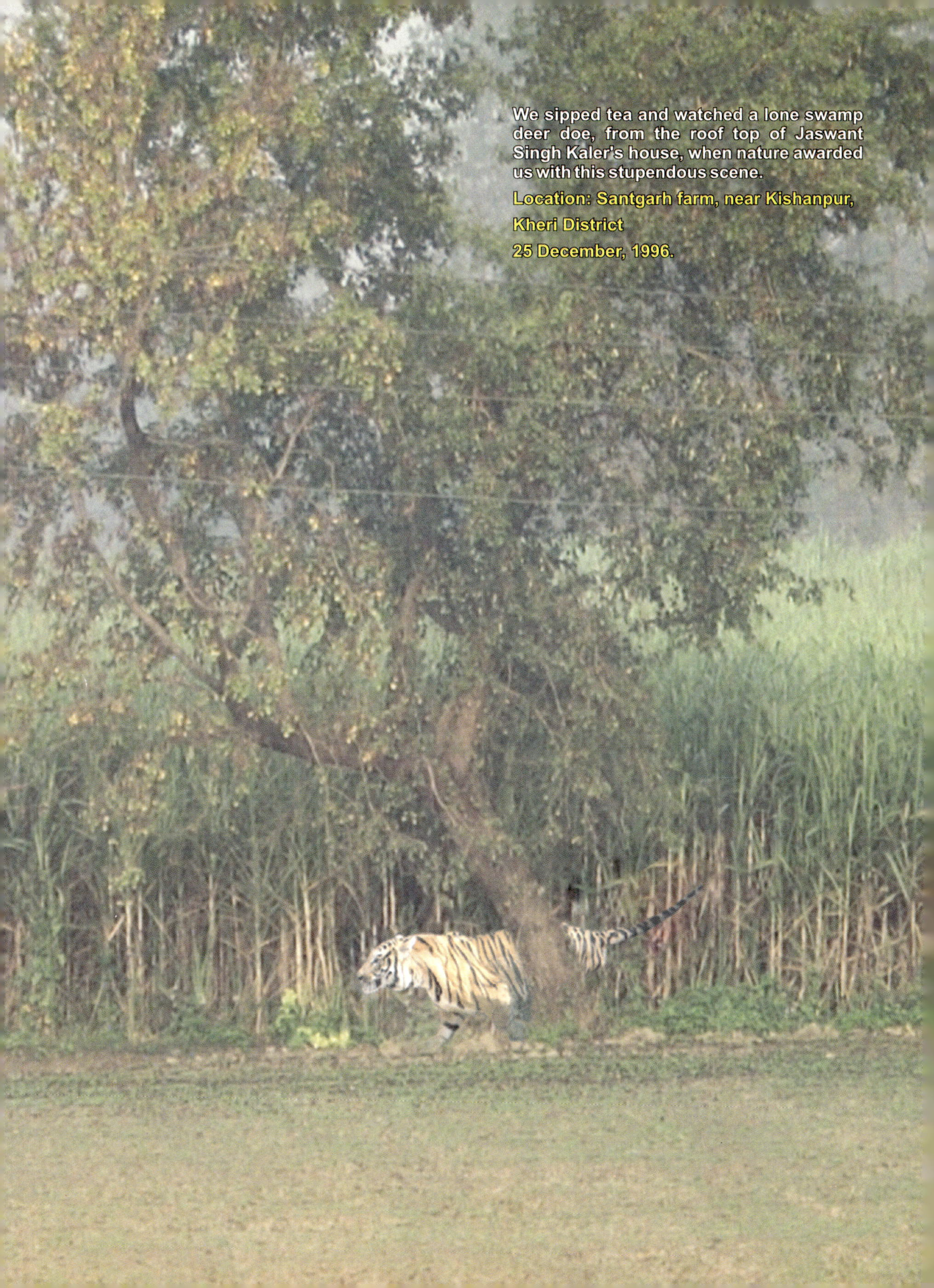

We sipped tea and watched a lone swamp deer doe, from the roof top of Jaswant Singh Kaler's house, when nature awarded us with this stupendous scene.

Location: Santgarh farm, near Kishanpur, Kheri District

25 December, 1996.

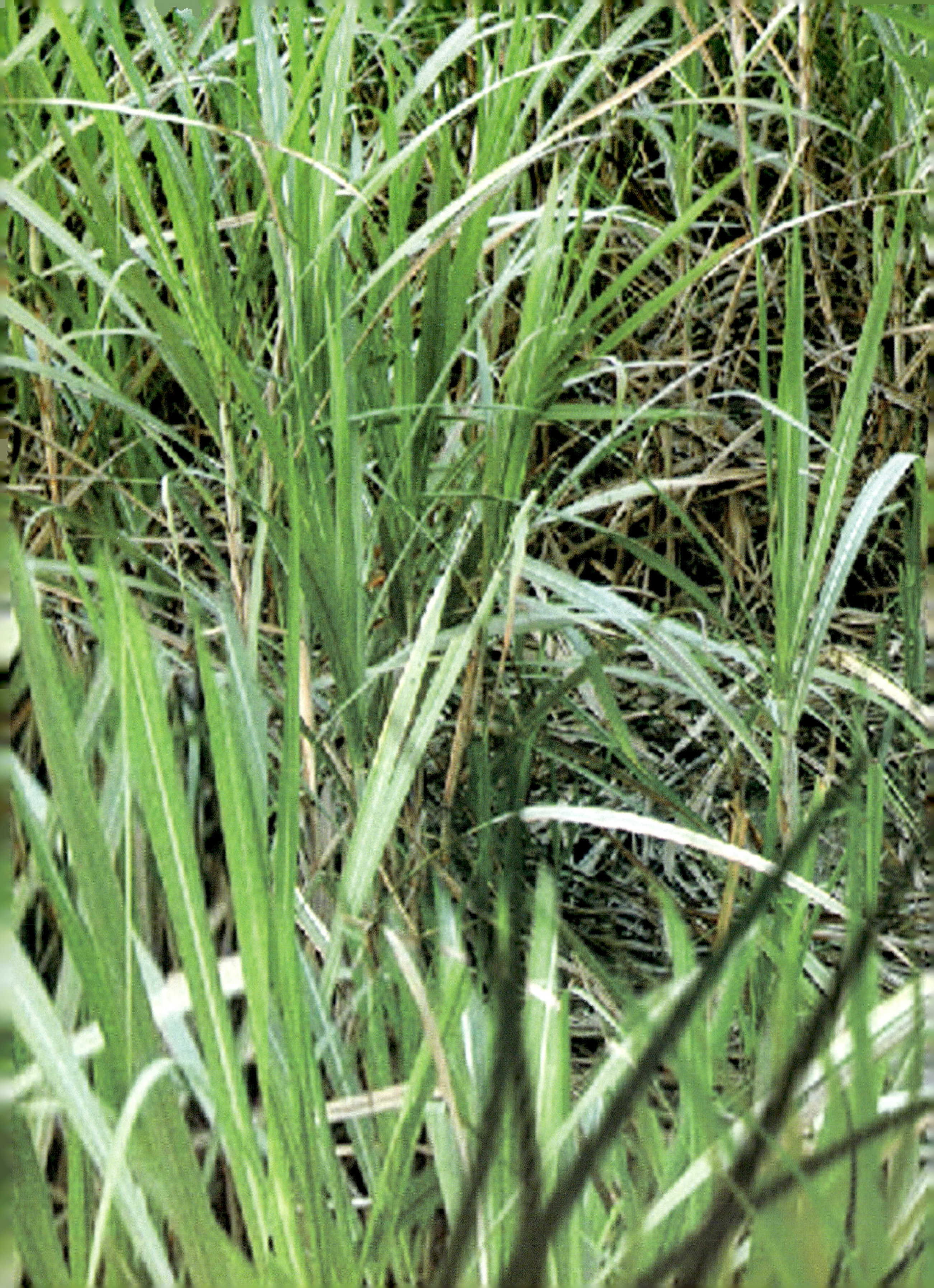

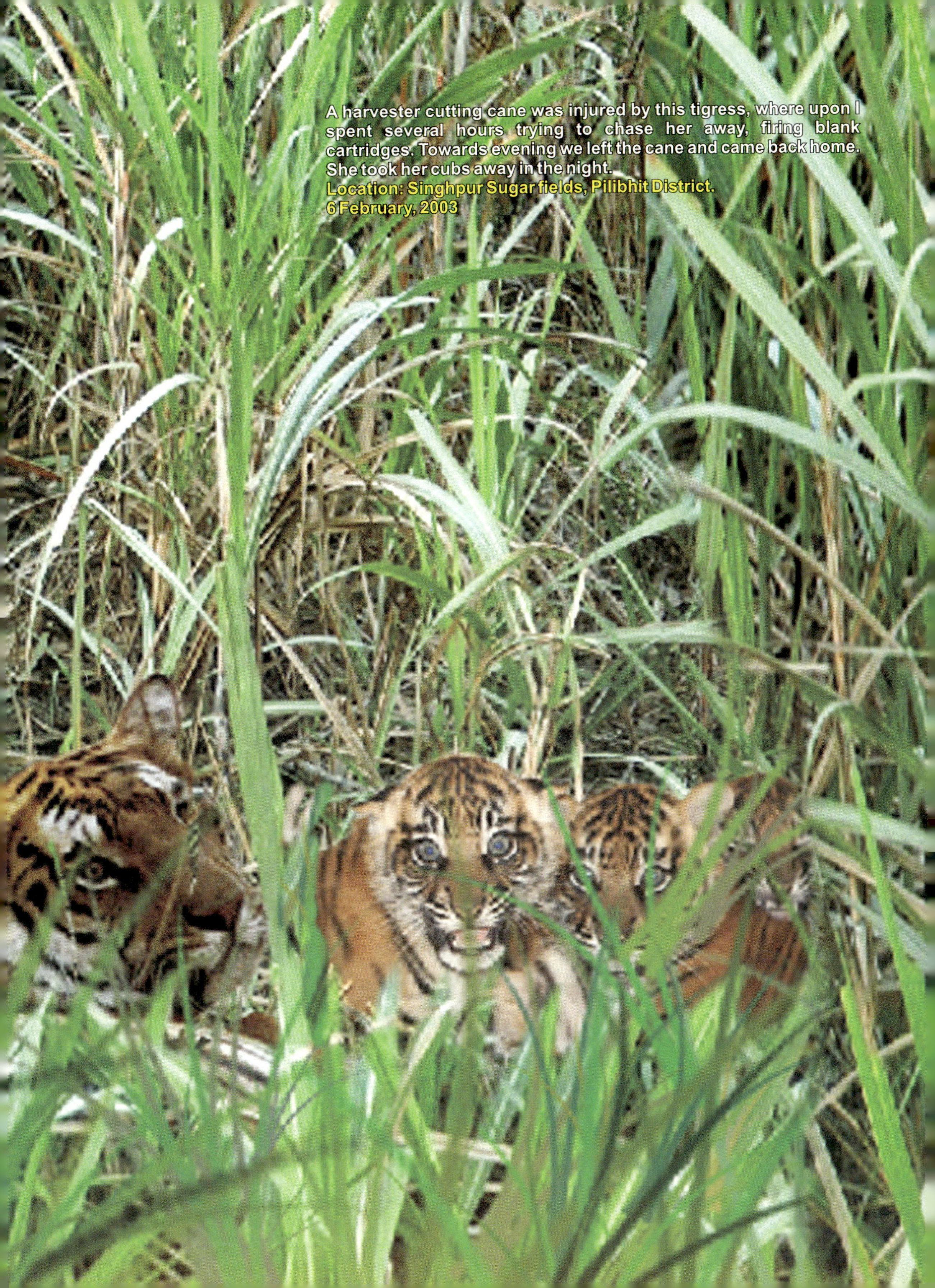

A harvester cutting cane was injured by this tigress, where upon I spent several hours trying to chase her away, firing blank cartridges. Towards evening we left the cane and came back home. She took her cubs away in the night.
Location: Singhpur Sugar fields, Pilibhit District.
6 February, 2003

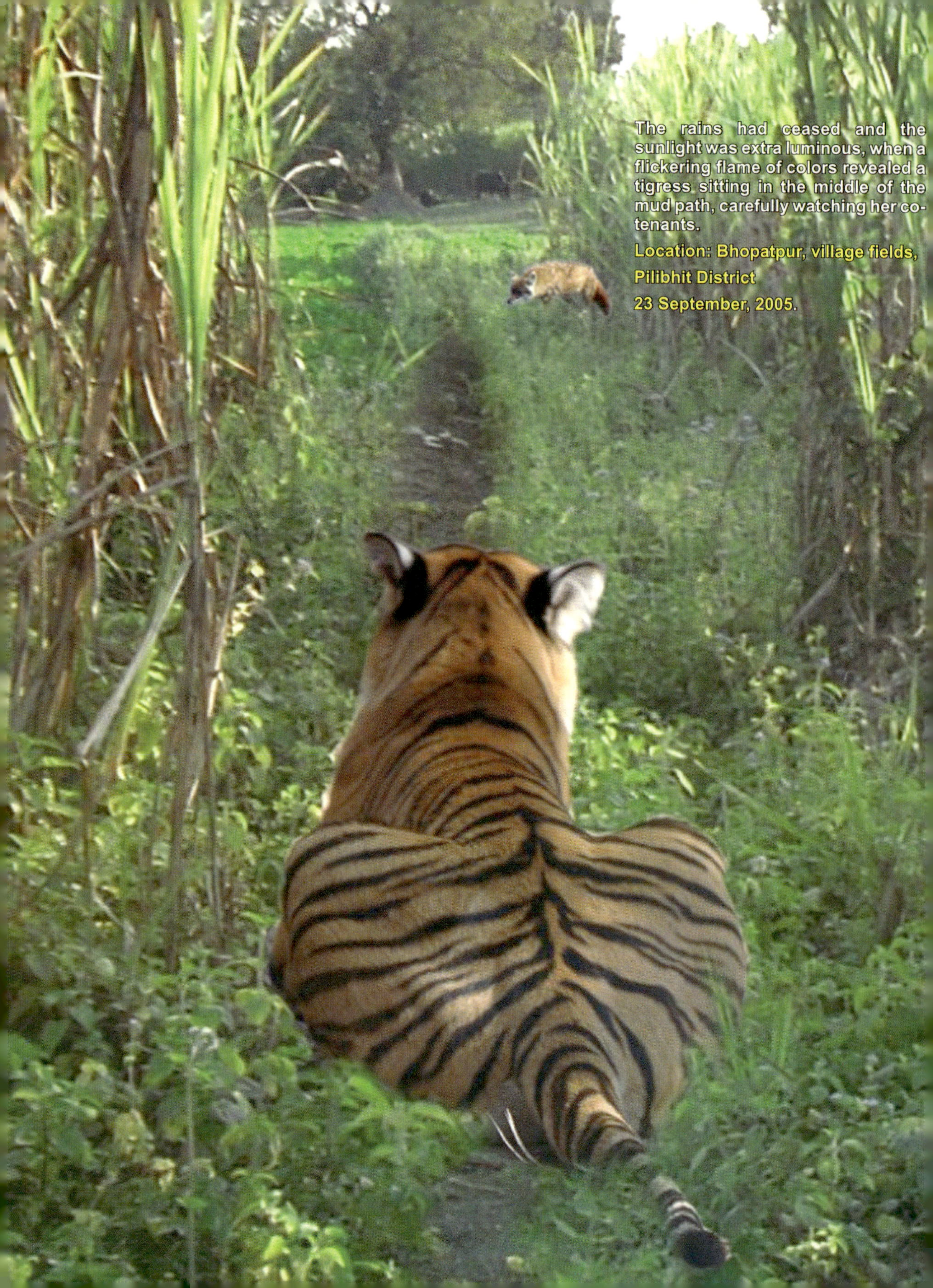

The rains had ceased and the sunlight was extra luminous, when a flickering flame of colors revealed a tigress sitting in the middle of the mud path, carefully watching her co-tenants.

Location: Bhopatpur, village fields, Pilibhit District

23 September, 2005.

through lands unknown, often more than a hundred miles from their homeland were essentially male tigers.

Tigers are mercurial animals; and great strays are certainly undertaken by confused transients. For jungle tigers as well as sugarcane tigers do not really migrate in true sense of the word. Rather, they keep extending their hunting ranges with habitat utilization differing from season to season. They also have an evolved mechanism to reduce possibilities of inter-species tensions. They just move out and leave the troubled zone. Under extreme circumstances their normal social system may also break down temporarily but the call of their own kind finally proves stronger and they return to fraternize and assume possession of resident females.

However, hunger and search of food is the prime mover of tigers. William Baze does not consent to the idea of tigers ever forgetting their directions. He says, "The tiger – who must follow his larder wherever he goes — is less likely than any other to lose his sense of direction. His compass is his stomach and it never leads him astray."

Nomads are sometimes encountered far from the usual haunts, wonderingly widely and without territory. Burton (1933) records a tiger that traveled fifty to sixty miles over cultivation. Perry (1964) records a tigress that appeared two hundred miles from the nearest known habitat. Some of the non-established animals are probably young adults, which having reached maturity are moving away from the area of their birth into unoccupied terrain.

This trait of "going astray" needs to be examined in detail, for it is certainly different from the standard dynamics of dispersal. Besides inevitable stresses, hunger, and intense competition, the acute tension of finding a breeding partner also seems to be a causative factor.

Breeding is a class of behaviour concerned with maintaining species integrity. No matter how much there is to eat, a great deal of energy consumed must go into the activity designed to maintain the species or food is wasted. On the other hand, no matter how prolific a species may be, the proliferation will snuff itself out if there is not enough energy to feed it. If all mature animals do the transmitting of genes the populations of progenies will contain a considerable portion of substandard material, simply by the laws of chance. In such condition, a genetic line is constantly at risk, for it can lose the struggle against an unfriendly environment at any stage in an animal's life cycle.

There is plenty of room for sugarcane tigers to maintain their genetic strength. To counter the adverse effects of inbreeding in small isolated populations, the translocation of just one unrelated breeding animal in each generation is sufficient. Is it possible that they take too long journeys under the dictates of nature to pass on their contribution to the gene pool of the population? It reduces the possibility of inbreeding caused by closely related females occupying a compact environment.

It is appropriate to mention that eearlier the scientists were worried about inbreeding depression, where highly inbred animals become sterile, susceptible to infections and lose their vitality. However, the recent experimental study by Chellam explains that inbreeding isn't a real problem unless the group shrinks to 50 individuals or less.

Once driven away by a rival male, the genetic vigor of young juveniles does not die down. Fired with a seasonal extra dose of male hormones they opportunistically foster ahead; where the chance of their acceptance would herald the genetic diversity lacking in most of our tiger areas. There may be a minuscule population of only one to two breeding tigresses, fated to extinction — by any rational extrapolative model — that may get a chance to recover by this courting and proliferate. I may add that the metapopulation paradigm is relevant to conservation, though metapopulations might not be common in nature, and that is why, empirical parameterization within the metapopulation paradigm is usually infeasible.

However, the possible model of a working tiger population normally based on studies in well–protected tiger habitats where human interference is negligible, cannot be established in sugar zones. Paul Errington, a biologist, calls this population of transient tigers as 'doomed surplus' that is bound to perish every year. Whereas in the jungles the reasons for death may be shortage of space and prey, territorial tensions and potentially dangerous clashes with resident tigers, the reasons in farmlands are largely due to man-tiger conflict where several kinds if pit traps, native contraptions, poisoning of kills and firearms pose danger for them. Thus, major disincentive to further immigration is ostensibly the human presence. Such tigers are liable to involuntarily interact more and more with human life-style. Their encounters with humans become more frequent and decisively tilt the balance against the tiger.

Recorded strays of sugar tigers

In the last thirty years, the state of Uttar Pradesh witnessed more than forty strays of sugarcane tigers into towns and cities, most of which took place only in winters. All through minor strays, the tigers covered up to 50 kilometers in farmlands but later returned to jungle edges or to their natal places in sugarcanes. The major cases in which tigers covered over 100 kilometers include the districts of Hardoi, Sitapur, Barabanki, Bahraich, Shahjahanpur, Shravasti, Balrampur, Gonda, Sultanpur and Ambedkar Nagar. Here the 'transient floaters' were found in secondary type of habitats, trying to share space with man. Lucknow district also witnessed the appearance of four tigers respectively in the years 1969, 1979 and 1989 and 2009. The first three beasts occupied the poor jungle of Kukrail picnic spot, a third grade sub-optimal track from a tiger's point of view and provided some thrill to the city dwellers at the cost of their lives.

The last animal was a tigress who achieved a high level of publicity. In November 2008, she strayed out of Pilibhit forests, traveled alongside the river through the scrub and grass providing ideal cover, and then through Shahjahanpur, Kheri,

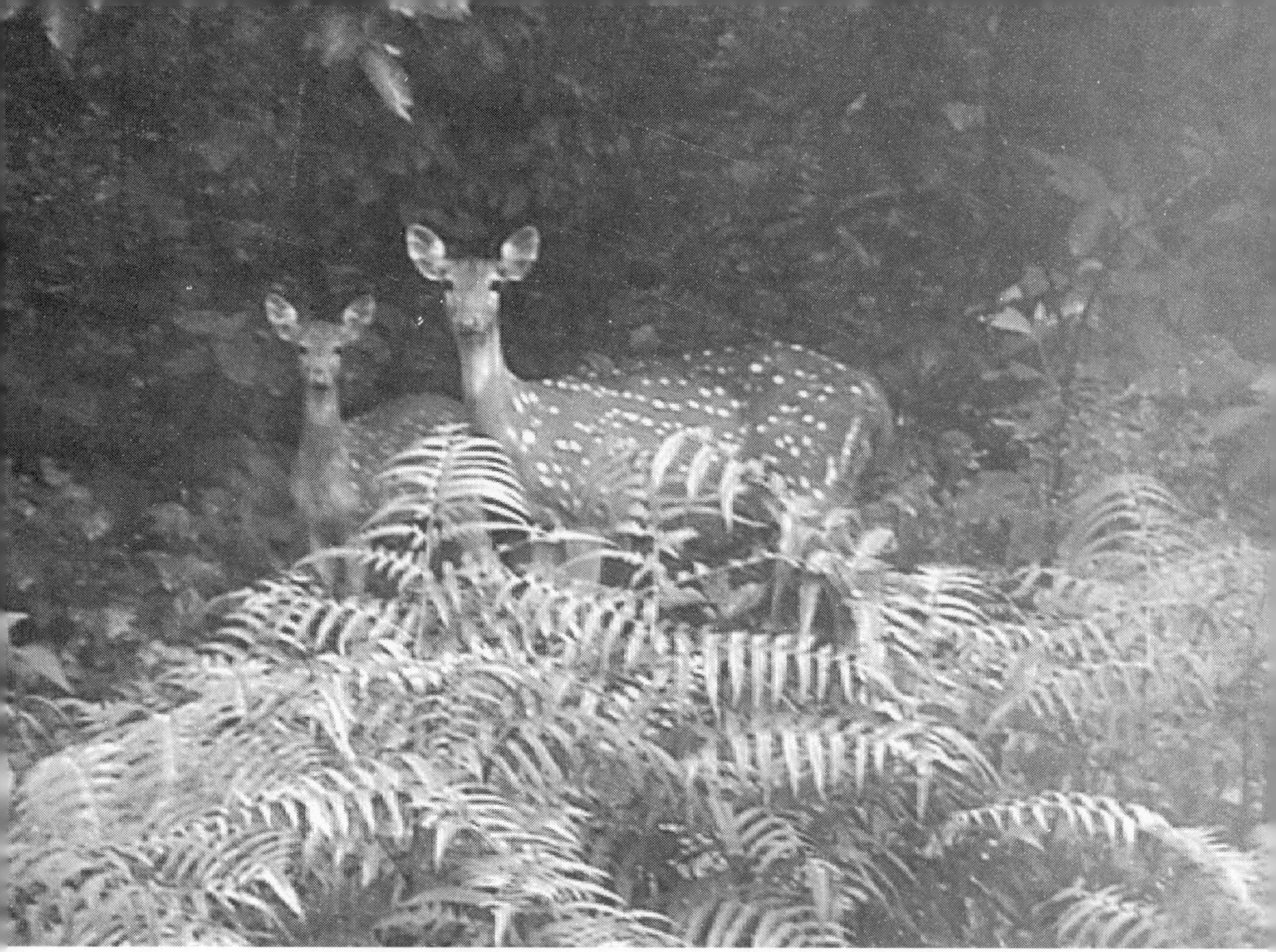

Spotted deer looking at the photographer

Sitapur, Lucknow and Barabanki reached Faizabad district. It covered more than 500 kilometers in five months and often moved at an average rate of 10 to 12 kilometers in the night, in which she seldom searched for prey or lay intermittently still as the tigers usually do in the jungle. Amazingly forest department identified her as a male. Despite the fact that she was seen nearly a hundred times at close quarters and thousands of her pugmarks were identified, the forest department submitted an affidavit that she was a young male.

Her extraordinary journey became a litmus test for the forest department. The case revealed that the department suffers from an acute lack of infrastructure, expertise and proper team leadership. This exposure also implied that on the performance curve they are nearer the bottom with most of their representatives appearing not to know their job well. The entire drama of capturing the animal alive went on for months. Circumstantial evidence suggested that the tigress was not a man-eater, though she was definitely guilty of injuring three men that died later but she had never fed on any of them. Perhaps under the pressure of media that was constantly questioning the competence of forest managers, the final orders for her elimination were issued in March 2009, and she was shot dead in Faizabad district.

Besides this unfortunate animal, as many as five more tigers were recorded to have strayed out in U.P between November 2008 and March 2009. One man-eater operating in sugarcanes of Kanp-Tanda in Kheri was later captured for the Lucknow Zoo. Two tigers took a vacation of three months to Sitapur district after which they went back on their own to Nanpara tehsil near Katarnia Ghat. One juvenile was reported from Ambedkar Nagar and another from Azamgarh district, both of these were supposed to have strayed out from Palamau National Park in Bihar.

Straying is abnormal behaviour. We have already seen that sexual restlessness in juveniles is one of the causes that triggers their long journeys which often result in straying. However "PSI (pressure per square inch) trailings" a term that Dr. Joseph Rhine of Duke University coined to refer to animal's psychic capacity of homing in, attempts to explain a cat's ability to travel a long distance to return to their home again. One theory to explain this ability is that felines have sensitivity to the earth's magnetic field. It is said that in the Time-Space Continuum they use the earth's gravity to determine "their place" in the world. Old cats are able to perform better, perhaps because as they age, more mettle is deposited in their brain to develop the ability to return "home" when necessary. This suggests that wandering off could very well be the result of human chase, forcing tigers to act against their grain.

Next to it is an interesting theory of the fog phenomenon. In winters, it seems to contribute as a critical determinant to tiger movements, and there is a definite correlation between the two. In the Tarai, two types of fog occur that are dubbed as Tule and Radiation fog. Both are formed by the cooling of land after sunset by thermal radiation. In perfect calm conditions, the fog layer can be less than a meter deep but turbulence can promote a thicker layer.

Siberian tigers have many adaptations to make them perfectly suited to hard winter conditions, but peninsular tigers being separated in time and space have little of that strain left in them. During December and January, the Tarai sky is generally covered by low stratus and stratocumulus clouds. This fog occasionally produces precipitation in the form of drizzle, when the humidity attains 100% and the minute cloud droplets begin to coalesce into larger droplets. Consequently, the cover of these clouds, overflowing with fog and haze on the ground, often becomes so extensive that it persists for a week or more, and reduces the visibility to only few meters.

A cat's world is three-dimensional. It includes anthills and tree branches and because mobility amongst tigers is an ever-changing phenomenon their world is largely mapped by smells which represent territorial boundaries or signposts. In case of human dominated landscape, agricultural implements left lying around, abandoned huts, trees, orchids, electric poles, tube wells, wayside hand pumps, small temples and other human interventions mark their regular route which they mark in their unique way. (In Deep Nagar and Barsola area, a tigress that patrolled its territory in the night, often used to spray mark the walls of a basic school and a dispensary at the outskirts of the villages. She did this for three consecutive winters and later even started marking a PCO that had sprung up on its beat). In case of any change in these signposts – such as a tree cut down, implements removed or huts demolished — confusion reigns in the tiger's mind in relation to predation and intra-specific sharing of the habitat.

Like most felids, tigers sustain a spatially and temporally dispersed social system, where adults essentially communicate. As cloudiness increases, they often suffer the loss of communication with their social organization and lose their way. Failing to differentiate between terrains, they go vagabonding in unknown directions, cross wide belts of agriculture and break out in unfamiliar countries. Such strays essentially occur in winters because a lower temperature and plentiful water helps the dispersal of prey species, which they follow. Such cases are from the midst of those whose social structure is disrupted and which live at correspondingly low level of interaction with other tigers. Stanly Breeden estimates that, it was most likely such transients that swelled the bags of last century hunters rather than the real forest dwellers.

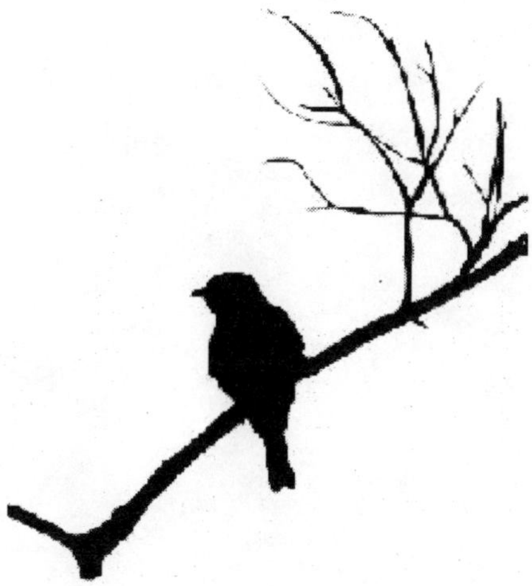

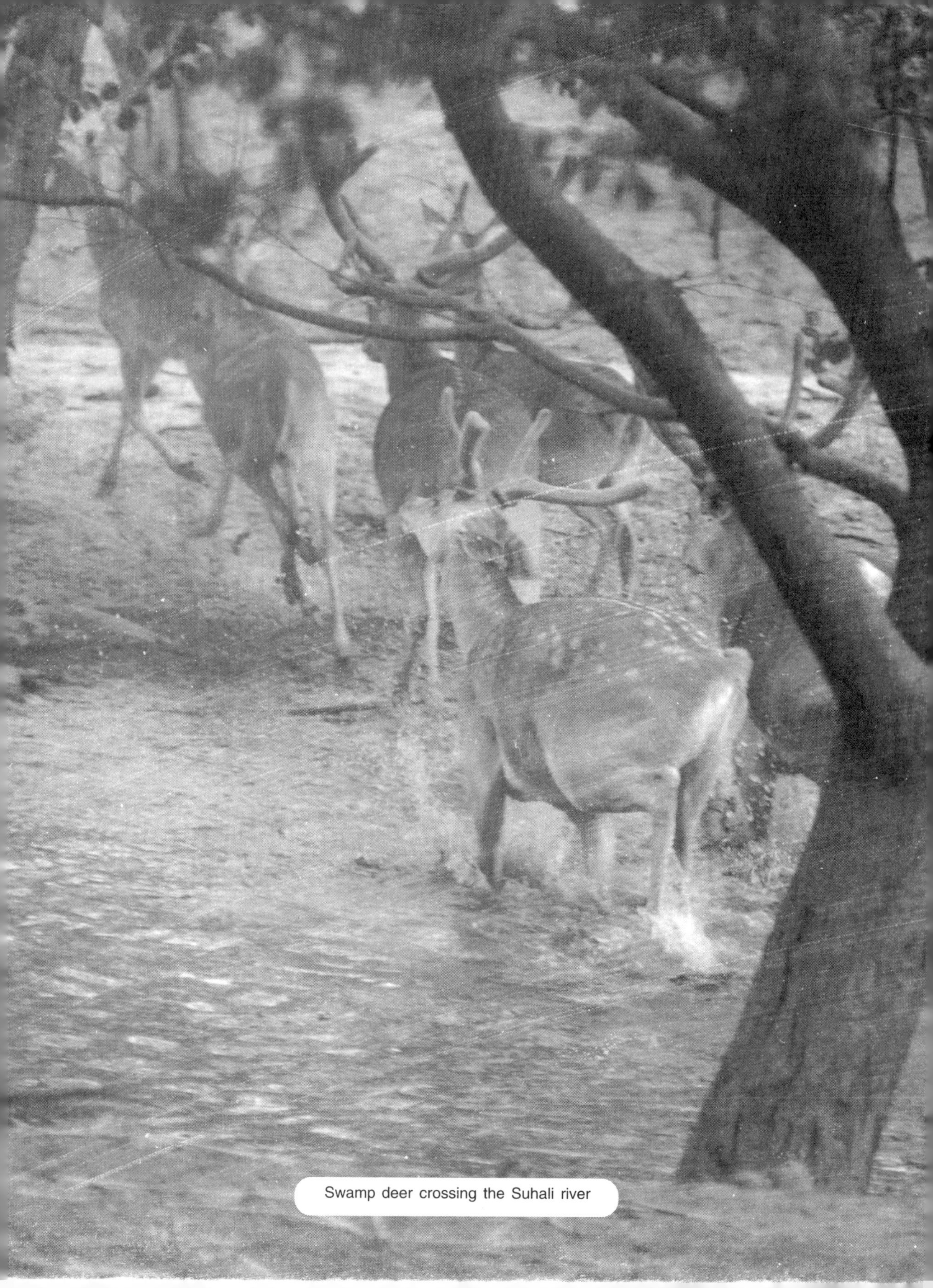

Swamp deer crossing the Suhali river

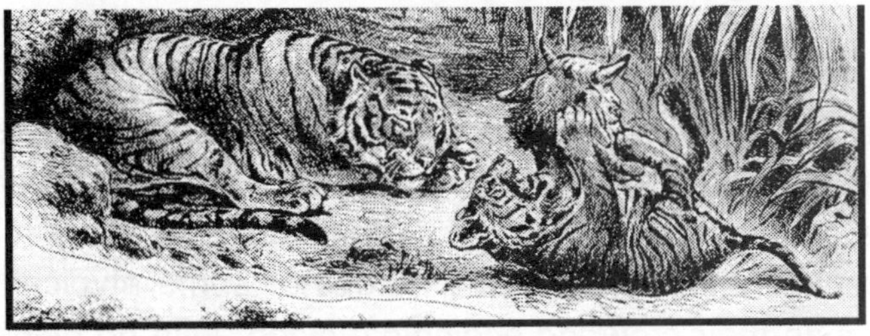

20

The Branding of Sugarcane Tiger

"A cat is a puzzle for which there is no solution."

- Hazel Nicholson

The immensity of sugarcane farms covering the Tarai needs to be seen to be believed. Stretching unabated for miles and miles on thousands of acres with death like stillness, the exuberant crops present a picturesque feature of wild and savage grandeur.

The view is eminently characteristic of an endless savannah. The appeal of the scenery varies from the distances; it is both historic and romantic, but always impressive even to the appeal of fascination. It is a luxuriant forest of grasslands, and a kind of canopied and monotonous ecosystem, which not only offers a strong larder and water to a range of indigenous wild species but also serves as a prosperous eco-tone zone (the area of integration between woodland and grassland) because of its propinquity to prime jungles.

Tarai farmlands cover approximately one quarter of Uttar Pradesh state's land mass and have historically provided a wide range of habitats for all the 'chota-shikar' -the standard wildlife, described in colonial memoires, comprising ungulate species like chital, Blackbuck and pig that breed outrageously large families and compete increasingly for with human beings for livelihood. These sugarcane farms, merging into jungles have long afforded perennial delight for the breeding of 'chota-shikar' and also offered ideal conditions as selective holding ground for the migrant big cats -which being unable to settle down in jungle because favorable niches are already occupied by residents- take to opportunistic lifestyle.

Thus while contemplating the problem of master predators in sugarcane that coexist with human competitors, we have to conceptualize it in its totality and discuss it from two principal prospective; historical and contextual. From natural history point of view the problem revolves round one fundamental question, is it a chance based non-systemic phenomenon or a systematic development based or matter specific phenomenon such as behavioral adaptableness of tigers to seasonal crops?

A rational approach to this puzzle would compel one to acquiesce that it was actually human expansion in forest areas that led to the foundation of farm tigers. Back in evolutionary course of natural history, when the tiger population reached the pinnacle of its territorial advancement and spilled out of the forest, their spread was controlled by human presence. The anthropogenic pressure, rendering their future both destructive and infructuous, must have naturally forced the core component to return to the forest, but all together some atypical scrawniness's preferring to change their crowded ecological niche -with no holds barred- must have taken to agrarian expansion. An important cause for this development must have been to avoid competition for using common food resources. Small wonder, this is a syndrome from which most of the tiger population that frequents the farmlands of Tarai suffers though it adds to their vulnerability. The challenge of living in human dominated landscape helped these tigers to ameliorate their skills and modify their hunting techniques in order to make best of the conditions; whether it was for camouflage or for attack and defense. In addition, local forests, presence of farmland wildlife and comfortable land use pattern with crops, such as maze and sugarcane naturally supported them to stay longer in farmlands.

It is a known fact that within a short time all populations of one species separated in specific spaces tend to become distinct 'eco-types'. So there was no denial to the fact that it is heritably an altered tiger, the plodding progression of which remained undiscovered for long so that very little was known about them.

Taking the history of Tarai into consideration, it is certain that farm tigers are the beasts of yore and sugarcane tigers that come down from the same lineage are perhaps at least a century old recorded beasts. They are a representative reminder of history's tangled webs, of the many strange ways in which the fates of people and wild animals intersect and what happens when man interferes with nature.

Large sugar farms created ecological opportunities for tigers to expand their ranges. Through eons of time, their ancestors had left their essential and stable jungles and intruded into human zones, adopting unstable farms in the beginning as their night-time home. These cliquey beasts were the ones who had never accepted barriers of buffer zones between jungles and human habitat and habitually violated their ecosystems. They had actively occupied farms under the demands of their own escalating population and by the same token aggravated by selected and enforced biological requirements, developed a penchant for a different prey composition because the farmlands essentially carry a separate biomass from the jungles. This behavioral adaptation to sugar-farms, led by a perplexing dilemma of circumstances, heralded an absolutely original chapter in the history of nature. Thus history is trapped in these tigers, and, they are as much trapped in history.

Here I must clarify that we should accept all the natural explanations (physical, biological, environmental, geographical and ecological) before we fall back upon such a theory as sugarcane tigers. I was endeavoring to trace these beasts to their source, in order to find if there was something peculiar which may account for their remarkable fate. Thus before I proceeded further with my survey, I had to rationalize as what I genuinely knew about these tigers, and make most of it to separate the essential from accidental.

My conjecture of a possible putative strain endorsed that natural selection does not create anything new; it only selects from the accessible genetic information. (It is the theory of the 'survival of the fittest' and not the 'arrival of the fittest'). With this judicious prudence in mind, the existence of sugarcane tiger appears no mystery. Evolution has done this in centuries. It is the old undiscovered imprecise natural history, viewed through skeptical eyes as new natural history. These tigers are the compelling evidence of their former continuity -- the progenies of genetic aberrations of positive 'eco-types' -- whose gamble to change their habitat proved to be of advantage to them and consequently their life style was hereditarily altered. They had been using the farm ranges, adapting to ever altering crop dynamics and land use change for hundreds of years, and that their numbers with minor variations had never multiplied to such an extent that they could seriously interfere with the environment. Their potential was only realized when sugarcane took over as a major crop in the Tarai, that their slender population suddenly swelled and became detectable.

Books written in colonial times by anthropologists, travel writers, missionaries and officials, invariably feature some reference to this tiger while natural history accounts of these animals are relatively poorly served in hunting literature. Old Persian memoirs of Avadh Court portray as how Nawab Siraj-ud-Daulah mowed down quite a few of these beasts on the outskirts of Lucknow city. The first modern record of farmland tigers dates back to a Victorian Englishman, Surgeon Daniel Johnson of East India Company, who published *Indian Field Sports* in 1823. He describes random instances of tigers -that flourished in sugar farms- and were shot by Nawab Vazir of Oudh between Lucknow and Sitapur.

In early nineteenth century they could be seen during the day on the roads just outside Calcutta, and sir John Hewett, a former governor general of United Provinces, recorded that the town of Gorakhpur, on the Indo-Nepalese border, had to be protected from their depredations by a line of fires kept alive all night.

Billy Arjan Singh also mentions about such local beasts. In his book *Tiger! Tiger!* he observes -- "the shooting in the forest was allocated by a system of ballot... to circumvent this restriction, one unsavory pair of sportsmen took to going after farm tigers, on which there was then no limit. After they had shot a few...the chief wildlife warden worked up a case against them.... although it failed but had the salutary effect of putting an end to that particular form of shooting and gave the local tigers a respite." The word local naturally refers to the tigers living outside the jungle.

It is reasonable to presume that a teensy genetic component coming down the ancestral line had made a selected group of tigers adopt sugarcanes as their basic home. It was neither deviation from the basics for them, nor any evolutionary stake to have put most of their bets on the abundance of a particular habitat of sugar crop. Once, on an online conversation with me, John Aspinall, a British conservationist addressed these tigers as 'ecological freaks'. It may sound uncharitable, but it may be true. Adaptations usually occur because a gene mutates or changes by accident! Some mutations can help an animal survive better than others from among the same species sans mutation. Hardcore sugar tigers might as well be 'ecological freaks' for such "freaks" like genetic freaks do not evolve according to the age-old laws of nature. They evolve abruptly and revolutionarily. It is something like dexterity in human beings, where left-handed people are not considered normal only in the sense that there are more right-handed people in the world.

The conservation of sugarcane tigers is indubitably a formidable business. Confusions are too many and convolutions need be tackled on large-scale imaginations. Eventually of course, every conservation venture is an experiment, even if it is an experiment conducted in much more complex and multifaceted laboratory environment that what scientists usually inhabit. Experience shows that conservationists would have to avoid a general reductionist approach and simplistic

A man mauler tigress trapped in Tikoniya sugarcane fields in nets (lying inside the cage)

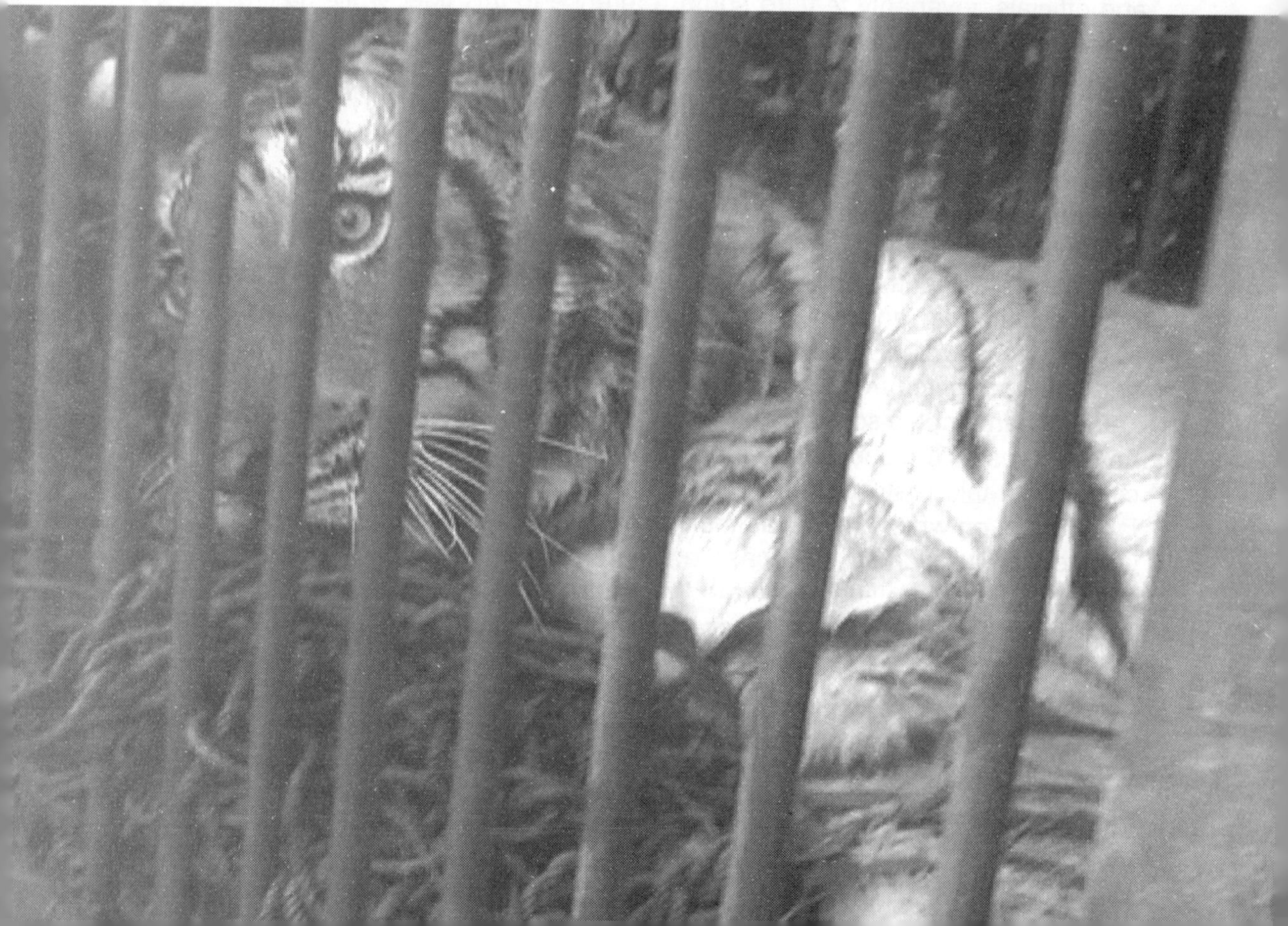

responses to the challenges of conservation. It is a time to embrace complexities by forgetting old line of reasoning and learning from past mistakes.

It is argued that sugarcanes are potentially dangerous innovation for it makes tigers too tolerant of human presence and increases chances of clashes between two species. Unfortunately, tigers don't understand the laws of man. On one hand they are punished for not abiding with the diktat of the master race, which at first itself dishonored all the laws of nature and then created its own laws to control it. On the other hand, human populations around tiger reserves are at much higher densities and these alpha killers too have not progressed to the top of food chain to turn vegetarian; they will eat anything they can catch so the clash is an inevitable consequence.

By 1990, it was for the last time that a steady population of tigers was registered throughout the sugar belt of Tarai. Their regular presence was noticed in many areas but as a most frustrating aspect of conservation any reliable data about them was not available with the forest department, except for G.C. Mishra's personal catalogue which recorded a ballpark estimate of over thirty tigers in the sugar fields of Kheri. It was a considerable number; a numeric indicator that enables researchers to track trends. The evidence was prepared through round-the-year polling of all spatial-temporal evidences, ensuring the sanctity of individual space for a tiger. I was sure that the juggernaut of this phenomenon was radically affecting the way in which the full-scale tiger protection programme was being perused inside the reserves and in which the majority of these tigers were not included.

My observations in farmlands of Dudhwa circle proved that tigers could live amongst high densities of people as low levels of conflict and the resident prey base could conceivably sustain them. However, on my part, I was never satisfied with the eyewitness account of villagers of merely seeing these tigers, until I had myself accounted for their presence and accumulated a good deal of information about them. This included their probable range, their favorite beats, prey choice whether wild or domestic, whether their wild prey was not stolen by villagers, the span of stay in the crop, details of their past activities if available, and in case of a tigress the number of its cubs. From these points the population trends of tigers could be worked out. If some estimates about their age and sex ratio, fecundity, mortality rates and population densities could be noted then some indication of the true status of tigers in the canes could be established.

I also studied the pattern of human casualties, time of operation of man-killers, their vast operational zone, areas of maximum human casualties, age of the victims and the percentage of primary and secondary prey base available in the canes.

Interestingly no humans traveling on some vehicle or even a bicycle were ever attacked by tigers. Only those who were walking or squatting were targeted. A large number of records showed that tigers usually took on humans who were in a crouching or sitting position, presumably mistaking them for quadrupeds. Such cases formed about 50% of human casualty figures. This knowledge later helped the forest staff and me to reduce human casualties from tigers by more than fifty percent.

To my mind the cane tigers displayed every characteristic of grass tigers. Their hunting behaviour was also typical of their kens inhabiting tall and dense grasslands and this habitat formation definitely had some relation to their man-eating propensities. Owing to the density of cane, the visibility inside the crop is almost zero. Neither can the tigers see properly nor can they be seen until the intruder almost bumps into them. These attacks were definitely made in error of man being mistaken for legitimate prey, since most victims were left uneaten. Even so this was dangerous as these chance killings were helping them overcome the reluctance to attack humans.

There were many instances in which the apparent victim had resisted and somehow fought for his life and the tiger had abandoned his attack and fled. The behavioral patterns of animals clearly indicated the embryonic stage of a new ecological relationship which demonstrated the changing adaptive cycles and bio-ecological traits of these tigers. For example, whereas in case of tigresses the aggression could be attributed to their maternal protectiveness, the males were

Poachers bag caught by SSP, STF Rajiv Ranjan Verma

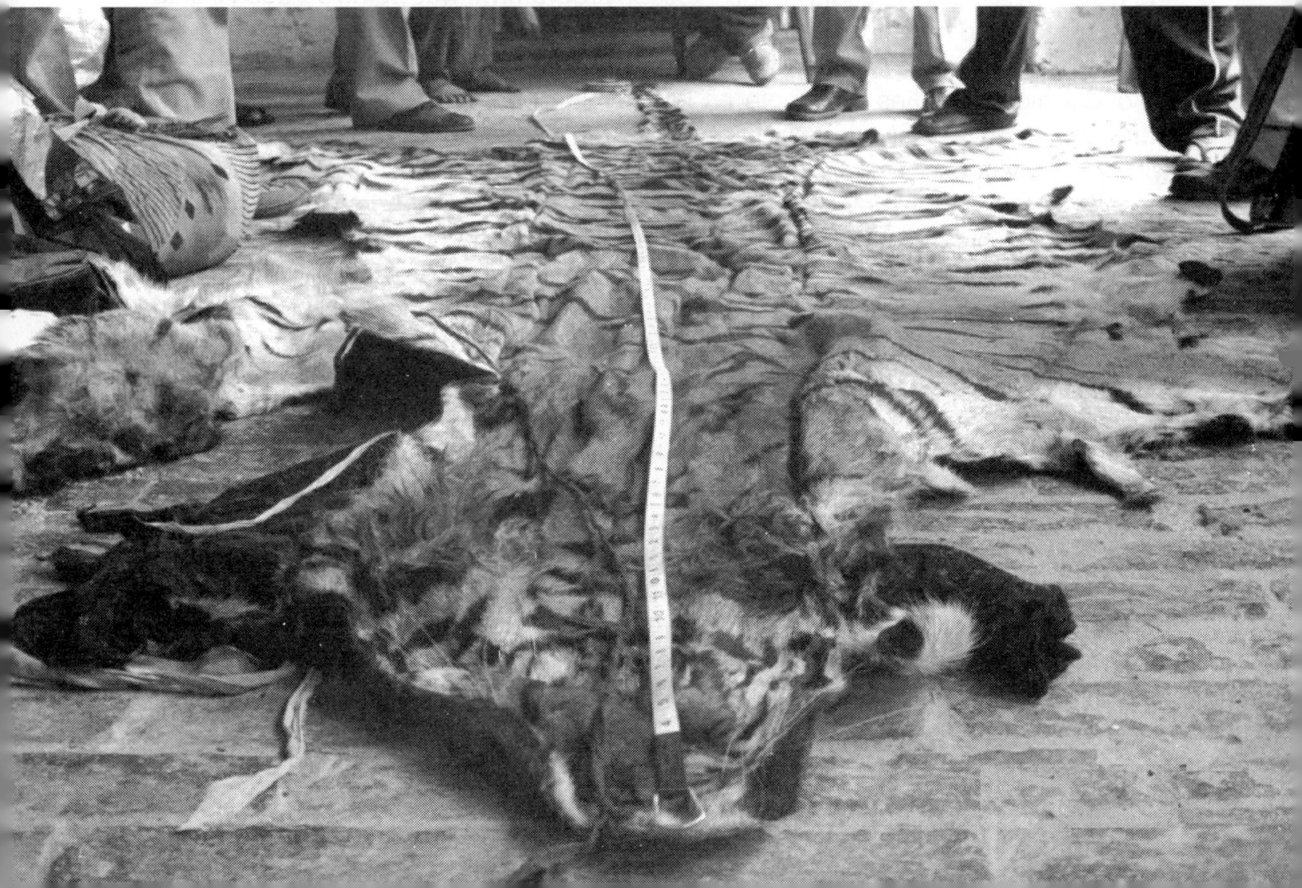

just reacting bitter about the erosion of their habitat. Such cases formed about 30% of human casualty figures.

Since there is no mechanism to achieve a proper separation between tigers and the villagers, most of the deaths result from accidental confrontation. But there had also emerged a fraction of tigers that appeared to hunt down humans opportunistically, just as they would hunt a cow, pig or a chital in the forest. Perhaps a small portion of big cats had acknowledged humans as a part of their food-chain for they were moving among them as their normal prey.

Such pressures of farmlands could induce more and more tigers to include human beings amongst their regular prey species and had even converted some individuals into habitual man-eaters.

I interviewed more than two hundred people, collected primary data through a structured questionnaire and recorded as many stories that gave an eloquent testimony of man-tiger interactions. Some sounded most exaggerated and unlikely. Finally when I sat down to write them, I looked for Om Bir's approval about their veracity.

"It appears that some of them are fictitious," I said, a little doubtful.

"No, they are quite true, because they have their basis in facts. Tigers can do anything; and anything can happen when tigers are around," he said in a tone of protest; his eyes gleaming bright with pride as if he owned Tarai.

The land-use change had evidently not only benefited the tiger but had also paved way to create an embryonic, incipient community of species for which the selective advantages of living in the sugarcane were much greater than the disadvantages. The most relevant aspect of their predation covers an exposure to the entire new world of submissive farm animals, along with the ability to move from food source to food source without being perceived and finally an escape away from danger with an equal ease. It was incredible to understand how marvelously the species had agreed itself to the antipodal change of its ecosystem into which their tribe is auto-genetically integrated.

The law of ultimate function tells that those organisms that are better adapted to life in their surroundings produce more young, bearing the very characteristics which gave their parents a survival edge. Thus the judge in the lottery of breeding and survival of this tiger was eventually and finally, the sugarcane environment.

On the basis of my experience in the field, I finally classified these tigers in three categories-

(1) The ones that come and go back;
(2) Those that have predilection to live in canes;
(3) And finally those that are here for more than a generation.

In the study of behavior, experts talk about nature versus nurture, meaning which behaviors are inbred (or instinct) and which are learned. It's an argument that will probably never be completely settled. Most experts, however agree that animals like cats have both kinds of behavior; some are predisposed ("prepared") to learn certain types of associations, and some are also predisposed not to learn at all ("contra-prepared"), Keping this in mind, I further classified these tigers into two more categories; the 'oriented' and the 'disoriented' ones.

It was the oriented ones that seemed to know the nuances of land. They knew that the humans are the worst predators, who use tools to exploit their environments. They knew that they use snares, clubs, spears, fishing gear, firearms to boats and motor vehicles. They knew that it is this agency which annually reshapes the huge expanses of their sugarcane world with different crop patterns and raises livestock, poultry, and fish to be eaten as meat. They even knew that humans use other predatory species, such as dogs in hunting and some people even enlist non-predatory beasts, like horses, oxen and elephants in getting approaches to prey. Thus these tigers hardly turned to livestock because it drew reprisals from people who then snared, shot and poisoned them and even burnt down their coverts to drive them out and kill them.

It was this oriented stuff, which navigated smoothly without impudence and without being registered much. I was sure that these tigers even changed the spatial and temporal use of landscape to avoid conflict with people whilst the disoriented ones -unfamiliar with the fine distinctions of habitat- such the complex mosaic of various crop fields, patches of grasslands and local forests and households dispersed across the landscape, generated chaos and failed to manipulate their behavioural traits. I may add that the behaviour of an animal is controlled by the endocrine and nervous system, hence it is affected by the environment the animal inhabits. Unstable environments repeatedly restrict wild animals from performing some species specific behaviours, which often manifest in abnormal behaviours usually termed as aberrations. Such tigers confronted village communities and even made the life of their innocent kens unduly difficult.

In Neurobiology and Darwinism, the former behaviour is described as instinctive urge for modification, which is purposeful and not random, because it helps survival to the hilt. I have already argued earlier that survival of the fittest is often misinterpreted to mean survival of the most aggressive; in fact fitness is a much broader term. Thus the very class of tigers that lived in the canes without any ruckus could be neatly compartmentalized as a true sugarcane tiger.

It is a truth that all populations of one species separated in habitat often just by a few miles, tend to become distinct 'ecotypes' or different strain of one species. These tigers were the classic example of this occurrence for they were behaviorally glued to this habitat for years. Away from the optimum jungles, sugar farms were their best home turfs. It was no mystery as to why they were using the territory of farm lands, asserting their dominance placidly, remarkably and quietly.

There was a tingling in my blood stream. I felt filled with the passion of an alchemist; the possessor of enigmatic facts; who had stealthily stalked these tigers and explored all the major dimensions about their habits and behavior and possibly also gathered every single biological explanations for their preference to this habitat. I felt comforted in the reflection of years, that whatever I had noticed about these tigers was an exceptional pack of knowledge, indeed 'only one of its kind'; so eventually, I branded them as sugarcane-tigers. This mint-fresh nomenclature first entered the conservation lexicon through my book *'Killing Grounds'* published in 1993.

Here I may add that speciation is a gradual process of divergence, until not only the form and behaviour differ, but the very structure of the genes often changes too far to allow a successful recombination. Though it was too early to say that any of the sugarcane tigers could pass the test of true speciation but one thing was certain that some of them were 'genetically and behaviorally compromised' and that the embryonic stage of a new strain had been achieved.

It is an irony that only a jungle tiger is considered a wild tiger in absolute terms of occupying a varied and complex biotype. When this regal animal takes residence in sugarcane plantations then its adaptability is not appreciated. Rather, the animal suddenly loses its honor and dignity and is taken akin an underdog, harassed and beaten, symbolizing the convoluted response of ecosystem against human surfeit. This prejudice has potentially closed our minds to other important aspects of the tiger's life. We must take a broader view. Our understanding and therefore our appreciation, of as what the tigers' do to stay alive in the world of sugarcane grass would make us look at its objects and events in their ecological prospective. Every ecosystem, howsoever haphazard collection of objects and events it may appear, has its own characteristics and as ecology is the science, which deals with the relationship between living organisms and their environment, the basic answer, which is really quite simple is not far off. This eternal phenomenon indeed explains as how some tigers adopt cane to aid their survival as a corollary to the axiom of survival of the fittest.

John Seidensticker, an ecologist of USA, identifies the key to changing human attitudes as 'making a living tiger worth more than a dead one to people.' This new *Gita* was more needed for the people of Project Tiger than the community villages falling abutting sugar fields. We have to look for an ecological rational of this tiger. A bold acceptance of facts is required and bolder imaginative steps to tackle it.

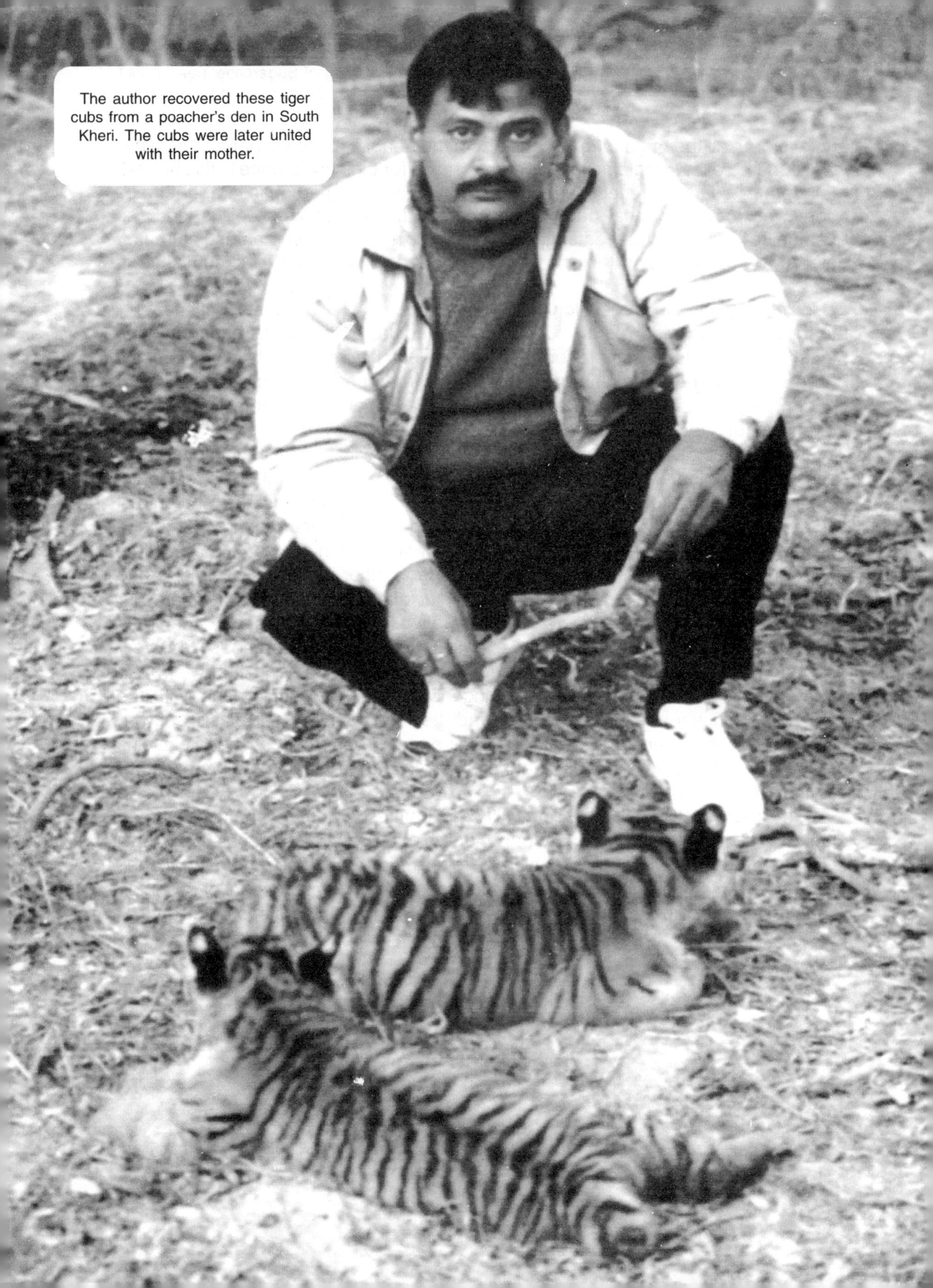

The author recovered these tiger cubs from a poacher's den in South Kheri. The cubs were later united with their mother.

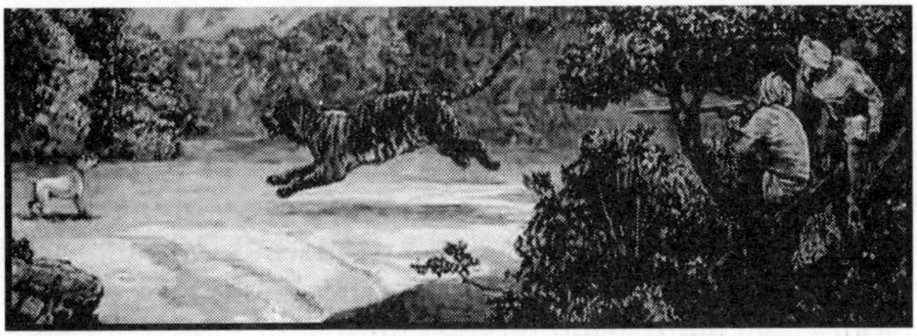

21

The Tiger Guardians

"Is not the intelligent preservation of game one of the most prominent signs of advancing civilizations?"

Robert Eliot 1834

With a plodding on beaten track for 30 years, it was evident that the Project Tiger was at cross-roads. Despite its solid foundation, its officers and advisers had very little say on the development policies of the government. Perhaps they had underpinned the efforts of Indian foresters in nurturing the project initiative. Even the World Bank had begun to influence as to what should and should not be done in the Project areas. Their growing perception that the tigers were being given higher priority than people had helped to create an on-going backlash against tigers that was very hard to counter.

Towards the end of last millennium the phenomenon of cane tiger was on the verge of decline. The man-tiger conflict and the outside influences impinged on wildlife had jeopardized the future of tigers in general and sugar-tigers in particular. I was worried that a great national asset was wasting away as the later were active in far-off lands, much outside the bounds of reserve, where being completely unguarded by foresters, they were vulnerable to poachers.

On April 15, 1997 I was talking to a group of villagers at Chaltua near Kishanpur Sanctuary, when I saw vultures alighting from the sky. A quick check revealed the carcass of a cow and lying dead close to it was a sub-adult tiger cub. There was no external injury on its body. I called the forest rangers Rajendra Prasad Saxena and Shyam Kishore on wireless line to collect the evidences and send the body away to the headquarters. It was a clear-cut case of insecticide poisoning but the autopsy revealed that the cervical vertebrae had been broken. Two days later I read an official statement of the Chief Wildlife Warden in a local newspaper that in the night two tigers had fought fiercely over a kill and the smaller female had killed the bigger male.

Fatal interactions amongst tigers do occur. In the *zamindari* forests of Larti, I had seen quite a few sites of encounters amongst tigers. Such places are essentially churned by unsheathed claws. A lot of hair is usually found where tigers have rolled in mortal combat. Blood smears, excreta and crushed undergrowth over a large area indicates struggle. Bites on hind and fore legs on are also common results of such fights. I remembered that there were no such signs at that place or on body. Yet the officers believed that the fight had taken place. I doubted if the autopsy reports were also being managed?

Kalupurva is a nondescript village at the eastern boundary of Dudhwa. On October 15, 1997 a bird trapper was killed by a tigress with three sub-adult cubs. They dragged the kill into a sugarcane field and devoured it there. A few days later a buffalo and four cows were killed by the same tiger family but no compensation was paid to the owner of cattle and dissatisfaction continued to simmer. On the eve of New Year, a village trader going on his cycle saw a tigress walking up the road which fell down unconscious. The trader raised an alarm and soon the news reached the wildlife guards. On January 1, 1998 the foresters discovered to their distress that not only the tigress but her three cubs had also died of poisoning.

I had known the particular beast for the last three years. She was a downright cane tigress for even in the mating season she was rarely known to go into the jungle close-by; on the contrary, the male tigers came out seeking her company in the cultivated haunts.

In my official capacity as Honorary Wildlife Warden, I was then camping at Indo-Nepalese border on the banks of Gaurva River, having fracas with a well armed gang of poachers from Nepal, when through a wireless link I received a call from the Forest Secretary, Dr. P.L. Punia to reach Dudhwa and take an appraisal of the whole story. I reached Kalupurva in the very evening. The news of tiger family's death had already spread like wild fire; the dusky forms of tens of natives thronged the vista. There was a queer poignancy in the atmosphere. The scene was glum and the foresters were silent. Hovering black clouds flickered in the sky, as the four grotesque figures of elephants lumbered silhouetted in the field of carnage. They looked like sinister monsters suddenly conjured out of the fog in a primeval landscape. The routine investigation was in progress and the formality of official statistics was being meticulously worked out to put the last touches on the government files.

All the recovered carcasses had been collected at a place. It was indeed a deplorable spectacle. A low cloud had thrown the vista into a deep shadow and in the gathering gloom of a foggy new year evening; the ill-fated spot looked even more gloomy. W. Longwa, the deputy director of Dudhwa and I walked the flat cinder covered surface of a dry Nala and watched the dead bodies of those three half grown tiger cubs and their mother. Lying on her side, with her paws together, and eyes half closed, the tigress still reflected a wild beauty and looked as if half asleep. Her cubs looked the same; very imposing and majestic even in their eternal slumber.

As a sportsman -if I may so dub myself- I had witnessed some disgusting manners of licensed butchers and their flagrant infringement of existing game laws but had truly never come across anything as revolting as this. I had no doubt that this was the tigress I had known before. I could only deeply regret the suffering that human wrath had inflected on the animals, I felt too aware of the terrible murderous hatred rising in my thoughts towards my own race. Stronger than anything was the feeling of helplessness that arose from the knowledge that now natural death for a sugarcane tiger is very rare.

Moments later a lugubrious fox yapped irritably at the sky. The long drawn, wailing notes of that most haunting of tunes came faintly from a distance, as if nodding in my approval, "oh yes, oh yes, oh yes"! It seemed to make a most striking and solemn ending to a very terrible tragedy of real life.

Things were yet not normal. On January 24 the same year, four more full-grown tigers were found dead at the outskirts of Corbett Park, one of them was riddled with lead and then on January 30, a tigress was killed near Santokhpur village in Nainital district. The death of nine tigers within one month was not motivated by any organized poaching gang but by agitated farmers whose domestic stock had been preyed upon by tigers; and who had been denied legitimate compensation by the forest department due to sluggish and tardy procedures. It was a disgraceful story in wildlife conservation. It was tragic for the tiger whose life went on so carelessly in sugarcanes and usually ended so cheaply and tragic for me that the battle which I had fought for over twenty years to save them seemed ending into a poor, regretful defeat.

Tigers are vulnerable because they do not cast a vote in a democratic nation and doing them good also does not win any vote either. They have no jurisprudence to support their claim to existence against the trauma of competition with man. Human ego goads a person to dabble in feats of vandalism to prove his mettle. Even if a single tiger is killed, it has far greater impact on their population. It changes the entire equation of the tiger demography in the area and affects the pattern of their movements. For example if a male is eliminated, his females are orphaned and then another male who is holding a different range would step into the scene. He might very well be courting two to three females, yet he would add the left-out females into his list and extend his range. He would first kill their cubs to bring them into season and then court. The consequence would be the death of many.

Over 95% of the farmers that I interviewed during a survey indicated that they had no idea of the problems facing the tigers' survival, or how important the sugarcane tiger population was to the species' survival. Therefore, it was imperative to re-evaluate and measure the entire gamut of man-tiger relationship in farmlands and put it into a proper prospective to cogitate about the immediate future of this animal.

Alarmed by the disheartening affair, the Governor of Uttar Pradesh Romesh Bhandari convened a meeting of tiger protection cell on February 10, 1998 at Lucknow' Raj Bhawan. It was largely a meeting of bureaucrats, where Billy Arjan Singh and I were the only outsiders. The former was a strange bunch of people with almost negligible understanding of tiger nuances. A director was emphatic that if the tigers were so fond of living in the sugarcane, then they must be provided with the similar "facilities" inside the principal jungles. The suggestion implied of creating considerable oasis of sugarcane plantations within the reserves so that the tigers should be happily contained 'indoors'. The ploy will prevent them from unnecessary 'outdoor-ventures' that risk their safety in human dominated areas and comply with their itch of dwelling in the canes. A railway official was extremely contented with the state's tiger conservation efforts. Only recently at Katarnia Ghat, he said to have seen a "herd" of tigers and many 'batches' of deer from the train.

An IFS officer's observations were so relevant that I was impressed. I heard him with appreciation and pleasure, I even started thinking that after all he has qualified a prestigious examination of India, and such officers should be posted in wildlife sectors. I was all laurels for him till he narrated a personal experience of his father-in-law in a jungle. "He had left his Ambassador car in the jungle to go up to a river site. When he returned he saw his car was all crushed and the engine rendered useless. The driver told him that a python had passed that way. Feeling angry at the car parked in his domain, he coiled round it and strangulated it out of shape."

The impression that man had cast upon me was washed off in an instant. Feeling silly and disillusioned, I wondered as how large misconceptions existed about wildlife and how such really intelligent people behaved so disoriented. They just do not rationalize things. Actually they are in such an awe of wildlife, so prone to exaggeration that they rather turn harebrained when the subject is talked about.

As the meeting proceeded, the report of 1997 tiger census in U.P was presented to the Governor. It showed that there were 71 tigers in the north complex of Dudhwa and 30 in Kishanpur reserve. Since the tiger family of Kalupurva was poisoned on December 31, I asked the Park Director to correct the error in his list and make it 67. To this he announced that Kalupurva tigress was purely of cane variety and the census was conducted only in jungle that did not include the cane fields.

To this I told him candidly that how desperately he had said this to change the facts and how interestingly the facts had come out. This was what I had wanted to prove for long and he had proved it by his own statement that there was a category of 'cane tigers' that needed a different management. And alas, while scientists and foresters have not been able to define the worth of this tiger, poachers understood it purely in economic terms. It was a ripe material to be cherry-picked any time.

Billy Arjan Singh disclosed from his personal knowledge that at present no less than nine tigresses were rearing their seventeen cubs in the cane-fields. It proved that the cane tiger problem by its very nature, explicitly defined the odds and prospects of wildlife conservation in future, and looked to the impending time instead of the past. It was the need of the hour that the conservation project for this tiger must also embrace disciplines scarcely known to the prophets of the past and wilderness in context of this tiger should be redefined.

In ecological sphere, the conflict between desirable extent of habitats for wildlife and undesirable extensions of reclamation for human occupation continues to be a problem. Wilderness is thereby recognized as an area where the earth and its communities of life are untrammeled by man and where man himself is a visitor. But here was a paradox. The commercial crop of sugar is indeed not a wilderness and it was an area where man and his works dominated the landscape. In the terrains of such nature, tigers are particularly disposed to prey on domestic stock and even develop into man-eaters. But since there are no short ways around to tiger conservation, and compatible human actions must matter decisively, hence my views were very specifically stated.

The idea coming to my mind was that once a royal hunting reserve, Chitwan became a national park in 1973. New economic incentives gave villagers a direct stake in this renowned tourist attraction, with more than a third of revenues from park entrance fees being returned to the 300,000 people living in 36 villages in the surrounding buffer zone. As a result, locals were now creating and managing tiger habitat and consider themselves guardians of their tigers similarly the families of landlords and cane farmers around Dudhwa, who had hunted tigers as a sport for centuries, can be assigned a parallel job with a slight modification and be appointed as 'Custodian of tigers'.

"Too good an advice to be ignored" said Romesh Bhandari smiling. P. L. Punia, the then state Forest Secretary, too was of similar opinion that like animals adopted by people in the zoos, cane tigers should also be adopted by farmers. The proposal was approved and 18 tiger guardians were appointed around Dudhwa National Park whose responsibility was to look after the well being of tigers.

Since then this innovative concept is gaining ground. These "guardian farmers," the new entrepreneurs of wildlife conservation, treat the tigers as their adopted children. Seeing the success of this practical context-specific model form the basis of conservation for the farmland wildlife in future- as it can also potentially serve as a powerful tool in refining terrestrial conservation methods which in most cases mandate the complete exclusion of people- the state forestry department has implemented a similar concept in the other reserve forests, not just for tigers but even other animals.

When I came out of the glittering arcades of Raj Bhawan, I felt a lot easier in my mind. It was a poignant moment for me, and a hot feel of victory was flaring in my blood. Although, it was too little and after too hard an input but it seemed that I had turned the wave in favour of tiger; our historic enemy, whose awe-inspiring presence electrifies the atmosphere and produces an apparition of fear; the race against his death had begun and it was to be saved for this century and beyond. That sort of thing seemed like a fairy tale, only very much more exciting. I hoped that I had not started too late.

Next morning, keen to read the arrant story, I excitedly picked up the newspaper. *Hindustan Times* had really done justice to the news. It wrote "It was inevitable that the paths of two strong conservationists, the Honorary Tiger of Dudhwa Billy Arjan Singh and Tiger-Champ Rahul Shukla both dealing in the affairs of Tarai's wildlife would cross sometimes. And cross they did, both publicly and privately; in fact now after this meeting their paths have merged on many conservation issues".

There was yet another paper which made the caricature of the historic meeting; its headlines read, "Cheetah to be protected by farmers'. There was a dynamic photograph of an African Cheetah with a Thomson's gazelle in his mouth, carrying a flashing title *'An Indian Cheetah in the Indian jungle'*. The off-track photograph was from the internet, which the mediocre correspondent had used thinking, that Cheetah and tiger are just two names of the same cat. Such is the paradox of wildlife conservation.

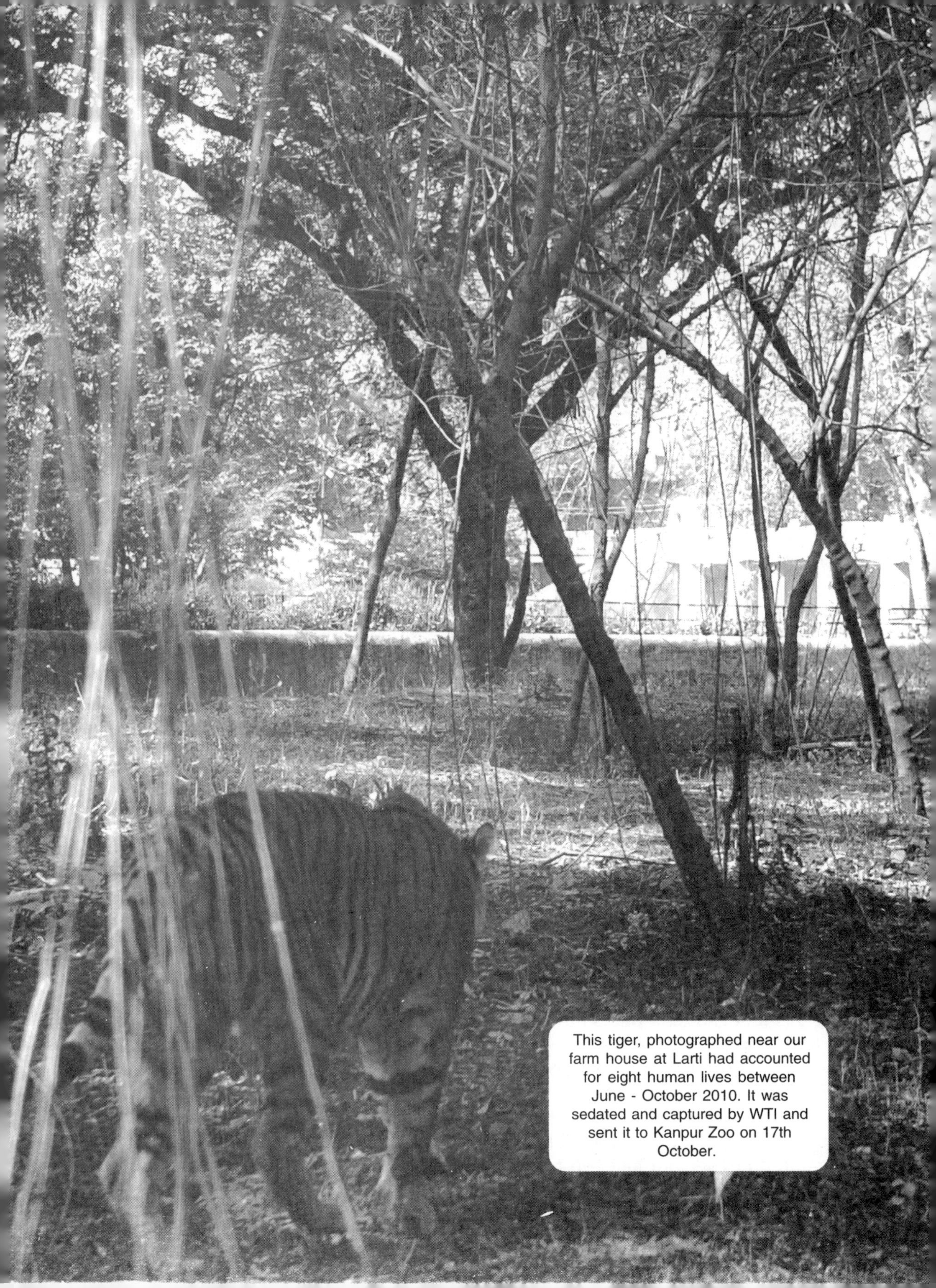

This tiger, photographed near our farm house at Larti had accounted for eight human lives between June - October 2010. It was sedated and captured by WTI and sent it to Kanpur Zoo on 17th October.

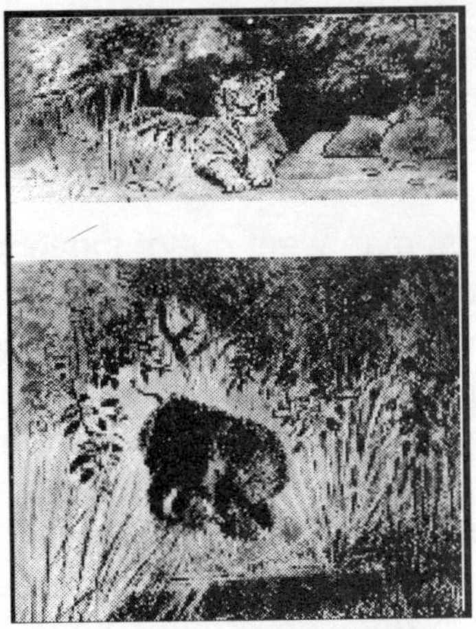

22

Man–Eaters and Saving Men from Tigers

One needs to study the people, that is desperately important; how tigers affect them. In the end, the tiger's fate depends on the people.

- Michiel, a Dutch environmentalist working at Vladivostok

Human beings have a mortal dread of the tiger. Regardless of the accumulated knowledge of mankind that only one tiger in a hundred may take to man-eating, the obvious reaction of a lay human upon confronting a tiger is to fear for his life. In this backdrop, the human reaction to a tiger living in sugarcane cannot be different. Therefore, the queer character called man-eater needs to be explored.

Species that do not adjust with the human being's game plan lose out and ultimately vanish. The impact of environmental conditions is inestimable as far as the predators are concerned and it is beguiling to hypothesize that the two master predators— the man and the tiger— can ever co-exist.

From the heights of his mental evolution, man sometimes forgets that he is an animal too; a primate with distant cousins among the lemurs and monkeys, and closer relations among the apes with whom he shares a common ancestry.

As an animal, man is governed by natural law just as much as every other living organism; he and his works are no less part of the earth's finite collection of materials than a termite and its mound.

While giraffes evolved their long necks, tigers sharpened their claws and antelopes learned to sprint, men developed their brains. It is a remarkable tool for living but makes man unique only so far as he can imagine the future, as well as consider the present and remember the past. Man is able to analyze cause and predict effects, and success of his species depends largely on his ability. At this stage, he is unlikely to evolve other physical adaptations to aid his survival. The cognitive brain is all he needs.

With the passage of years, man went out of the jungle to settle as a farmer and completely ceased to be the prey of tiger. The group living created a sense of security in man. But as civilization progressed, the sense of self-preservation in man got diluted over the ages by scientific development, but the tiger in his position as master predator remained the same — that can prey upon any other species. And when the tiger is forced by circumstances and hunger to wander in human areas, he can prove potentially dangerous to them.

Aberrant individual tigers that attack human beings because of hunger, inexperience or injuries or in defense of cubs have always existed. Dr. Karanth believes that such occasional manslaughter does not necessarily lead to persistent man-eating behaviour, but there is no doubt that some tigers that accidentally discover human vulnerability, might later become man-eaters.

Among the barrage of recaps about the last 30 years; the case studies of man-eater of Salukapur, Suheli tigress, Ghola Man-eater, Katna tigress, Tara the cocktail tigress, Mala man-eater and the last shot near my home town Mailani in 2006, together with over thirty others indicate that every man-eater is a unique animal. Their characteristics differ from every other individual of its species, including at least other man-eaters. Each one therefore must be studied separately and treated

The author and his favourite Uncle Blaster interacting with tiger harassed villegers

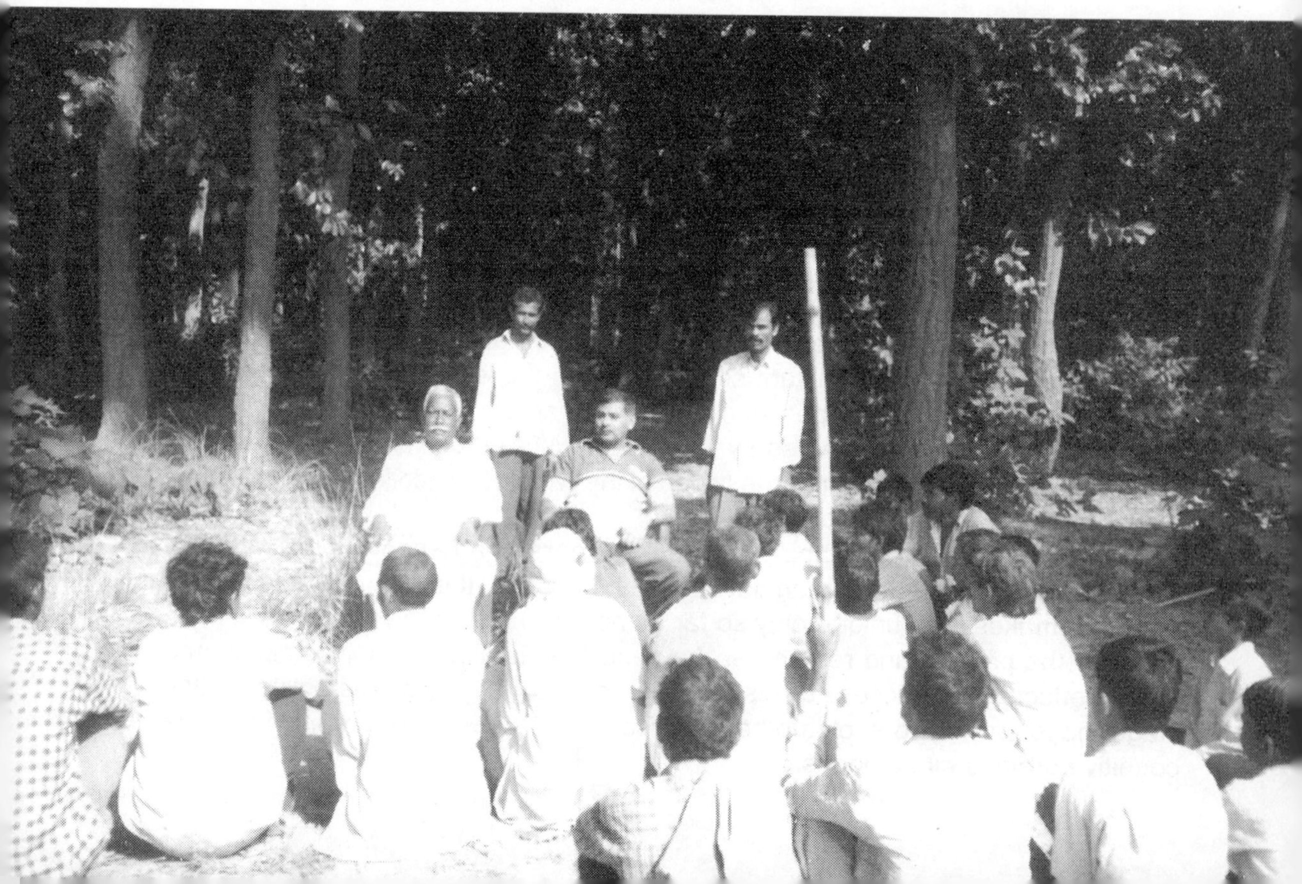

accordingly as an exclusive case. For these exceptional animals proved that to hunt them according to the familiar routine will do no good to anyone except the tiger. This idea could scarcely penetrate the head of an ordinary forester and some hunters were very slow to grasp it. That is why several innocent tigers were done to death while the real culprits invariably escaped.

The 42 established villages and 55 secondary villages around Dudhwa with nearly a thousand hamlets, whose croplands are carved out of forest, base their livelihood on their livestock, whether it is cattle or goat. The incessant activities of farmers, grass cutters and cattle grazers on foot increase their interactions with tiger. The movement of heavy traffic such as tractors and lorries severely impinges the normal activities of deer, antelope and wild pigs and others that come to share sugarcane habitat. It also disturbs the normal cycle of a tiger's life and compels him to adopt a different mode altogether with an increasing acceptance of changes as normal.

This unique anomaly had given rise to man-eaters in the area and little was understood as to why these killing had started in the first place. The fragmentation of habitats and resulting isolation of wildlife populations were primarily the results of increasing anthropogenic pressures. Consequently, even genuine wild tigers (the jungle dwellers) were using unbroken cane fields as corridors to cross over to other forested areas and getting exposed to collision course with humans.

Suggested causes for man-eating are...

1. Injury, causing problems in hunting the predator's normal prey
2. Absence of the normal prey species in an area
3. Graduation from scavenging
4. Learnt behaviour

Tigers that have excellent fitness for predatory life – a swift capture, killing and eating of living prey — are definitely more dangerous in sugar fields than their contemporaries in the jungle. We have not only already noticed that the sugar dwelling tigers display every characteristic of grass tigers; that owing to the inordinate density of grass cannot be seen beforehand, and paradoxically, nor can they see properly until the intruder almost bumps into them. They get no time to consider their action, and act upon their impulse to attack in self-defense or escape. The attacks are definitely made in error of man being mistaken for legitimate prey. This chance killing of man makes it easier for them to overcome the reluctance to attack human beings.

It is observed that prey animals are not always afraid of tiger though they sound an alarm at his sight but merely keep watching him as he moves in their domain. They instinctively know that he is not on hunting and thus they do not run away but the same animal always run away at the very sight of a man, they do not wait and watch him like tiger. It means that animals are more afraid of man than tigers and this also means that all animals are afraid of man including tiger; that is why even hardest man-eaters are not able to give up their shyness of man. Even if a tiger has realized the helplessness of man, it will still retain its innate fear that prevents him from attacking a man except when he is bending down in the manner of a quadruped.

A predator deprived of natural prey will turn to whatever is available. There are situations, where tigers were chased away from livestock kill resulting in deprivation of food and they perforce launched an attack on man. A few such instances embolden a tiger to take to man killing. All these human actions result in extending man-tiger conflict. He can acquire man-eating traits at any age and turn into an obsessive and uncontrolled man-eater.

Such man-eaters might generate more man-eaters. The offsprings of these beasts who compulsively and calculatedly seek human flesh are also extremely wary and intelligent since they deal with a prey with highest intelligence. They follow the example of their parents and become well versed of their prey's life-style. The life of a predator is not only an aggregate of its instincts, transference of practice and habits of countless ancestors, but in truth it is altered and modeled by the challenging circumstances and parental traditions. The deviousness and craftiness is born of the new experience that a tiger cub acquires in their association. Such man-eaters are never mangy or decrepit beasts, they are invariably as young, strong and lusty as normal tigers which prey on game and cattle. And finally owing to their knowledge of man they are difficult to trap.

Investigations prove that man-eating was more frequent in females than in males. The stress of long starvation and difficulty in finding food for their young ones initiates females into this bad habit. Early eighties were marked by an increase in the number of man-eating tigers in this area. Many villagers believed that the habit was taken up and continued by young cubs also born in sugarcane. Man-eating, like cattle killing, may also become a tradition passed on from parents to their younger generations. However, opinions on the fate of the cubs differ. For example, the Talla Desh man-eater, a tigress in Kumaon, was active over eight years during which she must have mothered several litters that fed on human flesh. Yet not one of them was recorded as man-eater in subsequent years. Jim Corbett himself held the view that the cubs do not necessarily become man-eaters because they have been weaned on human flesh.

One more cause can be traced to the origin of this new brand of man-eaters. I have already stated that sub-adult tigers who have left the area where they were raised and have emigrated elsewhere are fraught with dangers. Firstly because they are on unfamiliar ground and can no longer depend on their mothers. And secondly the slots in which they establish themselves are mostly sub-optimal and marginal and invariably degraded in quality prey. (The slots of prime prey are invariably under the control of large adults, who do not allow intruders). Consequently the high population build up on the fringes of the jungle, slowly immigrate into sugarcane farms.

These young tigers are conscious of their growing strength and bubbling energy. But it is unsafe time for they are not prudent enough to have learnt of good judgments in corresponding degree and the real art of survival. As Forsyth puts it; "Young tigers seem to rejoice in the exercise of the growing strength, springing up against trees, and scratching the bark as high as they can by way of gymnastics, and if they get among a herd of cattle, striking down as many as they can get hold off". Brander also endorses the view, "Sometimes a tiger will rush into a herd of cattle and down three or four beasts.... this is generally the work of a young tiger proud of his skill and rejoicing in the ease with which he kills".

Such tigers often abruptly turn man killers, act aggressively or even sometimes feast on human corpse but as humans do not fall into their normal prey species, they are prone to be restored to a normal existence expeditiously, if left in peace. On a December morning in 2001, I had an occasion to track such an aberrant beast when an inebriated elderly Sikh Banot Singh was killed at Bijaria in Chaltua sugar fields, district Shajahanpur. The director of Dudhwa Park, G.C. Mishra and DFO area were already present in Mailani and as there was no appropriate person around to go after an aberrant tiger, I was summoned in my official capacity as Honorary Wildlife Warden for guidance and helping foresters in recovery of relics. It was already late afternoon and there was no point to wait for the arrival of the elephants which the DFO had called from Dudhwa. I asked the forest guards to reach the site of the kill and arrange for some domestic buffaloes.

When I arrived, I found that the pugmarks were those of a male and the kill had taken place in the open; there was no cover and water near so the tiger had dragged its prey to a considerable distance. I acquired a .300 Ramington Ultra Magnum rifle from a Sikh *Granthi*, fired a couple of test shots and set out on foot, using a herd of a dozen tame buffaloes. These cattle with their large formidable horns and great powers of resistance are very useful in tracking destructive tigers, as in case of an attack on search party, they are invariably in some position to present an obstacle to the seizure of men. Two armed guards and a ranger, Rajendra Prasad Saxena also followed me to lend a helping hand. They were armed with an arsenal of .12 bore shot guns and a .315 rifle of Indian Ordinanace. The trail, went a long way through a dense sugarcane farm and through a *Nala,* and was copiously marked with blood. The killer had taken the boy 20 feet high, up a steep knoll and then entered another arable land.

Everything was obstinately silent. The cattle were moving sluggishly and the evening was setting in haste. Having followed the trail for a couple of miles and with single mindedness we began to feel the anxiety of expanding gloom, when I heard the sound of a bone cracking and something large suddenly jumped out and disappeared. The dumb buffaloes' took no notice of it and remained unaffected; but the ranger was quick to register the movement. He said the tiger was in the process of dinning; perhaps eating uninterruptedly for quite some time to finish his meal, when upon perceiving our arrival he suddenly leapt up and ran away. He had clearly seen it fleeing.

I cocked the rifle and sandwiched between two buffalos, drawing them by their reins, reached the place which was marked by a few bones and a big clotted dab of blood; a further on by the pale moon light we found the remains of unfortunate man. All that was left of him for cremation was -his head and rib cage- which the killer had perhaps discarded. It was quite dark now and the tiger being near it was not advisable to stay there. We collected the relics in a rucksack and returned.

Chaltua is only six miles distant from Larti, where I live to accomplish my duties as Hon. wildlife warden. I entrusted my native crew to monitor this tiger, while I returned to Lucknow. The ruddy animal lived till February in the area on feral cattle and farm dogs but never made a second human kill, and finally when the crop was harvested, disappeared in the jungle.

To my mind this category of tigers, aged from one to three years, forced to live in the sugarcanes becomes vulnerable to aberrations. In its self-indulgent rhapsody, it might, thoughtlessly and imprudently, may well first turn to man killing, which could be closely followed by man-eating. That is why most of the man-eaters killed in Kheri district during last thirty years were healthy and able bodied tigers with not even a single natural deformity like those described by Jim Corbett in his books, such as old age, injuries by porcupine quills or faulty or deteriorated dentures etc.

Indeed any sound ecological explanation does not exist for the pattern of man-eating observed in Tarai during the last four decades. But it gives a strong indication that the initiation of the aberrative behavior comes from a conflict with man, even if the cause is an indirect one. I contend that cats are hunters by nature. Unlike other predators, their desire to hunt is not suppressed by adequate supplemental food. Keep your house cat well fed, still it will kill bird and lizards at first opportunity but may not eat it. A cat kills its prey because of its motivation to hunt is based on movement, but may not necessarily recognize that prey as food. Realizing that prey is food is a learned behavior. It is obvious that it takes a prolonged period of recruitment for a tiger to become a cattle-lifter and maybe even a longer period to become a circumstantial man-killer and finally a motivated man-eater, because it takes a long journey for him to lose fear of the 'super animal' that man is.

In the January of 2009, I was invited by the Director of Dudhwa Park, Uma Shanker Singh to deal with a man-eater at Kanp-Tanda area, an agricultural country, bordering the Sharda River. This tiger had his beat among the rudely cultivated tracts of cane, where he appeared sometimes in broad daylight, carried off his human prey and retired into the fastness of sugarcanes, which afforded him almost inviolable sanctuary. It was one of most tiring operations I ever managed, in which I marched for nearly 250 kilometers in a fortnight, and when the culprit was finally steel caged by Anjan Talukdar, a tranquillizing drug expert of WTI, it turned out to be a robust male of three years. In the case of this tiger the abundance or scarcity of prey animals was not directly related to human causality figures and he had no physical deformities to account for his fatal predilection. The captive animal was subsequently sent to Lucknow zoo.

To my mind, besides inherent and designing man eaters, which is a class by

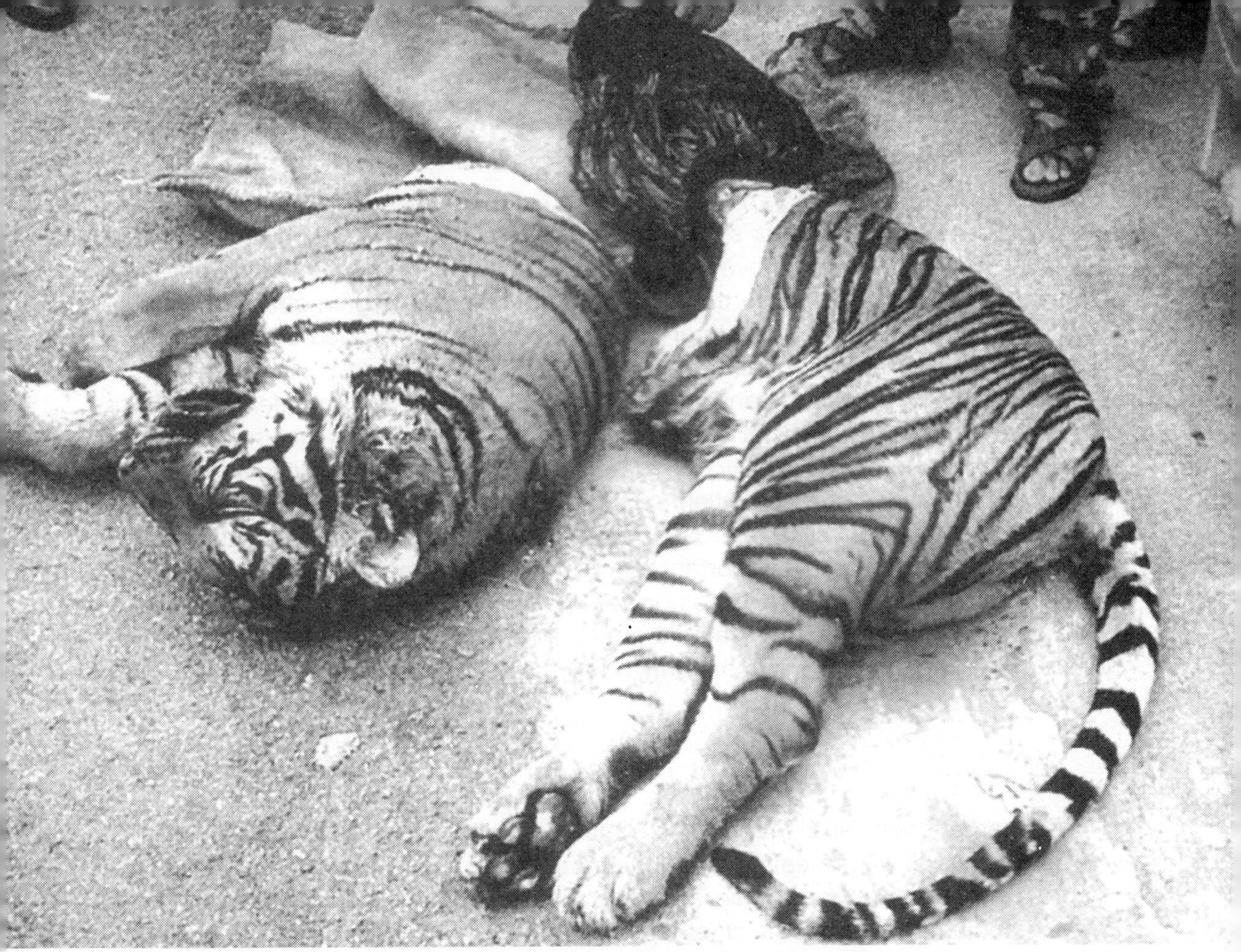

This decapitated tiger, killed of poisoning, was discovered on Katarniaghat-Dudhwa railway track, where it was placed to appear as train accident

itself, behavior patterns of predators with man-eating urge are classified as aggressive, lusty and adventurous, undesigning and eventually circumstantial. This tiger, now named as Krishna, represented the lusty and adventurous category, which is an aberration of highest kind. He had surprisingly snatched three victims from inside the village at the entrances of the houses in broad daylight. It is revealed only by the tigers that nurture condescension towards human beings and also possess immense power and confidence, in which normal fear of two legged animal is overruled by the contempt. And finally, my code of belief maintains that no established man-eater, even if kept and treated in captivity under controlled conditions, can ever be restored to normal existence.

On December 7, 2009, a tiger struck at Azad Nagar-Bishunpuri area, killing a boy named Sabloo. By his sister's account, having delivered lunch to his father he was returning home when the tigress with two large three-quarter grown cubs stalked and ambushed him through canes. It was not an accidental confrontation; I surmise that the family must have been starved for weeks before embarking on such a reprehensible maneuver. The entire body was consumed and the mother too had fed on the kill as well. The grim relics contained of few bones and a chewed head, cleaned of all hair by predator's rasping tongue. The tigress was known to locals as Mausi (mother's sister) for over a year, which had never demonstrated or roared. On January 4, 2010, her large cubs, hunting on their own, again attacked a girl Rinki, stripping cane and injured her before she could be rescued by the labors. Now there was a clamor for her immediate elimination.

It seems that man-eating behavior gets established from the complex interplay of several ecological and social factors. Dr. Ullas Karanth believes that the number of tigers, natural prey availability, topography and hunter accessibility, amount of interference between human settlements and tiger habitats, human density, local decimation of prey, physical retardation in the tiger, potential for quick retaliation and sheer chances, play an important role in making of a man-eater.

We realize that it is not always easy to resolve the competition between man and wildlife. The prognosis is grim; an old jungle adage says, 'Even Man Eaters are justified in killing humans if it is the only way left for them to eat to live'.

(II)

In the large forests at the foot of the Himalayas, where there is plenty of game, the occurrence of a man-eating tiger is comparatively rare. But farmlands offer a different proposition, where a tigress with cubs finds herself driven to resort to preying on human beings. The chief reasons for man-tiger conflict can be covered in three major points. These are: human pressure on tiger habitat, gradual shrinkage of habitat and the reduction of prey animals. The very points also stand for the abrupt appearance of entirely new pattern of man-eating, besides human socio-economic situations that are chiefly responsible for creating the collision course between the two species and also the depletion in tiger population brought on by ecological crisis.

Previously, the farmers did not mind the presence of tigers in their canes as they were considered the 'unpaid guards' keeping herbivores at bay. It was a sort of symbiotic relationship in which both the species — the farmer and the tiger — were mutually benefited. However, in context of the peripheries of Dudhwa, where the maximum cases of man-eating had occurred, the most important point was the disappearance or in some cases the loss of the natural ability to hunt in some wild tigers, which later set the trend of man-eating.

After the loss of Tara, Billy Arjan Singh was left with no big cats to manage demonstrations for his foreign clients. His all showpieces including leopards were dead, so he started running a sort of 'canteen' for all the Dudhwa tigers around his Tiger Heaven farm. He created a feeding station near the twin lake point, where he provided tigers with regular buffalo baits in order to localize them within his vicinity. His intention was to offer managed shows and attract foreign clients once again to make commercial films and write about his jungle settlement, where the tigers wandered past in the night. Baiting is also an expedient method for drawing predators out of reserve and parks by poachers. The temptation of bait attracted many tigers -from the heart of their range- into the peripheral area and as they became hooked on baiting, they became showpieces for his clients.

During the peak tourist season, Billy generated as many as three feeding stations namely Juliet point, Jungle Fowl Jetty and Twin Lakes where baits were often found tied by the Park staff, un-tethered and taken away. The availability of an easy prey slowly deprived many tigers of their natural ability to kill a normal wild prey. When the rains broke out in Dudhwa and the feeding stations got flooded, Billy stopped baiting and the tigers began to wonder extensively. The Old Crooked Foot and Long Toes, the wild tigers described in his books, when never endowed with enough baits switched over to grazers' buffaloes and plow oxen. They even attacked horses used for carting forest products.

I personally believe that many tigers that had become used to easy prey, possibly because the buffalo calves are more tender and taste better, later took to cattle killing and some even progressed further to acquiring man-eating traits. This triggered the man-eating phenomenon grow recklessly on the borders of the park, which Billy addressed as nature's reaction. A fat tiger had become so inept by regular baiting that he never bothered to kill the tethered calf at all, he rather begun to dine on it straight away. If the calf protested hard, only then he was obliged to kill it otherwise he would go on, eating it live as the hyenas or wild dogs do, with no specialized skill to kill a big prey and rather eat to kill. Sometime later this tiger —unable to subdue enough wild prey to satisfy his appetite— is suspected to have become Ghola man-eater.

It is significant that Billy's unsuccessful experiment regarding the rehabilitation of his pet tigress Tara had also vitiated the old friendly relationship between man and tiger beyond repair. Being largely fed on hand by her caretakers Tara had never learnt the hunting nuances as the wild tigers learn from their parents through observation and practice; and thus unable to kill the potentially dangerous wild game, the inept killer had finally switched over to the meek prey of human beings.

Guy Mountfort's observation in this regard stands important. He writes, "Returning social animals such as ungulates and even lions to the wild is possible, but for the solitary tiger, which depends for survival on a two year tutelage by its mother, this is virtually impossible."

At another place he writes that "Introducing large captive bred carnivores to the wild is fraught with difficulties. They need parental training in capturing prey. They may continue to try to be familiar with people. This can be alarming, and might lead to accidents. Adverse public reaction can hamper conservation efforts."

To my mind, Tara was an inbred, human imprinted and psychologically damaged pet which had absolutely no conservation value. She could not be rehabilitated into the wilds; she was a danger to pure-blooded Indian tiger because of her Siberian

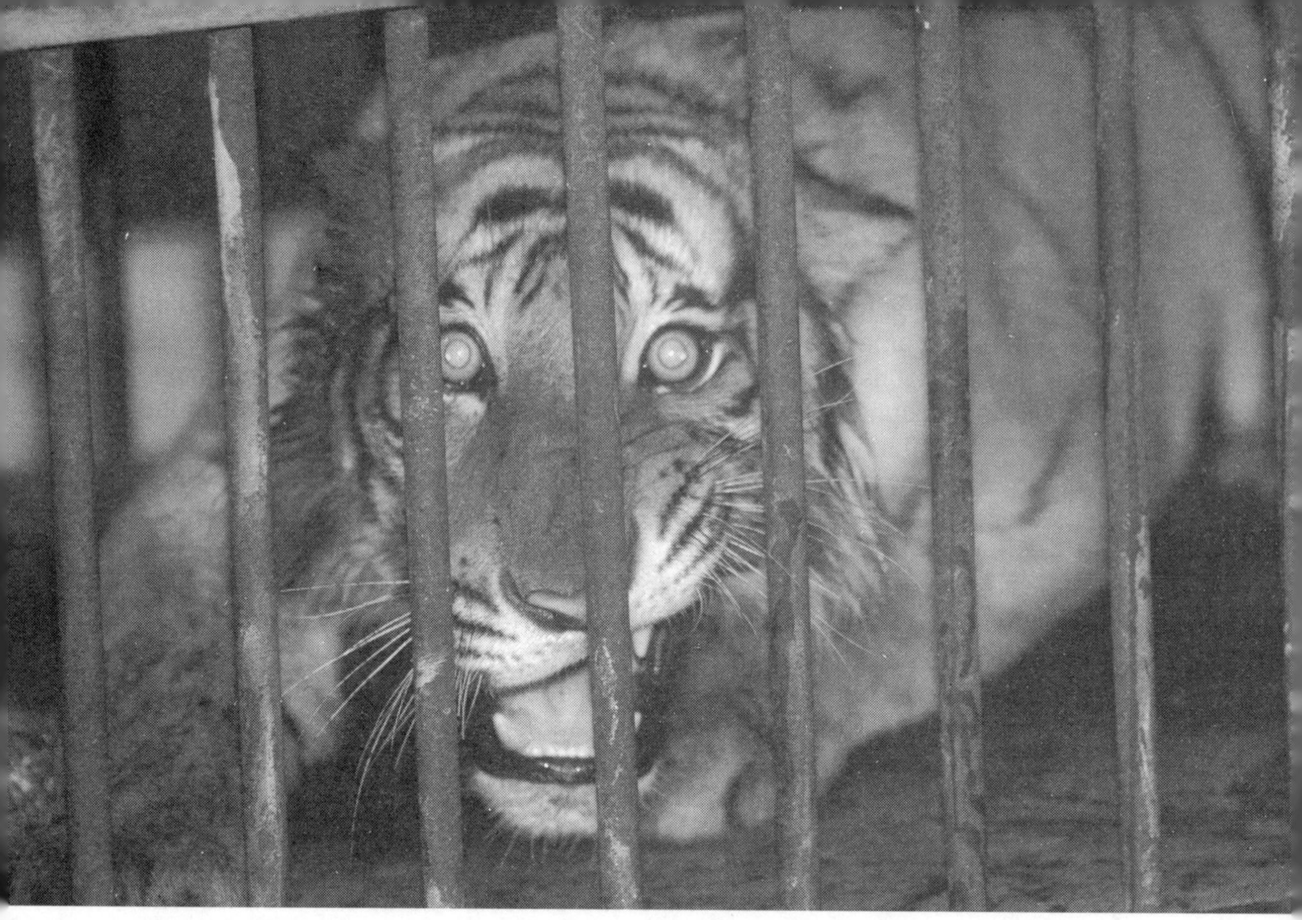

The caged man-eater of Kanp Tanda. In Jan 2009, the authour and his tiny crew of ten reformed poachers chased this tiger for a fortnight

strain, and could never be useful to supplement dwindling wild populations. She had not only killed 22 human beings inefficiently, making a mess of them, but had destroyed the old symbiotic relationship between man and tiger in the area. She had generated such a fear that farmers even stopped trusting the normal tigers that had made their territories on their farms for years.

In fact man-eating had only begun around Dudhwa since Billy had released Tara. In last months of her life her appetite was purely anthropophagous. She no doubt preferred the flavor of better-nourished flesh of man. It was a point blank assertion of some experts that at some moment the human kills of this hardened offender were also shared by her wild companions. Therefore, even the inoffensive tigers colonizing agriculture fields were regarded with suspicion and many of them were eliminated by irate villagers for their own perceived safety at the first opportunity. R. L. Singh describes the funeral scene of the half-eaten body of Labh Singh, a Sikh *Granthi* (priest) of a local Gurdwara who was killed by Tara. He writes in his book *Tara; the cocktail tigress* that "None of the well wishers who had gathered at his cremation was unarmed. Some had small arms, others wielded rifles. The crowd felt that the tigress had committed an unpardonable sin by killing such a religious man..." while his Warden told him that, "They will gun down any tiger wandering in the fields as well as forest workers entrusted with the protection of big cats." It was also confirmed by the district magistrate who told the author, "If the man-eater was not killed, they will finish off all the tigers hiding in the sugarcane fields."

Billy had confused the whole situation, though to a great degree Dudhwa was his creation and the last herds of swamp deer were saved from being hunted into oblivion solely through his intervention, but now his obsessed-enthusiasm had prepared the coffin of Dudhwa tigers, set the nails in it and made the Park a gloomy cuss of land; the Frankenstein monster he had created was surely out of control.

I am sure that in the west, any such offender would have been held guilty and tried in court for three offences- killing of a large number of human beings by his pet tigress Tara; the heinous act of spreading genetic pollution and furthermore as an offshoot of the first reason for generating an excruciating panic amongst masses that is responsible for the killing of several innocent tigers. Thanks to Tara! She had won Billy a constant blaze of publicity, offering virtually unlimited fodder for wildlife junkies to debate on, whereas the blameless Dudhwa tigers were paying immeasurable penalty for the culprit, falling prey to the hatred of people. Hatred is not the same as disapproval, contempt or anger. Hatred is loathing combined with fear, and with the desire to lash out at the hated object, to wound, to disfigure, to destroy it and this was being done to tigers by the natives.

Tara may have incited negative emotions in the village communities but every attention-seeking junkie knows that there is no such thing as bad publicity, "except your own obituary", as a writer Brendan Behan has said. The emotional setback of Tara's death had changed Billy's life and he was now a different man. A rabid tunnel-visioned conservationist had rather become a man hater. He issued statements against the government with brutal selfishness to which a gullible and willing-to-be-used media fell for. Though he farmed near the jungle but he failed to come up with any practical programme to help people and control these killings. He never went to any village to listen to the plight of people, or ever counseled a single man as to how to evade tigers or to dilute their smoldering bitterness against the beast and treat their actual physical pain.

There was nothing reticent about him. People were reduced to a state of nervous wrecks, bordering on hysteria, and at every human kill he blatantly stated that 'man has tasted tiger's blood for centuries without having been tasted much in return. Now it is their turn'. I think he was right, perhaps Tara had become a man-eater not out of necessity but more for 'sport' and the old man was quite content to feed his fellow human beings to his preferred species - the ferocious tigress with which he had spent his life trying to 'bond."

Without attempting to be a discursive critique, I shall give a pertinent example of a PIL (Public Interest Litigation) that I filed in June 2007 in Lucknow bench of Allahabad High Court, in which I prayed that the forest property in the possession of land sharks should also be identified and evacuated. On the order of the High Court, chunks of land were identified and I was surprised to see that Billy Arjan Singh's name appeared fourth in the list of land-grabbers. The foresters got over a hundred acre of cultivated land that contained mature cane crops over it evacuated from his possession. Billy denied that he ever owned this land but the Palia sugar factory revealed that loads of sugarcane were received in their factory on the name of Billy and naturally the payment of particular sugar chunk was being made to him for many decades.

The same farmers, who were once the friends of tigers, had now taken the law into their hands and were deciding the fate of cats by exterminating them. Tigers living in the neighborhood of villages were poisoned and found lying next to domestic stock often surrounded by dying scavengers, vultures and jackals, who had fed on the fatal cadaver. Three corpses were found floating down the Sharda canal while two were discovered mutilated on railway tracks. Every cheap gunman in the country was now after them. They were shot and electrocuted by stretching live wire along cultivation fields and crude bombs exploded in their jaws as they fed on their cattle kills. Worst was the year of 1986, when fourteen tiger carcasses were found in the cane fields around Dudhwa. Under practical and significant considerations, this payback had to start somewhere as it could not be postponed indefinitely.

In April 1984, I had gone to Dudhwa to take a stock of the situation. I was surprised to see the way things were working there. Man-eating had become endemic. A tigress with cubs was declared man-eater outside Dudhwa. She had killed two shepherds and lately mauled one who was attempting to plunder her wild boar kill. A tiger was shot over a cow kill whose incisors had been blown out by buckshot and he was now chasing passers-by. A woman was killed in a cane field; a tiger was declared man-eater and later shot. In addition to all this sycophantic officers were declaring tigers as man-eaters on the least pretext and using it as an excuse to cover their failures of management. It was worst than nonsense.

Just in a fortnight, I saw the carcasses of a dozen cattle and five human beings, all killed by tigers. The body of a village grocer Bhairav Prasad was totally consumed, only his skull, palms of the hands and feet were left by the killer who seemed to dislike these parts. I also saw a captured man-eater injuring himself badly in an iron cage in its struggle to escape and a poisoned carcass of a tiger. Later the autopsy showed five bullets in its body including one of .450/.500 cordite rifle. How had he managed to survive this wound greatly puzzled me. However, one thing was certain that the whirlwind of misfortune was raging over Dudhwa and things were left to themselves, no attempt was being made by official agencies to protect either tiger or humans.

The cane tiger problem was also spreading, throwing a spanner in the works of the conservationists and I was feeling tired and dispirited about their fate. I wondered what was the use of all life's success, personal ambitions and urban pursuits, if I had no power to protect such a magnificent creation of god which had given me so much of thrill and happiness in life? Such feelings deepened every time I saw a tiger in the canes. There was great tension in the area; extremists were advocating more measures against tigers and the situation had acquired a lunatic fringe. It raised a question in my mind, is the project Tiger really working, and if it is, then how come the tiger is becoming endangered? How come the poaching and killing is not reduced? Perhaps we had failed to involve the most important human angle into tiger conservation and demonstrate a special concern for the natives, whose farms these beasts used as ranges.

The first worrisome facet of this development was that the governments much hyped conservation efforts were being defeated at the grassroots by villagers unconvinced of the needs to preserve the countries dwindling wildlife. Secondly, steady encroachments of animal habitats was resulting in their migration out of sanctuaries, enhancing the chances of more frequent confrontations between villagers and animals in desperate search of food. Thus the supposed man-animal conflict had become a one sided affair with a variety of wild creatures being regularly bludgeoned to death. Unfortunately it was a melancholy fact that unless some effective form of legislation was brought in by the government concerned, this unique state of plenty was doomed to disappear in the very near future. This gave me a strange premonitory feeling that each tiger in sugar fields was reduced to the status of a goat in a butcher's shop, waiting for an inevitable fate.

After examining all the incidents of tiger attacks, which had largely occurred due to human mistakes, I asked myself two things. Why our response is supportive to destroy predators that attack? And why do we need to be reassured that this has happened? In defense of the predators, they are just doing what their instincts tell them to do, and most often their only mistake is that they selected their prey poorly. But the reality was, as the government statistics suggested that there were only 30-35 tiger attacks per year and only 28 fatalities over the past 2 years. It is estimated that some ten million people inhabit the peripheries of principal tiger belt only in Uttar Pradesh and thus are vulnerable to man animal conflict. Looking at this gargantuan number of people occupying the periphery of reserves, the segment killed by tiger attacks was just insignificant. Incidentally the number of deaths caused by snake bites in these villages was much higher whereas the probability of a man getting killed by tiger, while working at his farm was one in thousand.

Then why do we fear such a low probability event, in contrast to automobile accidents those are the leading cause of death amongst young people. Thousands of people die and millions are injured in car accidents every year all over the world. Recently, in Lucknow, where I live, 16 pedestrians were killed in 6 days. Personally I find vehicles far more dangerous than tigers, yet I do not feel nervous when I cross a street. If our fears and responses to human injury and death reflected the actual major risks, we would invoke restrictive rules regarding automobile use but we do not seem to care much.

On the similar line of reasoning, when India's 35,000 annual deaths by rabies don't lead to a moratorium on stray dogs then why tigers are victimized for every misdemeanor from mauling man and lifting livestock to wandering into fields or merely being seen? While six billion people scratch and nibble at the earth's surface, our creatures of pre-historic antiquity are threatened and in another few years they will be gone for good. I needed to save their lives, save them by saving people who were constantly harassed, intimidated, and hounded by their presence near their villages.

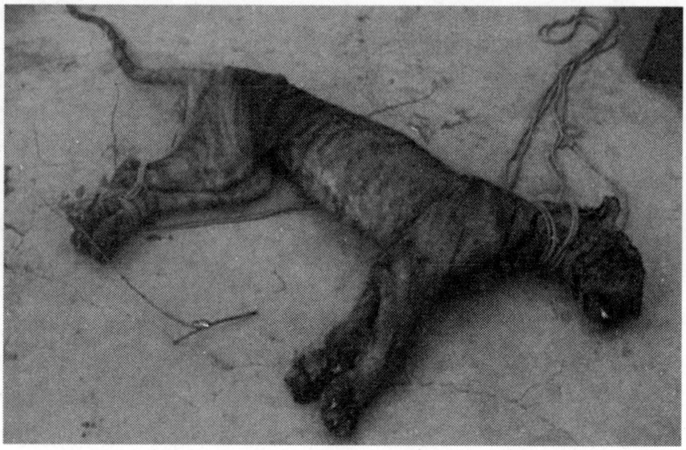

This mangy beast was killer of seven human beings but not a man eater it was eliminated in August in 2006 near my village Larti at Mailani

The very next day, I was attending the college chapel and as usual pre-occupied with my thought when I heard the speaker say "Blessed are the peacemakers for they shall be called the children of God." Peacemaker? The word clicked in my mind. Could I be this in the Tarai somehow? Could I achieve that somehow in the man-tiger battle? Prevent the tigers from becoming the hunters of humanity, bail-out as well, forgive them and realize the ways to co-exist.

Yes, a simple mechanism could save them. The villagers must learn as how to avoid tigers and not to be deceived by their calm presence; for some of them were also opportunistic and aberrant; so what to do in case of a confrontation? An awareness campaign had to be initiated to address this issue. Could I design one successfully? Well, why not? I couldn't go to a temple and worship Shakti, the Mother Goddess, -the terminator of all false prophets and the ultimate champion of several Armageddons- if I didn't try to help those men and also save the Goddesses mighty vehicle from obliteration.

(III)

On a still winter morning and I was at peace with the soft silky sun when dramatic events overtook the idyllic scenario. I was sipping coffee that my servant had set on a mud parapet at my side when I was told that a tiger had just killed a farmer in Navrangpur sugar fields and help was needed there. I finished the coffee and rushed to the spot. A crowd had already gathered at the site. We immediately set out to find the body of the victim. Tracks led us to the human kill lying in a harvested field. The tiger had chewed off its left hand by a strong bite, it lay hardly a meter away. A bunch of hair had been torn off from the head and both the ears were missing. Right thigh was also eaten up and leg severed from the knee. The sight was unbearably gory. We brought the mortal remains back home and the same day it was cremated.

It was the first day when I collected nearly 200 villagers and talked to them at length about the crisis. Natives displayed a great dread of tigers and found it hard to believe that they could co-exist with them. Their large size and predatory life style posed a big problem. Natives told me that even if they find a tiger moving in the fields in a calmest and friendliest mood, they run like hares for safety. I told them that this was the greatest fault. Usually, the sight of any fleeing figure would prompt any carnivore animal to give a chase. Even a domestic dog would chase anyone who runs from him. It makes the tiger interested in them.

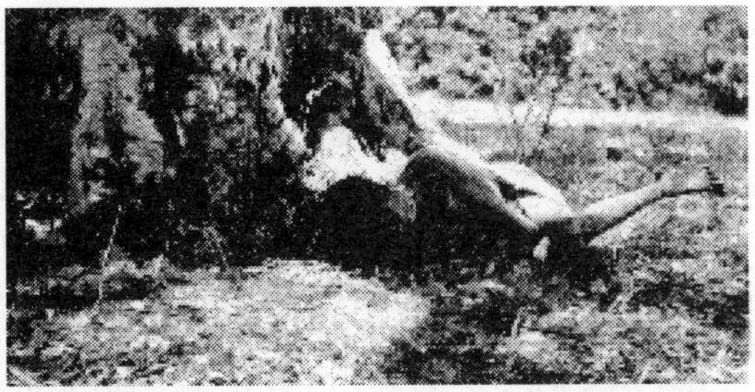

A human kill by Baraucha nala man eater

I emphasized the importance of dogs. They can smell a tiger and give a timely alarm. A waiting tiger will prefer to catch a dog rather than a man, for in spite of everything dog is his normal food.

Reports of desultory human kills were coming in from scattered areas. One of my uncles from Larti whom I affectionately called Uncle Blaster was getting interested in them. One day, he took out his Jeep and we proceeded to confirm the truth in news and if possible to help the victims. We visited a chain of 22 small hamlets in south Kheri where tigers had taken a big human toll. It was godforsaken country where small farmer families were living in isolation and reeling under tiger fear. They were most defenseless and vulnerable to man-eaters. I inspected their *Jhalas*, pointed out ineffectual defenses, asked people to not to move at all during the night, move in compact groups, avoid moving in single file, keep a fire burning in the night, never sleep outside and raise noise at first apprehension of the tiger's approach. I asked the Gram Pradhan to promote the idea of group living in the area and consolidate the isolated hutments into the main village as this would help humans to separate themselves from nocturnal activities of tigers.

Everywhere we went people reported confrontations with tigers and wanted us to shoot them. At places we were given the names of missing villagers and it was presumed that tigers had devoured them, even though there was no definite evidence to corroborate that presumption. Dogma maintained that the man-eaters could not be restored to a normal existence and efforts to reform them was a waste of time, whereas we tried to convince villagers that many of these tigers are not habitual man-eaters and a little bit of precaution would avoid the tragedy.

Forest department officials are generally unpopular in these parts. They are feared but sometimes badly confronted on defaults. At one village we met a chief who was adamant on poisoning a tiger which had lifted several goats and cows. That morning the brute had been seen in a nearby field. We counseled the chief but he appeared very rigid. "What are these foresters doing?' he continued questioning.

The magnitude of the problem was large; it covered thousands of square kilometers and was not easy to deal with. My efforts to tackle the crisis also demanded a formidable organization and expense so I called my friends to help me. Yogesh Kumar, Prabhas K. Jha, N. Ravi Shanker — all civil servants — along with B.K. Bhalla and Vijay Kumar, stalwarts from Indian Police Service, offered to join hands with me. Their companionship and resourcefulness made my task much easier. With their invaluable help I penetrated into deeper zones of Tarai, where the man-eaters were scoring high and where fatal accidents had been accepted as necessary for living in a tiger country mainly because of the neglect of some basic rules.

It is very difficult for a reader to imagine what it is like to be living in the domain of a man-eater. These villages were a picture of abject misery. People could not go out and herd their cows, go to the river to draw water or wash clothes, go to gather fodder, firewood, and visit nearest temple or bazaar or to answer a call of nature or even to step out of doors at dusk. They seemed to live under the shadow of sudden and violent death. Earthen pots filled with green chili, honey and lime and in some cases even half-burnt human bones, picked purposely from the pyres, hung on the trees as charms to ward off the evil effect of tigers.

In Balhipur area of south Kheri a tigress with three large cubs had kept a village under siege for a fortnight. The budding predators, having learnt hunting techniques from their mother had conducted excess livestock killings in enthusiasm. They had admirably knocked down nearly a dozen cattle in the past two weeks. They rampaged roaring through sugar fields in the night and paced the roads approaching the village during the day. It was found on two occasions in the morning, that they had come quiet close to the cattle enclosure but fortunately for some reason had quit the idea of entering it. In nights there was little sound sleep in this village. Every man was anxiously watchful and on his feet. Bright fires were kept burning all through the hours of darkness and time to time natives kept clattering empty oil canes that were conveniently suspended on various trees.

A village grocer had dangled an empty can at the entrance of his house. It was manipulated with help of pulleys and a long rope that ran up to his room. He was compelled to make the gadget because once he opened the door of his house in the night and was horrified to see a tiger standing a few yards away from him. Now sitting in the safety of his bed room, he pulled it in the night at frequent intervals. The horrific sounds thus produced were supposed to terrify the marauders and keep them away.

Near Katarnia Ghat a large vista between Tewaripurwa and Pathakpurwa villages was the hot-spot of man-tiger conflict. It was a favorite breeding ground of tigresses, where once I had found two abandoned tigers cubs that were later sent to Lucknow zoo. The area harbored dozens of men who had been mauled by tigers. Some had been crippled for life, while others were slowly dying of septic and gangrene for lack of proper medical aid. Some of them were okay, but had lost an arm or hand. I met a brawny man Dhukkoo whose body was mauled and biceps were chewed by a tiger but he survived. A woman Debuka Bua, whose left shoulder was pierced by canine holes and her breast was badly clawed. All her wounds were filled with pus and covered with flies. I washed, disinfected and bandaged her wounds and helped her with money, clothes and medicine.

The silence of these villages struck me. I even missed the usual clamor of the dogs as they had been devoured by the tigers. I met a man Girdhar who had survived a tiger attack, he ran high temperature for months with regular fits of nervousness and kept shouting, 'Tiger! Tiger!' in his delirium, "The tiger has seized me again! Save me sahib, save me! I feel his teeth in my throat! My breath is stopped! Ah-ah", he gasped like a person drowning. I remember nocturnal visits of a black robed, veiled old woman going from hut to hut, who murmured incantations which may have some connection with magic.

She was accompanied by an old butcher who carefully splattered the blood of a pig on door posts. As a historian of Ancient Civilizations, I knew it as a Jewish ritualistic rite that dates back to Biblical times. I could never determine how this Semitic rite had filtered into the folk ways of this remote Indian village. It was late 20th century but in Tarai the century had to live side by side with many queer ghosts of past centuries.

I accepted the old woman's blessings and asked the butcher to apply some more pig blood on the door of my hut or rather make a double coat of it. I even ordered for a pot of chilly-honey and bones to be kept by my side during the night and all that gree-gree that puts a stop to being eaten by tigers, be hoarded in my room. Though I don't belong to that part of Tarai but the bug of superstition had eaten deep into my mind, and I was merely taking precautions.

I arrived at a hamlet where tiger scare had imposed a curfew. Only two days ago, it had crushed a man's skull like a walnut and since then his body was lying in the back of a hut. There was an unpleasant odor at the place yet people had no courage to go out and cremate the decomposing cadaver. The tiger was still in the area because his growls had been heard on the track to the village for past two nights.

I accompanied the family to the banks of the Ull River and stood guard with a sport rifle while the body was cremated. The smell was so pungent that a pack of jackals swirled excitedly around the place, chattering with anticipation but without the courage to approach the body.

During my varied experience in tiger-infested sugarcanes, I was always conscious of the fact that these fields are silent spectators of the ceaseless fight for survival between prey and predators where some win and some bite the dust. These are the sinister turfs of tigers, which have long maintained the evil reputation with its ferocious wild beasts. In their depths all is stillness and no movement is discernable, and hiding amongst them are the bravura figures of tigers, some of which nurture man-eating proclivities. In the villages, I heard the stories and mournful cries of family members of untold tiger victims. Their lives had become eternal struggles against the big cats yet the land always seemed innocuously calm as if nothing had actually happened to disturb its unending tranquility.

I held a series of meetings with the villagers and was welcomed in every settlement. The story of one small hamlet was the story of many. It was a quaint world. I felt very close to the ebb and surge of native life, the desperate fight back for survival, joy and despair. There was a frantic sense of nightmarish fear and urgency in some villages while some were just peacefully tranquil without any air of agony. On a couple of occasions while attending the festive ceremonies, I at once, heard from a distance the rhythmic chanting of funeral procession of yet another tiger victim.

As I saw the drama of human struggle and suffering -- not to be looked on lightly and then forgotten -- I could not help but think that the Tarai is a world that exists in its own right and natural law is not based on a concept of right or wrong; it existed before man and to it man's laws are quite superfluous. Her all creatures are strictly subject to the law of the survival of the fittest. From this law, rise the strange facts that exemplify the insensitivity, greed and heartlessness on account of every animal as well as man.

However, as the past, present and the future of these villages are closely tied up with their animal neighbours, our primary interest was to make them familiar with a few measures to protect themselves against tigers. These were like simplified traffic rules, easy to grasp but potent enough to make the difference between life and death. Our suggestions were something like this:

1. Do not run at the sight of a tiger. This natural reaction awakes attack instinct in animal, and may result in mauling and killing of man.
2. Do not plough your field alone; always stay in a group of four to five men.
3. Move only during day light and in groups, keep to the main roads. Talk loudly and wear colourful clothes.
4. A couple of watchmen must be stationed in the field to guard the working labours. This discourages tigers from attacking.
5. Do not sit on haunches for longer times, for a tiger then mistakes the man to be a quadruped and attacks.
6. Take a dog along. It forewarns a tiger's presence and in the event of attack the predator will prefer it to a man.

7. While moving alone keep beating an empty tin can. Loud sounds drive animals away.
8. Wear a human mask at the back of your face. For a tiger seldom faces its perspective prey but seizes it unaware from behind. The mask makes it feel that you are looking at it and then it abandons the attack.

And when the aberration is limited only to cattle killing, an understanding human response allowing the dead cattle to be eaten is necessary. It prevents unnecessary killing. A tiger chased away from the kill would soon raid somewhere again till he appeases his hunger properly. As the process goes on, he becomes bold enough to retain his game when confronted. This is a warning sign that should not be overlooked and foresters be immediately informed.

Saving men from tigers is a gigantic step forward in tiger conservation efforts. In trying to save sugarcane tiger I have presented some possible formulas that may address the needs of developing villages while enabling them to co-exist with the big carnivores. I have taken on this formidable task of social service to make natives understand that they can promote a viable conservation because their livelihood and culture has always intimately shared its space with the big cats. I know that until we adopt a bold and imaginative step in our attempt to meet its requirements and put an end to retaliation and persecution of wildlife, including the hideous abuse of poisoning, we are going to lose the battle. But one of the most important aspects of this project is that since its inception, many villagers have actively prevented retaliation killings of predators by their fellow beings including chasing away several poaching parties that often raided their areas for big game shooting. I have a satisfying feeling that this campaign embraces traditional knowledge and culture as a driving force on the way to sustainability which aims to provide substantial components towards co-existence.

My struggle to minimize man-tiger conflict was immensely appreciated by His Excellency Suraj Bhan, the Governor of Uttar Pradesh. He made a successful trip with me to Dudhwa National park. There is little doubt that I immensely enjoyed the company of this lively personality though there was a certain amount of worry in the burden of responsibility attached to the honorable assignment. Later at the behest of his Principal Secretary, Shri G.B. Patnaik, whose understanding and sympathy for my cause now stood him in invaluable stead; the Excellency was pleased to honor me with an official missive of appreciation at a function in Raj Bhawan. This gift acknowledged my work as an aggressive social intervention and acted as a timely rainfall that produces a valuable harvest. It became balm to my wounded pride, set my crawling campaign almost flying and silenced those chattering hurtful voices which had long reverberated against me.

The Governor's Letter of Honour to Dr. Rahul Shukla For Meritorious Social Service and Tiger Conservation

Suraj Bhan
Governor U.P.

સત્યમેવ જયતે

RAJ BHAVAN
Lucknow - 227 132

10.10.1999

At the turn of this century vast tracks of the country were covered with a variety of forest that provided a flourshing home for the tigers and the number of mankind was much less. Today when we get ready to enter the 21st century the official figure of tiger census has gone staggeringly low. Leaving sufficient margin for error it is more likely to be less than three thousand where as the human population has crossed 950 million with a livestock of 2 billion. Life and death issues confront project tiger today. More than twenty-five years have passed since the project was launched, the threat still looms large over tiger. Human demands on jungle have increased. The incredible pressure on natural resources seems to have further diluted the chances of tiger's long term survival as the forests have reduced to mere 8% threatening the ecosystem. Tarai areas of U.P. are one of the worst examples of man's tampering with the ecosystem where the profuse cane cultivation along the jungle borders stretches for miles and as the crops lie unattended for many months, tigers have started living in them more or less on permanent basis, emerging as a unique phenomenon.

The research work on cane tiger done by Dr. Rahul Shukla, is a path breaking study and has been recognized by the forest department of U.P. It has also for the first time highlighted the major cause for the tigers presence outside the protected zones that has given way to the man - tiger conflict which is now being rated as the greatest socio-ecological problem of Tarai. The peripheral communities of forest are directly affected by cane tiger problem. Their cattle are essentially killed by the tigers and their close interactions often result in serious injuries and deaths and even man-eating. The bane of confrontation is that villagers also kill tigers by poisoning the left overs of their prey. Only in last three year (Jan 97 - Jan 99) ten tigers had been found dead in cane crops of U.P. Tarai.

In the decade of 80s, nearly thirty tigers in all became man-eaters in successive years in Lakhimpur Kheri and Bahraich districts. As soon one man-eater was killed the other replaced it. In June '84 seven different man eating tigers operating within 100 sq. km areas outside Dudhwa National Park were known to have killed more than 200 people and the number was moving inexorably high. At such time of trouble, Rahul Shukla conceptualized the idea of **"saving men from tigers"**. He called his friend Sri Yogesh Kumar, IAS for the purpose of photography & Govt. assistance and with an aim to serve humanity, went into the remote areas of Tarai, to locate tigers in canes, mapping their movements in human zones, to inform forest department about their whereabouts and orient villages how to deal with them.

Dr. Rahul Shukla visited seventy-eight fear stricken villages, where the man-eaters had taken their toll. Most of the villagers belonged to Scheduled Castes and Tribes such as Chamar, Pasi, Mallah, Lonia and Tharus whose economic status was very poor and who hardly had any means to protect themselves against tigers. He spent nights in the villages, inspected their flimsy houses and pointed out weak points. He organized small groups of villagers to keep vigil, briefing men not to sleep outside the house or in open in the night and must move in groups, keep crackers and matchsticks in pocket must take a dog along as it will fore warn the presence of tiger and in the event of attack a tiger will prefer to take it than man. Rahul advised men to wear a human mask at the back of the head as it makes a tiger feel it is being watched and discourages him from attack and many other useful tips.

The outstanding field project of Dr. Rahul Shukla & Yogesh Kumar **"Saving men from tigers"** is still continuing in the Tarai areas Newspapers and magazines have already highlighted their efforts to achieve natural balance between man and wildlife and their commendable selfless public service. It is interesting to note that their work is fully self motivated and is not financed by any corporate or Govt. body. And in all their twenty years of service, they have never been posted in the area, like Kheri, Bahraich or Pilibhit District, in which they did the life saving service to public.

The field project started in 1984 is now 15 years old and the orientation for the protection from tigers, that was zestfully pursued in mid 80s is now more of a preventional measure due to its earlier success. Even today, cane tigers prowl round the villages at night and lie up all the day in the cane watching the population unseen and unsuspected. Fortunately, there is no man eating tiger on the record but repeated encounters with human beings can make even a normal tiger a man-eater.

The awareness campaign lead by Dr. Shukla and his friends is undoubtedly of great environmental significance as it also lays emphasis on the necessity for the protection of tiger's environment as why the prey base should not be destroyed and the forests not eradicated. Such measures will definitely prevent tigers from straying out of the jungle into human areas in search of food. The campaign has successfully resulted in a two way achievement. They have not only saved men from tigers, but it is also vice versa.

This field work has also inspired a commitment for tiger conservation in the areas of the Tarai. A number of farmers, whose cane crops, the tigers occupy, feel indebted to these friends for having given them the correct picture of tiger conservation and it is by their recommendation that the U.P. State Wildlife Department appointed several cane farmers of Tarai as Tiger Guardians. Dr. Shukla is trying to comprehend the plight of such villagers who are destinated to live in the close proximity of tigers, and saving them from the tigers is more necessary, only then in turn they will actively participate and save the big cats and their environment.

Suraj Bhan

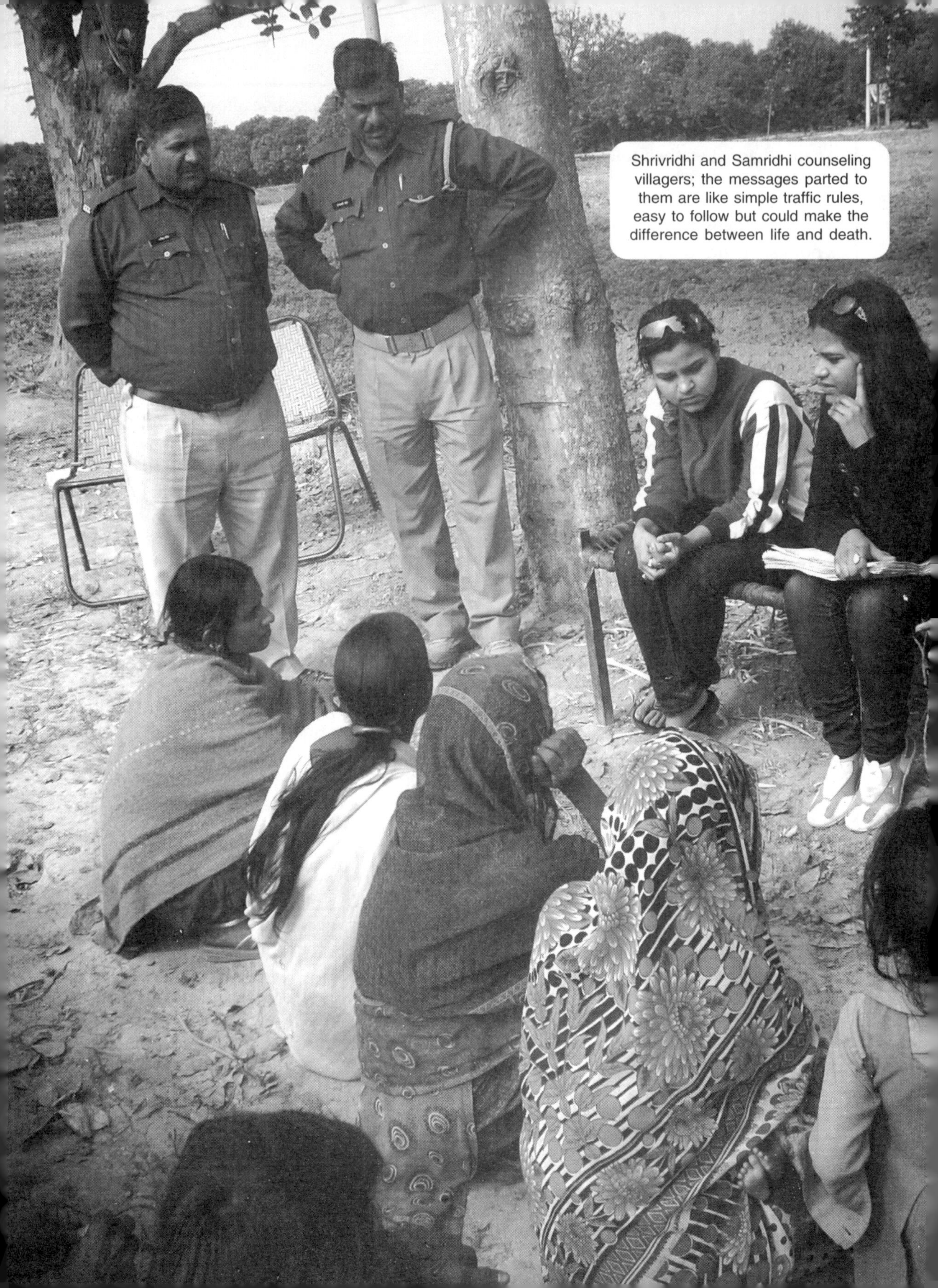

Shrivridhi and Samridhi counseling villagers; the messages parted to them are like simple traffic rules, easy to follow but could make the difference between life and death.

Appendix To Chapter 22

In Defense Of Heritage

IMPARTING OF A LEGACY

An Introduction to Determining the Future of the Experiment, 'Saving Men from Tigers through Traditional Knowledge', to conserve fierce animals in densely populated landscapes.

On March 16, 1997, I received a phone call from my old friend N. Ravi Shanker, Secretary Home to the Government of Uttar Pradesh, that a tigress had been creating problem around a village called Khanjanpurva (Maurhawa - Burkharya) in Bahraich district. She was an audacious animal, had killed over a dozen livestock and was frequently seen moving in the open fields during the day time. Livestock is monetary asset to every villager. I knew that in the face of such conflict, when the surge of carnivore attack follows on tended livestock, retaliatory killings are bound to take place. Though, till 1997 it was possible for the administrators to punctuate wild animals with accurate bullets that had become dangerous for human lives but post '97 a shift in political ideology towards the welfare of individuals had made lethal control of even problem carnivores almost impossible. The area was remote, lacking in development and politically marginalized. There were no tiger guardians and administration, having full knowledge of these disgraceful state of affairs, feared that this might set her fate soon so Ravi wanted me to reach there urgently and manage the situation.

My daughters Shrivridhi and Samridhi, ever ready to company me, did not miss the opportunity. Having driven for 240 kilometers over rough roads our team reached the village at about two in the afternoon. The administration wanted to help me so the Station House Officer of the area had already arrived and there was enough Police force waiting to assist me. I was informed that the very day in the morning the tigress had killed a couple of goats and devouring them then and there had entered an isolated pastoral coppice of *Narkul.* On hearing the occurrence I called those half a dozen herders, who had witnessed the scene and took a firsthand account from them.

One of the key components of successful conservation is communication; I encouraged some open dialogue with them and learnt that the killer was still sheltering in the cover. Two herders even admitted that this time, having become fed up of her mischief's they had made up their mind to have their revenge upon her. They had brought a bottle of pesticide called *Lintof* and were determined to sprinkle it on the remains of the goat. This was an immediate cause for alarm. Normally the predominant response to the problem of a carnivore is its removal, and when herders are highly vulnerable to chronic poverty with such a high rate of livestock killings, it seems more imminent. Furthermore, no economic incentive was being used as a conservation tool in the area so if I had to save her, I had to rid the villagers of her menacing presence. It was difficult decision but I decided to drive her away into the jungle that was some eight kilometers away.

The presence of police made things easy. A throng of over hundred people collected at my call. After sharing the information with all transparency, I appreciated their tolerance and counseled them briefly that their culture is tempered entirely to meet the demands of the tough life into which they have been born, even their forefathers had faced similar situations but never acknowledged tigers as their enemy to be slain by guns or poisoning. Their proven solution of the problem lay in pushing away the tigers from their area so we will do what their ancestors had always done.

The idea clicked the crowd. They agreed to help me for the cause; some of them even claimed that they were tolerant towards carnivores and already knew how to live with tigers. We soon set on a beat. Bicycle runners were sent in advance to the neighboring villages to inform that the beat might follow across their area and they should be prepared to participate. In the beleaguered arena of conservation techniques, all history of wildlife had swirled its way back to the present, the guns, spears and staves and excitement of people, triggering memories of sporting days when such forces were utilized in destruction of big cats but now the exotic scene seemed like a large scale local community participation programme for the protection of a problematic tiger.

Much of the sugarcane had been harvested, save for the scattered plots of wheat and lintel and the fields lay bare. The kids wanted to obtain moving pictures of tigress and this they believed could be best accomplished from my black Gypsy King.

The beat started and the tigress flushed out from the narkul retreat. It ran through the open country looking for the thick cover around but there was none for over a mile. I sped after her going about thirty to thirty five miles an hour. I knew from the past experience the difficulty in getting near a tiger in the open terrain. I crossed a wheat plot and maneuvered the vehicle close to her, whilst enduring bumps and bounces, the kids continued clicking their cameras.

By a stroke of luck, the tigress entered a flat vista of pastoral land where the grass was knee high. The cat increased her speed and so did I, following her with the hot zest. Finally we actually came alongside her at a distance of less than 20 yards and the classic situation lasted for more than half a minute. The way she concentrated on the race was a mesmerizing sight. She threw every ounce of strength into her great stride and literally flew along. Her neck was protruded, ears laid back, almost touching the head, her tail was straight and every hair along her back was rigid. With mouth wide open and her metabolism working at an entirely different tempo, she bounced like a ruddy leather ball. Every movement showing the flashing grace of her rippling muscles and straining tendons, she looked infinitely wild in her flight.

Small coveys of snipes and partridges burst out into flights between us. A pair of 'did-you-do-it' plovers, screeching eccentrically flew over the tigress, diving time to time, to prod their beaks. The spectators were breathless with admiration and the children determinedly enraptured by all the new impressions of a fugitive, flooding lavishly before them.

It was a gigantic undertaking. It took a complete exercise of four hours in which a strong crowd of six to seven villages joined the enterprise in the way. It was much like a rally race, where the crowd of one village took over from the other. Quite a few hog deer galloped out of the crops and even a pair of black bucks took to flight in their steeping and floating action. People working in their fields kept informing us about the latest location of the tigress; finally with the sunset the crowd managed to push her into the jungle. On our part, we took off our hats with a cheer to her departing hindquarters as she vanished into the jumble of dark trees.

Girls were ecstatic; 'it was simply splendid', they told the media reporters, 'the feeling of one sailing through the air with a tiger by his side is most exhilarating. Papa managed to drive with effortless ease; talked to us all the way and was not a bit nervous'.

This was one of the first really good events in their outdoor life. The unique experience initiated my daughters into the ways of the wild and whetted their appetite for more tiger adventures. Until now they had often joined my expeditions in a picnic mode and nothing had left a landmark impression on them but since then they became determined to know more about tigers and their visits to the Tarai became more frequent. I encouraged a sense of natural history in them, identifying the animals and birds, explaining the reasons for their migratory flights. It evoked too many keen memories as I shared my teen age venture with them.

Just like a doctor's child plays with the stethoscope and gives mock shots of injections they learnt to handle my rifles with élan and my book-lined room that houses my personal collection of over a thousand books on Africana and Indian Shikar became their pet retreat after dinner. The early awareness of tiger affairs and the subtlety of its nuances enlivened their inherent love of wildlife and while my wife felt excluded and superfluous in my conservation endeavors, the children shared a rapturous time and promptly came to occupy an important place in my field work.

Tiger tracking, like old time big game hunting, is a severe test of compatibility. Everything is unpredictable. Adverse conditions, ignorance, fear and fatigue of partners who track the great beasts can act as tripwires in successful ventures but as growing teenagers the girls learnt their lessons of patience and perseverance with the big cats rather well, walking on game tracks at full moon with their father. Their short conversations mixed with the doleful wail of a night heron or the sharp foxy bark of the jackal, all the while there would be the drowsy tune of the little nightjar. In some measure, it was very much on the lines as I had received my jungle training with the native hunters in Larti.

Now, the keen amateur photographers, ever eager to go after tigers comfortably manipulated cameras and their attention centered exclusively on wildlife. I have no real knowledge of the art of photography -but I believe it is a more refined sport than shooting provided you can make the tiger join the spirit of the sport without bloodshed and finally -when the clicking session is over- part like civilized beings! The gaze through the lenses of the camera on the tiger is platonic and the results immortalized on celluloid are exultant.

Rural areas of Tarai rank low in human development index, with high population density and accelerated rates of growth. The girls displayed an increasing awareness of the social consequences of protecting large cats in such landscapes and with a detached sense of professionalism tried to find scientific solutions to this situation; focusing on essentials to understand the initial motivations of natives for killing tigers in order to accurately propose viable mitigation measures that might help reduce the conflict and increase their tolerance towards carnivores. This quality which distinguished them from the crowed in childhood increased with maturity. The elder one even maintained a diary. Among her notes is a chronology of dates connected with sugar tigers where first entry is small but significant "4 tigers poisoned at Kalupurva, Dudhwa, 31.12.97. Papa is on official duty, dealing with the poachers".

The girls would record personal tales of native encounters with big cats and roam about distributing pamphlets in the mob, helped by a lady whose face was disfigured by the loss of an ear and nose in a tiger attack. In the process, they had now begun contributing new points to my old blackboard with the measures that addressed man-tiger conflict in a scientific way. This became a valuable booster in the development of my campaign and encouraged communities to participate unreservedly in the process of conservation in a proactive manner.

Despite the incredible stories told about tigers, the people who have survived their strikes and often proudly sport the scars of mauling, maintain that tigers are not necessarily vicious. They are pleased to mind their own business and let man mind his. At Tulsipur village in Pilibhit district, a tiger killed and devoured a cow just outside a residential hut near the village well. The witness told the amateur naturalists that he had heard the sounds of bone cracking in the darkness and then tearing of large chunks of flesh, which were masticated and swallowed. The killer was accompanied by a partner. The duo continued their gruesome feast uninterruptedly for quite a few hours, performing a sort of blood chilling concert at intervals. For the entire night, the shocking dreadful sounds raged within the earshot of the victim's family. Finally they left towards dawn when the cock crowed. The tigers frequented the area for months but never harmed humans.

One tiger was known to strike men down in one blow with a paw, stand over the victim and then after a few minutes, walk haughtily away without attempting to kill. He had done this with some half a dozen people.

All good conservationists study the rhythm of the wild and the culture of social communities that live in its neighborhoods. I had imposed this discipline upon myself and taught the children to do the same. Reviewing tiger attacks and reasoning scientifically we came to the conclusion that capriciousness of the tiger was the key to his powerful reputation where imagination and superstition have greatly contributed to this image. It is only when we recognize the value of the natural peaceful temperament of big cats as how they come to adapt their lives in human landscapes without creating problems we would be able to understand these aberrations.

For several years now, our work has focused on man-tiger conflict in human dominated landscapes inhabited by large number of people and essentially a few wildest of the wild cats- the tigers. These are the crisis-prone places of Tarai, where abounding marauders menace the farmers and where my family and I visit periodically, distributing pamphlets and asking the villagers to learn the incisive instructions by heart, which if acted with expediency offer a promising solution to their problem. At this instance, I have served the cause for over 27 years. The spirit of this irresistible adventure that had once entered my soul has now also taken over Shrivridhi and Samridhi. They regard tigers and their haunted zones with happy indulgent affection -the natural result of their parental legacy and happy childhood memories- and are thrilled that just by providing a few guidelines of self protection to village communities; they can deliver people from the predators, without firearms, without harming or killing them.

To reveal art and conceal artist is the arts aim, so the campaign goes on. I have a gratifying feeling that the forest sector too has started orientation programmes for the native. This appears a pro-people instance at first sight, but our effort has been as much to save tigers as it has been to save human beings.

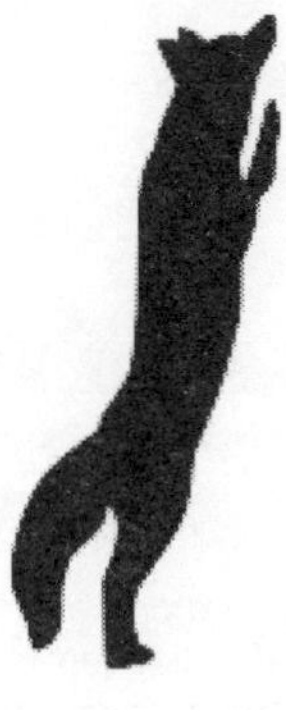

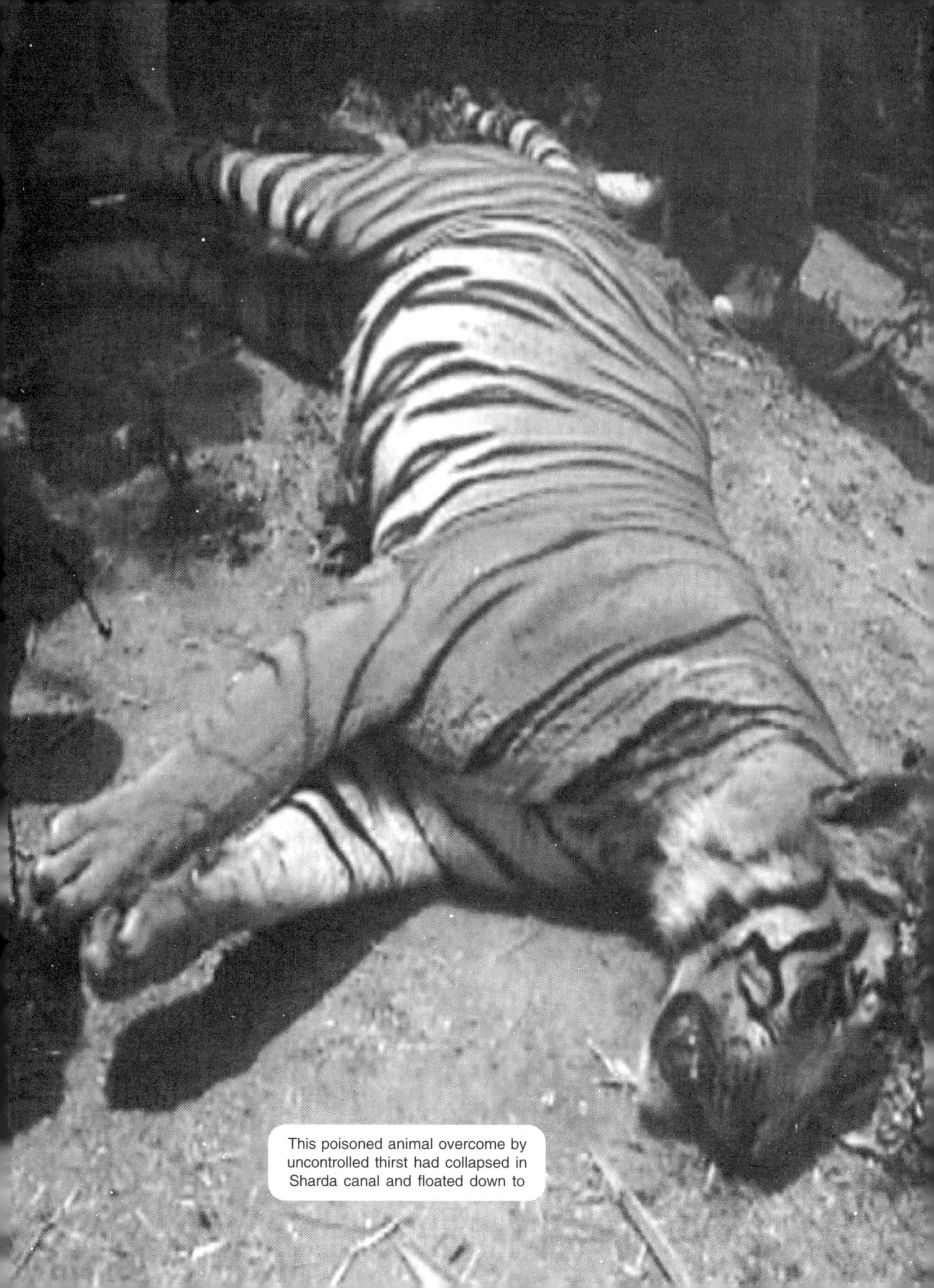

This poisoned animal overcome by uncontrolled thirst had collapsed in Sharda canal and floated down to

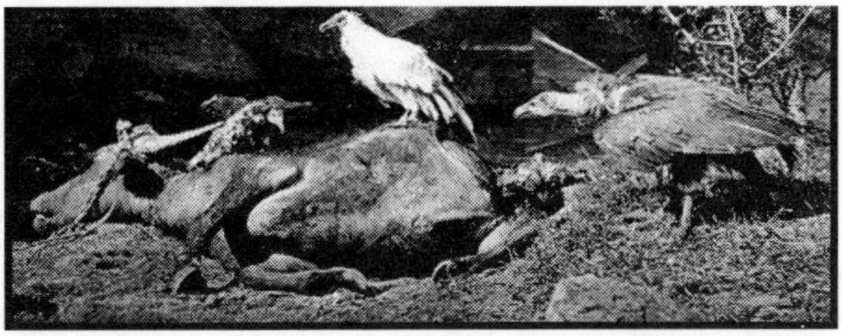

23

The Decline of Sugarcane Tiger

Tigers pay a heavy price for their role in human fantasy. They are casualty of symbolism.

- Ruth Padel

George Marsh's book, *Man and Nature,* written long ago in 1864 was a clear bugle call to mankind for conservation action. He warned the protagonists of civilization that when the balance of nature is disturbed without calculating the consequences, then man could expect all kinds of disaster. Marsh described life as a web made up of every single organism; where the destruction of any part of web could disrupt the whole biological community. It has been only less than one hundred years that the value of wildlife has been fully appreciated and wildlife specialists have come to know much about animals and their relationship to each other within their complex environment. Ecology of living things is now an important branch of biology, in which the original core of wildlife scientist tries to explore more about the ecology of wildlife and its multifaceted relationship with man on priority. It tries to do so by deriving a simple index that tracks ups and downs of biological matrix under the influence of the forces of nature and largely the cumulative impact of human civilization. The human societies that surround the animal are undergoing dramatic and rapid changes. That is why if wildlife is to be saved fresh strategies and tactics are needed to be invented.

In the 1940s, an American forester Aldo Leopold had first generated the idea of modern wildlife management which was approvingly hailed for its utility in sustainable harvest of abundant species and regulation of wildlife pests. In 1960s a wildlife scientist, Professor Bernhard Grzimek pioneered the idea of grass-root conservation, followed by Dr. George Schaller, who fostered a new approach to conservation, now termed as "Conservation Biology"; still a step further Dr. Ullas Karanth mooted the idea of conservation through technical science, which has become a new tool to explore the world of the tiger and safeguard its biological diversity on a multiple scale.

Wildlife conservation is a vast enterprise. An average person is bewildered by the wide range of conservation activities, many of them in places he never heard of and most of them are of a complicated nature. Correspondingly, conservation of sugarcane tiger is decidedly a complex matter, it encompasses many major and minor problems in the preservation and management of natural resources within human surroundings, which are practically not workable and where its many capricious proposals are affected by chance and human will. The only workable conservation plans will be those that improve conditions for both tigers and people.

Unlike America, we do not have leaders in farmland conservation, which might battle to find ways of helping wildlife of countryside. The scientists at the farms, who understand the pressure farmers undergo to produce more food for us, also know about modern farming compulsions that hasten the decline of wildlife. They know that now their work is more vital than ever if they have to halt this decline.

My past experience of wildlife related issues had taught me that with each passing year, tiger conservation is going to become even more problematic than it has been earlier, because it is not an easy task to decide as to which human interventions might be wise to save tigers and which might not. Actually the lack of trustworthy information is a major handicap in rationalizing the issue of tiger conservation in farmlands.

I had a sour feeling that I was losing time, so I tried making an effort to shape a consumable concept of conservation in this framework, thinking in terms of long term practices in favor of both humans and tigers. Both ways it was essentially a pro-tiger campaign.

The major problems facing the protection of sugarcane tiger are related to people and their livestock. Thus, my first solution was to hit upon the root of the problem so that the sugarcane tiger phenomenon is first contained and then gradually brought to a natural end. It was utterly realistic and based on the basic principle of achieving large scale separation measures between man and the wild animal. If humans can be removed from tiger zones such as in Ranthambhore and Simlipal sanctuary then the tiger should also be removed from human zones, howsoever enormous the operations may be.

This was nipping the problem in the bud. It was unfortunate, but definitely a pragmatic conclusion to a queer chapter of natural history, because on scientific parameters, creation of a wildlife refuge within cane farms is neither practical nor financially viable. Conserving tigers, ecologically in the sugarcane is an irrational thing because sooner or later it will become counterproductive and lead to a catastrophe. I was sure that this strategy would assuage anti-tiger forces that represented a formidable aggregate of pressure groups. I suggested that a buffer zone devoid of sugarcane that should not be less than ten kilometers in length, be instituted around forest trails of Tarai and especially around Dudhwa National Park. Here, the farmers should be given full compensation for not growing sugarcane. As an alternative income-generating opportunity they should be encouraged to grow other staples such as wheat, barley, mustard and other short crops, which tigers do not relish.

This serious conservation option was sure to dilute the trouble as a specific solution to the problem, for then the sugarcane tigers will return to the restricted space of jungles and their automatic systems of population control will adjust their numbers. It is plain and simple — if we cannot adjust with or look after something that has come down to us in nature we have to plug its growth before a clash occurs under the baleful influence of man and the mentally inferior species loses its final battle. This way a putative creed might wane, but an ecological catastrophe will come to an end and the future of the Tarai tiger will be safe in the wilds.

The situation normatively seemed ideal, but it was bound to deal with severe challenges on grounds of impracticality. The motivating factor in all this is of course money. And the solution to the problem of saving tigers is also a matter of money. If adequate compensation was not awarded to the farmers, the cultivation of sugarcane would continue along the jungle and with it the tricky phenomenon would again regenerate, to go on unabated. In this case, the second solution of conserving this tiger within human landscape had to be applied. We needed to think bigger on these lines because it was a formidable task and involved grave risks; people not only interacted with tigers but also impinged the normal movement of their natural prey like deer, antelopes and wild boar, and this disturbance was now in fact a part of the ecology for this tiger, who was now well adapted to it. In this way, until the authorities were prepared to embrace bold and imaginative steps, the conservation of this animal was not possible.

Human intervention invariably plays a greater role but often even good intentions prove bad in practice. Thus, the whole exercise had to be based on solid scientific grounds as well as rational understanding of the social context and intensified conservation educational work among local communities and also the land management policies of farmers. A timely, purposeful and rational action can facilitate reduced human impact on these animals, forestall man-tiger conflict and help their survival.

Unquestionably, if we hope to preserve an assortment of wildlife, we must continue to research for ways by which man and wildlife can coexist. The inevitable future of this earth is a burgeoning growth of human population and less and less space for wildlife. It needs to be understood that the issues of tiger's survival involve philosophy as much as conservation issues and that when human progress and economic development of villages cannot be halted, the survival needs of the tiger in the sugar-fields will always rival the needs of people. Therefore, we cannot view these protected areas in isolation from the surrounding socio-economic realities and developmental priorities of the Government. This calls for a cross-sectoral and cross-disciplinary approach.

A long-term conservation consciousness was needed to perform this job. As the phenomenon was to continue indefinitely in the human area, I phrased this consciousness as 'strategic conservation', where wildlife conservation should no longer be the concern of a few specialists; it is and should be everybody's business.

Finally, the key to successful conservation of cane tiger will be an informed villager and the government focusing on settling the compensation of the villagers who lose their cattle. It was for the natives to decide whether they believed in this conservation movement and felt proud about it.

My idea of creating tiger guardians was the first step in this crisis management and at least in North Kheri the template had partially succeeded. In five years I was to know whether I had succeeded in winning the battle or not. Tiger guardian is not a panacea for conservation but I am sure in accord with the whole paradoxical nature of animal predation this incentive-driven ploy could make an important contribution towards safety of the sugar tigers everywhere and even for the sugar leopards in the state of Maharashtra. It was built on ancient knowledge and belief that local people have the motivation to tolerate rather than kill predators. The campaign was intended to promote and remind villagers that they already know how to live with tigers. The involvement of just one dedicated volunteer naturalist from each village could mark an important approach to monitoring big cats. Then on the basis of the data collected from the field he could assist the managers to make the best decisions for the animal's welfare that will facilitate their eventual survival.

It is said that conservation is invariably a compromise between the need to protect wildlife and the aspirations of local human population. I sometimes wondered when at present, several reserves protect aborigines and wildlife as a part of the same ecosystem, despite the fact that the aborigine's life is contaminated by modern civilization and its inventions, then why a similar rhythm cannot be generated between sugarcane tiger and farmers.

However, a niggling time for the tigers had once again begun in earnest. Perhaps the bounty hunting of tigers for many past centuries had parted us with tons of excuses, and the macho psyche had trickled down the time unconsciously.

Politicians were constantly asserting that the Kheri district had the most acute man-eating problem to date and most of the sugar tigers were obsessive man-eaters, whereas my observations at Bishunpurva, Barotha and then Nighasan glens were encouraging proof that the big cats on no account regarded humans as prey species even at the places where they had grown accustomed to the presence of humans. Apart from a few minor demonstrations put up by cub rearing tigresses - that too at the time of harvesting of crops- they had never attacked human beings at liberty. I could confidently count a few tigers that even in the excitement of hunting a stray cattle, had deliberately avoided aggression on herders and other human intruders.

For this purpose, I suggested that before the season, when conflicts are anticipated, due publicity should be given and education programs be launched through newspapers and by distributing pamphlets. I also suggested launching a scheme to organize anti-depredation watch committees in the line of Village Forest Protection Committees. These committees should keep track of problem animals or females rearing cubs and inform the villagers and the Forest Department in case of approaching emergencies. Measures must be taken to ward off the problem-causing animals from the site which must include the use of high-intensity focus light, crackers, drums and fire-torches. Whenever some particular animal is linked with a series of incidents, it should be immediately removed from the site.

Towards the end of my tenure as member of State Wildlife Advisory Board by 1997, I recommended to the government to give complete protection to this tiger till its ecological status is established by necessary research investigations. I emphasized that tiger is undeniably a dangerous hunter but equally undeniable is its goodness and restraint regarding humans. For every day, hundreds of farmers, school going children, laborers, honey gatherers, grazers, grass cutters and small time traders pass through arable fields and all return home alive and well. One may not see tigers during the day for they rest in thickets; yet lumbering human beings do blunder past them safely. It means that tigers tolerate human presence, both in jungle and sugarcanes and thus they qualify to be protected.

I even stated that in last thirty years, save for man-eaters, most of which were created by human error, we would fail to collect even half dozen genuine accounts of deliberate attack by sugar tigers whereas in the meantime hundreds of sugar tigers must have fallen prey to poachers in their home. I also pointed out some key human use areas and farmlands, which are still biologically exceptionally endowed regions and which despite the human use of resources, could still be declared as Sites of Special Scientific Interests (SSSIs), if their present characteristic is truthfully maintained and preserved for research.

One such landholding, for example, is a four thousand acre agrarian patch of Ghola. Bounded to the south by Naudha Baghar and to the west and north by Soheli stream with a lake in its centre, this human dominated landscape is situated on Sampurna Nagar road. Once a favored stomping ground of swamp deer, it has now been entirely de-grassed for cultivation. I am constantly amazed at the way the tigers invariably linger in this habitat niche of sugar fields, unmindful of human competitors. For last thirty years, without any break of season, one tiger, or a tigress with cubs, have essentially lived in this area, paying a visit in the night even during pinch period. Here the self imposed barrier is voluntarily maintained, which is seldom trespassed. This country stretching in the rotund shape of a cup is seemingly equipped with a stop- valve, which only allows one tiger at a time.

Another example is the Kanp-Tanda area, a low-lying ten thousand acre stretch of uninterrupted sugarcane plantations. This flood vulnerable landscape is bounded to the west by river Sharda and to the east by a high rise of running mounds and Kishanpur sanctuary and is in the shape of a crescent moon. Here tigers mostly females effectively hold stable ranges all through the year and the visit of males from jungle is not a subject to stringent seasonal schedules.

To back up my proposal for practical purposes, I presented pictures of cane tigers and submitted the clippings of my newspaper articles to the board, emphasizing that we have a plethora of studies related to the pattern of tiger attacks on livestock and people but nobody has ever conducted a study which could tell as how the majority of dangerous animals manage themselves in farmlands and live near humans without causing any harm. There were leopards in Mahrashtra that lived amongst high densities of people without inflicting any harm to people. A radio collared leopardess, living in sugar fields in Gujarat, was within 50 meter of people most of the time, yet the cane strippers were not aware of her presence and when her cubs died due to human nuisance she just left the area without creating any problem.

But it was sad to know that everyone had some kind of objection for the carnivorous animals. I may be pardoned for saying that many members of the then Board were inspired by the false reputation for ferocity ascribed to wild beasts. They believed in the established tradition that all the predators are dangerous and exhibited an inordinate terror of tigers. In particular cases, this terror may not be altogether unfounded, for rogues exist in every species, including the human, but it is certainly groundless in connection with tigers in general and one cannot let their atypical behavior vilify their whole race. However, the members confidently held the prevailing notion on the subject, confusion and fear reigned supreme and my project was consigned to sidelines. As anticipated, no budget was allotted and no research was mooted for the cause.

I wrote several protesting letters to sympathetic people in authority but nothing happened. In fact anybody who attempts to interfere with the existing order is immediately obstructed by politicians because the system protects the vested interests of powerful people. I had not thought that I would not get even a little help from the establishment whose trustworthiness rests in protecting wildlife, whereas any research on this phenomenon might have dispelled many canards and stochastic factors associated with the small population of these animals.

It had been a long struggle and I was crestfallen. There was no supporting advance at the end than there had been at the beginning. I was left without help to guard my sugar tigers; an unofficial factotum to carry out the duties of forest department in the farmland.

More than ever I felt that I was alone in my efforts.

(II)

Things had certainly moved full circle by now and the magnificent sugar-cats were indeed back on the danger list. The future of cane tiger was threatened. Though I had set clear timelines for the animal that at current levels of output, this historical legacy was not expected to last for more than ten years, and due to rampant poaching and vengeful killings, its red list status had seemingly dipped down from Endangered to Critically Endangered, which meant that it was just one

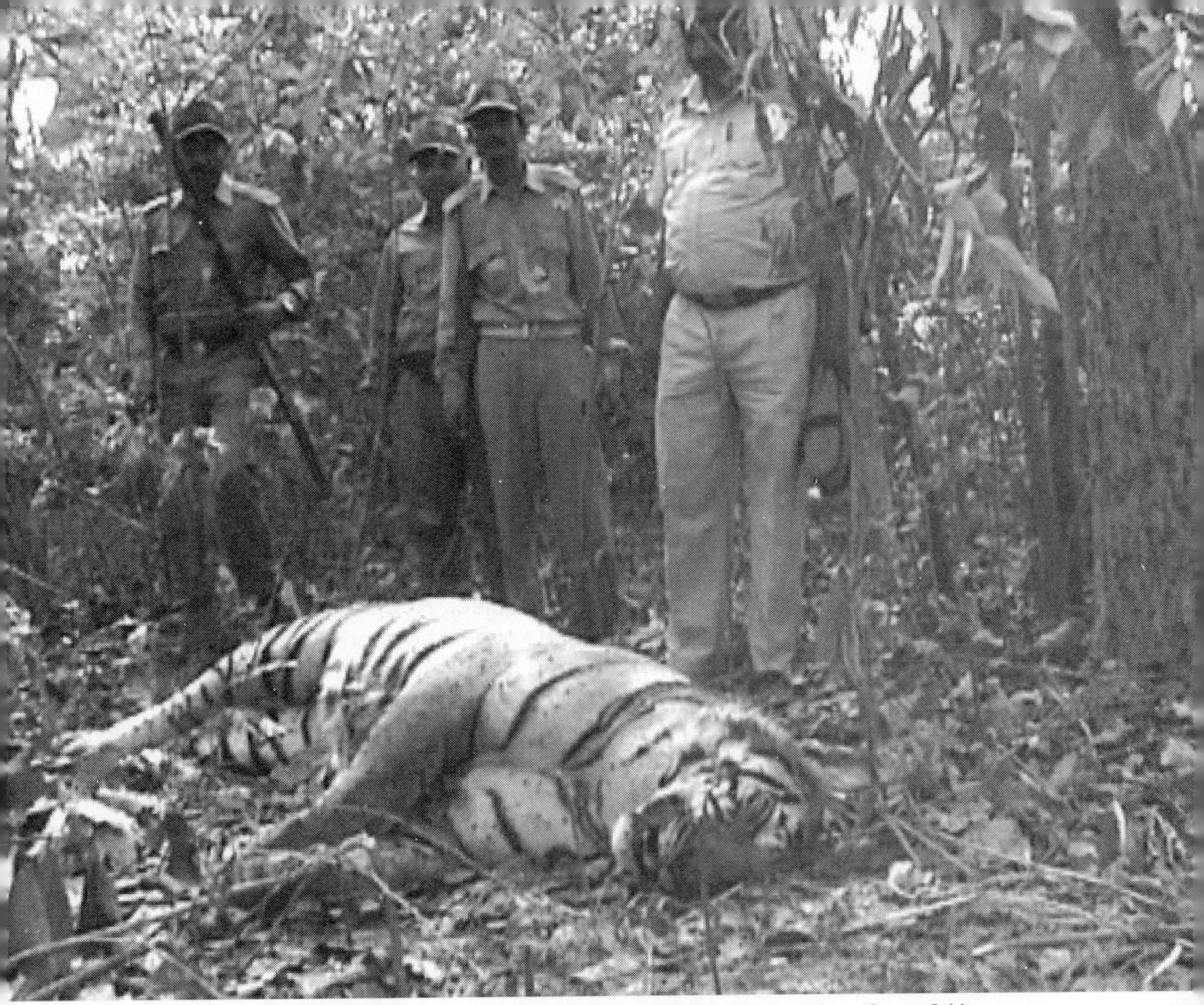

This tiger was electrocuted by stretching live wire along the boundary of sugar field near Paraspur on 6 Jan 2010

stop away from extinction, yet as usual, the foresters had preferred to look right through the scale of imbroglio. As a result, there was nothing like so many tigers as it used to be at the earlier times. The sound of guns and man's role of predator had taught them afresh to be on defensive. The bad lesson had changed their perception of man and they moved under the cover of darkness. These were beleaguered tigers, which had been hunted and fired at on some occasion during their life, and such a partly molested or a missed tiger, when recovers from an injury or mental shock never forgets such a horrendous occurrence. Therefore there was no guarantee of seeing a tiger in the farms now, in fact sugar farms seemed to be losing their tiger tag.

The reasons for the decline of sugar tigers were several, that I observed with exasperation and helplessness. One of the major reasons was the unfortunate change in attitude of the bureaucracy supervising the project. Influenced by the so-called man-eating phenomenon, the state had shifted its center of emphasis from saving the tiger to saving the ecosystem first. The spectacular beast was no longer the symbol of a healthy environment; its presence in the sugarcane was rather taken as debasing factor in the normal environment, which was affecting the entire ecosystem like a malignant growth. Hence, Project Tiger had changed direction and the sugarcane tiger was the first casualty.

There were many factors threatening the survival of their population. There was no tiger management in sugar fields and no game patrols to protect these animals, there were no scientists either. Tiger numbers are hugely important metric, it was essential to know how many were dying naturally, how many were being shot and trapped each year, and how many cubs were surviving to offset this mortality rate. All this was too cumbersome a calisthenics to work out for an individual like me, lacking in funds, equipments and resources. I had no means to reckon the calculation of tiger population in sugarcane fields; I had adopted an awkward method of counting dead tigers to keep a track on my subject. Hopelessly and haplessly, during the nineties, I was merely counting dead animals hit upon randomly in sugar fields; whatever the actual number, my 'reverse counting' was proof that the tigers were still established there.

Natural causes for the death of a tiger are not many. Disease either does not appear to be a prominent cause of death in tigers. Burton reported two cases of rabies in tigers while E.P. Gee noted a tigress heavily infested with ticks. Belding reported of tigers becoming infected with cystode by eating an excessive frog diet. And even Moniez, the parasite of cows, had been found in the faces of cattle lifting tigers. Tigers were also reported of dying of oriental lung fluke. Cat, dog, goat, pig and of course man is a definitive host of this fluke. And if these are part of a tiger's diet, including snail, the disease can be a prominent cause of death. Adult tigers addicted to putrescent flesh also die of infestation of tapeworms. Billy Arjan Singh notes that tiger cubs are susceptible to intestinal and liver ailments.

Pinch period landscapes function as islands of conservation for the sugar tigers. These bits of capital cover, scattered here and there, appear to have favoured their survival for decades. But as, ever since the founding of the refugee colonies, the forestlands of Tarai have been subjected to continuous exploitation; the rapid disappearance of such cover continues to be the chief reason for depletion of sugar tigers. These privately owned haunts served as umbilical cords in the proximity of sugar farms, representing an array of diverse ecosystems outside the protected zone. These include alluvial grasslands, tree forests, shrub lands, sub-montane forests, thorn forests, swamps, glens etc, where a number of shrubs, herbs and grasses grow — the most common being *Cannabis sativa* or *bhang*, *Lantana camara* and elephant grass. Large bamboo strands also occur frequently near villages in several blocks.

During my early expeditions in Kheri and Pilibhit districts, I saw quite a few such wooded fragments of natural Tarai in the neighborhood of farms; Sonasar, Bharkaliganj, Benda, Lohangapur, Machahera and Sauraha, Haripur, Besalganj,

Digia were such great vistas that alternated with unbeatable bogs and dense cover that held a fairly bright promise as a suitable home for sugar tigers, supporting a compact biota for the perpetual maintenance of an integrated ecological fabric in nature.

Many great chunks of marsh and grasslands, which were leased to large scale farmers, had not been cultivated for many decades because of the government's policy of imposing a ceiling on the size of holdings and distributing the surplus land to landless labour. Till the end of the last millennium, they were fairly free from the pressure of advancing human settlements. Many of them were of true wild character, where I had seen the marks of monitor lizard, mouse deer, four horned antelopes and panthers and even heard a sambhar bell one night.

In 1998, the scenario drastically changed. The state government cleared a populist bill that thoughtlessly allowed the annual contract system for the peasantry to cultivate the additional land. The tightly packed and fine spans of grasslands were leased out to landless people for the opening up new agricultural frontiers and several such forest patches were exacerbated under the heavy pressure of animal husbandry and wood poaching.

The old Forest Act provides people living in and around a protected area a right to collect and remove forest produce for 'bona fide needs' but unfortunately there is no definition of what the phrase means. From the vantage point of the outside world, the forests offer a more concrete and wholesome support system for man and livestock alike, in terms of edible vegetation and fodder availability, so it is natural for the villagers to impinge upon them.

The environmentalism of the poor sees the environment as a source of livelihood. In many villages of Tarai government aided 'Gobar Gas Plants' have sprung up, where dung producing animals are maintained in large numbers. Their number often becomes disproportionate to the actual forage of the area. The cattle degrade the forest chunks by overgrazing the favoured fodder plants while natives denude the trees of their foliage in search of fire wood. Herders also climb trees to the top branches to cut fodder to feed their hungry livestock. The excessive density of cattle reduces the fertility and productivity of the soil and the local forest, unable to regenerate its old character, gradually dies. Thus one more shelter that had protected generations of sugarcane tigers and 'where they had lived determined to return into the long grass of canes when the opportunity arose' is removed for their itinerary.

Some unsavory villagers are in the habit of appropriating tiger's natural kills. When a tiger brings down an antelope or a wild boar, the squeals and squeaks of dying victim often advertise its position to farmers working near-by. They create a din, drive the tiger away and collect an inexpensive supply of fresh meat. In the northern area of Pilibhit district, where cane tigers occur, I estimated that five out of every ten wild preys brought down by tigers, are eaten by human scavengers. As a growing teenager in Larti, I remember having participated in the native feasts

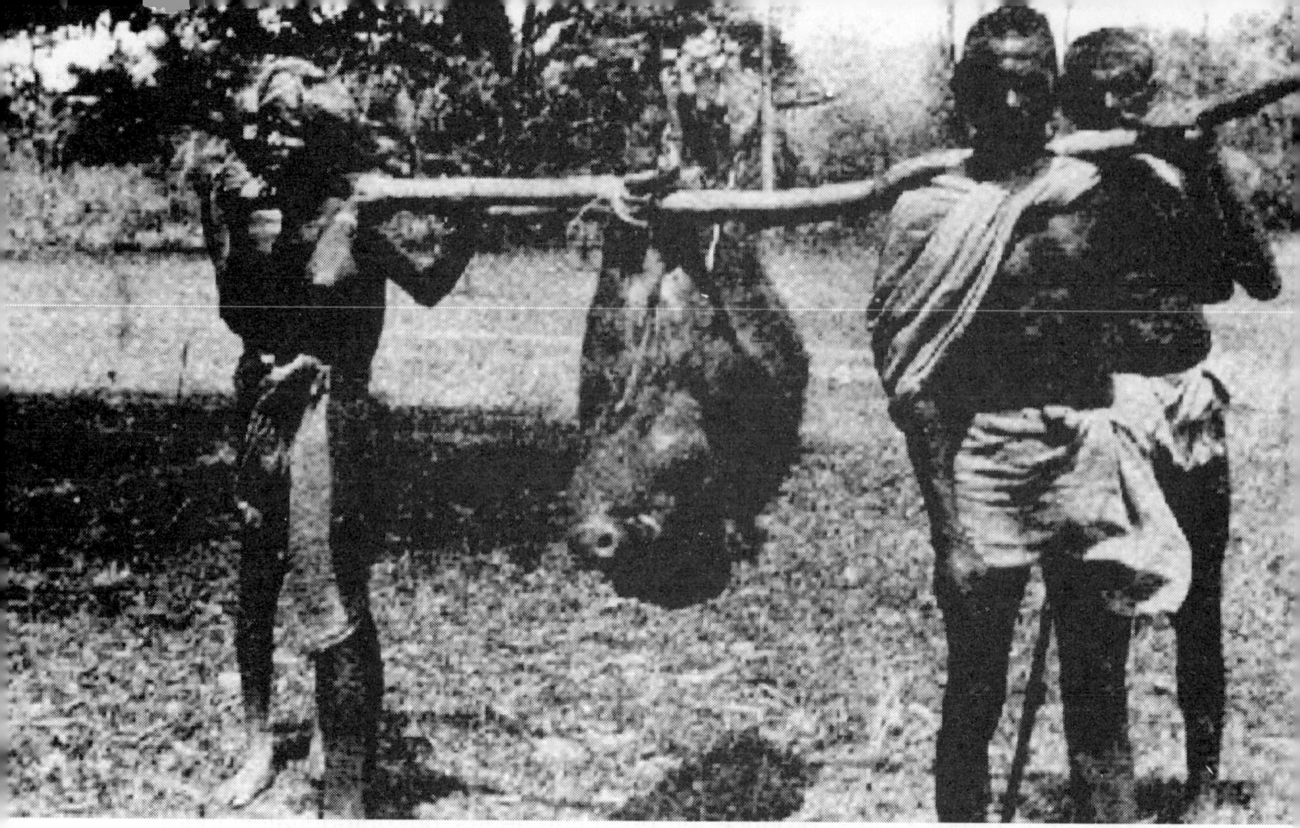

An appropriated tiger kill by villagers

of stolen meat, a hog deer, chital or a wild boar. It was a badge of honor to dine on a tiger's kill that made wonderful curries. Now, as I judge in retrospect the brutality and the callousness of the act it is easy to assume that many tiger cubs die of starvation as the milk production of their mothers is drastically reduced when their well-merited prey is stolen.

The epidemic of revengeful killing by locals is another significant cause. Hungry tigers strike down cattle and their owner sprays poisonous chemicals on the carcass, using pesticides namely Carbofuran, BHC Gamma, Lindane, Lintaf, Hepta Chlorine and Paradon etc which are freely available for crop protection from pests. Tigers feed upon them, fall unconscious and die.

However, as far as I know cats are sensitive to smells and tastes, and, normally it is very difficult to poison a cat by chemical poisoning. It will instantly spit the morsel at any unfamiliar smell unless a sophisticated substance with minimum taste and smell is used. Such poisons are naturally not available to villagers. In the case of tigers dying of pesticide poisoning the only possible explanation is that by living in canes they are so accustomed to the smells of sprinkled pesticides that their olfactory and gustatory senses dilute and they turn insensitive even to such chemicals in their food that kill them.

Often to execute vengeance on the enemy, the natives bury crude home-made bombs in livestock carcass which blow away the jaws of tiger that feeds on it.

Electrocution is yet another technique to poach wildlife. High-voltage electricity wires illegally tapped from the running power poles are used to charge the hidden stumble wires laid across the beaten paths of animals. Tigers and other wildlife using these paths are easily electrocuted.

The recurrent monsoon floods have also become a major contributing factor to the decline of tiger numbers in Tarai. The flood situation worseness dramatically when the bordering state of Nepal releases hundreds of thousands of cusecs of water into Indian rivers and the entire tiger habitat in Pilibhit, Kheri and Bahraich districts gets submerged under two meters of water. Survival poses a tough challenge to tiger cubs and prey animals both in the jungle and farmlands. The sudden deluge leaves thousands of the villages totally marooned and as rescue and evacuation of villagers takes precedence for local administration, tiger cubs and deer fawns are helplessly swept away in water currents. Villagers often spot them speeding along with water current, while the animals reaching the bank are slaughtered by lathi blows.

In 2007, Nepal released 11 lakh cusecs of water from Girja barrage. Next year, it let off 17 lakh cusecs and in 2009 it reached a record 21 lakh cusecs of water, disturbing the ecology of the region beyond repair. Human beings can be rushed to safety under emergencies but evacuation of wild animals in disaster is still an unknown art to mankind.

It is not be an exaggeration to state that human-caused mortality accounts for most of the tigers in sugarcanes than natural deaths. Males, females and young cubs are destroyed indiscriminately by villagers. They die as a result of having been snared, speared, electrocuted or poisoned than through any other cause. They remain vulnerable to human predation and certainly do not live their full life cycle.

Human populations around tiger reserves are now easily connected to global markets through local and regional markets and poaching is always a cost-effective option for a villager to ignore. Consider the price of a bullet, Jin-trap, net or snare to kill a tiger, against an estimated US$ 50,000 that the skin and bones fetch in the market or the venison of a chital, which can sell for around five thousand rupees.

Changing this trajectory of wildlife extinction is a challenging task. The proportion of such professional netters and poachers may be quite small in rural populace but their success rate is very high. The toll taken by them is never ceasing. Day in, day out, through all seasons and from year to year, they keep active. It attacks the fountainhead of animal life — females, immature and young. This throws a tremendous impact on tigers' principal prey, which consequently manipulates tiger populations; in effect toward depletion.

The encumbrance of population control of wild animals rests in the hands of nature. They are inured to routine of a flood or famine, and death by drought or starvation, which work as modalities of population hold back, whereas humans are practically immune to these processes of oppression mooted by Mother Nature. They are not governed by natural conditions; they have complete control of their

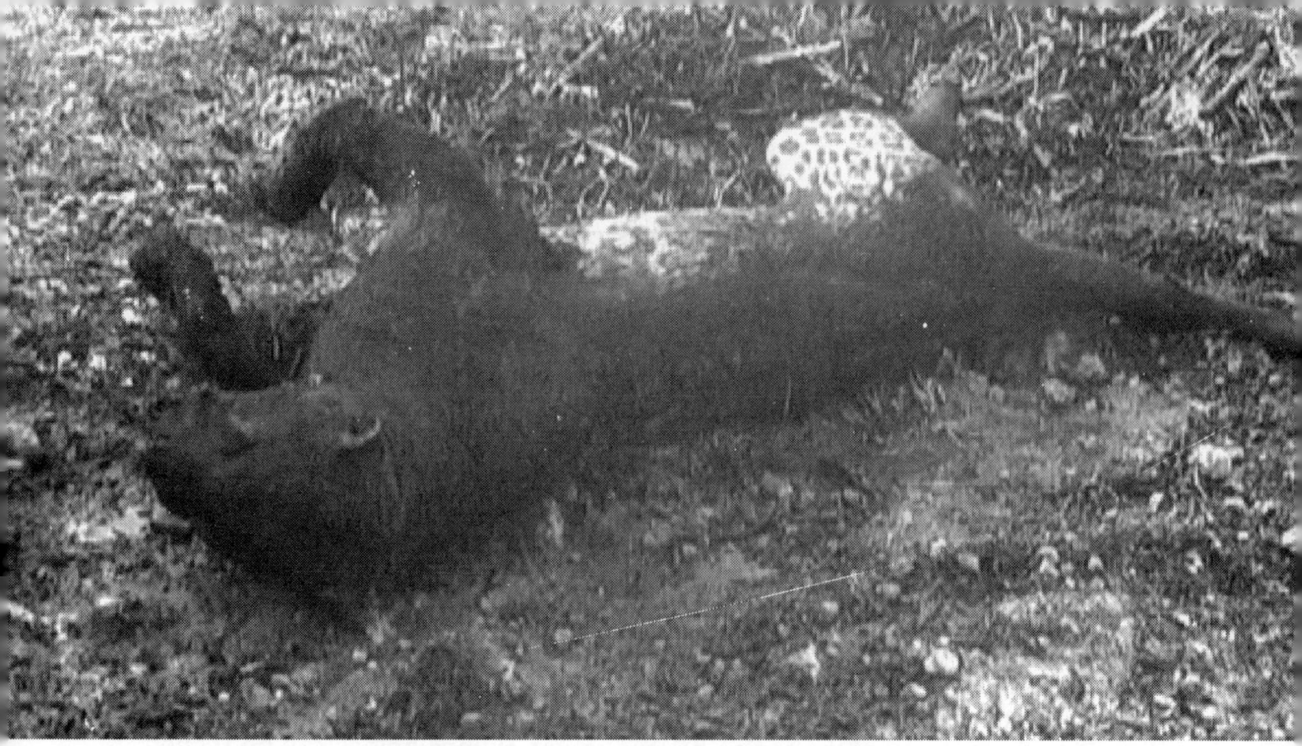

A leopard burnt down by villagers in the cane fields near Isanagar township, district Kheri in 2006

own destiny. Any potential limitation posed by the natural world is surpassable using human ingenuity.

Consequently, their contemporary population, resulting from advanced medical treatment and technological improvements in industry and agriculture, has radically affected the guard of nature.

In last thirty years, I have seen small hamlets of a dozen people turning into full standard villages of over two to three hundred people, where contemporary child population is more than half of the adult population. India's burgeoning population has been hampering overall growth in all sectors. Due to this, we have failed miserably in checking the disappearance of our forests, shrinking agricultural land and natural resources. This has created an ecological mismatch between numbers of consumers and its poor biological resource base, the truly scientific description of which will be more alarming and drastic to understand.

The material aspiration of unskilled, uneducated and often unintelligent people of remote areas, where the booming market economy has penetrated is yet another dangerous signal for wildlife. Everywhere there is evidence of the altered economic equation and many a traditionally poor have become new riches of the area; because there are commercial interests that spend millions of dollars to destroy our environment.

Even if overly optimistic notions about tigers' continued existence are proclaimed and the entire mankind decides that the tiger should be saved for posterity, ultimately his fate will depend on whether or not the lunatic speed of human population is checked and checked soon. Before the social order is swamped by ill-bred, ill-fed swarms of socio-economically unproductive-citizens, we have to start conserving whatever resources are left and strictly control the growth of this ill-rated population if we want our country to progress.

(III)

In contrast to the jungle tigers, which are relatively safe, the cane dwellers are freely available to poachers. Their exceeding vulnerability is undeniably the single-most important cause for the decline of their population. However, from time to time, newspapers were inviting debate on the recurrent phenomena and it had attracted the attention of poaching networks. While the pseudo wildlife pundits in Delhi tried to rationalize in their AC rooms whether tigers can find breeding cover in sugar crops and whether the cane tigers can really exist, the poachers understood the distilled essence of news and lost no time to appearing in the cane fields.

I am a historian by profession and the most cogent analogy that comes in my mind to illustrate this contradiction in terms, is from my own discipline. Strangely, the honor of being first archaeologist goes to the petty band of criminals, the burglars and robbers, who plundered the Egyptian Pyramids and the Roman cities of Pompeii and Herculaneum, which were destroyed by volcanic ash-rains of Vesuvius and lay burried for over a thousand years. Mustafa, Yuheed, Oscar Esecpano, Suprono and Sungon are a few names that are acknowledged as the first ever known excavators of these lost civilizations. They were thieves and murderers on lookout for easy money; they brought magnificent curios from the buried cities and sold them for a cheap price in the fourteenth century French and Italian markets. The flux of such antiques gradually created popular interest of European elite in their history and focused the eyes of the world on these ancient settlements, which were centuries later declared as protected sites and brought to light by qualified archaeologists.

Similarly, the poachers were the first conscientious believers in my cane tiger theory. The kingpins alerted their commands and like the 'honorable thieves' of archaeology the bands of poachers arrived in the fields and started collecting the booty. Sugarcane plantations became their paradise. All this happened because there were no means to prevent the destruction of wildlife outside the forest areas, there was no patrolling and no means to enforce the legislation. This continued for years, till one fine morning the truck loads of contraband products were caught by Ghaziabad police near Delhi. The subsequent interrogation of culprits revealed that a larger chunk of confiscated tiger skins was collected from the farmlands of Tarai. The catch sounded an alarm bell. One thing was simple that cane tigers were on their way to nemesis; much like the reminiscent of stray chickens in the world of foxes.

It bears remembering to late S.R. Chaudhary's suggestion that a 'Tiger Watch' force should be raised by the forest department to monitor farm tigers in the Tarai but the advice was never seriously heeded. It was an unrewarding posting for a forest officer and there were no takers for it. The proposal is still gathering dust in government files and traffickers are continuing having a blast.

The massive hatred built up against the tigers also contributed to their large scale poisoning and poaching. The involvement of local communities in commercial poaching ultimately became the genesis for the chaos, causing an irreversible plummeting of their population. An unpleasant name that recurrently enunciates for nearly twenty years is that of Bheema Bawaria. This notorious criminal operates between Uttarakhand and Uttar Pradesh and is a killer of tigers. Villagers fear him because he is tough and looks like a mad booboo, who cannot think beyond death and violence. He is absconding for many years, and perhaps still active, he is said to have dispatched over a fifty tigers single handedly.

Repeat offenders are a serious problem. Om Prakash, a tiger poacher was arrested in Corbett Tiger Reserve in 2003, with a number of tiger traps in his possession. He is believed to have killed as many as fifteen tigers since then and was arrested again for killing of three tigers in 2009. Deen Dayal Bilwal, a leading poacher who shoots tiger for pleasure of sport near Corbett and then sells their skins has been arrested thrice. Another criminal is Dariya, arrested four times with tiger skins at Palamu, Bihar, Katarnia Ghat and Bandhvgarh. He was recently prosecuted in a fresh case and was punished with a fine of Rs 10,000 and 3 months' rigorous imprisonment.

With the boom in information technology, cheap mobile phones have become available to common villagers and as its result global market forces have penetrated deep into Tarai. There are no laws and no patrolling by foresters in cultivation fields and the enforcement is at its lowest ebb. The poachers invariably keep each other informed about occasional patrols and make a field day. Touring gangs of such poachers are regular visitors to Tarai fields, where harassed villagers happily co-operate with anybody who attempts to exonerate the menace. Forest authorities claim that poaching has leveled off as there are no captures occurring inside the Park while statistics implies that the pressure on the Park would only increase when the game is exterminated outside its boundaries.

Animals are no longer killed in order to gain room to live, they are not hunted to feed hungry people, they are now slaughtered for money. A group of poachers from Allahabad with political connections has had a great time killing around 30-35 tigers in every winter season. Shabbir Quarishi confessed of having smuggled over 600 tiger skins during his two decade long unlawful business. Wanted by CBI, Shabbir, the guiding power behind the poaching ring and 15 others were arrested by Special Task Force (STF) from his house in Kareli locality of Allahabad where three tiger skins and a complete skeleton was recovered from his possession. Investigators believed that Shabbir was the pointsman of Tsering Atup Tamang and Wong Kim Quee -- ethnically Tibetan and Napalese citizens who happen to be a resident of Humla near Chinese border. Tamang is also accused in Ghaziabad and Khaga seizures of UP in 1999 and 2000. He was till now doing business with Sansar Chand and is supposed to be one of the biggest buyers of animal hides and bones from India.

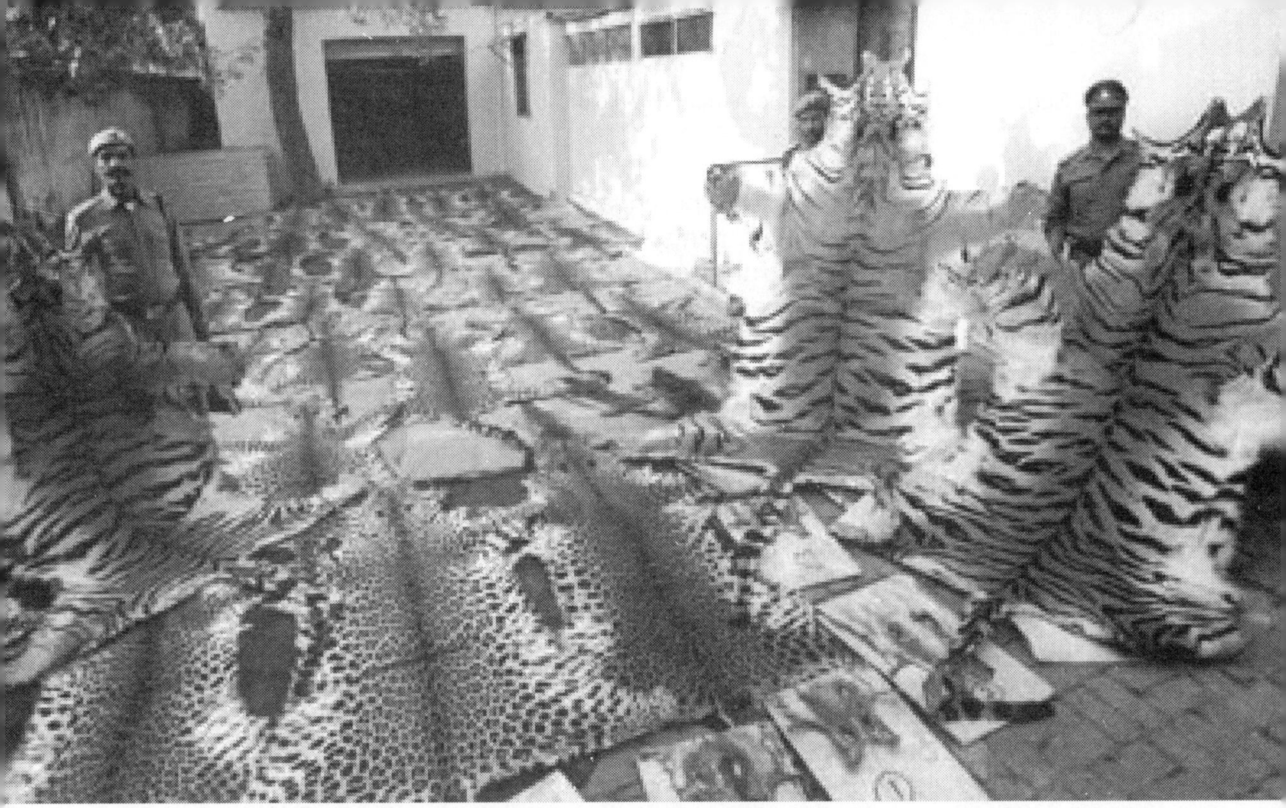

Police officers Rajeev Ranjan Verma and Dr. Arvind Chaturvedi confiscated these tiger & leopard skins from illegal trafficars at Allahabad in 2003

The signature of Tsering found on skins seized in Ghaziabad and Khaga was cross referenced with the signatures of the guests staying in hotels in Siliguri and Fatehpur at the time of seizures. It was confirmed that the signatures on the skins were same as that of the man calling himself Tashi Tsering.

Wong Kim Quee is the main accused in Siliguri case where two rhino horns were seized. Kim stockpiled his goods in Bhutan and was apparently the man who allegedly supplied 22 rhino horns to the princess of Bhutan (the king's sister). The 1999 seizure in Ghaziabad was booked by Shabbir's son Sarfaraz and was to be delivered at Siliguri apparently for Kim.

Shabbir confessed during investigation that he was also present when police raided the Khaga premises in 2000 and seized four tiger skins, 70 leopard skins and, 18,000 leopard claws and 150 kilograms of bones. He, however, managed to slip away leaving his wife behind who was arrested. The Khaga seizure has been identified as the biggest in a single raid ever in India having multimillion dollar affiliations in Europe.

Seizure from the house of Shabbir also shed some light on the latest modus operandi of poachers. Police recovered around 150 pieces of burqa (veils worn by Muslim women) from the house and some very narrow strips of clothes stitched at one end and open at the other, like pillow cover. The superintendent of Police, Dr. Arvind Chaturvedi, who has recently been decorated with the President's medal for gallantry, led the ground operation. He told me that these were used to carry stacks of currency notes. It is noteworthy that in two of the cases lodged against

Shabbir, his two sons and his brother-in-law Ayub, thousands of US dollars were also recovered along with other items.

The man also revealed to the team in charge Amitabh Yash that the gang used a special net which was spread over the ditch near the point where tigers generally come to drink water. The net is made of steel rings that tightens the moment pressure is put on them. The poachers preferred to kill the cat by hitting it with lathis to avoid any tampering of the skin. One arrested tribal woman from Madhya Pradesh identified as Chillo, was also a prize catch, as she was an expert in killing a tiger by slashing its throat with a chopper in one go, that too in a manner that the skin of the animal is not damaged. She said she used to hit in the middle of the lower jaw, shoving the chopper up to cut the main vein. By looking at her, one would not suspect that she possesses such a fatal skill. It is she to whose chopper Panna National Park in Madhya Pradesh has lost all its resident striped cats.

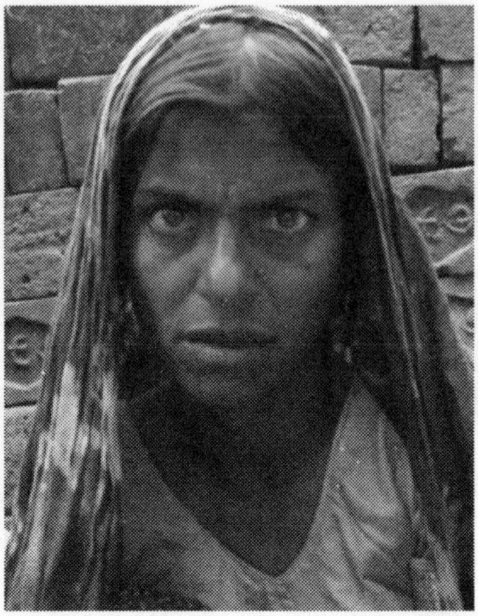

Chillo

Recently a Lakhimpur Kheri court awarded five-year jail term to a 55-year old, Bawariya woman poacher Dilepoo. Her entire family - daughter Kamla, son Jitmal, and brother Tota Ram - is into poaching and trading of animal parts. They have been active in Tarai areas killing tigers in Utter Pradesh and Uttarakhand for many years. She was arrested twice in the past, at Pilibhit and Katarnia Ghat but after being released on bail, remained untraceable, when one fine day she was again found involved in tiger poaching at Kishanpur sanctuary and was arrested. The precision with which the family kills their victims makes them most sought after in the trade. Having set the traps, they revisit the place and make the trapped tiger to roar by nudging it with a long stick. As soon as it opens the mouth they force the stick in its mouth and asphyxiate it.

In the absence of proper records wildlife trade is galloping unchecked. After narcotics, wildlife trade is the second booming illegal industry, but, questioning government on the extent and turnout of wildlife trade may not provide one with answers. And this is because there is no specific agency to monitor this trade. There are certainly some NGOs who periodically raise a hue and cry about the trade but they just talk and issue statements as soon a seizure comes to light. Their names triumph in the newspapers and the real soldiers who carry out the feat of catching poachers and contraband gradually fade into the background. There are a few wildlife historians who easily capture public platform and count the record of such seizures on their fingertips, and also selected information bureaus that feed such news on dotcoms and become the first informers.

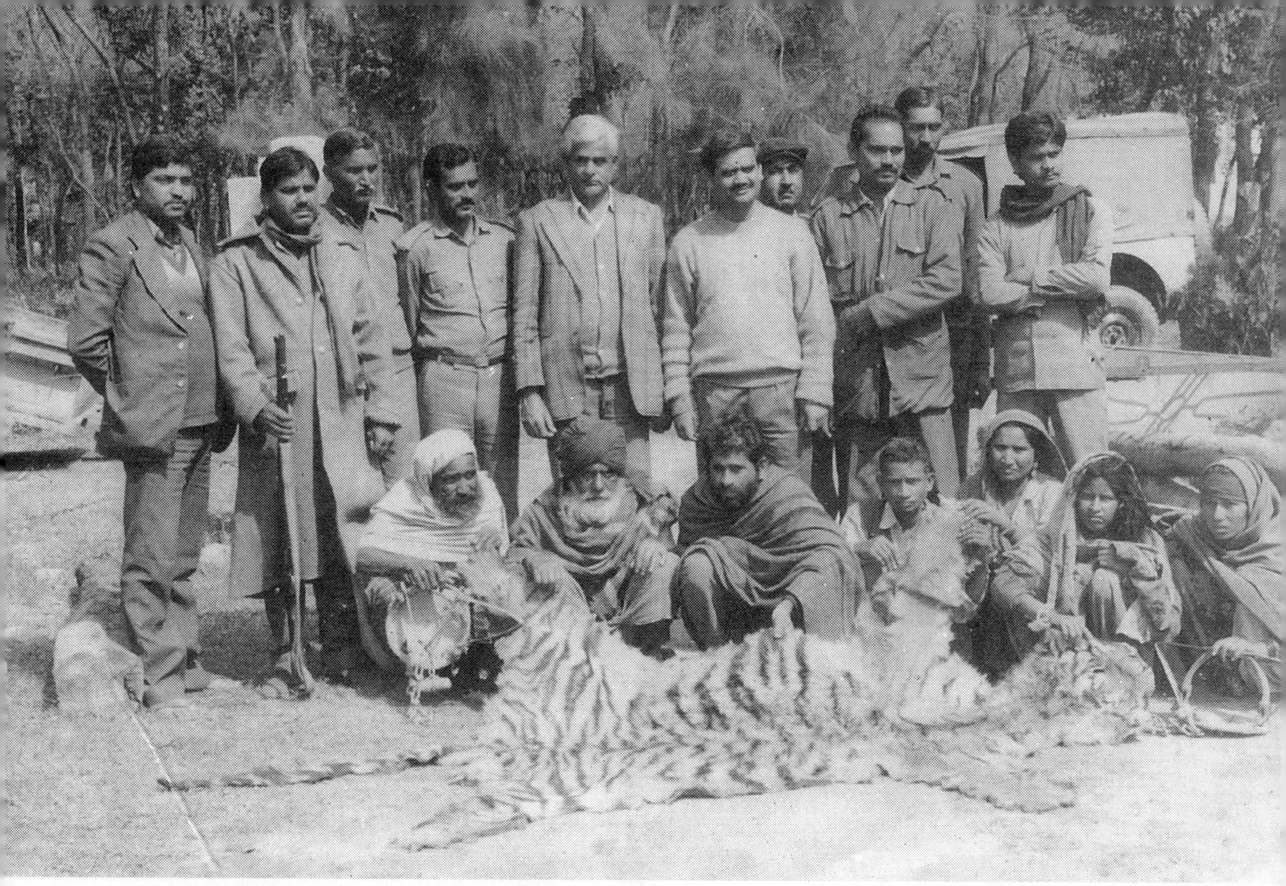

This Bawaria gang was caught near Kishanpur tiger reserve. The recovered skin was of a cub rearing tigress

There has never been any attempt to evaluate this trade by any government. Trade in wildlife is not permitted and it is not recorded. When actually any sale and exchange beyond the quota sanctioned by commerce is "illegal" and as most of the wildlife trade in India is prohibited, it is difficult to quantify such trade and many figures keep floating around. Experts and voices within the government agree that the entire exalted talk about saving wildlife or earmarking excess funds for conservation is as ineffectual as opening an umbrella in a typhoon in the backdrop of the fact that we do not have basics to work on.

It is true that serious effort on the part of the government is missing. No wonder, till date we do not have any nationalized wildlife crime database when there is an urgent need for one. Wildlife scientists estimate that 10-35% of the annual mortality can be derived from poaching. Poaching limits the population increase in large carnivore populations and if the menace is not dealt with, it risks expanding both in proportion and range. It is assumed that out of ten tiger poaching cases all over India, only one case is cracked by authorities.

By pretending that cane tigers do not exist at all, the then Project Tiger and now NTCA have solved the problem and absolved themselves from the need to protect them. This raises a more fundamental question -- is there anything like long-term survival for the sugarcane tigers? The major problems facing tiger conservation in farm fields are related to people and their livestock. The tiger population may

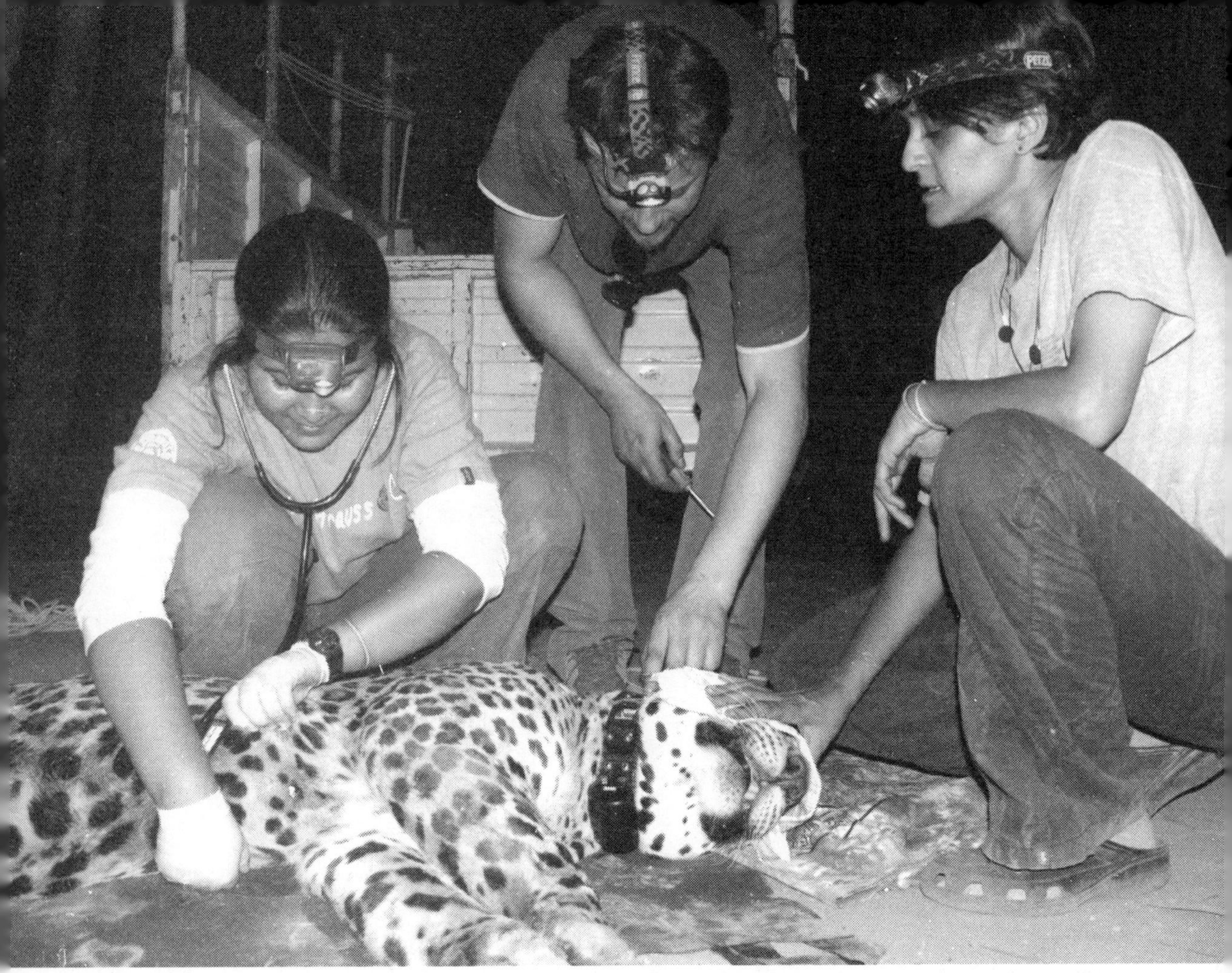

Vidya Atraya with her team, handling a Tranqualized Leopard caught in sugar fields

show a temporary upward trend in the crops but the kind of ruthless man-tiger conflict it generates, it is bound to become counterproductive for any conservation schemes and loom large over the future of the species.

Tigers cannot live longer as competitors to humans. Any attempt at an integration with human interest would border on serious ramifications. The principal reason for intermittent emergence of man-eaters is unquestionably the pressure of human population on tiger habitat, which has spiraled out of control to well over one billion people. I recall the words of a pseudo-Sikh hero, who had accounted for a couple of the great predators by the means of chemical pesticides, "Any tiger can become a killer of human beings, in localities where they are numerous, it is essential in the interest of inhabitants to keep their numbers in check".

Large and dangerous mammals have profound influence on the systems in which they exist, but regrettably our knowledge base -as how they live around human dominated systems without becoming a problem- is very scanty; alongside the studies related to attacks on people do tell that the methods, the villagers employ to deal with dangerous animals often result in an increased danger to the community as it goads even a complacent predator to change its mind and attack. Thus it is very difficult to define a tiger landscape within farmlands for coexistence. It is also difficult for man to find a reprieved room for the predators of such razor-sharp reflexes and of considerable proportions by his side; because an accustomed predator may soon discover humans as the most prolific prey species, which is easiest to kill and may entice him to hanker after human diet. It will result in a ruthless and perennial conflict and the tiger will eventually be wiped out. And finally, as the order of priority tells that everything must be subservient to human interest, the answer is very difficult.

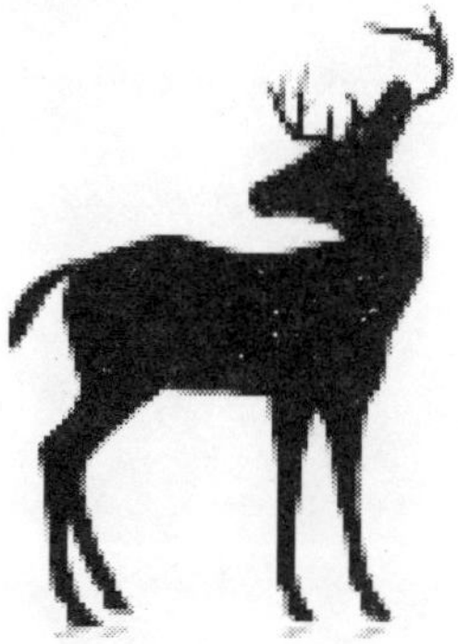

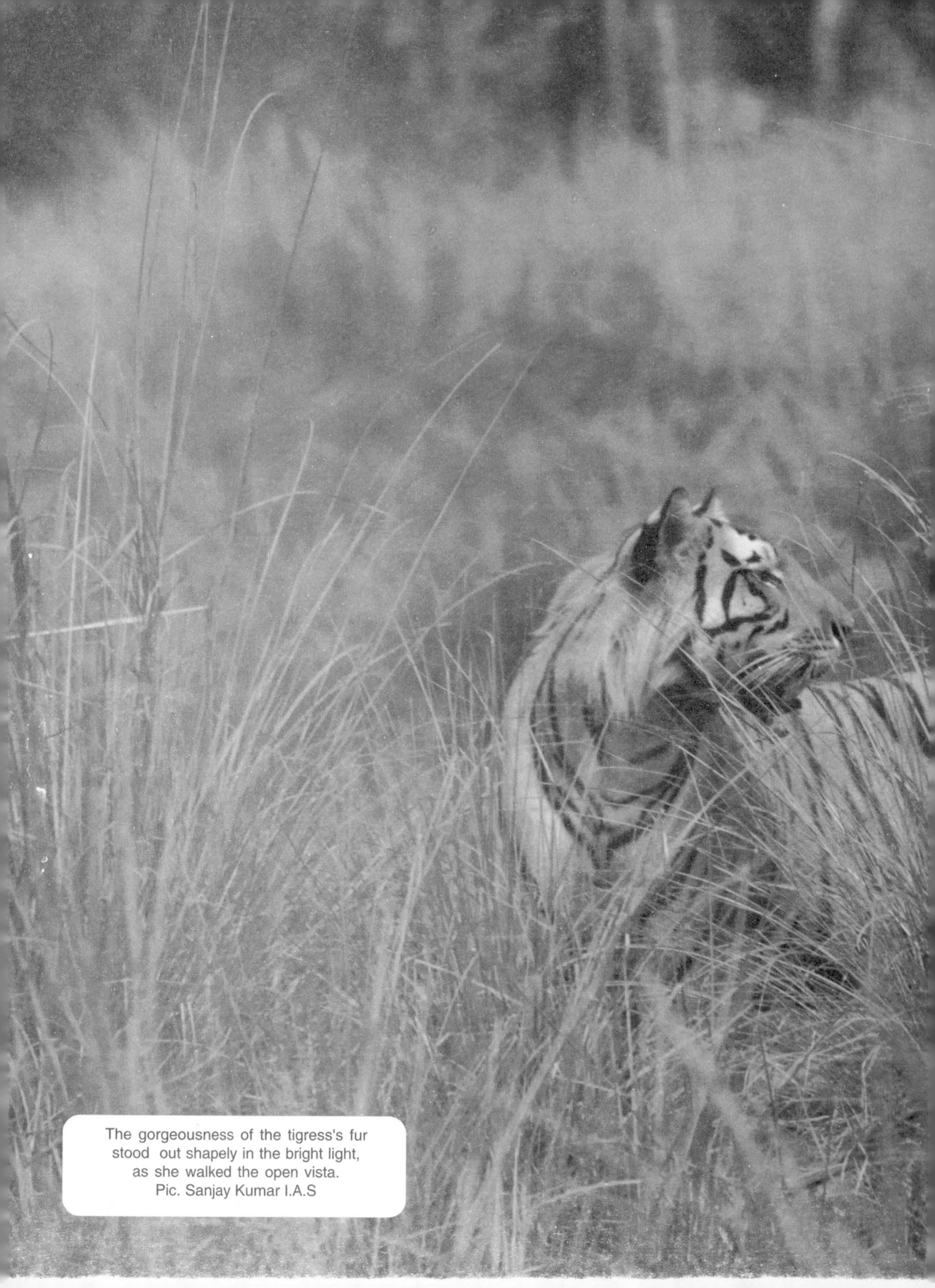

The gorgeousness of the tigress's fur stood out shapely in the bright light, as she walked the open vista.
Pic. Sanjay Kumar I.A.S

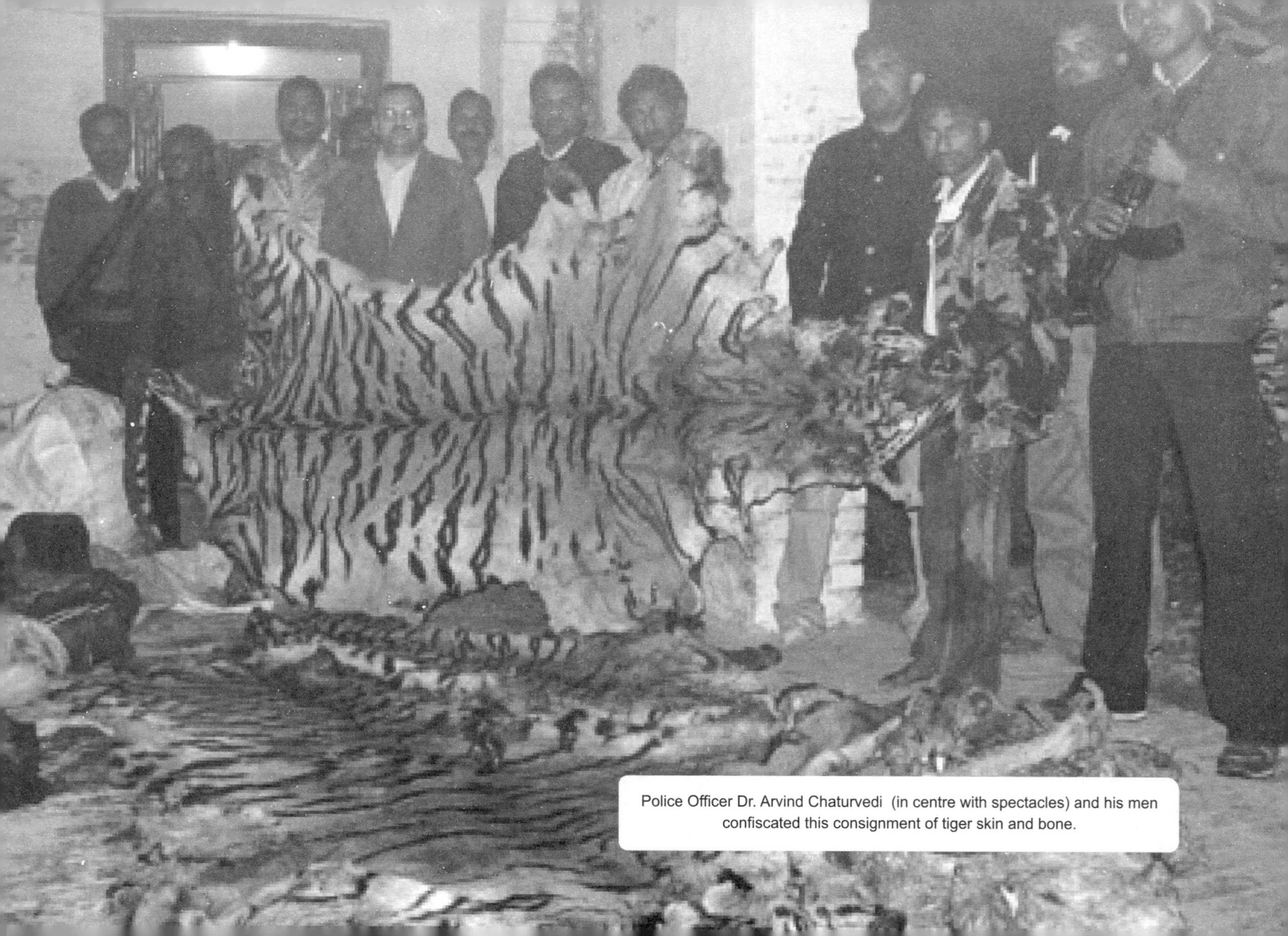

Police Officer Dr. Arvind Chaturvedi (in centre with spectacles) and his men confiscated this consignment of tiger skin and bone.

Epilogue

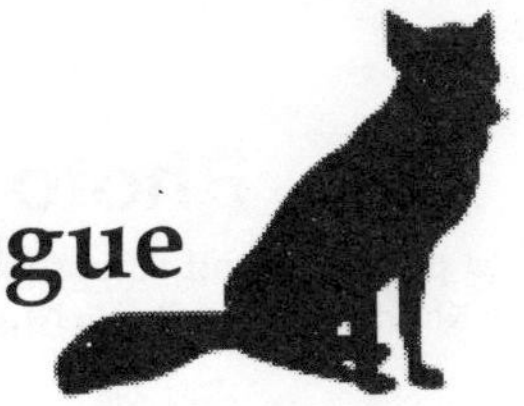

I wanted movement and not a calm course of existence. I wanted excitement and danger and the chance to sacrifice myself for my love. I felt in myself a superabundance of energy which found no outlet in our quiet life.

- Leo Tolstoy

Now as years have passed and amid the present-day sanity, I look back on my youthful days when I had wandered after tigers, all by my own, and where adventures were a simple matter of fact, I am scarcely able to understand them myself. All that I can account for was the powerful desire to escape from the confinement of city walls and go far beyond its limits.

There is something suffocating about the city life, which I find hard to endure. It is a world devoid of innocence. All around me, I see people deceiving themselves, deceiving their emotions, their passions and their desires. There is something hollow in the whole scenario. You laugh when you are expected to and you cry because it is meant to be so: these are the standards of urbanization, neither of the heart nor soul. I can never thrive on this make-believe world. All I ever want is to go to a place, which welcomes you with a quaint tranquility, unknown to minds sunk in the rut of the civilized life, where winds do not blow so strange and where you feel a raw throb of existence.

Such places are the tiger lands of Himalayan Tarai, where I enjoy lovely long marches through the wonderful scenery, seeing cheery friendly persons and my amusing receptions in the villages and where sunsets have an atmosphere of rest and content about them. They create magic in everyday life; fulfill my little dreams and my angels guide me well through most rough patches when the colours of the day fade out above the darkening belt of the forests and the moon floodlights the landscape with its cold metallic gleam, making the night overwhelming and mysterious. The night sounds that predominate in an atmosphere of great peace are conducive to confessions.

There is a tremendous energy in that atmosphere. The Tarai has given me great spectacles and great experiences that will remain unforgettable forever. It is this fundamental enchantment of the place that made me a naturalist and a conservationist and finally culminated in the generation of this manuscript.

Photo Credits

The old photographs, oil paintings and lithographs reproduced in this book are taken from the private collection of M. H. Mamman Khan and Raja Ranjit Bhargav, including old books and internet sites listed below.

Publications

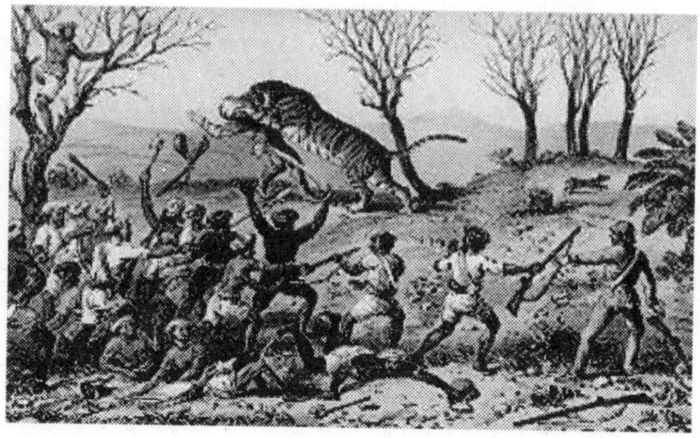

Baker E. B, *Sport in Bengal*, London, 1888

Baldwin, J.A, *The Large and Small game of Bengal*, London, 1877

Best, J.W, *Indian Shikar Notes*; London 1931

—*Forest Life in India,* London, 1935

Brown, J, Moray, *Shikar Sketches*, London, 1887

Denial Johnson, Surgeon, *Indian Field Sports*, 1823,

E. Smyth's, *Big Game Shooting in Nepal*, London, 1942

Eardley Wilmot, S. *Forest Life and Sport in India*, London, 1910

Simpson, Frank.B, *Letters on Sport in Eastern Bengal*, London 1886

Hicks F.C. *Forty Years among Wild Animals in India*, Allahabad, 1910

Ingles James, *Tent Life in Tigerland*, London, 1888

Forsyth, J. *The Highlands of Central India*, London, 1872

Glasfurd A.I.R, *Rifle and Romance in the Indian Jungle*, London, 1905

Glasfurd A.I.R, *Musings of an Old Shikari*, London, 1928.

Gordon Cumming, W, *Wild Men and Beasts*, Edinburgh, 1871

Wray. J.W. *With rifle and Spear in India*, London, 1925

Illustrated London News, March 1876

Websites

save-tigers.co.cc

logoi.com, farmingpathogens.word, pictures-of-cats.org, outlookindia.com, columbia.edu, manimal-world.com

burntorangenation.com, picasaweb.google.com, africahunting.com, geh.org, laughing1wolf.blogspot, outdoors.webshots.com,

oldindianphotos.in, ethnologica.com, prints-4-all.com. girls-143. blogspot.com, savethetigers62.blogsp, odysseustrunk.blogspot, dakotaboo-vintage-post, dakotaboo-vintage-post.. artnet.com, forums.civfanatics.com,

mediastorehouse.com, squidoo.com

davidrumsey.com, lyricsdog.eu, ssplprints.com, tiger. pictures-of-cats, old-print.com, vustv.com, wheretobuyairsoft.com,

Heritage-images.com, Hulton Archive/Getty Images, Underwood & Underwood/CORBIS/MAGMA. Swim Ink/ CORBIS/MAGMA

Color photographs contributed by Shrivridhi & Samridhi Shukla.

Black & White photographs contributed by :

Abhishek Verma 'Vikky'
Arvind Chaturvedi
Billy Arjan Singh
Delip Chhatwani
Daphne Stuart
Dillon Wheatley
Gaurav Mishra
M. Haider Mamman Khan
Prabal WTI
Ranjit Bhargav
Rajiv Ranjan Verma
R.L. Singh
Sanjay Kumar, I.A.S.
Sanjay Narain

Postscript

Large carnivores' illicit strong emotions and their management is more socio-political than biological. The large carnivores think there is enough space for them to return to many areas. The key element to their recovery is whether people are willing to share that space with them.

Dr Alistair Bath, WWF Consultant

All these years while tracking golden cats in the Tarai, I have enjoyed a wild spirit of enthusiasm and romance. I characterize this phase as a series of surprising discoveries about tigers and their behaviour, but now that flutter of achievement and inner happiness is replaced by a sagging feeling of disappointment for the real sugarcane tiger that I knew of is no more. The sugarcane turf of the Tarai may be considered a landscape of low conservation value, for it does not fit into the way ecosystems are valued and governed. Instead, it has been both the birth place and graveyard of many, perhaps hundreds of tigers; breathing and watching as a silent witness to too many outstanding stories.

The phenomenon of sugarcane tigers gathered force in the later half of the 20th century when the species flourished here, overflowed and reached its elegiac glow. And then, it slowly faded out. In fact it was rather allowed to fade out in the hands of poachers, natives and vengeance killers. Inapt bullets from poachers transformed more and more of the big cats into chance hunters of humanity. The treasure of nature was first converted into curse of nature and then looted and ravaged. This animal of farmlands, which had first begun on friendly terms with farmers as an unpaid watchman of crops against graminivorous ungulates, and on whose mercy husbandmen's and natives had slept carefree in the nights, gradually earned a bad name of being a bloodthirsty monster and was done away with by the hands of their one-time friends.

I regret to say that despite my work spanning nearly four decades, believed by many, disbelieved by a few, and acknowledged by all, the actual sugarcane tiger, which had a complete heritable constitution to live in the canes has vanished even though there may be some tigers still living in the sugarcane. The extinction of sugarcane tiger shows that we have failed spactacularly. The phenomenon was a vehicle to infuse a sense of urgency and energy into tiger conservation, seeking to bring about a paradigm shift. Extinct animals cannot live again. With this is gone an opportunity to observe a chapter in natural history that was yet to unfold.

R.I.P., sugarcane tiger!

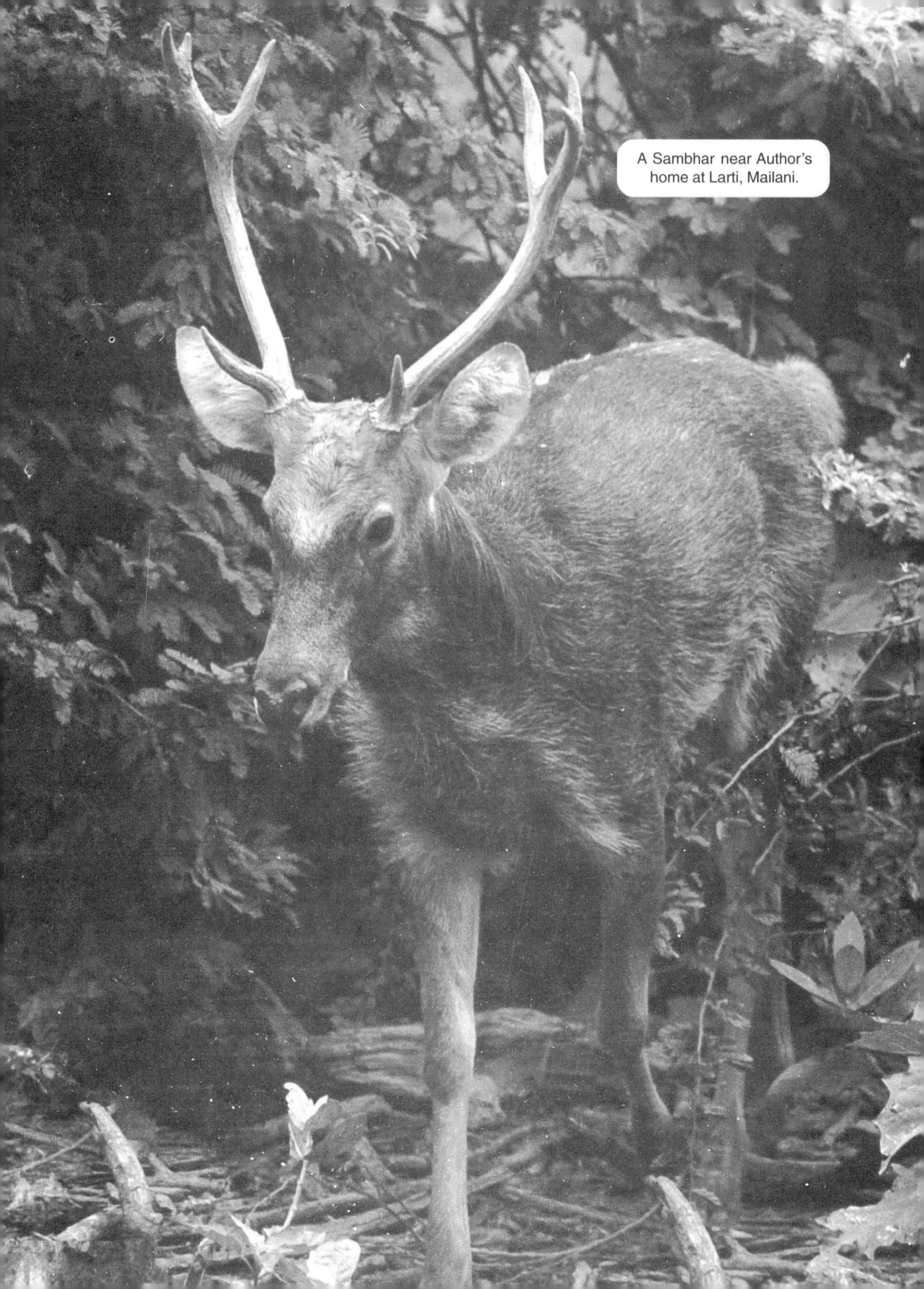

A Sambhar near Author's home at Larti, Mailani.

The ecological niche of an organism depends not only on where it lives but also on what it does. By analogy, it may be said that the habitat is the organism's "address", and the niche is its "profession", biologically speaking.

— **W B Saunders 1959**

ADDENDUM

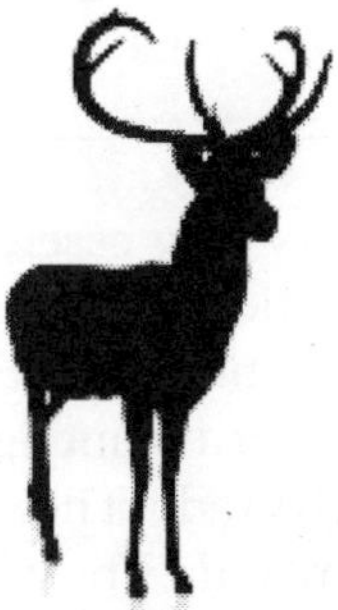

An Insight into Putative Strain; A Comparative Analysis

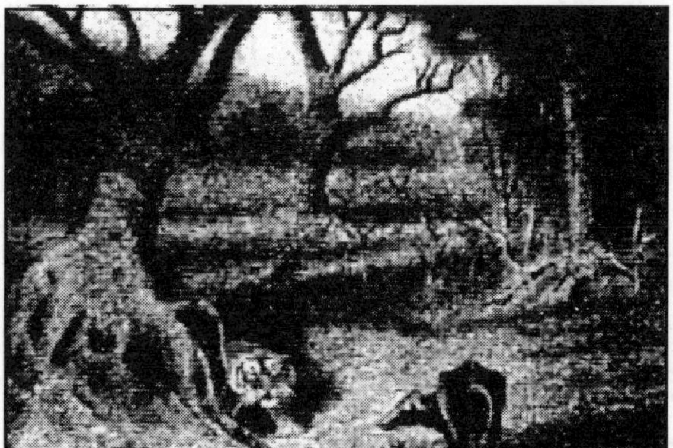

The "control of nature" is a phrase conceived in arrogance, born of the Neanderthal Age of biology and the convenience of man.

— Rachel Carson

An Insight into Putative Strain: A Comparative Analysis

In its very essence, sugarcane tiger is an adventure and an expression of summation of my life experience. It is an attempt to question the world of conservation practitioners who take rigid and logo-centric scientific dogmas as the final truth and ignore the complex patterning of reality. Tigers are flexible enough to adopt new environmental changes including anthropogenic pressures of farmlands. The whole story of my observations is an acceptance of this chaos that encourages a play with meaning, and makes my sugarcane tiger theory, an attempt to find a new and more truthful version of changing facts about tigers, in their farm-range land based existence. (**Author in a meeting of State Wildlife Advisory Board of U.P. Government. Lucknow, 1997)**

This addendum is a sequel to the introduction of this book. In this narrative, I propose my own experiences of tigers in the sugarcane ecosystem and the conclusions gathered from them. In the process, I was ever conscious of the boundaries of my subject and limitations of my statements and even prior to the promulgation of my sugarcane tiger theory, I had successfully drawn the finish lines before I had begun.

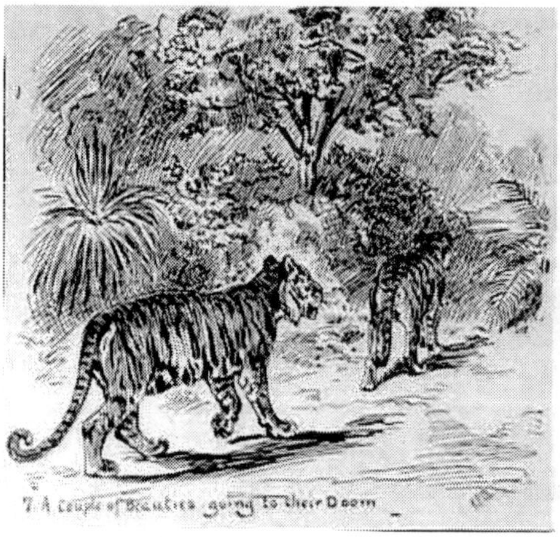

7. A Couple of Beauties going to their Doom

To understand the milieu and matrix of wildlife in the Tarai farmlands, I have radically interrogated natural history records, spanning last two centuries, beliefs, conservation strategies and world views, often crossing over into territories of different disciplines, going across the Tarai and back and forth in time. I have evaluated all types of anthropogenic pressures and forces of market driven commerce that effect agrarian lands, despoliation of local forests, encroachment of pastoral habitat areas and also the present status of conflict between farmers and large carnivores. While synthesizing every historical detail connected with this tiger, I have put the entire scenario of prevailing conditions and almost everything into question. Sugarcane tiger is not an ecological disaster as viewed by some skeptics; it is in fact an incidental by-product, an achievement by default that opens up a window for the future conservation experiments.

I must emphasize once again that wild carnivores exist at the top of the food chain and are extremely scarce. They have long intervals between litters and deliver a small number of cubs, out of which only some survive adulthood. Starvation remains the most important factor for mortality. This combined with human induced factors such as habitat destruction and active persecution severely depress their number. However, farmlands also serve as a vital linkage for numerous wide-ranging species and there are many carnivore species, such as foxes, hyenas, jackals, king cobra, monitor lizard and others that continue to flourish outside the forest in human dominated landscape. Two lethal predators, namely leopards and tigers, represent the flagship species of this great fleet. This proves that human interventions not always necessarily jeopardize the survival of large carnivores but sometimes play a greater role in it.

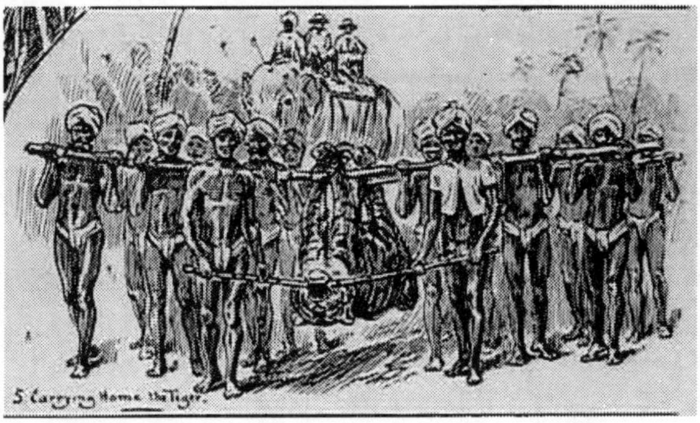

This book admits that human actions matter decisively for this tiger, and in no way, detracts from the central idea that the current pattern of land use change, occurring throughout Tarai, has favored the return of large carnivore's populations. The sugarcane plantations that can better be described as a climax vegetation terrain do fulfill the ecological needs of large predators. It is a manmade biome that has received small consideration from scientists and needs to be understood for its potentialities as a wildlife habitat. I have worked hard in this volume to state that subjectivity cannot be absolutely separated from objectivity, and, when many tigers are living in the sugarcane eco-system some of them must be hardcore sugarcane tigers.

The controversy that raged for years amongst tiger buffs over the identity of sugarcane tiger helped me to improve and upgrade the quality of my research and enabled me to continue my work with doubled enthusiasm. The more I heard different perspectives of the debate, the more I heard my own echo with dissonant opinions. It rather made me believe that an appreciation for the ecological roles of large carnivores cannot be expected to improve if the correct information is lacking and misconceptions persist.

Human initiatives have immense capacity to do more harm than good to this tiger and do not seem to hold much promise for its future survival, yet the catalytic role played by human agency in the production of this tiger is widely acknowledged and the putative strain of sugarcane tiger, is more or less, a man made product. All that we need is to save this tiger through a sensible course of action that should be based on this animal's social and biological history.

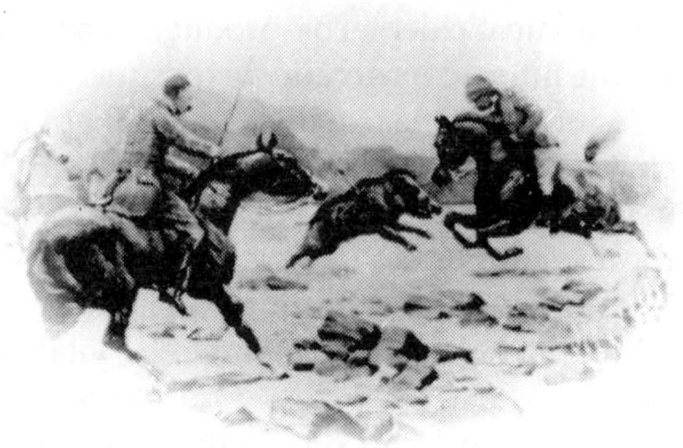

To revisit the question of this book; whether sugarcane tiger is a putative strain and how could I promote the concept of putative strain, without including all the source populations of tigers in the farmlands?

This question, with all its complexity and possible excesses had arisen due to the lack of scientific understanding of my concept. My answer was that the entire tiger population operating in the sugarcane farms characterized a phenomenon of tigers, which shifted between different ecosystems as each offered the scattered bonanzas of high quality food. But alongside, a small pack of animals within that tribe was of authentic sugarcane tigers, which were here by their predilection to cane. Though there must be too much of connectivity and intermixing between tigers in sugarcane and hardcore sugarcane tigers but if you ask me there existed a cluster of breeding females which had its rangeland in better prey rich areas, which was perhaps producing a dramatic surplus of wild tigers. Much of this surplus was surviving to maturity with reduced mortality rate due to mother's success to hunt sufficient food with in her home range and this food was largely made up of buffer food of feral cattle.

During seventies, when my studies were in the nascent stage, I had carefully chosen to address this very segment as a feasible strain because in biological definitions; the true sub-speciation is caused by geographical isolation and separate evolution. Now years after, as the quotidian phenomenon was continuing and copious generations of tigers had been born in the canes, I had no doubt left but to believe that far from the initial stage, there was now a fully formed strain of such animals. If human disturbance is minimized and normal tigers are not distracted into deviant ways by human misbehavior, and nature is allowed to play its part fully, the reactions were bound to be favorable for these animals which were getting bracket together as a putative sugarcane brand, whose all corporeal and mental

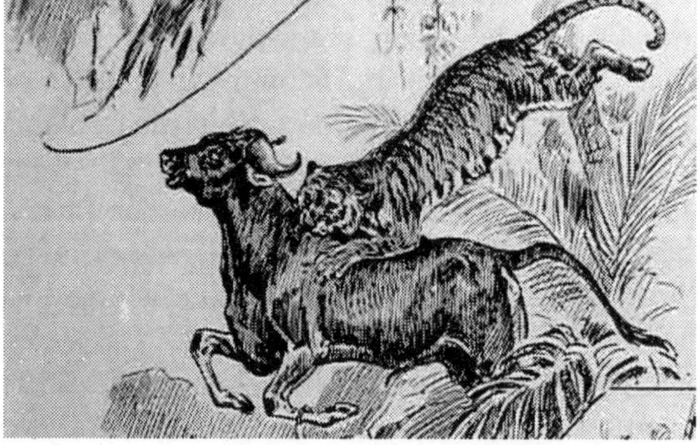

endowments were tending to progress towards aptness.

The *Dictionary of Biological Terms* describes strain as a group of organisms within a species or variety, distinguished by one or more minor characteristics. On the basis of this thesis, as some tigers confirmed their predilection for sugar habitat, I had formed my concept of sugarcane tiger. I had deliberately used this arcane scientific phrase that also synthesizes eco-preferences of living organisms with small separations, which is reasonably explained by established principles of zoology and ecology. It was a pellucid point, for which I had categorically and unwaveringly, stood forever.

The size of tiger family is controlled mainly, I believe, by habitat conditions. In poor habitats tigers survive briefly without being able to produce, whereas good habitats with large amount of prey can potently produce a 'surplus'. Sugarcane crops and jungles are two different mosaics of land with two completely different environments. Was this not a totally unusual conservation dilemma that tigers were becoming extinct in the pristine environments but flourishing in sugar plantations? Thus the design of their population recovery in farmlands, needed to be understood by the book. It is estimated that in the jungle usually only one cub from each litter survives to maturity and even the natural process of litter in a tigress is often retarded due to the stress of solitary living and constant search for food. Now when the tigers' extirpation over most of their proper ranges is straightaway ascribed to the incompatible human activities, then what was the mechanism of their population resurgence in the sugar crops, where the optimum conditions for supporting a viable tiger population by maintaining their new and entire eco-system, were practically not possible?

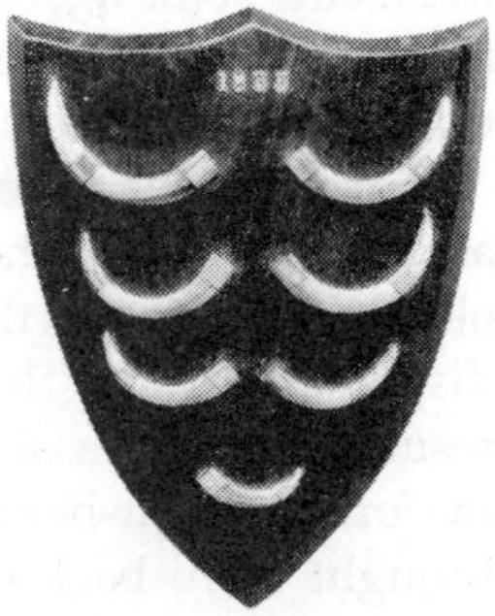

I was perplexed by the fact of this remarkable growth rate that was accompanied by starvation, by anthropogenic pressure and by man-tiger conflict. Two Victorian hunters, Rice (1857) and Gordon Cumming (1872), who shot a reported total of 71 tigresses in the central highlands, state that about one-third of these did not appear to have any cubs. This figure indicates that a large percentage of adult jungle tigress do not have cubs. On this line of information, to understand the population graph of sugar tigers, we have to first understand the parameters of two different habitats, viz. of jungle and cane in order to explain the contradictions. I stated that these tigers perhaps knew how to utilize farmland resources for survival, they qualified to vital life history parameters such as fortitude, exigencies of prey base utilization, sustaining the impact of human activities and proper dispersal of their population, and hence the demographic escalation was registered. A further research was also needed to discover the features that serve as linchpin to this ecosystem and the fragile ecological webs that bind a tiger to sugar habitat. It was an awkward fact which the forest department ignored and the hassle of their scientific dogma continued to cast its shade on this tiger beyond the shadow of doubt.

In Chapter 6 of this book I have already explained the possible causes of baby boom in sugar crops. Survival is only one component of selection, and reproduction is another. For example, where a number of males survive to reproductive age, yet only a few ever mate, the difference in reproductive success would stem from factors other than the ability to survive, such as an ability to successfully attract mates. In an evolutionary reproductive sense, fitness is the average reproductive output of a class of genetic variants in a gene pool, and should not be confused with meaning physically fit - biggest, fastest or strongest - and which does not necessarily lead to reproductive success.

Howsoever exaggerated it may seem, some wild tigers that had been driven in the crops by stress of circumstances and even though surrounded by an ever increasing human population where they were, had seemingly learnt to share in the existence of civilization around them. It is worth mentioning that many scientists studying the highly dangerous animals like elephants, tigers and snakes have lauded the deep-rooted forbearance of rural Indian communities even in the face of conflict. Due to this factor, some tigers were not only settled over the fringes of cultivation fields, but in some cases were well established in the plantations near villages much inside the transition zones of civilization.

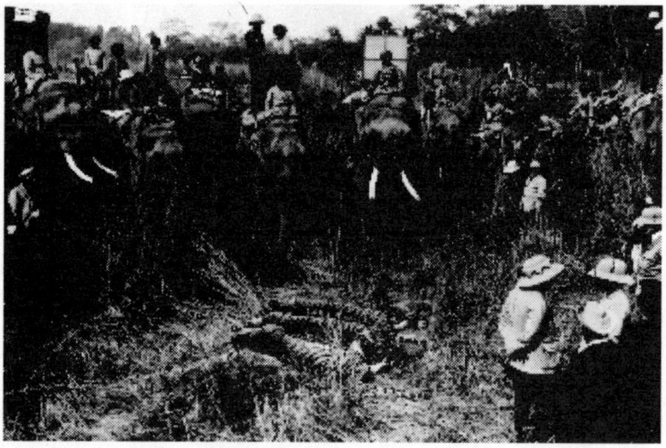

Formerly the process of attrition had cleared their age old home and forced them to disperse but now the vast resurgence of grassland in the form of sugar-biome had brought them back on the very soil; at times uncomfortably close to humans. The animal which had always shunned humans now lived on by self orientation of co-existence with them. People hardly ever saw them during day time and they were unlikely to be much affected by accidental deaths and injury. Their acceptance of prey was controlled and inhabited by many additional constrains. Towards dusk when the cattle return to the village and their bells tinkle merrily, it is a peculiarly fascinating sound to a tiger. Seeing cows pacing slowly forward with rhythmically nodding head, even a jungle tiger starts following them, yet these legendary predators in the canes, safely differentiated between domestic and feral cattle and never chased them.

This cliquey strain -determined according to the distillate wisdom of nature- as even under the baleful conditions of human influence nature's infinite wisdom is adaptable and not wasteful- had indeed, added a new chapter in the natural history of species, also meaning thereby that the cover of sugar crops was idyllically suitable to carnivore ecology, of which a sound breeding nucleus is the chief component.

As regards 'clinal' variation, it was too small a span of time to say that any such distinction may have taken place in these tigers -for this force of natural selection operates on a huge evolutionary time scale-and on no account with a revolutionary magnitude.

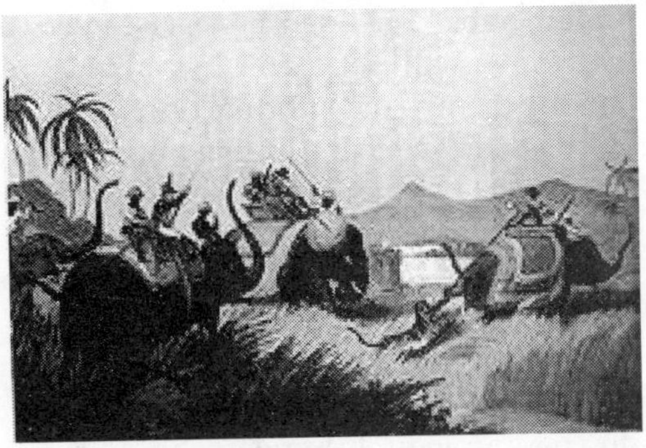

In upper echelons, this lack of knowledge was a bit worrying. The bureaucrats in charge of tiger welfare had no room for their own growth and seemed adamant to leave no room for my growth too. These men, whose introduction in Indian Forest Services is more by default than by any design who are otherwise called 'experts', simply through holding a status in the department and whose evergreen naiveté is compulsorily helped and guided by reading the archaic books of old-timers, perceived a hopelessly distorted and anthropocentric view of the problem. Their wisdom seemed limited by the wisdom of guide authors. Impervious of their stance, I continued to disseminate my 'acuity of an idiot' that sugarcane is a dynamic habitat, the basic essence of which, contains a salubrious life support system to big cats. It is certainly far better than inhospitable mangrove forests of Sunderbans in the Bay of Bengal. This riparian delta is the pneumatophore-studded mangrove swamp, an extremely poor quality habitat with ostensibly low densities of prey; where scarcity of diverse forms of larger mammals results due to the specialized nature of habitat, where every animal must either survive the rigors of hostile environment or die trying to do so.

Sunderbans are one of densest and most impenetrable forests in the world. Studded closely with fantastic labyrinths, bifurcations, interlacing and looping of rivers around tiny flats, here the flow of fresh water is virtually negligible and tigers generally show characteristics like many estuarine beings. They live in swampy coverts of high salinity, walk mud between the toes, depend on brackish and turbid water that damages their liver and kidneys, and consume floating food such as mudskippers and crabs on opportunity. During high tidal waves, when their entire island is submerged, they swim down wide stretches in quest of elevated lands above inundation levels in search of prey animals. Even tigresses do so with cubs, negotiating creeks and channels as wide as five kilometers or more. In such situations the aquatic predators like salt crocodiles and sharks move into land terrain and pose a threat to land animals, which tigers must fight to protect themselves.

Tiger is a multi-habitat animal and when the harsh, insalubrious ecological conditions in Sunderbans delta can evolve the local tigers into an almost a separate sub-species of semi-aquatic marsh-dwellers, then why the comparatively congenial salubrious conditions in sugarcane fields could not favor the making of a unique strain of tigers, despite inhabiting the landscape for several decades? When some of the Sunderbans tigers uniquely treat human beings as normal prey and accept the innumerable fishermen, honey gatherers, and woodcutters, who move in the islands as their normal diet, then why can't sugarcane tigers accept feral cattle, which move among them as their normal prey?

It is believed that effective conservation is possible only where human intrusions are minimal; otherwise the entire ecological balance is disturbed. But if the tiger continues to survive in these interrupted conditions and even breeds successfully, and when driven away, repeatedly comes back to live in farmlands, then what should it be called, an assemblage of some mad beasts or it must be accepted as their acclimatization to a new ecology? In Sunderbans man-eating is called a way of ensuring survival, whereas in sugarcane even cattle killing is called aberration. Why should it not be treated as illustrative of an 'anomalous adjustment' achieved all the way through ecological response to flagrant over-exploitation of natural resources carried out by humans? In lexicon of understanding, it is not as much of a reaction as much it is a response of helpless and hapless animals to disconcerting consequences; a corollary of acquiescence and tolerance to inevitable human factor as an equipment of survival.

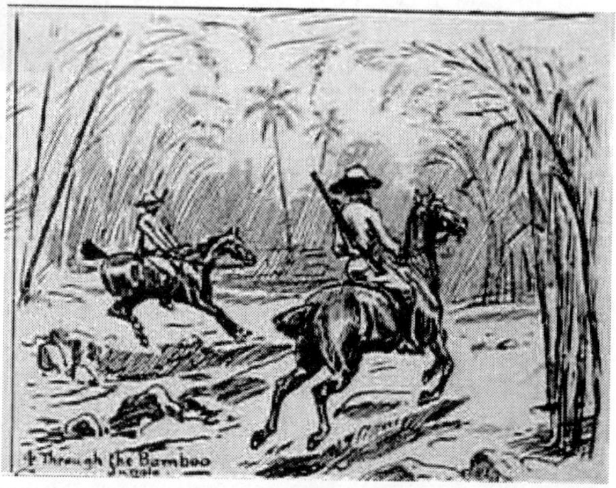

The degree of anthropogenic pressure, which generates a different type of ecological crisis in both the zones -- Sunderbans and sugar plantations of Tarai - therefore remains the same, besides the bearing of bio-geographic factors that are so distinctive to zones. Ostensibly on different scales nature is tending its own wards in both the zones, thus the tigers in these areas show immense tenacity in overcoming the odds of anthropogenic pressure and manage to survive in the face of their impending downfall. Both of these wretched segments -basically singular in nature and eminently adaptable- need a measure of commiseration yet one is protected under NTCA and later is reprimanded with impulsive avidity.

I was a layman and a lot of scientific dimensions are meaningless to a layman. But I knew from my limited knowledge that there is nothing superfluous in the natural world. Nature encompasses all the objects and events with their ecological perspective. The foremost principle of this perspective is the Rule of Non-Randomness. Sugarcane tiger was not a random isolated event around Dudhwa only, similar conditions existed in the greater Tarai, all along the 500-odd miles of Indo-Nepalese border in Uttar Pradesh; and since this tiger has continued to flourish for so long, it is surely and invariably a part of the system, a part of a biological process that is both measurable and predictable.

If the niches become over-crowded as the number of big cats using common resources increases; one way to avoid conflict is for one of the contestants to change its taste. If the divergence increases its chance of survival, it is on its way to becoming a new species, and over the eons, will slip into another ecological niche.

The sugarcane tiger required to be envisaged under this fact of science. Their behavior pattern had to be closely studied, monitored and investigated to unveil their biological properties. The effect of their prey selection, such as feral cattle and even jackals, was to reduce competition between the members of species, to increase the quotient of survival and of course to exploit the number of paths energy takes through the ecosystem. The hypothesis that this tiger was behaviorally adapted to the sugarcanes in no way lessened the importance of this animal. The pinchbeck and condescending attitude of foresters was gratuitous. We must even take care of those wild animals that are down on their luck from human point of view because their habitat selection is of wrong nature, though ecologically it is not so.

I knew that I had made these observations with an intrinsic scientific passion, with a firm belief that in all sciences the procedure of refining earlier knowledge is essentially a quest for truth and with no end. Routine knowledge or work is enemy of innovation. But I was not a qualified scientist, no degree holder from a university and the verticality of disciplines were inaccessible to me. That is why I had intentionally refrained from calling my observations as study, un-desirous of encumbering it with torrential scientific lingo. I had cogently and faithfully told what I had seen with single-mindedness. And since ecological research is subject to stringent seasonal timetable, delays in data collection by even a few months can result in loss of data for an entire year. Such constrains had apparently kept me on tenterhooks and I had never failed to meet my schedules that required information at specific times of the year, viz during winters in canes and during peak summers in local jungles.

To my surprise, this repository of facts was so much in volume and of such a specialized nature that it made a profound difference to me. A serious observation was obviously required by field-technocrats to cross-examine my theory. It was an unrefined crude package of information which threw a challenge to the biologist to modify their old ideas and still better to abandon them. For on my part, instead of twisting the facts to suit the old theories, I had twisted

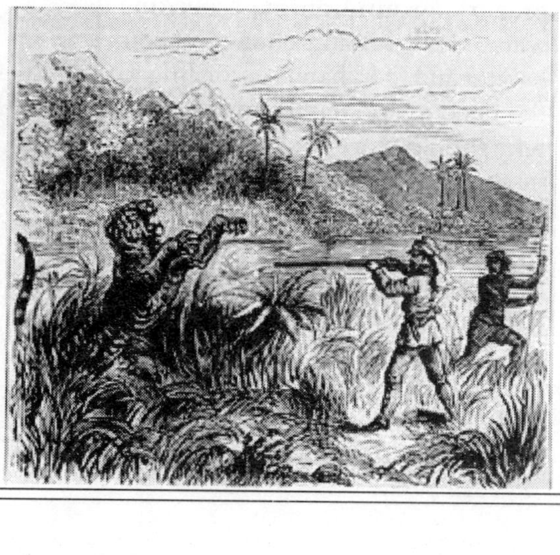

theories to suit facts and smashed the old beliefs to smithereens.

Attack on knowledge production systems, marginalizing independent researchers and even making them subservient to the needs of government is a somewhat xenophobic and unfortunate trend. I would have appreciated, if, some heroic ethologist, a connoisseur of natural history or a capable cadre of biologists had once accepted this challenge and made an impartial reappraisal of my theory. The rebuttal of sugarcane tiger needed qualifications of sustained and trenchant field observations of years and years, which unfortunately none of my detractors possessed.

A niche is a tricky thing to describe since the exercise demands an intimate knowledge of an animal's way of life to define everything it does for survival. In my book it is similar to the concept of human vocations. Given just a little more knowledge and experience the sugarcane tiger could tell us quite a lot about other aspects of its fascinating system, where the induced land-use change, in some way seemed designed to benefit the survival of species.

Interestingly, the hard ground swamp deer of Kanha are genetically the same as the marsh inhabitants of Dudhwa; and when sambhar, supposed to be shy and secluded occupants of deep forests, have gregariously adapted water-based life in Ranthambhore, feeding on water plants, these are accepted as exceedingly malleable animals. Ranthambhore is the only place where sambhar -- habitually the lonely deep forest deer -- congregate in large numbers than anywhere else in India. Even the continuous predation by tigers has not dissuaded the deer from their obsession to the water and its plants. Young sambhar fawns are seen following their mothers into the water, developing as 'water deer', as naturalist Valmik Thapar has called them.

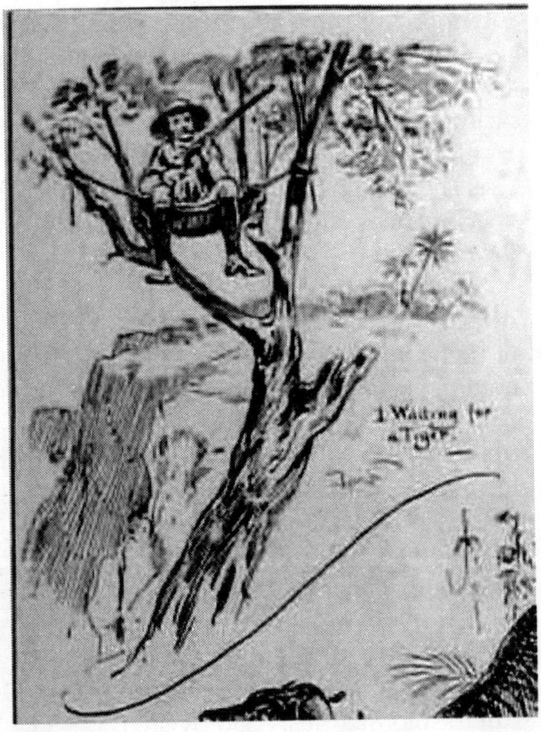

When browsers can become grazers, ground animals become water deer, having changed their habitat and food habits according to the need of the environment, then why should there be such hesitation in acceptance of the fact that some jungle tigers can become hardcore sugarcane dwellers, and there is a rough breed of them that likes to live exclusively in the crops, and that it has discovered other sources of food and opted for other forms of life maintenance as ordained by nature. This behavioral pattern not only indicates an accomplished ecological relationship with the new habitat but clearly demonstrates the changing bio-ecological traits of some tigers.

One can never easily reach conclusions with wildlife and its inherent changing cycles. It was clear that our mistakes had arisen from quick generalizations. The denial of sugarcane tiger should have come from a qualified lobby which had at least once conducted a scientific field survey and studied the phenomenon at length and brought it to a logical conclusion that no tiger can be behaviorally and rudimentarily adapted to live in the cane. There was no report or even a single reference on the topic anywhere, not even a single published source anywhere other than mine but there were plenty of confuting raucous voices and the eventual denunciation of the beast by the people, some of whom had never seen the Tarai and never glimpsed its wild tigers. It was against this, a decidedly hostile, argumentative background that I was trying to trigger the measures aimed at preserving this incorrigible beast.

Those who lack the opportunity of forming their own opinion on any particular subject are apt to accept the opinion of others, and in no case it is more apparent than in the case of tigers. In this research I had challenged the dogmas of science, fought for a cause and paradigmatically searched out the biological causes for the occurrence of this phenomenon, which provided ample evidence for an alternative understanding of tigers' behavior, because, despite a century of its lauded existence our knowledge about this animal was still sketchy; entwined in confusions of fact and fiction.

The study had molded my part-time hobby into my quasi-religion. I had not only taken up the idea but made it my life, thought and dreamt of it. If I abandoned the cause I could never live with myself.

It was universally accepted that tigers stay in the sugar crops for good nine months from July to March. Then the question was: how do they manage to live? It was a riddle to naturalists and called for new lines of investigations. These could be: (1) Remarkable ecological flexibility, (2) Deep understanding of human psyche, (3) Capacity for manipulating itself, (4) Intricate patterns of predation such as eating jackals, (5) Tremendous mobility often resulting in strays, (6) Extra killing of cattle, (7) The impact of crop harvesting on tiger populations, (8) Diurnal habits to reach for food, (9) Consumption of vulture operated kill, (10) Land tenure patterns, (11) Aptitude to absorb the stress of adverse connection with man, (12) Dynamics of meta-populations, (13) Consumption of standing crop biomass viz. primary/ secondary prey including domestic livestock and so on.

In case of man-eaters, these would be: (1) Peak hours of attacking human prey, (2) Entry into human settlements during frosty nights, (3) Preference for squatting man perceived as prey.

The animals that live in the savannas of sugar farmlands are adapted to a great deal of variability in the food supply throughout the year; there are times of plenty (during and after the wet season) and times of almost no food or water (during the dry season). Many animals migrate to deal with this problem and so do the tigers

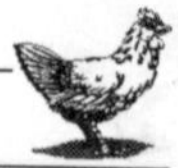

that know how to keep pace with seasonal changes. My last argument that a small segment of these tigers even under the pressure of pinch period stayed out of the principal jungles remained contentious.

I had clearly stated that because of the convoluted problem of their mal-adjustment with resident tigers, the real sugarcane tigers preferred to rehabilitate themselves into local jungles and swamps rather than the regular ones. The reasoning was very much on the lines of translocation of an outside tiger into a new environment, which runs the risk of con-specific aggression by other tigers into whose territory it happens to stray. But my testimony was miscomprehended and their final remark that 'it is not a feasible conjecture because all the local jungles are under siege from fecund settlers', seemed to gratuitously seal the fate of this tiger.

While admitting that the habitat had been desecrated and the prey species decimated, I had submitted a list of nearly 35 large natural areas and 59 subsidiary habitats with over 100 outlying water bodies within the cane zone of Kheri district only, with which I was fairly acquainted and where the cane tigers could possibly be found during pinch periods. I had personally inspected and appreciated the capacity of such wild vistas to harbor tigers in summers. It was prudent to assume that the entire tract of Tarai still held several 'valuable tigerine' localities outside the forest, and moving into them was just one point in the graph of sugar tiger's routine. There was nothing haphazard about it, for the hardened tigers were well entrenched into the system and it was just one significant step in the whole organization of events which followed a chronological order.

I needed to stop repeating nonsense about the uncertainty of sugarcane tiger and start talking seriously about the right approach to address this issue. But my findings were taken with skepticism. Even their scat samples were never examined to determine their food range and the frequency of their depredations on the phlegmatic cattle, in addition to monitor lizards, monkeys and rodents, which my own experience had led me to believe was the staple food of farmland tigers. It is appropriate to mention here some cursory non-laboratory examination of feces, done by my Shikari crew, namely Chottey, Phagunia and Kakaria Kanjar. I do not know as how they interpreted the contents in a digested matter yet the feces was like basic currency to them and they confirmed that in more than 50 percent samples, the remains of cattle were

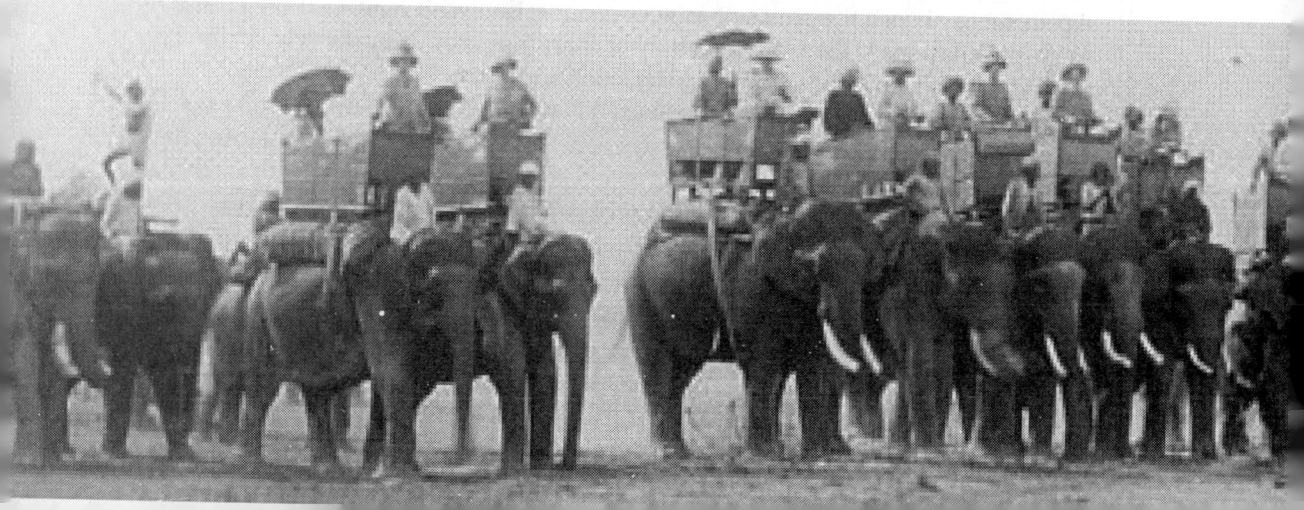

present, though there were no means to confirm that whether this represented the scavenged food or the prey killed by tigers themselves. I hang back to call these claims as futile and misleading for these men were constantly in touch with this animal and were able to understand it differently and accurately.

Finally when in 1995, I submitted my project to CWLW for approval, I was in high spirits that examining feces for food contents is an empirical science and soon the curtain would lift from the old construal's, the explication of which had remained speculative on every occasion, but which I had believed, because of my deep-rooted faith in my Shikari crew. However the begrudging bureaucrat, a scurvy old reprobate, who had also been the director of Dudhwa Park, shrewdly refused my request. He thought that in due course I would also get hold of reports and if this scientific data confirms my hypothesis, I would capitalize on it without delay and it would help me to establish the cane tiger theory more decisively, to the detriment of his department, which he had been hostilely opposing for years. So as if to take revenge on me he prioritized other things and launched a kind of delaying action of which only a malingerer was capable. It was futile to allay his animosity. Even the pressure from the media failed to kick-start the program.

I don't know if this approach was also prompted by inaction or by the knowledge vacuum in tiger conservation strategies which needed to be addressed with still more solid science - against orthodox science -- in the defense of sugarcane tigers. In contradiction of my findings the forest department showed an unexpectedly regressive attitude on the part of the establishment that is supposed to care for wildlife assiduously.

We have noted in previous chapters that the worst of man-tiger conflict had happened in the sugarcane fields; and all that happened in the Tarai had never happened in the modern annals of natural history in any of the thirteen tiger range countries. Cane tigers had temporarily trounced the man-killers of Sunderbans and were rudely eliminated by natives. By a blanket order of CWLW, many of them were either shot or captured in baited shut down cages and sent to zoo. I think if the right policies toward sugar tigers were pursued, they would not have gone to zoos. In fact if the right policies toward nature are pursued; we would need no zoos at all.

Project Tiger seemed limited to a scientific consciousness of a specific nature,

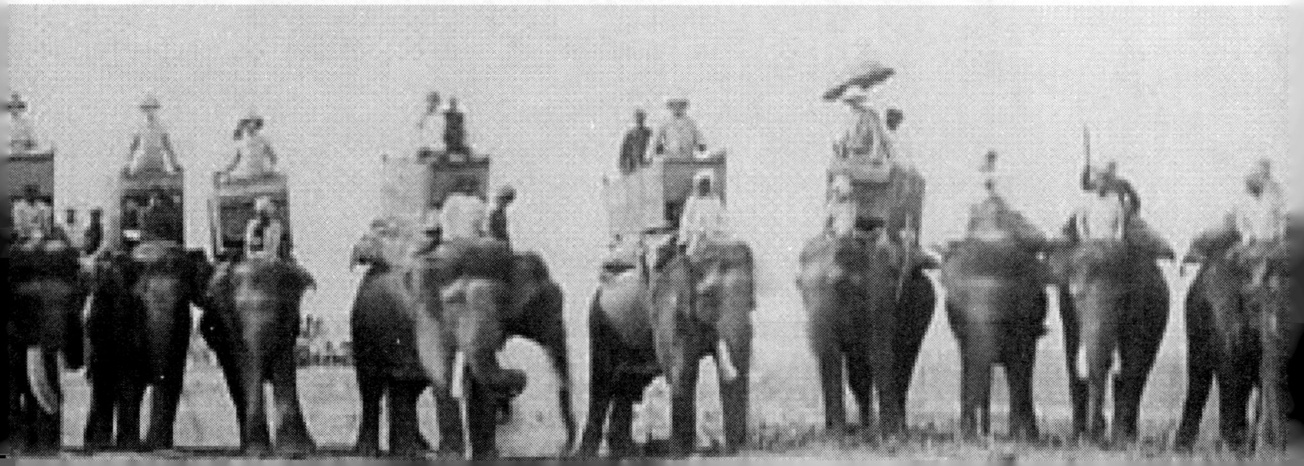

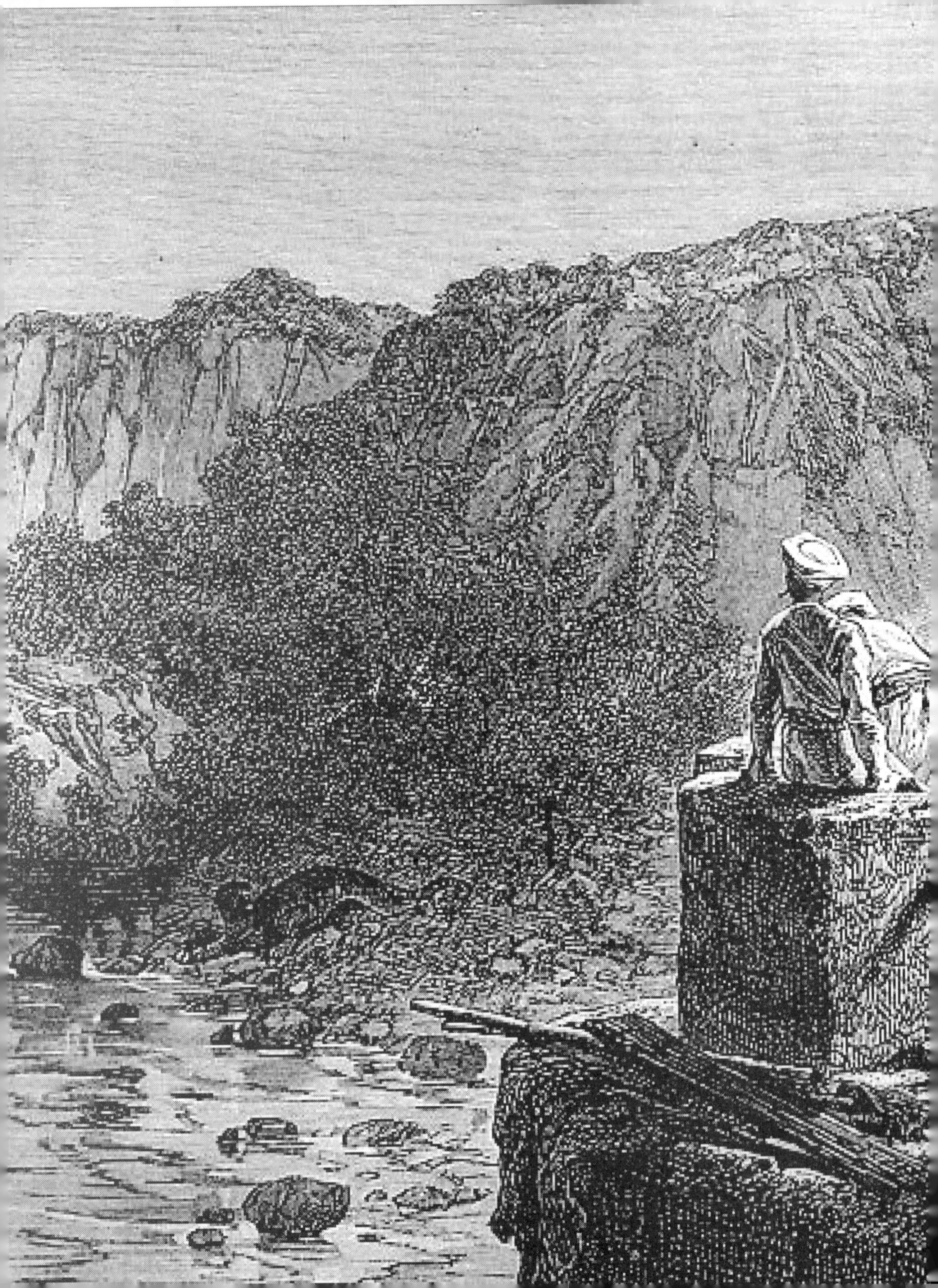

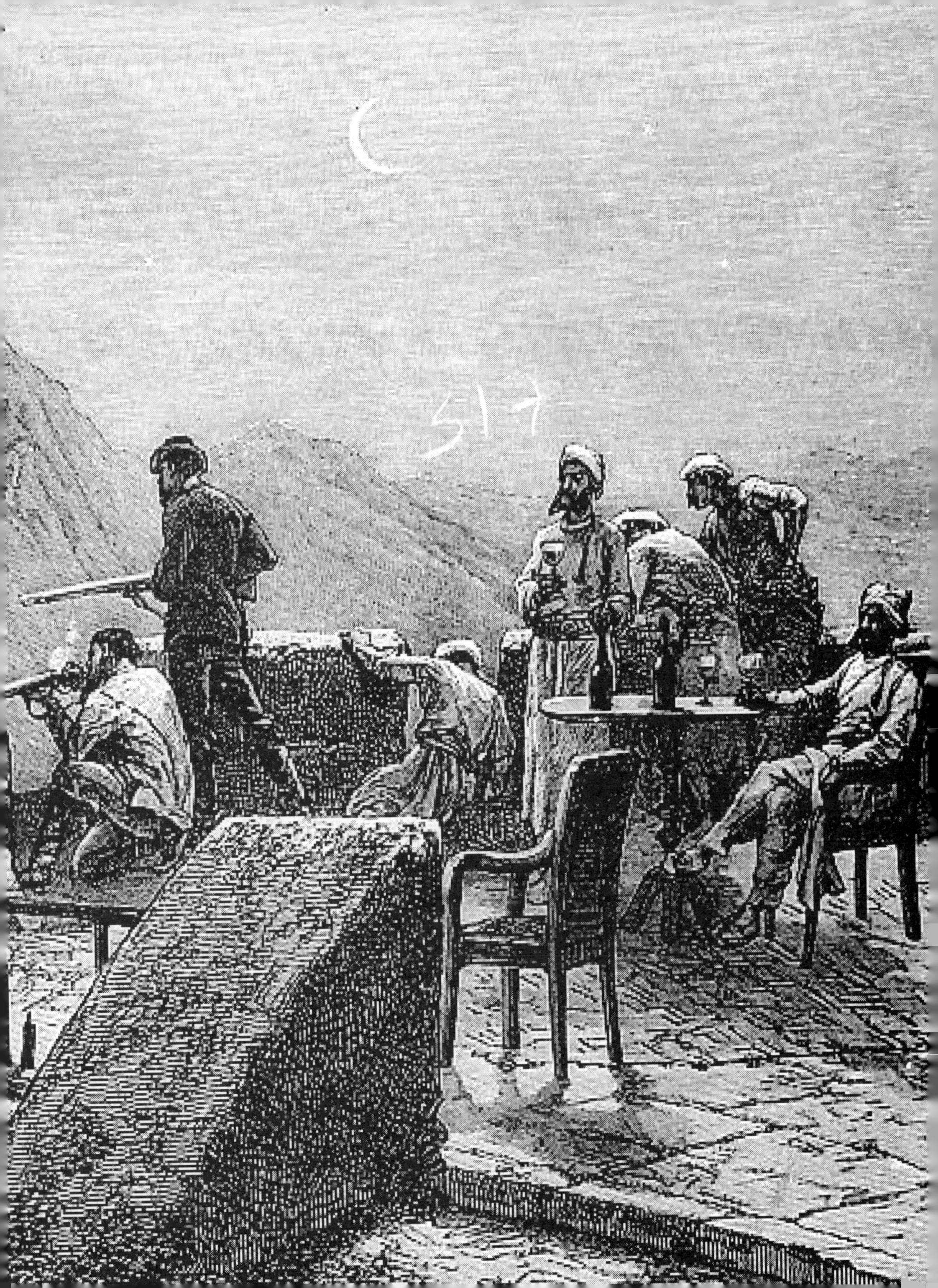

which they perceived by specific means and no others and which had made them ignorant about existing reality, and, exceedingly prone to capital mistake of speculating things in their favor without data. For years the succession of events, with an overwhelming force, had cried out loudly about the presence of tigers in cane. Despite this gargantuan loss of tigers in farmlands, through poisoning, poaching and dispersal, their population had held steady through four decades and many sugarcane fields were still noteworthy tiger watching sites. Then what was the problem with experts I did not know. Perhaps the exaggerated accounts of sufferers had added widespread misconception about the cat's response to man and fear inspired by a few man-eating individuals had contributed to belief that tigers attack without provocation, which had also added to their reputation of innate savagery. In such an ominous situation, any talk about tiger protection in cane zone was an extremely touchy matter and a lone crusader's voice that it was de facto the tiger, which was in crisis, was not more than the plummeting piping of a bird in a storm.

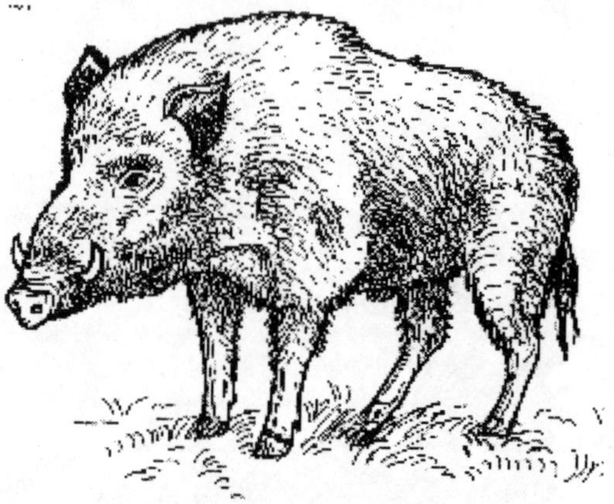

It was disgusting that I had to fight my own government to save this tiger.

Such indifference to the plight of cane tigers must be treated as a heinous crime against wildlife. It was grossly wrong to say that tiger hounding had been bunged; only the ways had changed; and indeed the old contours still appeared the same. Now the executive custodians of this animal were cheerfully telling me that tigers in the farms were essentially man-killers and how they hoped to contribute to the destruction of all that I was working hard to protect. It was easy to discredit me than to face the grueling facts because it was more comfortable that way. Through batter and negligence -we have but exterminated the tiger. One officer remarked that there are nearly six hundred parks and sanctuaries in our country and we are unable to protect them properly. There is a need to defuse this situation and short list some key places. The query was: "What is the use of adding your sugar tiger in this already protracted list?"

I was aghast at the morass of his bureaucratic apathy. Everyone is entitled to be stupid, but there are some who abuse the privilege. Surprisingly when in India the British Government could successfully manage 40% forests of the total land mass with its teeming wildlife; our modern forester has problems in managing only 3% chunk of forests with hardly any wildlife. Perhaps the officer had forgotten that he was getting his salary because the tiger was still there. It gave the department an aura of glamour and helped them to obtain more government funds than it deserved or knew what to do with. Indeed it had given him a job. Indirectly this animal was putting bread in this joker's mouth. Perhaps he had never thought that his job as a forester will be transformed into a mutant of itself if this natural wonder fades away? Such an odious approach of foresters is a more culpable wildlife abuse than culling for sport, for it burns their own foundations. The sin of this genocide must squarely rest on the shoulders of such authorities, on whom the onus of tiger management rests.

A member of Project Tiger steering committee unscrupulously declared that as my project was never formally sanctioned by the government and no NGO had funded it even with a shoestring budget, thus it was not a binding upon them to consider my suggestions. Moreover, it was impossible for an individual to accomplish such a gargantuan feat of field research single-handedly; so to a great extent my views, so definitely expressed were highly subjective in approach and could not be taken as correct.

The whole claim was apparent nonsense. They had forgotten three fundamental points. First, although opposition was built up against me in my effort to save tigers in the sugar farms, yet the trial had endorsement of the Governor of Uttar Pradesh in consent with CWLW. It was not me but the state government which had appointed eighteen farmers as Tiger Guardians around Dudhwa. And if there were no tigers on these farms then what for the guardians were chosen and what for CWLW was pleased to acknowledge the hard work of farmers, whose struggle to save tigers in farmlands seemed to have been paying off.

The second point is my locus standi. For last many generations the maternal side of my family is deeply-rooted in the Tarai. My maternal grandmother's father Pundit Chhotey Lal Dixit, owned Zamindari of more than eighty villages at the borders of Kishanpur tiger reserve while my maternal grandfather Pundit Ganga Prashad Bajpae, was the officiating chairperson of the confederation of 36 princely states of Tarai, having inherited the chair from his elder brother Rai Bahaur Sankata Prashad Bajpae, to represent the union at Dilli Darbar of 1911. Therefore my relations with many former feudals, whose farms harbored tigers, have been most cordial. Though at no stage, I had ever availed any infrastructural facilities or monetary favours from the apex body, but my privileged background and the earnest support of locals had been deeply instrumental in culmination of my research.

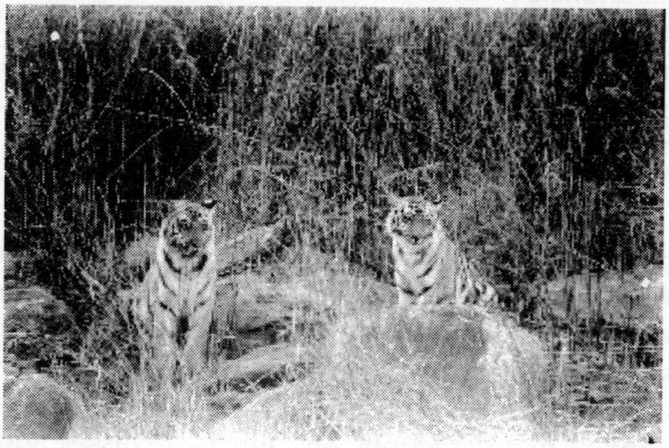

And thirdly, I had never abandoned my project. I had always thought about it as 'worth the effort to try' as each component of it had allowed me to learn more about these animals and reach quite different conclusions. I admit

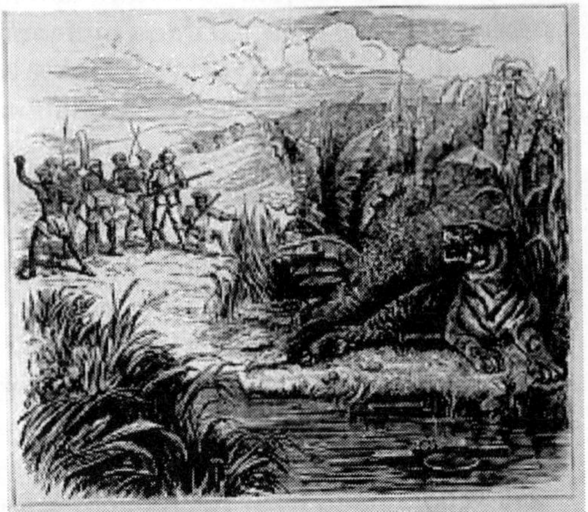

WOUNDED TIGER BEING DRIVEN FROM LAIR BY NATIVES

that all aspects of my research were conducted in cooperation with the farmers, since it was on their lands that the tigers had their ranges and it was in their farmhouses and hamlets that I had stayed on to pursue these cats unabated for weeks. Personally I recall these simple peasants, including my *shikaries* and other supporters with admiration and grateful remembrance.

Soon it became apparent that the authorities were not prepared to accept my reports as well as my requests. But alas! As no organization can function without a bureaucratic structure of some kind, the decision to save this tiger was up to them. I may be forgiven for saying that you cannot educate someone beyond his intelligence and I could easily make out a mass of uninitiated and incompetent officials at the bottom of it all. Many of them had joined the service to get a good government job like any other and could not develop a keen passion to serve wildlife. At times I wondered if such a collective creates the final opinion then it is logical to conclude that the collective must be the source of right. But all this out-pouring of luddite unscientific mind-set was a dangerous assignation, which finally meant that the collective was the source of wrong. As for the foresters it was much easier to get the tigers killed than to kill their rigid scientific article of faith, which frowned at my observations with confident assertions. I am sure the ancillary of this dogma was the intangible notion that abstractedly believed in tiger's disinclination to inhabit human dominated landscapes, than by any generous endorsement realized by a long-standing modern study, through the application of scientific tools.

This book of mine is not the last word on the tigers of the Tarai but it is certainly the ultimate verdict on sugarcane tigers because strategically I am stationed on ground zero, the historical game board of sugar-tigers, where these spectacular cats are involved as quaint players; and where, as it portends, I can document their ending games, advantageously and authoritatively to their last-ditch battle for survival and may also perhaps procrastinate the exodus of a few still extant by my steadfast frontline actions.

The rabid credo of scientists must move out of its comfort zone and respect the poignant notion of conservationist. It is believed that you only grow when you are willing to feel awkward and uncomfortable when you try something new. It is a wonder that scientists never issued a public apology for this howler whereas they should have gone for a penance in caves for the rest of their lives.

Scientists are funny people, now when some very little is left of dodo, a piece of wing, a few depictions on Dutch canvasses and just one stuffed specimen in

Mauritius, there is a Japanese researcher who has spent his whole life studying dodo without ever having seen a living sample. It is remarkable that the zoologists of nineteenth century, some of them quite eminent like Georges Cuvier, let many evidences of this extinct birds go waste by doubting their existence.

My blow by blow account of sugarcane tiger controversy, and of its rise and fall, is a poignant example of how the unique beast, which had agreed to environmental transformation with noteworthy aplomb, was crowded against the wall by sheer neglect of administrators and how by their excessive nefarious intrusion natives played havoc with a putative strain which might have been evolving. This sometimes makes me wonder what would be the future of these grand animals of the sugar farms. Whether the new professional agency, National Tiger Conservation Authority (NTCA) that replaces Project Tiger as a statutorily empowered decision-making body with several functions towards tiger conservation- would ever acknowledge the predicament of few animals' predilection to sugarcane or only behave in the unruffled manner as its predecessors did, and let this miracle of nature fade away or else recognize it only when they are finally gone?

YES, IF WE DO NOT UNDERSTAND SOMETHING, WE DON'T CARE IF IT GOES.

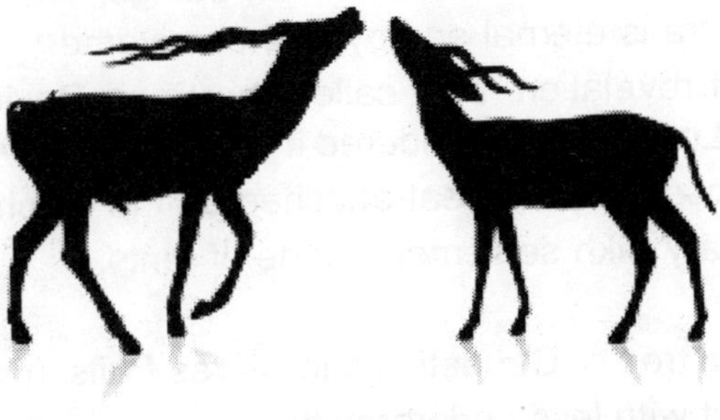

Glossary of Indian words

Aloo-Pakori: Indian fast-food -deep fried gram paste and potato balls.
Arahiya Wali Beyar: A March wind that blows for two and a half days.
Baghaar: Low lying marsh land
Babool: The Indian acacia tree
Bhaiya: Brotherly junior master
Brahmin: A high caste Hindu.
Chota-shikar: small game weighing up to 100 pounds.
Churia: Shiwalik hills in Nepal, which is outermost of the Himalayan ranges, characterized by unconsolidated nature of its rocks.
Dashera: Hindu religious festival-October
Deccan: central south India
Gadaniya: Dense jungle
Gayatri Mantra: Hinduism was not founded by any human being. It is believed to have been founded by God himself for the welfare of his creations. He gave this religion to the angels of heaven in form of Gayatri mantra which makes the worshipper one with the extraterrestrial consciousness and grants salvation. Angels passed it on to the human beings. The radiant energy resulting from the mantra is eternal energy of the universe.
Gita: The book of revelation, also called the Song Devine is an acknowledged Hindu Bible. Lord Krishna rendered it to his disciple Arjun.
Howdah: an enclosed cot like seat attached on the elephant's back
Jhala: the temporary Sikh settlement made of tents.
Jheel: Local Lakes
Jamun: A common tree of Gangetic plains gives fruits in rains.
Kapis: a thin forest with less undergrowth
Khalihans: temporary go downs
Khalla: a low lying area
Khar: Thach grass
Laati: The trail of the wild animal
Lathi: a staff or bamboo stave, fondly kept by Indian peasants
Lehru: wooden ox cart
Maharaja: King of a large state
Mahua: A common tree of Gangatic plains its flowers and fruits are very popular with wild animals and human beings.
Machan: A raised platform, used as shooting post or watch tower.
Mahauts: Hereditary elephant trainers.

Maha-Mratunjay Mantra: A holy chant of Lord Shiva that averts untimely death.

Neem: A popular tree of medicinal use

Nala: Dry stream bed

Peepal: A common tree with strong roots. The spirits of dead are believed to live on it.

Pundit: A scholar of high repute.

Pujari: A priest of Hindu temple.

Raj: the period of British rule in India.

Raja: The king of Indian state.

Sahib: Master

Sal: A major timber tree in north India.

Shakti: In Sanatan Hindu thought the mother goddess is supreme consciousness of Godhood and this endless universe created by her will never come to an end completely. Life is forever and her energy prevails through entire cosmos through the gigantic phases of time, divided into Satyug, Treta, Dwaper and Kalyug. Since the creation of cosmos, this set of all the four Yugas that runs into a seasonal cycle amounting to 12,30,00,000 years in one set have been repeated 261 times. This roughly corresponds to the age of this universe, as being 31,000000000 plus years old, which is closer to Stefan Hawking's calculation specified in his book "*The Theory of Time*'.

At the end of each Yuga, the entire cosmos becomes the cosmic body of the mother Goddesses as she eliminates the false prophets and harvests the souls that have been harvested by them on the fictitious promise of salvation and grants them the salvation. She is the ultimate champion of several Armageddon's that essentially occur, when the old order having joined the Gadarene rush, ends, and a new order begins afresh.

Shikar: Hunting - used mainly with reference to big game.

Shikari: Village based hunter.

Shiva: the foremost God of the Hindu trinity and the Lord of Northern sky.

Sikh: a follower of Sikh religion

Tarai: the country that lies immediately below the outer foothills of Himlayas is known as the Tarai. It is full of sluggish meandering streams, marshes, swamps and lush Sal forests.

Tharu: indigenous people of Mongoloid origins, living in the area of the Tarai.

Thakur: A term of respect, specially applied to master.

Wahe-Guru: God the supreme guide

Zamindar: Owners of large lands.

Zamindari: large landholdings

Glossary of of Scientific Terms, Principal Animals, Birds and Reptiles

Anthropogenic Pressures-The anthropogenic pressures include the conversion of woodlands into fields and pastures, diversion of surface and groundwater, ground water salinization due to inadequate drainage. pollution of soil and water by chemicals found in fertilizer and pesticides, the human alteration of plants by breeding and selection, removal of topsoil and creation of spoil piles, diversion of groundwater by mine shafts, surface runoff bearing mining wastes, release of air pollution by refining processes. removal of natural habitats by grading, diversion of groundwater, filling in marshes, bays, swamps, ponds, stream beds and finally concentration of human activities in discrete zones and concentration of waste products, sewage, and debris.

Androus pheromone; male sexual hormone

Asian elephants (Elephas maximus) :More compact than the African elephant . Most tractable, famous for its services to mankind.

Black Buck (Antelopa cervicapra)**:** Handsome antelope on verge of extinction.

Brahminy Duck (Tadorna ferruginea) A large orange brown duck with paler head.

Bush Rat (Golunda ellioti) a small size brown and black rat fairly common in Kishanpur sanctuary.

Cheetah, (Acinonyx jubatus) now extinct in India.

Chital (Axis axis): Strongly spotted deer, weighing up to 200 lbs. Favourite prey of leopard.

Chinkara (Gazella gazella) a full grown male antelope weighs upto 50 lbs.

Clouded Leopard (Neofelis Nebulosa)

Commom Mangoose (Herpestes edwardsi)

Common Teal (Anas crecca) Perhaps commonest migratory and an excellent sporting duck.

Contra-prepared ; a term used in behavioral sciences, which means predisposed not to learn at all.

Con-specific aggression; territorial species like cats are likely to fight con-specifics to maintain their territories.

Crow pheasant; (Centropus sinesis) A meat eating Common bird in Kishanpur.

Dhole (Cuon alpinus)A red colored dog weighing upto forty ilbs. Once common in Dudhwa now extinct.

Eco-tone zone; The area of integration between woodland and grassland.

Ecologically surplus abilities; The aptitude that permits animals to cope with rapid or unexpected change in the environment,

Gavial (Gavialis gangeticus) Also known as the gharial. The most seriously endangered of India's crocodiles; protected since 1972.

Grey Langoor (Presbytis entellus) Long tailed monkey up to 40 lbs.

Fishing Cat (Felis Viverrina) Rare over all but fairly common in Dudhwa area.

Fulvous fruit Bat (Rousettus leschenaulti)

Goose Barheaded (Anser indicus) Gaggles on rivers and Jheels and about young winter cultivation.

Goose Greyleg (Anser anser) A common winter visitor .Believed to be ancestor of our domestic breed.

Hare Rufoustailed (Lepus nigricollis ruficaudatus)Fairly common in Kishanpur and Dudhwa area, weighing up to five lbs.

Hog Deer (Axis porcinus) solid looking , short legged deer weighing up to 125 lbs.

Horn Bill Grey (Tockus birostirs) A clumsy brownish grey bird commonly living on fig ladden Banyan and Pepal trees near villages.

Hyena, (Hyaena hyaena) a carrion eater and hunter inhabits scrub lands , now rare in Dudhwa area. **Hyena ,spotted** (Crocuta crocuta) found all over Central and South Africa.

Indian Mangoose (Herpestes griseus) A great killer of snakes and rats.

Indian Tiger (Panthera tigris tigris) One of the seven sub species of the tiger which survive in the world . some 2000 now live in India's parks and reserves, where they are fully protected.

Indian Fox :(Vulpes bengalensis) A slender limbed animal of grey color with black tail .Common in the interiors of Tarai.

Jackal (Canis aureus) Fox sized predator , common in Kishanpur sanctuary and Dudhwa.

Jungle Cat (Felis Chaus) Common in Dudhwa area.

Keystone species; Predators that help increase the biodiversity of communities by preventing a single species from becoming dominant. Such predators are known as keystone species that have a profound influence on the balance of organisms in a particular ecosystem.

King cobra (Ophiophagus hannah) a deadly snake with neurotoxic poison upto twelve feet. **Indian cobra**(Naja naja) highly venomous but a little short in length from king cobra.

Lammergeier (Gypaetus barbatus) Bearded vulture with wingspan up to 10 feet.

Langur common (Presbytis entellus) Mainly arborial in their habits.Common in Kishanpur,

Leopard (Panthera pardus) Three sub-species of leopard survive in India. All are now protected but numbers have decreased alarmingly.

Leopard Cat (Felis bengalensis) Its color and markings give it the aspect of a miniature panther weighing upto eight lb.

Lion(Panthera leo) A highly endangered animal found only in Gir forest of Junagarh district.

Little Egret (Egretta alba) Fairly common in Dudhwa area.

Mallard (Anas platyrhynchos) A typical dabbling duck largely vegetarian.

Marsh Crocodile (Crocodylus palustris) An endangered species which has disappeared from most of India, also known as the mugger. Now legally protected but still subject to poaching for its skin.

Mongoose (Herpestes edwardsi) Famous for tackling snakes, they also have natural resistance to snake venom.

Monitor Lizard (Varanus monitor) Agile lizard up to 5 feet long.

Muntjac (Muntiacus muntjac) Barking deer also known as the Kakar up to 40 lbs.

Nilgai, Bluebull. (Boselaphustragocamelus)Large, ungainly antelope which inhabits open plains.

Partridge, Black (Francolinus francolinus) A black stub tailed game bird with white spots, lives in tall grass and well watered scrub.

Partridge Grey (Francolinus pondicerianus) Avoids heavy forest and lives in thorn scrub and open grass countery.Fairly common in Tarai

Peacock (Pavo Cristatus) The national bird of India.

Pheall cry: a tremulous P-i-a-a-o-o, P-i-a-a-a-o-o-o cry given by the jackal at the sight of tiger.

Pintail (Anas acuta) A duck of chocolate color head with white bands on either side of body.

Pochard White eyed (Aythya nyroca) A blakish brown color duck with whitish wing bar conspicuous in flight.

Pond Heron (Ardeola grayii) and **Night Heron**(Nycticorax nycticorax) both common in Kishanpur

Porcupine (Hystrix Indica) Preyed on by tigers and leopards. Weighs up to 40 lbs.

PSI trailings (Pressure per square inch) Cats have sensitivity to earth's magnetici field in time-space-continuum, they use the earth's gravity to determine their place in the world.

Python (Pybon molorus) Large snake fairly common in Dudhwa.

Redwattled Lapwing (Vanellus indicus) The common did- you –do- it bird.

Rhesus Monkey (Macaca mulatta) Favourite prey of leopards. Weighs up to 40 lbs.

Sambhar (Cervus unicolor) The largest deer in India . Weighs up to 700 lbs.

Shoveller (Anas clypeata) A duck with white breast and glossy dark green head and neck.

SSSI ; Sites of Special Scientific Interests

Sloth Beer (Melursus ursinus) Partially protected in India , Nepal and Sri Lanka but still endangered.

Smooth Indian Otter (Lutra perpicillata) Fairly common in Dudhwa and Kishanpur.

Squirrel Three Striped (Funambulus pennanti) A forest animal and a persistent egg robber.

Swamp Deer (Cervus duvauceli} an endangered species, now protected. The Kishanpur sanctuary of Dudhwa National Park is one of its main strongholds in Northern India. It weighs up to 500 lbs.

Symbiosis :the living together of two dissimilar organisms, as in mutualism, commensalism, amensalism, or parasitism.

Symbiotic relationship: A close, prolonged association between two or more different organisms of different species that may, but does not necessarily, benefit each member. .

Termites (Isoptra) Known as white ants but do not belong to ant family. Rich in Protein eaten by tribes and sloth beer. Common in Kishanpur.

Tufted Pochard (Aythya fuligula) one of the commonest migratory diving duck.

Vulture King (Sarcogyps calvus)A huge turkey like vulture with deep scarlet naked head.

Vulture White backed A heavy dirty blackish brown vulture with scrawny naked head and neck.

Wild boar {Sus scrofa }Favorite prey of the tiger.

Wigeon (Anas panalope) winter visitor duck frequents shallow jheels and marshes

Wolf {Canis lupus} partially protected in India since 1972.

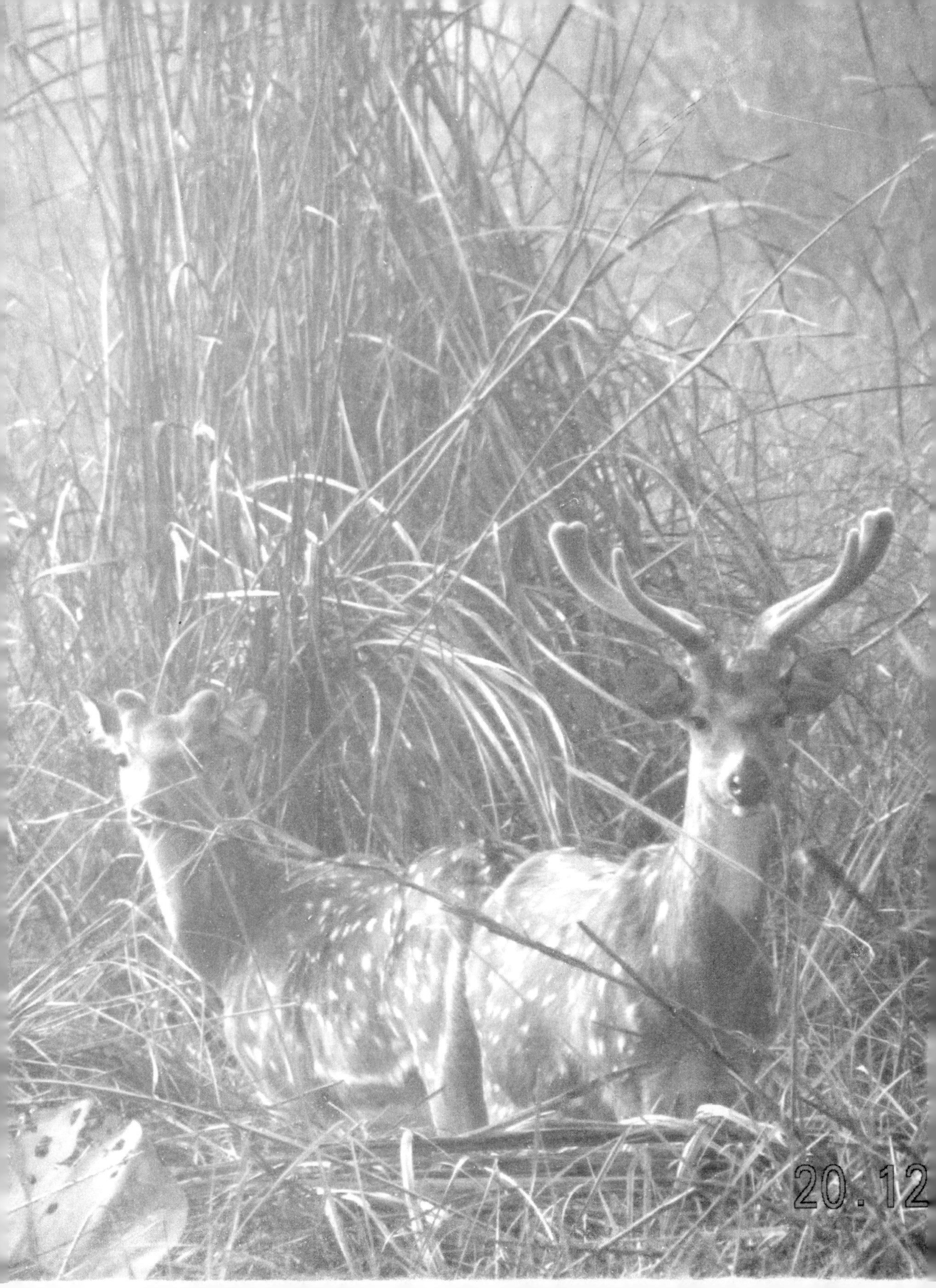
20.12

Tiger connection bookshelf

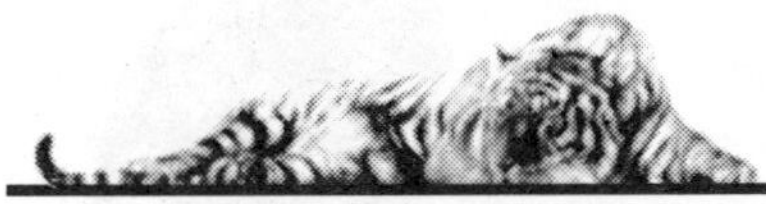

There have been several celebrated hunters, naturalists, scientists, conservationists and wildlife managers in past decades who have made remarkable contributions to wildlife conservation. It is largely because of their information and interpretations that we have a better understanding of forests and their dwellers. I salute those whose views I have quoted in the text and also those whose ideas and information have been incorporated in this work.

- Author

Select Bibliography

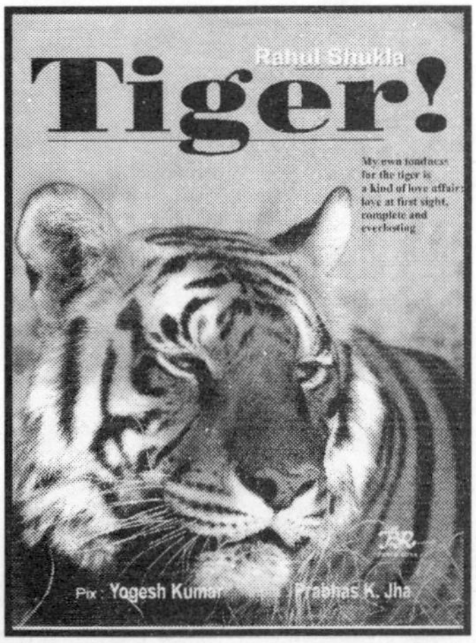

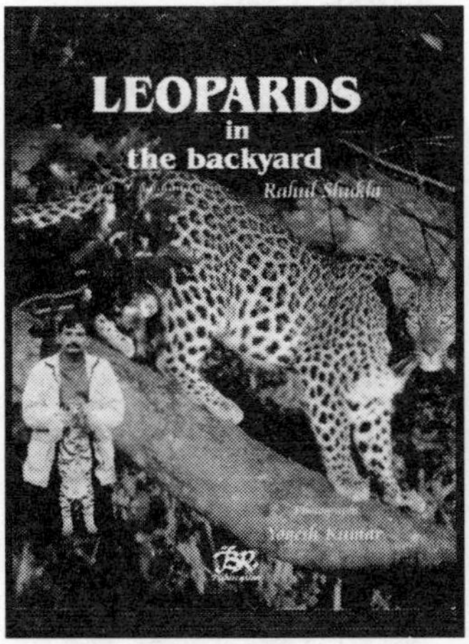

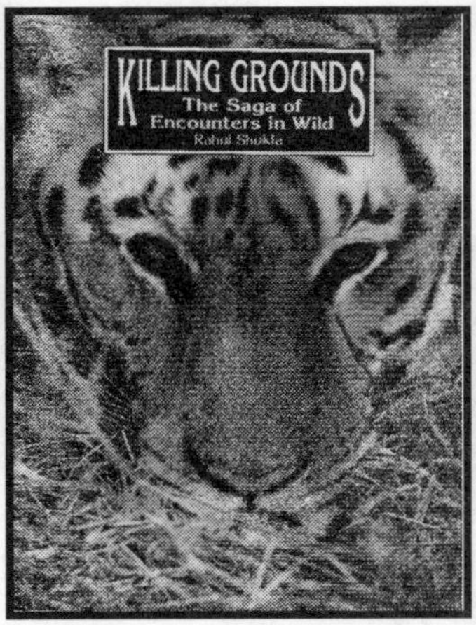

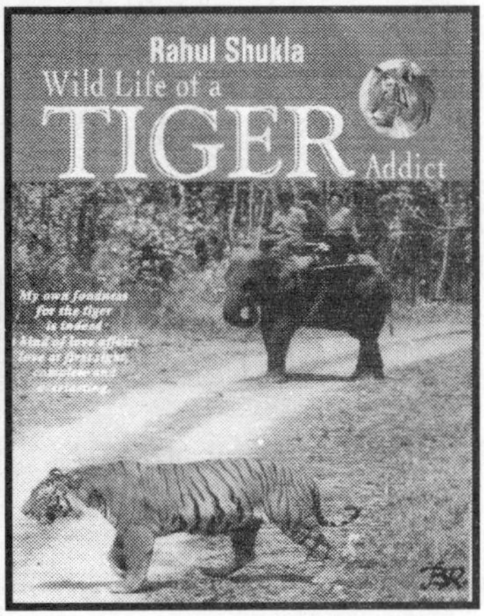

Bibliography

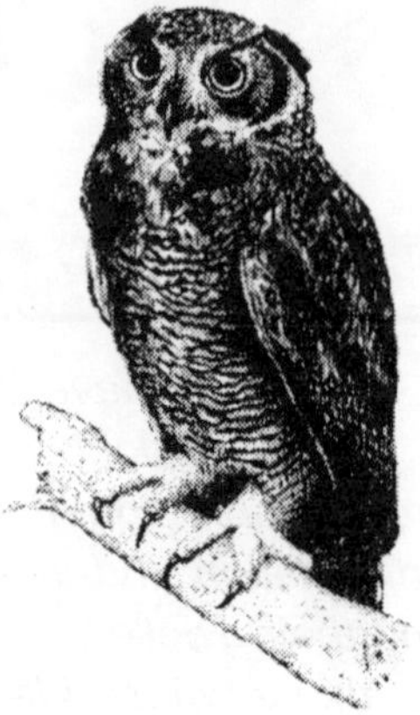

American Zoo and Aquarium Association. Communiqué, *"Save the Tiger Fund."* November 1995.

Baker E. B, *Sport in Bengal*, London, 1888

Baldwin, J.A, *The Large and Small game of Bengal*, London, 1877

Baze W, *Tiger! Tiger!* London, 1957

Best, J.W, *Indian Shikar Notes*; London 1931

—*Forest Life in India*, London, 1935

Bolton, W, *Royal Chitwan National Park Management Plan*,

Katmandu, 1979

Brakefield, Tom. *Big Cats Kingdom of Might*. Stillwater, MN: Voyageur Press, 1993.

Brander A. A Dunbar, *Wild Animals of Central India*, London, 1923

Brown, J, Moray, *Shikar Sketches*, London, 1887

Burton R.G. *The Book of Tiger*, London, 1933

Campbell, Major Walter, *The old Forest Ranger*, London, 1843

Champion, F.W, *With a Camera in Tiger Land*,

—*The Jungle in Sunlight and Shadow*,

Christie, Jackson and Seidensticker, eds, *Riding the Tiger; Tiger Conservation in Human Landscapes*, Cambridge University Press, 1999.

Corbett Jim, *Man-eaters of Kumaon*, New York and Bombay, 1944

The Temple Tiger, 1954

Jungle Lore, London, 1953

Tree Tops, London, 1955

De., Rathendranath, *The Sunderbans*, Oxford University Press, Calutta, 1990

Denial Johnson, Surgeon, *Indian Field Sports,* 1823,

Dockin, R, *The Selfish Gene*, Oxford University Press, 1976

Eardley Wilmot, S. *Forest Life and Sport in India*, London, 1910

Forsyth, J. *The Highlands of Central India*, London, 1872

Glasfurd A.I.R, Rifle and

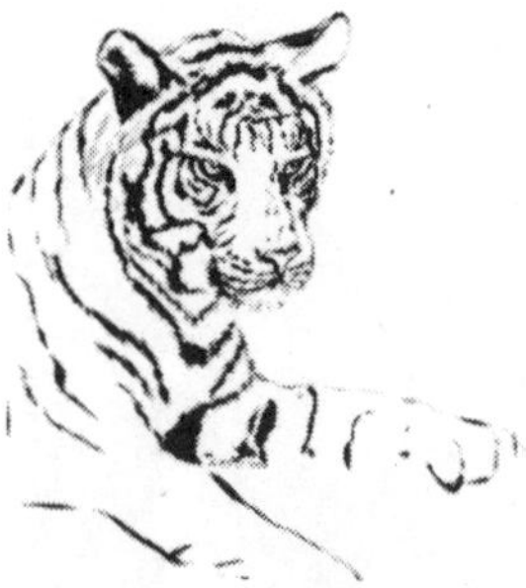

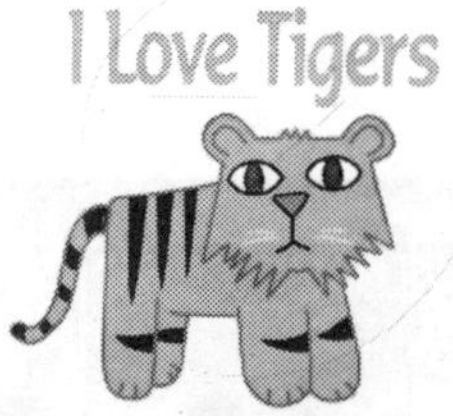

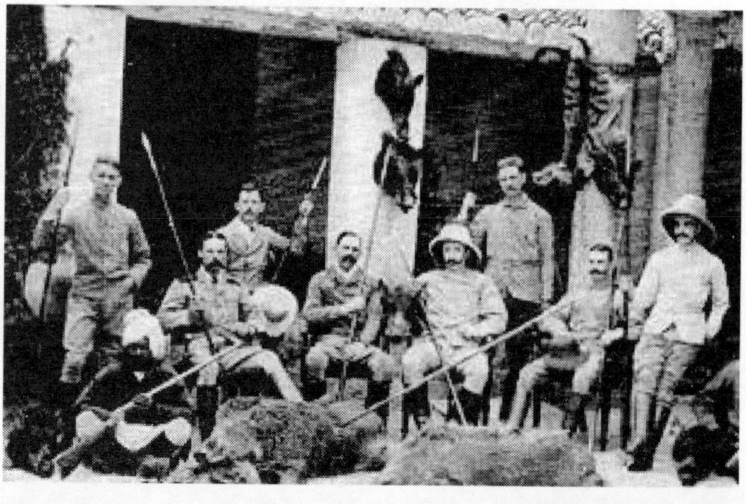

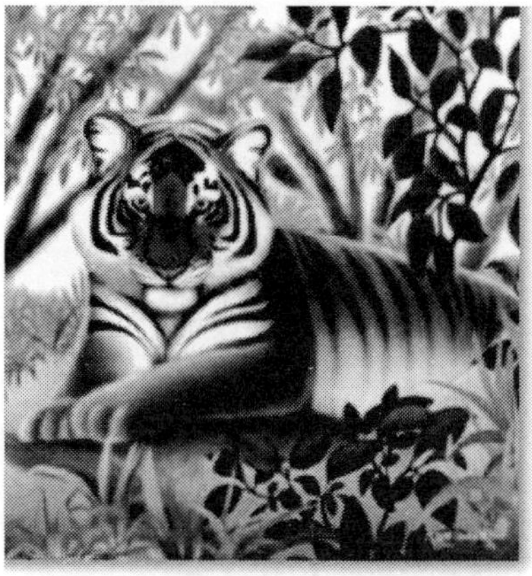

Romance in the Indian Jungle, London, 1905
Gordon Cumming, W, Wild Men and Beasts, Edinburgh, 1871
Gause, G. F, The Struggle for Existence, Williams

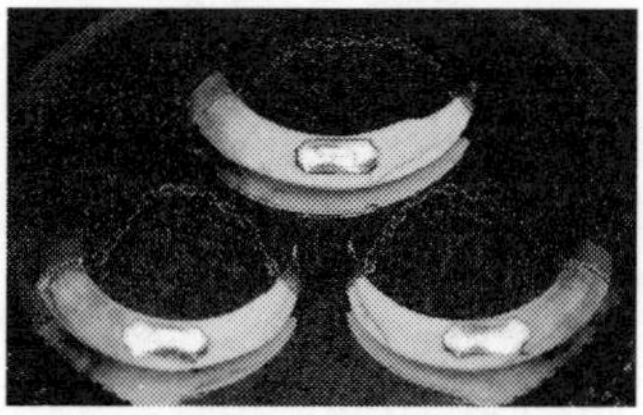

& Wilkins, Baltimore, Md, USA, 1934.
Hamilton, D. Records of Sport in Southern India, London, 1892
Hewett John, Jungle Trails in North India, London, 1938
Hanely, P. Tiger Trails in Assam, 1961
Hicks F.C. Forty Years among Wild Animals in India, Allahabad, 1910
Inglis James, Tent Life in

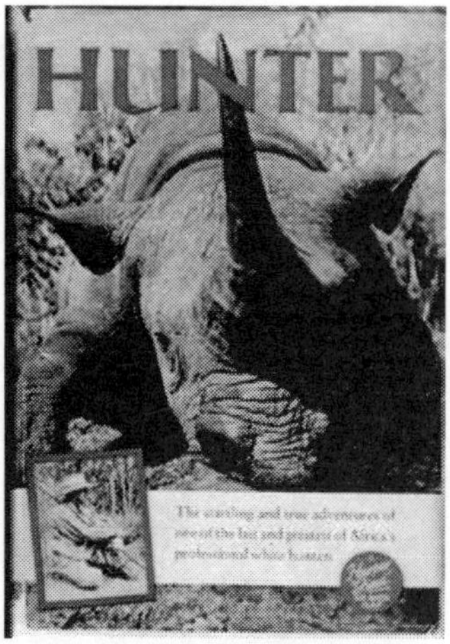

Tigerland, London, 1888
Jackson, Peter. *Endangered Species. Tigers.* London: Quintet Publishing Limited, 1990.
Jackson, Peter. *Status of the Tigers of the World.* CBSG News 4(4) 1993, pp. 12-14.(4)
Karan, P.P. and Myron

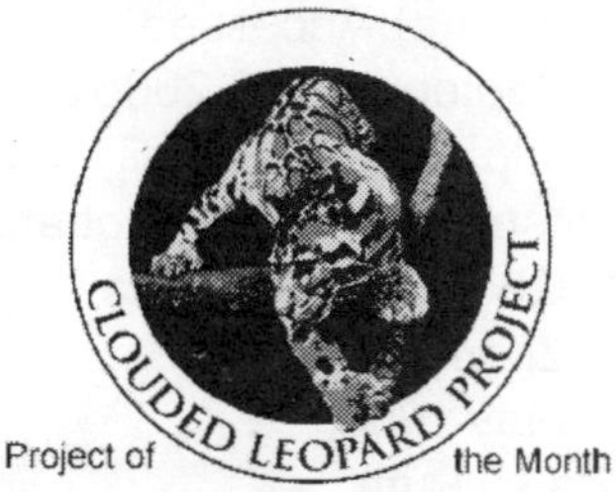

Weiner. "India." The World Book Encyclopedia. Volume 10. Chicago: World Book, Inc., 1995, pp. 108-135. (17)
Kitchener, Andrew. *The Natural History of the Wild Cats.* Ithaca, NY: Comstock Publishing Associates, 1991. (3)
Mac Dougal, Charls, The Face of the Tiger, London, 1977
MacDonald, David, ed. *The Encyclopedia of Mammals.* New York: Facts on File, Inc., 1993. (8)
Matthiessen, Peter. *Tigers in the Snow*. North Point

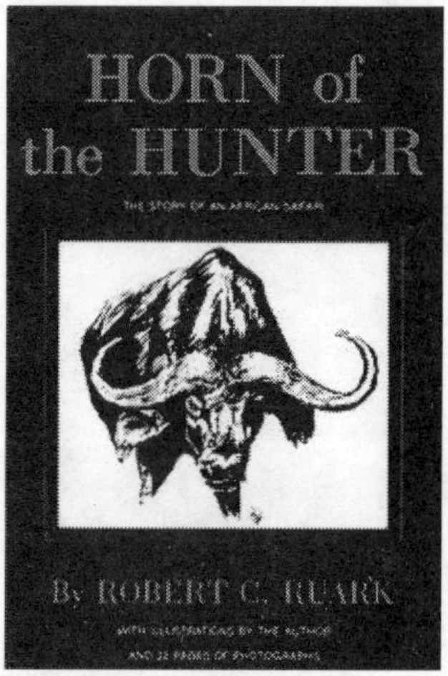

Press, 2000.
McDougal, Charles. *The Face of the Tiger.* London: Rivington Books and Andre Deutsch, 1977. (14)
Myers, P., R. Espinosa, C.

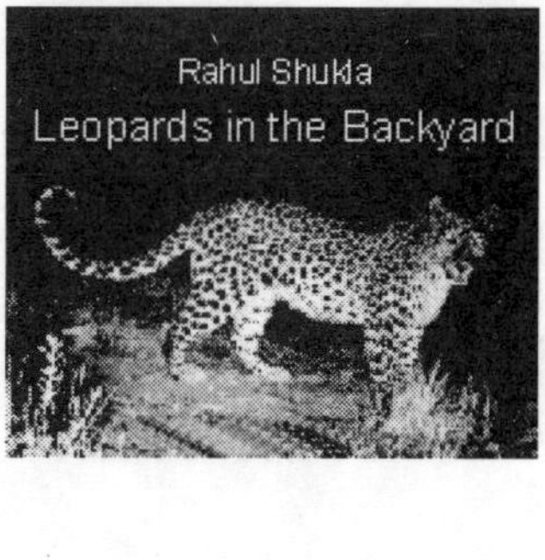

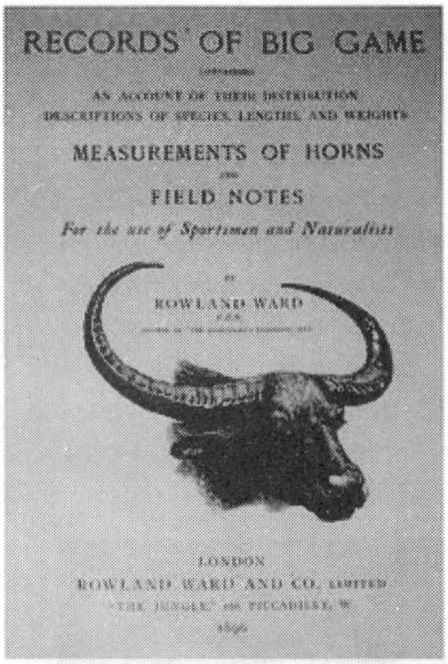

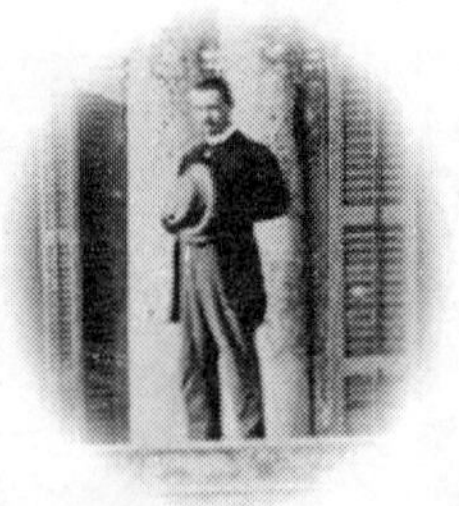

Wildlife photographer Carl McGrager in Lucknow

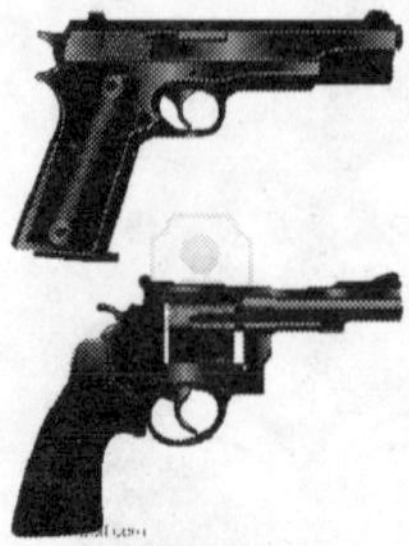

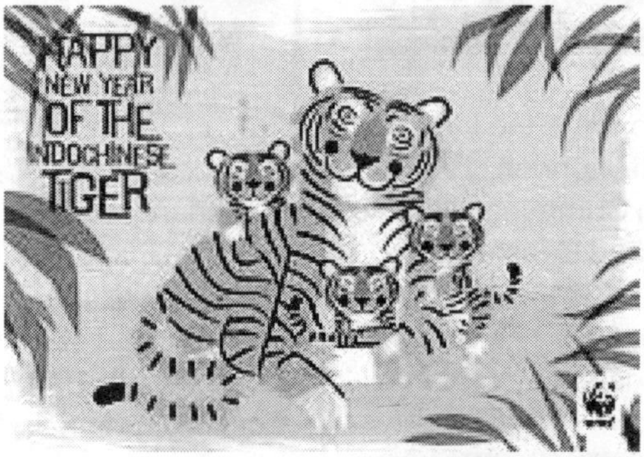

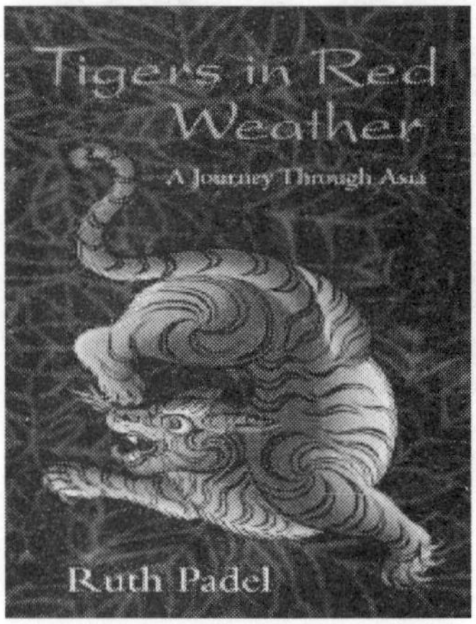

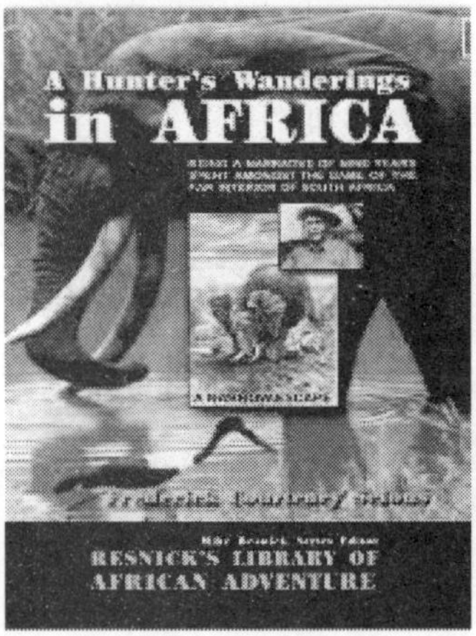

S. Parr, T. Jones, G. S. Hammond, and T. A. Dewey. 2006. The Animal Diversity Web (online). Accessed September 27, 2005 at http://animaldiversity.org.

Nostrand, Mary L. "Mohan, Ghost Tiger of Rewa." *Zoonooz* May 1984,

Padel Ruth, *Tigers in Red Weather*, Little Brown, London, 2005

Quammen, D, *Monster of God; The Man-eating Predator in the Jungles of History and the Mind*, Norton, 2003.

Shukla, Rahul, *Killing Grounds*, Deryaganj Delhi, 1994

— *Leopards in the Backyard*, 2002

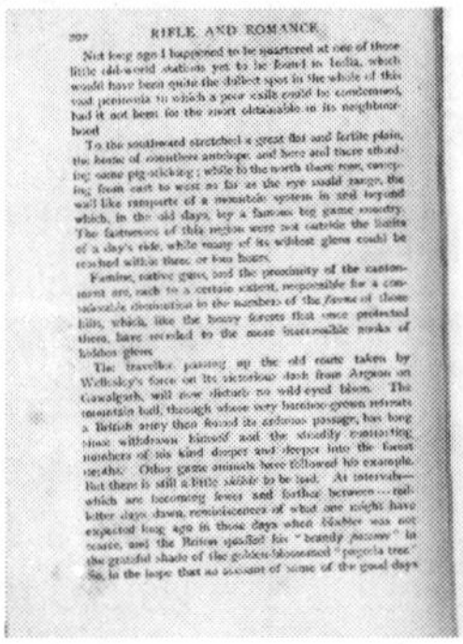

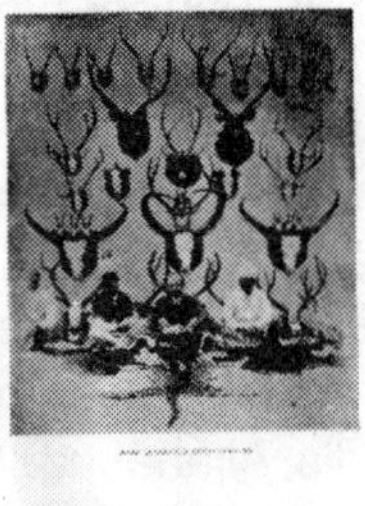

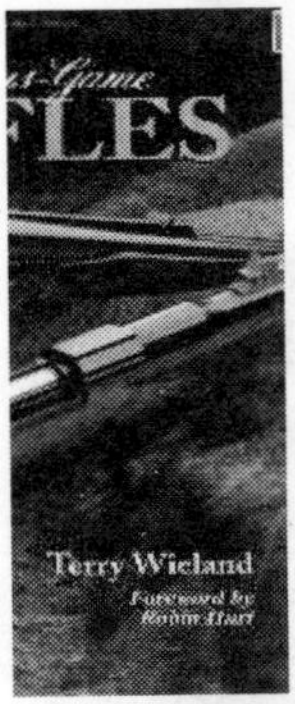

—*Tiger*, 2008

Simpson, Frank.B, *Letters on Sport in Eastern Bengal*, London 1886

Singh Arjan, *Tiger Heaven*, London, 1973

——— *Tara the Tigress*, London,

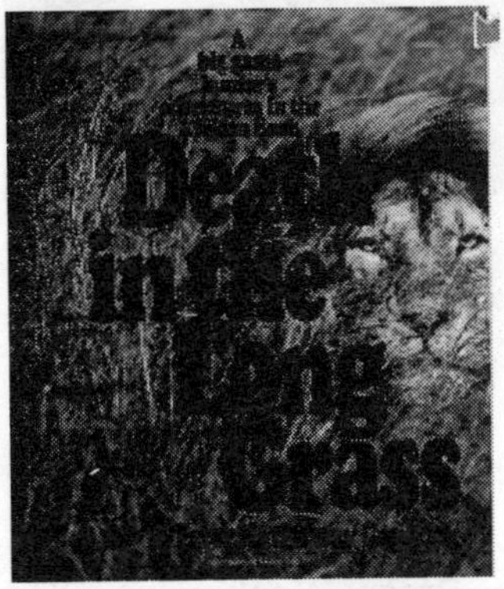

1981

—— *The Legend of Maneater*, Delhi, 1999

Singh R. L, *Tara the Cocktail Tigress*, Allahabad, 2000

Seidensticker, John. *Tigers (World Life Library)*. Stillwater, MN: Voyageur Press, 1996.

Seidensticker and Susan Lumpkin. *Smithsonian Answer Book Cats*. Washington: Smithsonian Books, 2004.

Stanley Breeden & Belinda Wright; *Through the Tigers Eyes*, California 1996

Storer J.H, *The Web of Life*, New York, 1953

Sunquist, Mel. *Wildcats of the World*. Chicago: University of Chicago Press, 2002.

Tobias.J. Lanz, *The Life and Fate of the Indian Tiger*, Praeger Publishers, 2009

Sanquist, F and M; *Tiger Moon; Tracking the Great Cats in Nepal*, University of Chicago Press, 1989

Thaper Valmik, *Secret Life of Tigers*, Oxford,

\- *Tiger; the Predator*, London, 1986

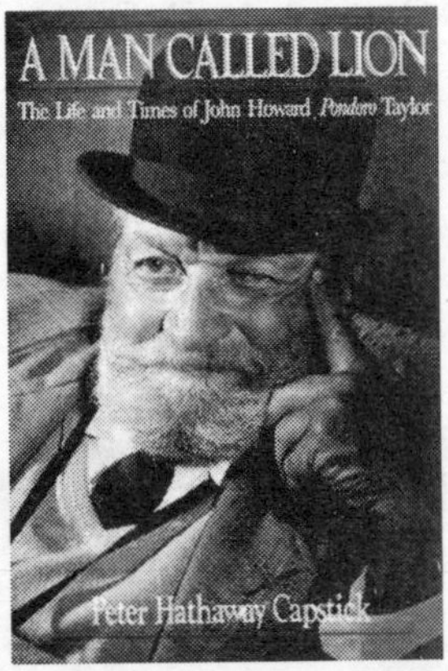

Thomas Kuhn, *The Structure of Scientific Revolutions*, University of Chicago Press, Chicago, Ill, USA, 2nd edition, 1970.

Tilson, Ronald L. and

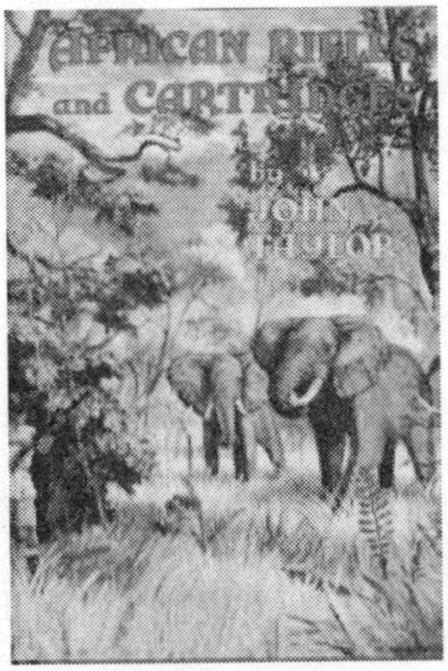

Ulysses S. Seal, ed. *Tigers of the World.* Park Ridge, NJ: Noyes Publications, 1987. (5)

Ullas Karanth, "Understanding Tigers." Wildlife Conservation June 1995, pp. 26-37. (9)

Ullas Karanth, *The Way of the Tiger*, 2001

Williamson, Thomas, *Oriental field Sports,* London, 1807

Wilson, E.O, *Sociobiology*, Harvard University Press, 1975

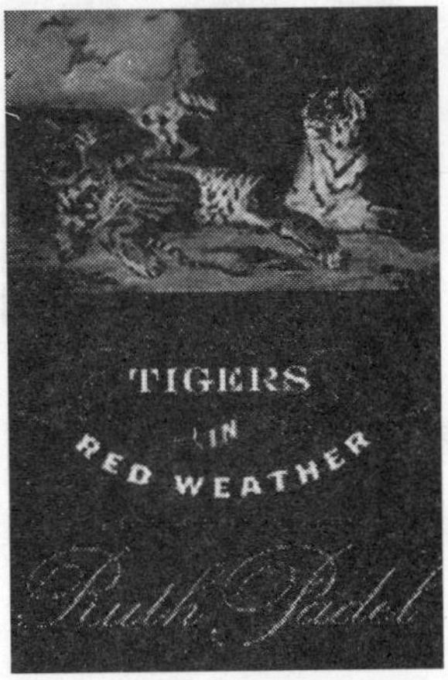

Research Papers and Scientific Articles

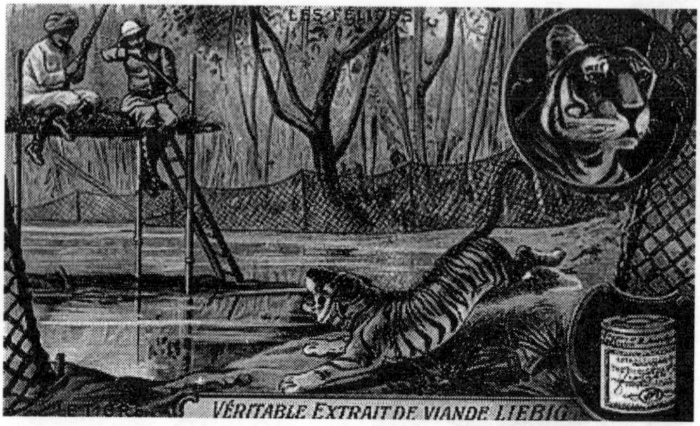

Berger. D, '*Wildlife Extension; Participatory Conservation by the Masai of Kenya*'. English Press, Ltd, Narobi, Kenya, 1993.

Bhatt. N, "*Kings as Wardens and Wardens as Kings; Post-Rana Ties between Nepali Royalty and Park Staff*', Conservation and Society1,2003,240-270.

Bowdoin, Julia, et al., ed. *AZA Annual Report on Conservation and Science*. Bethesda, MD: American Association of Zoological Parks and

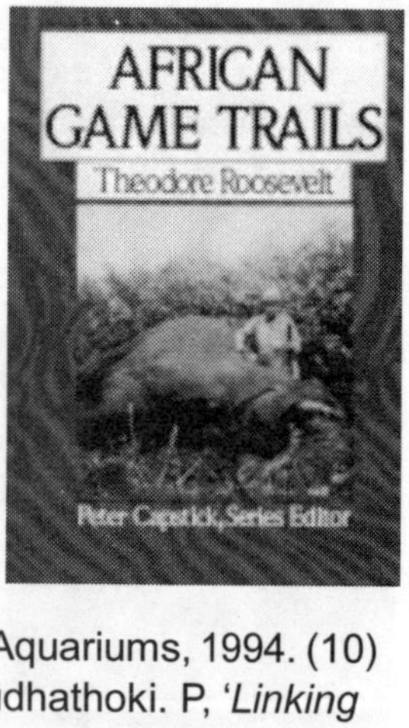

Aquariums, 1994. (10)

Budhathoki. P, '*Linking Communities with conservation in Developing Countries; Buffar Zone Management Initiatives in Nepal*', Oryx 38, 2004, 330-340; Baral et.al, op.cit, 2007.

Dinerstein,E.,E Wikramanayake, J. Robinson, U Karanth, A Rabinowitz, D. Olson, T. Mathew, P.Heddao, M, Conner, G. Hamley, and D.Bloze, ' *A Framework for Identifying High-Priority Areas and Actions for the Conservations of Tigers in the Wilds'*, WWF- US, 1997

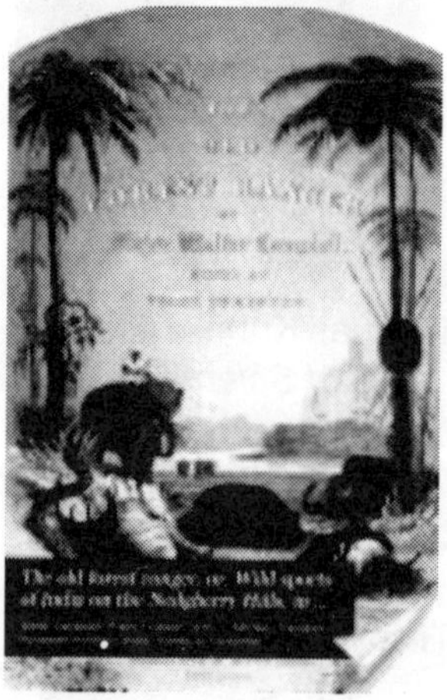

D. R. McCullough, *Metapopulations in Wildlife Conservation*, Ed., pp. 187–216, Island Press, Washington, DC, USA; 1996.

Goodrich J. L Kerley, D Miquelle, E Smirnove, H Quigley and M Harnocker ' *Effects of Roads and Human*

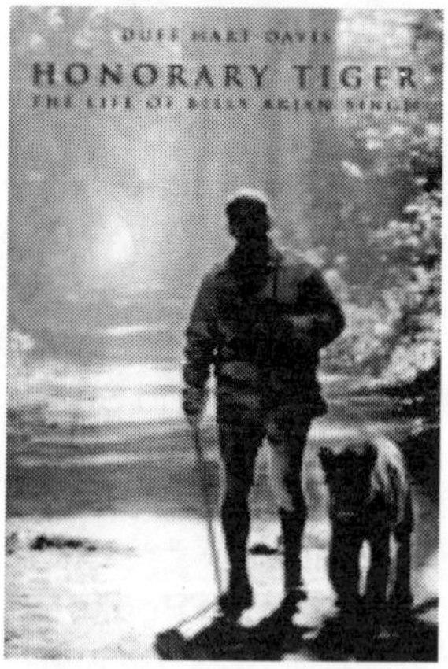

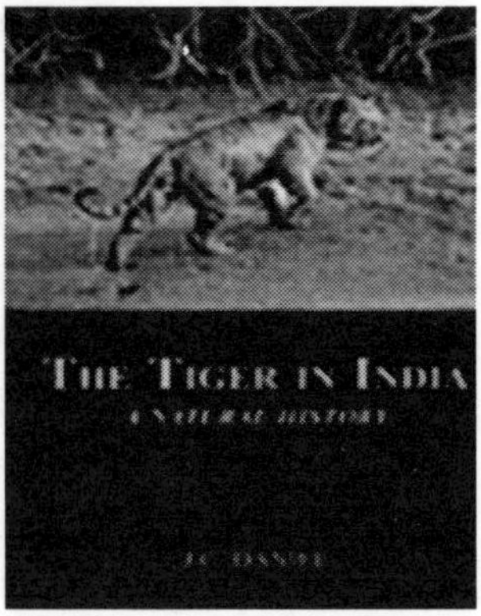

Disturbance on Amur Tigers' Conservation biology16,(1) Feb 2002, page 92-109

—*Reproductive Parameters of wild female Amur Tigers*' Journal of Mammology, 84(1) 2003

H. MacGregor, *The economic value of deer hunting and its distribution in the Fundy Model Forest- 1994*, M.S.

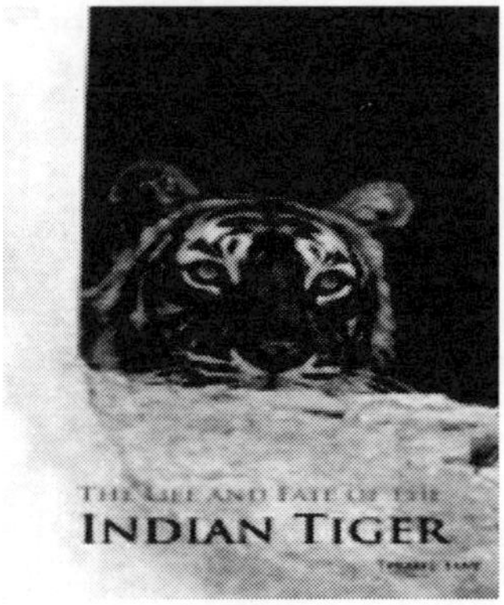

thesis, University of New Brunswick, New Brunswick, Canada, 1998

J. S. Brashares, P. Arcese, M. K. Sam, P. B. Coppolillo, A. R. E. Sinclair, and A. Balmford, *"Bushmeat hunting, wildlife declines, and fish supply in West Africa,"* Science, vol. 306, no. 5699, pp. 1180–1183, 2004.

J. S. Brashares, P. Arcese, and M. K. Sam,

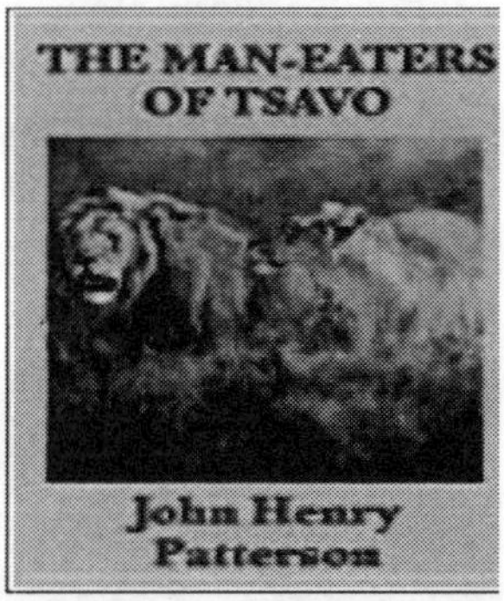

"Human demography and reserve size predict wildlife extinction in West Africa," Proceedings of the Royal Society *B*, vol. 268, no. 1484, pp

IUCN/SSC Cat Specialist Group (The World

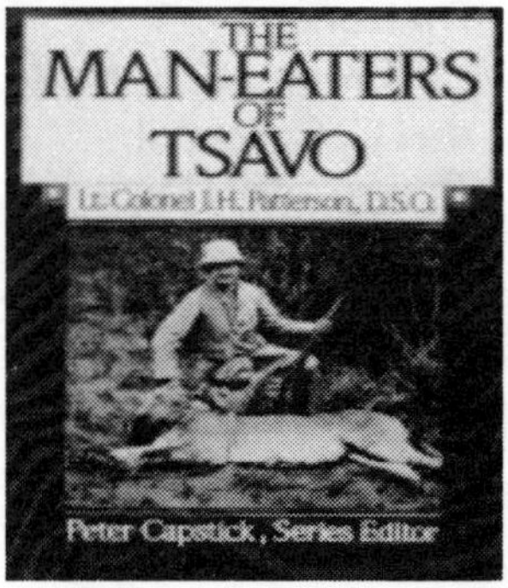

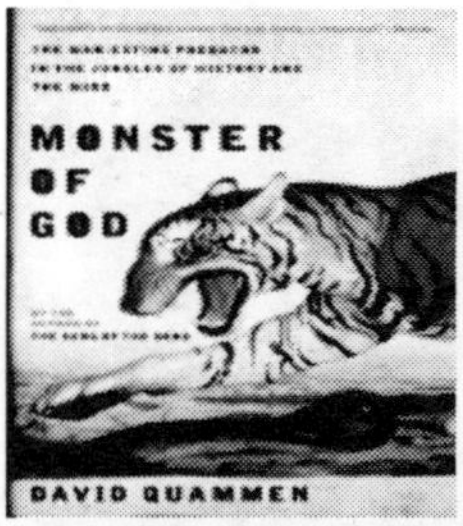

Conservation Union). *Status Survey and Conservation Action Plan Wild Cats*. IUCN: Switzerland, 1996.

Karanth U, with W.A Link, *'Correction for Over dispersion in Tests of Prey Selectivity'*, Ecology, 75(8) 1994

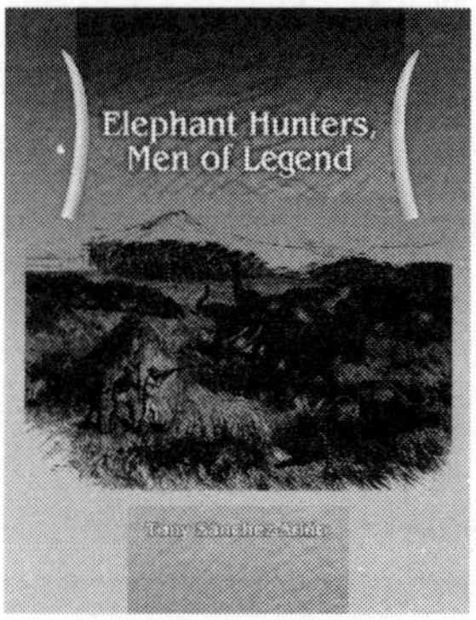

——*'Estimating Tiger Populations from Camera Trap Data Using Capture and Recapture Methods'* Biological Conservation, 71, 1995

Karanth U, with B M Stith, *'Prey Depletion as Critical Determent of Tiger Population Viability'* in Christie, *et al, 1999*

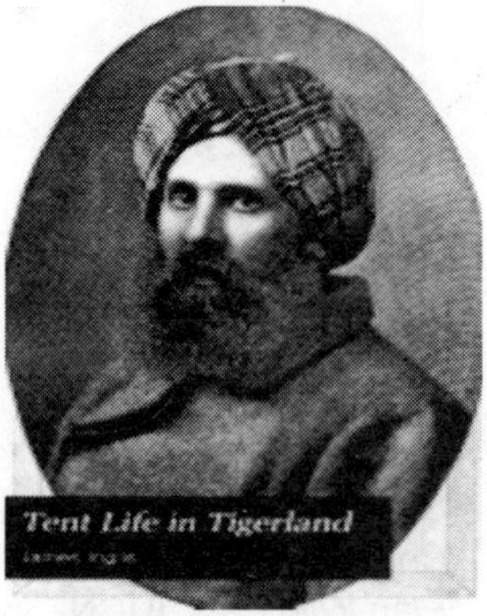

—'*Debating Conservation as if Reality Matters*', Conservation and Society,1, 2003

—*Science Deficiency in Conservation Practice; The Monitoring of Tiger Populations in India*' Animal Conservation, 6, 2003

Lever C, *'The Impact of Traditional Chinese Medicine on Threatened Species,* 'Oryx, 38, January 2004.

Leela Hazzah, Nelson Institute of Environmental Studies, University of Wisconsin, Madison; and Stephen Dolrenry, Living with Lions, Nanyuki, Kenya. *Coexisting with Predators*, Seminar, New Delhi, 2007

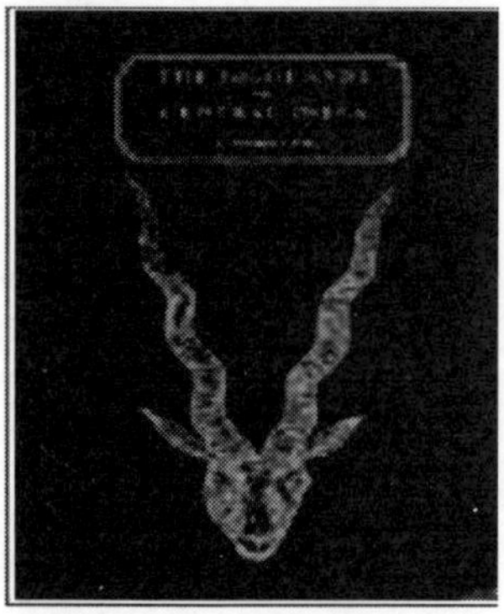

Linden, Eugene. "Tigers on the Brink." *Time* 143(13) 1994, pp. 44-51.

M.D Madhusudan and Rohan Arthur, *Succeeding Poorly or Failing Better*, Seminar, New Delhi, 2007

MacDougal, C., "*Tiger and Human Conflict Increase in Chitwan Reserve Buffer Zone*" Cat News, 40, 2004, IUCN, Berne, Switzerland.

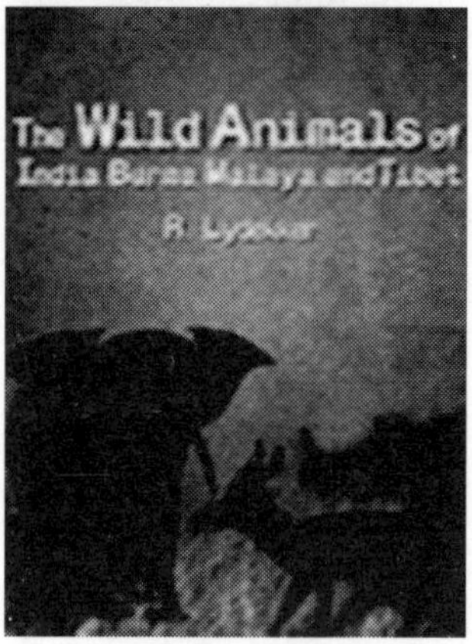

M. J. Groom, G. K. Meffe, and C. R. Carroll, *Principles of Conservation Biology*, Sinauer Associates, Sunderland, UK, 3rd edition, 2006.

S. Harrison, *"Local extinction in a metapopulation context: an empirical evaluation,"* Biological Journal of the Linnean Society, vol. 42, no. 1-2, pp. 73–88, 1991.

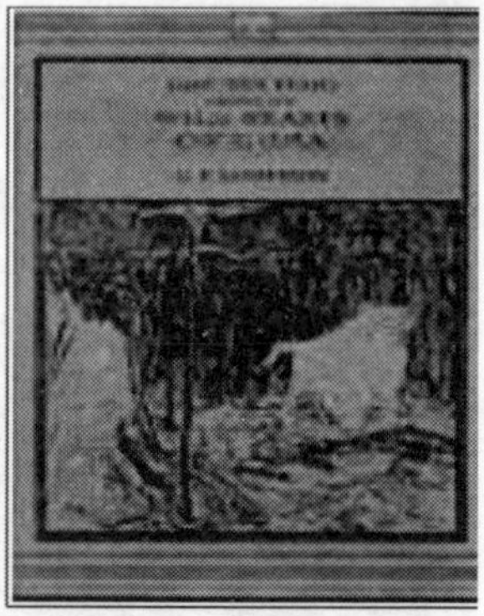

Smith, James L., et al. "*Scent Marking in Free-ranging Tigers, Panthera tigris.*" *Animal Behaviour* 37(1) 1989, pp. 1-10. (13)

Smith, James L. and Charles McDougal. "*The Contribution of Variance in Lifetime Reproduction to Effective Population Size in Tigers.*" Conservation Biology 5(4) 1991, pp. 484-490.

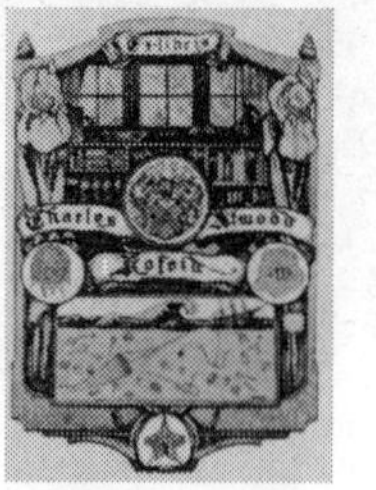

Smith, James L. "The Role of Dispersal in Structuring the Chitwan Tiger Population." *Behaviour* 124(3-4) 1993, pp. 165-

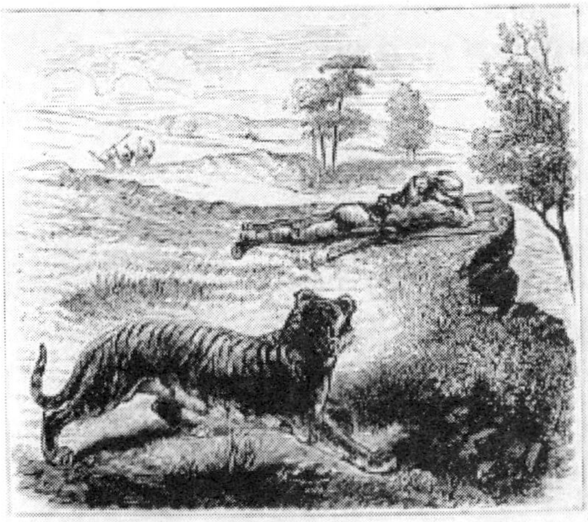

FROM AN UNEXPECTED POINT

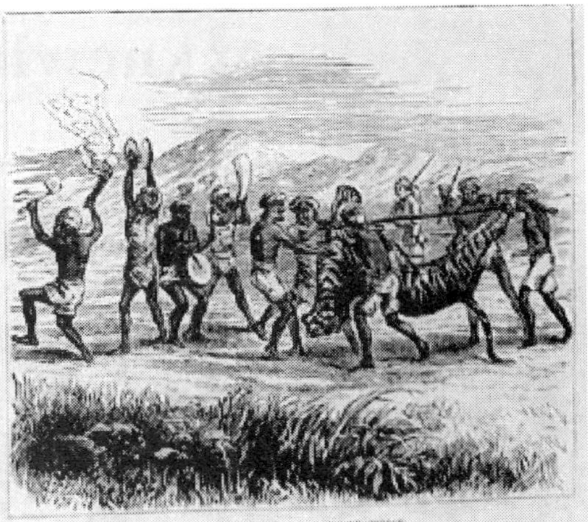

BRINGING THE DEAD TIGER HOME

195. (15)

Sunquist, Melvin E. *The Social Organization of Tigers (Panthera tigris) in Royal Chitawan National Park, Nepal.* Smithsonian Contributions to Zoology Number 336. Washington DC: Smithsonian Institution Press, 1981. (6)

Shakeshpear, H. Wild Sports of India (London, 1862).

Sheffield, F. How I Killed the Tiger (London, 1902)

Vidya Athreya, Kaati Trust, Pune; Centre for Wildlife Studies Banglore, *Living with Dangerous Animals*, Seminar, New Delhi, 2007

Ward, Geoffrey C. "*The People and the Tiger.*" Audubon July/August 1994, pp.62-69. (16)

Webber, T.W. The Forests of Upper India (London, 1902).

Woodyatt, N. My Sporting Memories (London, 1923)

World Wildlife Fund. "*U.S. Gives Notice to China and Taiwan to Stop Rhino and Tiger Trade.*" Traffic *USA* 13(1) 1994, pp. 1-3. (11)

World Wildlife Fund. *"Species of Special Concern."* *Focus*. Vol. 17 No. 6. November/ December 1995, p. 4.

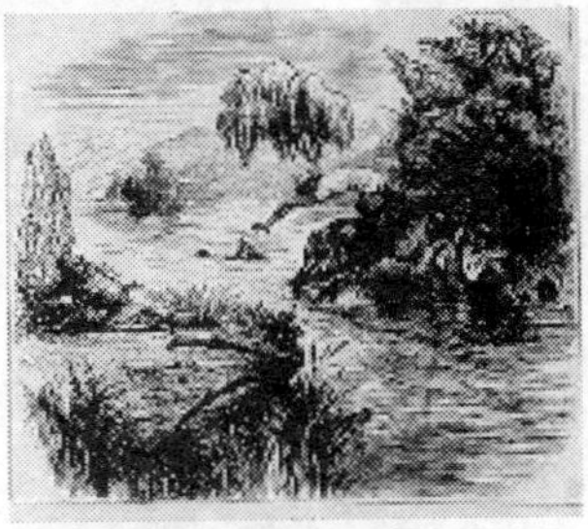

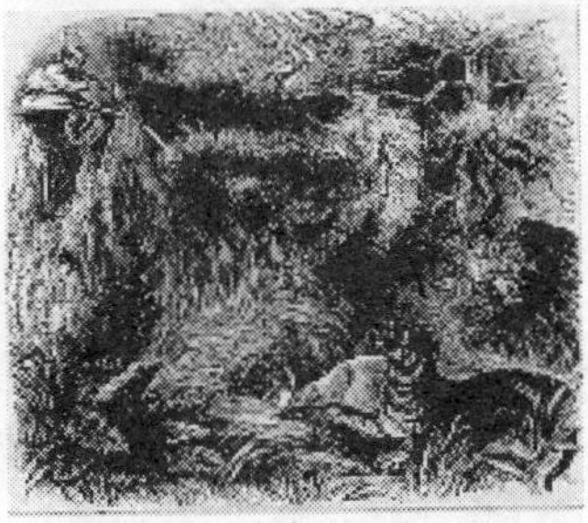

****

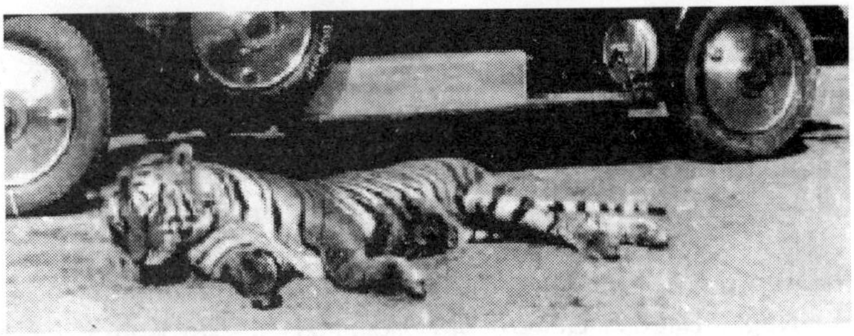

Acknowledgement

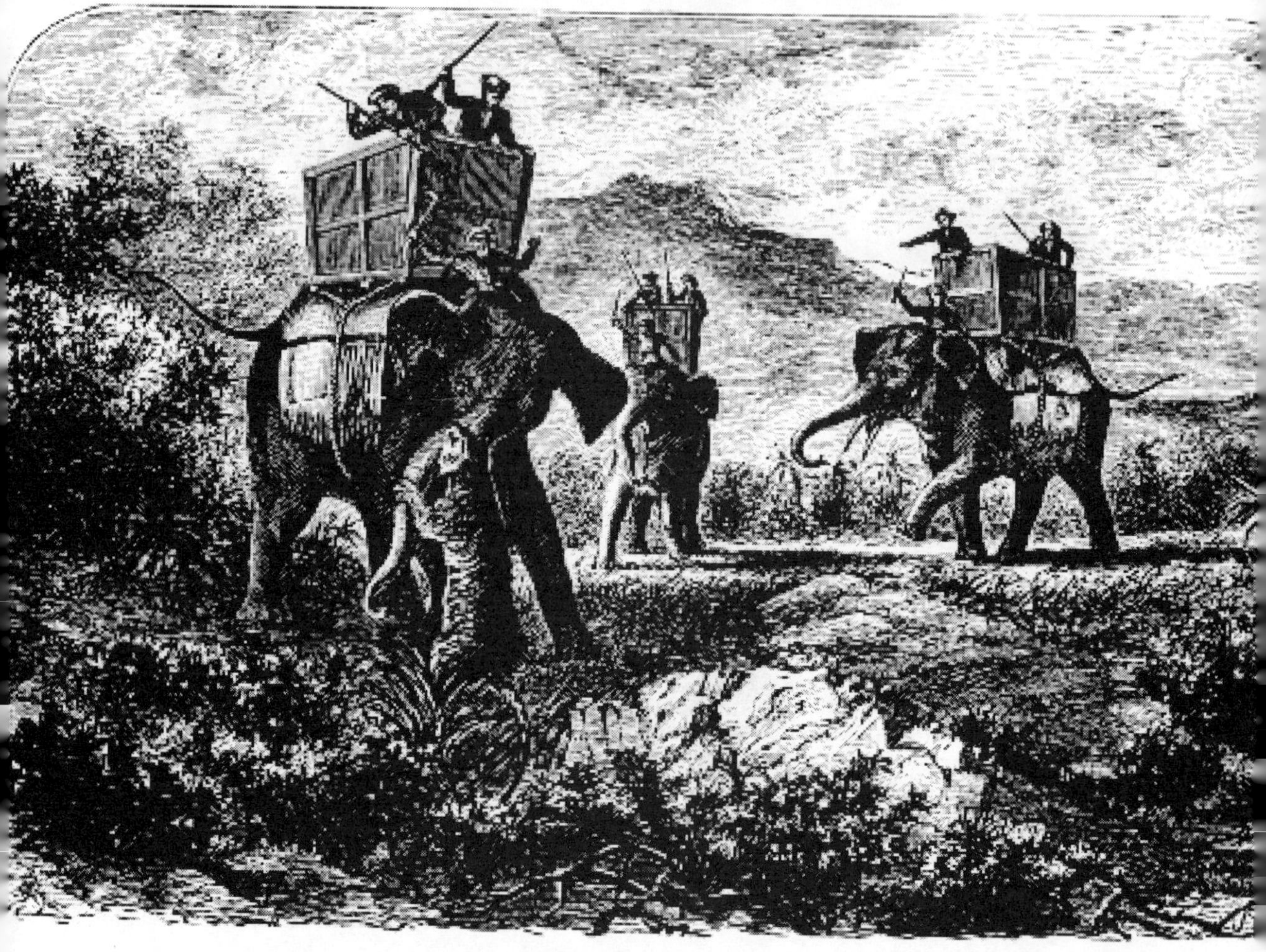

This is one of the most difficult books of my entire career and without the assistance of many people its research and writing would not have been possible. Firstly, I thank my daughters Shrivridhi and Samridhi, who have with utmost patience and dedication assisted me throughout the process of writing this book. My grateful thanks are due to my friends whose names are mentioned in this book and also those who are not mentioned but who believed in my work and stood by me as solid rock, in spite of the popular opposition to my theory and lack of cooperation by Project Tiger. G.B. Patnaik, N. Ravi Shankar, Dr. Har Sharan Das, Yogesh Kumar, Avnish Avasthi, Ravindra Nayak, Sanjay Kumar and Mutto Swami Balasubramanyam are a few names, who taught me what true friendship is. I owe them much more than they will ever realize.

Rashmi Kant Shukla, R.C. Jha, K.K. Singh, Sanjay Pathak all dedicated foresters, provided me with unfailing moral and material support in the defense of this magnificent animal. Mr. Dev Raj Nagar, Director General of Police, P.A.C., Vijay Kumar, Rajeev Ranjan Verma and Jai Narain

Singh of Indian Police Services gave much valid segmentation in preparation of this work.

My thanks are due to my cousin brother Ajay Mishra (I.A.S) former Chief Secretary of Jharkhand for accompanying me on my outdoor ventures. My thanks are also due to Dr. Nirmala and Ms Ishita Basu, who typed my manuscript and Prof. Kumkum Kishore who did the proof-reading, Sanjay Narain who gave me several interesting suggestions and to Ratan Mani Lal, who finally edited this manuscript. Long online discussions with Vidya Athreya provided me with much insight into the problem of large carnivores that inhabit the human dominated landscape. I've incorporated several suggestions given by her in this book.

I am also thankful to Shri Suneel Gomber, Prashant Gupta and Ritesh Sharma who imaginatively and meticuliously designed this book for publication.

I owe an immense debt of gratitude to the putative creed of supreme predators that are the stars of this book whom I have fondly dubbed as sugarcane tigers. It is in fact a tribute to their patience, and tolerance towards the pressures built up by mankind in their existence.

And finally I thank the incorrigible old man of Dudhwa, Billy Arjan Singh, who was after all a maverick of sorts, and mavericks create no dynasties, or worse, they leave a greater chaos behind than they were themselves able to generate and take the advantage of it.

However to error is human, his dedication to wildlife cannot be disputed. Indeed I will miss him, so will many; I salute him.

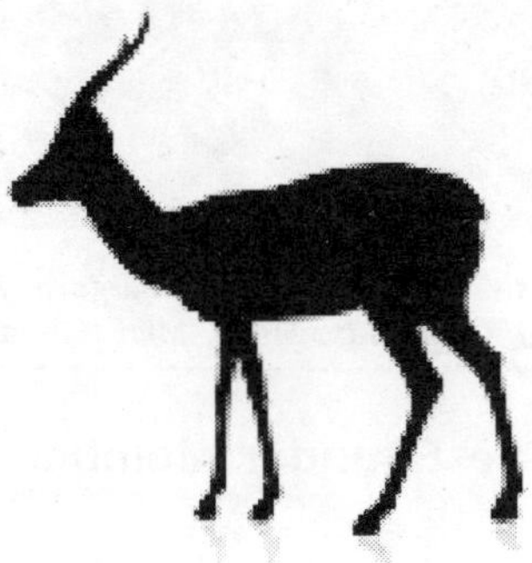

Tiger & Terrain

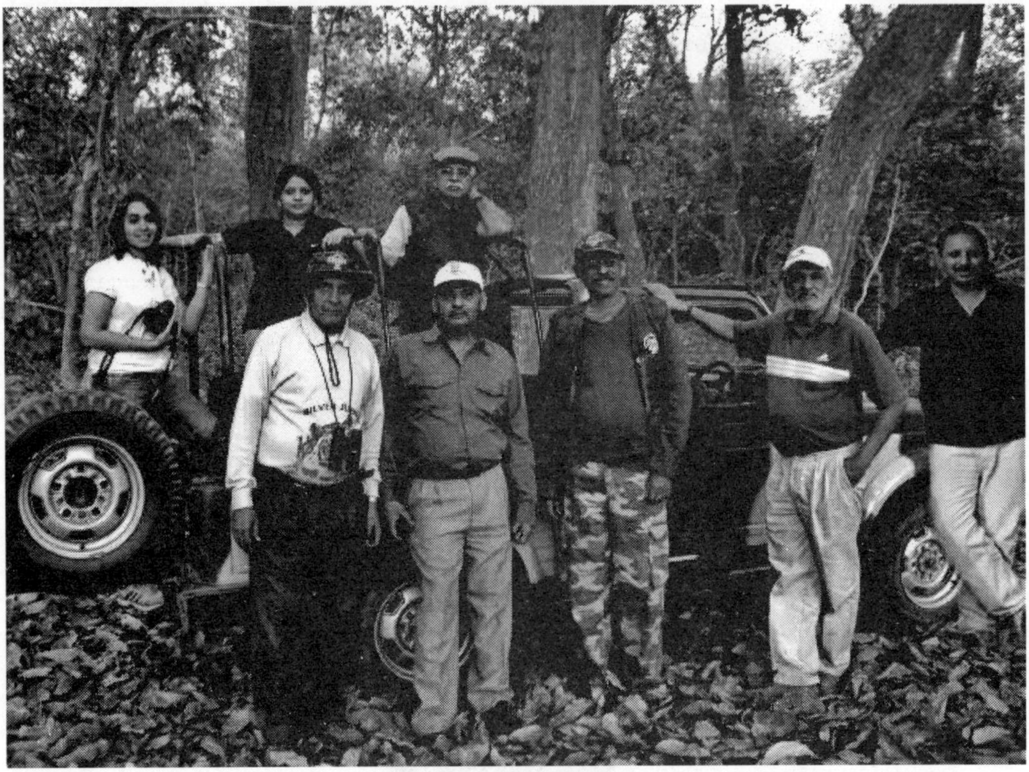

Standing on the ground (L to R) G.C. Mishra, Author, Ranjit Bhargava, Raghvendra Singh, and Sanjay Narain. On the Gypsy (R to L) Kaushlendra Singh, Mini Narain and Radhika Singh

The Founder Members

G.C.Mishra

A retired member of the Indian Forest Service, he first served as Wildlife Warden and then twice as Director of Dudhwa National Park. He has also worked as **Forestry Consultant to the European Commission** for the **Ravine Stabilization Project**, a pilot trial in the ravines of river Yamuna in six districts of UP. The project envisaged six components, viz. Soil Conservation, Agriculture Extension, Animal Husbandry, Social Forestry, Horticulture and Community Organization.

Rahul Shukla; Author

Can be contacted at - tigersoftarai@gmail.com

Padma Shri Ranjit Bhargava

He is among the pioneers of India's environment movement and a relentless environmental activist. Dr Bhargava is Honorary Advisor foe Ecology, Environment and Heritage to the Army Central Command (1991-2007), in which capacity he has shown exceptional vision, experience and determination in planning and monitoring a variety of environment and Heritage betterment schemes.

Raghvendra Singh

Former member of state wildlife advisory board and an avid tiger activist who continues to work on behalf of tiger habitat and species preservation.

Sanjay Narain

A specialist in the areas of wild life protection, conservation and fighting for animal rights while protecting the fragile Eco System, rehabilitation and integration of local population (Tribals, Ethnic communities) into the main stream of Ecotourism to provide Commercial opportunities for self sustenance. He has both national and international exposure in the field of wild life and has been associated with the author in quiet a few tiger rescue operations in the Tarai.

narainsanjay@gmail.com

Kaushlendra Singh

Former Member, Wild Life Advisory Board, Uttranchal Government. Having learnt the pheasant breeding techniques especially artificial insemination and Eco-ducts for wild animals at Belgium, he is an acclaimed breeder of captive Pheasants in the country. He also assisted Billy Arjan Singh, who passed on the baton appreciating his efforts and understanding of tiger problems and its solutions.

Mrs. Mini Narain Kumar

Daughter of Late Sri. R.S Narain (I.P.S), is a highly motivated individual, having lived in Kenya near Masai Mara National Park for decades, she acquired a strong interest in wild life and conservation.

Radhika Singh

Serves as secretary to the organization.

The Tiger &Terrain is a non-profit organization dedicated to protecting and providing shelter for all animals. Its mission is to educate the public about the humane care and treatment of animals, promote spay/neuter and encourage the adoption of homeless animals. It is going through our various charitable programs for humans as well as for the domestic and Wild Animals. The organization relies on donations from its members and other donors in the community in order to fund these programs and is deeply concerned about environmental hazards, diminishing forest and vanishing wild life. T&T is known for acting on sound science. Science leads and guides our strategies and approaches, from the best way to restore tigers and other animals in viable, breeding populations to deciding which areas need protection the most.

Index

Firearms

A

B

E

F

G

H

I

J

K

L

T

U

V

W

Y

Z